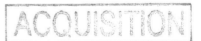

Lecture Notes

Human Physiology

EDITED BY

Ole H. Petersen
MD FRCP FRS
The Physiological Laboratory
School of Biomedical Sciences
University of Liverpool
UK

Fifth Edition

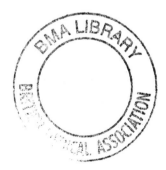

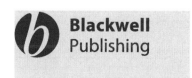

Blackwell
Publishing

© 1986, 1989, 1994, 1999 by Blackwell Science Ltd
© 2007 by Blackwell Publishing Ltd
Blackwell Publishing, Inc., 350 Main Street, Malden, Massachusetts 02148-5020, USA
Blackwell Publishing Ltd, 9600 Garsington Road, Oxford OX4 2DQ, UK
Blackwell Publishing Asia Pty Ltd, 550 Swanston Street, Carlton, Victoria 3053, Australia

First published 1986
Second edition 1989
Third edition 1994
Fourth edition 1999
Fifth edition 2007
4   2012

Library of Congress Cataloging-in-Publication Data

Lecture notes. Human physiology / edited by Ole H. Petersen. – 5th ed.
p. ; cm.
Rev. ed. of: Lecture notes on human physiology. 4th ed. 1999.
Includes bibliographical references and index.
ISBN 978-1-4051-3651-8 (alk. paper)
1. Human physiology.   I. Petersen, O. H. (Ole Holger)
II. Lecture notes on human physiology.
III. Title: Human physiology.
[DNLM: 1. Physiology. QT 104 L4705 2007]
QP34.5.L44 2007
612–dc22

2006020168

A catalogue record for this title is available from the British Library

Set in 8 on 12 pt Stone Serif by SNP Best-set Typesetter Ltd., Hong Kong

Commissioning Editor: Martin Sugden
Editorial Assistant: Eleanor Bonnet
Development Editors: Mirjana Misina, Hayley Salter
Production Controller: Kate Charman

For further information on Blackwell Publishing, visit our website: http://www.blackwellpublishing.com

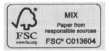

Contents

Contributors

Ole H. Petersen
FRS, FMedSci
Vice-President of The Royal Society
MRC Research Professor
George Holt Professor of Physiology
Department of Physiology
University of Liverpool
UK
Chapters 1, 2, 20, 24

Alexei Verkhratsky
MD, PhD, Mem. Acad Eur.
Professor
Faculty of Life Sciences
University of Manchester
UK
Chapter 3

Emil C. Toescu
MD, DPhil
Senior Lecturer
Department of Physiology
Division of Medical Sciences
Medical School
University of Birmingham
UK
Chapter 4

Susan Wray
PhD, FRCOG
Professor of Physiology
Department of Physiology
University of Liverpool
UK
Chapter 5

Carl C.H. Petersen
PhD
Professor
Laboratory of Sensory Processing

Brain Mind Institute
Ecole Polytechnique Federale de Lausanne (EPFL)
Switzerland
Chapters 6, 9

Roger W.A. Linden
BDS, PhD, MFDS RCS
Professor of Craniofacial Biology
Head of Department of Physiology
School of Biomedical and Health Sciences
King's College London
UK
Chapter 7

Serge Rossignol
MD, PhD
Professor
Department of Physiology
Center for Research in Neurological sciences
Université de Montréal
Canada
Chapter 8

Allan M. Smith
PhD
Professor and Director
Department of Physiology
Center for Research in Neurological Sciences
Université de Montréal
Canada
Chapter 8

Anita Holdcroft
MB ChB, MD, FRCA
Reader in Anaesthesia and Honorary Consultant Anaesthetist
Department of Anaesthetics, Pain Medicine and Intensive Care
Division of Surgery, Oncology, Reproductive Biology and Anaesthetics (SORA)

Faculty of Medicine
Imperial College London
UK
Chapter 10

Andras Spät
MD, PhD
Professor
Department of Physiology
Faculty of Medicine
Semmelweis University
Budapest, Hungary
Chapter 11

David M. de Kretser
MBBS, MD, FRACP, FAA, FTSE
Emeritus Professor, Monash Institute of Medical
Research
Monash University
Melbourne, Australia
Chapter 12

Virgilio L. Lew
MD
Director of Research
Department of Physiology, Development and
Neuroscience
University of Cambridge
UK
Chapter 13

Teresa Tiffert
MD
Lecturer
Department of Physiology, Development and
Neuroscience
University of Cambridge
UK
Chapter 13

Bruce H. Smaill
Associate Professor, Department of Physiology
Deputy Director, The Bioengineering Institute
University of Auckland
Australia
Chapter 14

Peter Kohl
MD, PhD
Reader in Cardiac Physiology
Director of the Cardiac Mechano-Electric
Feedback Laboratory
Department of Physiology, Anatomy and Genetics
University of Oxford
UK
Chapter 15

Michiel Helmes
PhD
Senior Scientist, Cardiac Mechano-Electric
Feedback Laboratory
Department of Physiology, Anatomy and Genetics
University of Oxford
UK
Chapter 15

Christopher J. Garland
BSc, PhD, FBPharmacolS
Professor and Head of Pharmacology
Department of Pharmacy and Pharmacology
University of Bath
UK
Chapter 16

Roger A.L. Dampney
PhD, DSc
Professor of Cardiovascular Neuroscience
Department of Physiology, School of Medical
Sciences
University of Sydney
Australia
Chapter 17

Mary Morrell
PhD
Reader, Respiratory Physiology
Clinical and Academic Unit of Sleep and
Breathing
National Heart and Lung Institute
School of Medicine
Imperial College London
UK
Chapter 18

Rod Dimaline
PhD
Professor
Department of Physiology
School of Biomedical Sciences
University of Liverpool
UK
Chapter 19

Peter Bie
MD, DMSc
Professor
Department of Physiology and Pharmacology
Institute of Medical Biology
University of Southern Denmark
Odense, Denmark
Chapter 21

Anthony J. Hulbert
PhD, DSc
Professor
Metabolic Research Centre
University of Wollongong
Australia
Chapter 22

Andrej A. Romanovsky
MD, PhD
Senior Staff Scientist and Director, Systemic
Inflammation Laboratory
Trauma Research
St Joseph's Hospital and Medical Center
Phoenix, Arizona
USA
Chapter 23

Preface

After four very successful editions of *Lecture Notes on Human Physiology*, Tony Macknight and his team, from the School of Medicine at Otago University in New Zealand, decided that due to many other pressures they would be unable to proceed with a fifth edition. I was asked to take over this project and accepted because of the great respect I have always had for this textbook. Indeed, as it so happens, I reviewed the first edition for *Nature* many years ago and praised the book highly!

It is important to stress that, although there has been a complete change of colleagues revising the individual chapters, this fifth edition is very much based on Tony Macknight's original concept and has retained substantial amounts of the detail present in the fourth edition. Physiology has of course progressed enormously since the last edition was published in 1999, but a large part of the basic material most relevant to undergraduate physiology studies has not changed dramatically and I saw no reason to 'reinvent the wheel' by changing elements that seemed to me to have been presented perfectly by Tony Macknight and his team. I am extremely grateful to Tony for allowing me and my co-authors to retain from the fourth edition those parts we particularly liked. As will become apparent, some chapters have been changed radically, whereas others have simply been up-dated and only modified to a minor degree.

The task I inherited was to up-date *Lecture Notes on Human Physiology*, simplify its structure and introduce more pathophysiology. All this had to be achieved without any major expansion of the book, in order to continue to make this text relevant, practical and useful for a wide range of undergraduate physiology courses. Considering the enormous increase in the amount of physiological knowledge, which we have acquired in recent years, this was not an easy task and—needless to say—not everyone will agree fully with my selection.

Whereas the first four editions were all created by a team of authors from New Zealand, this fifth edition has contributors from many parts of the world. In selecting the revising authors I was much helped by the many contacts I have built up in recent years as Secretary General of the International Union of Physiological Sciences (IUPS) and European Editor of *Physiological Reviews*. In a university world that often appears to be dominated by intense research competition, I was pleasantly surprised to find that a number of outstanding scientists and teachers were willing to help me create this fifth edition of a textbook we have all admired and used for many years. I am extremely grateful to my co-author colleagues, who spent a lot of their valuable research time in order to contribute to this edition.

Throughout the planning and execution of this project, I have had an excellent collaboration with Blackwell Publishing. It is a pleasure here to acknowledge the very effective and friendly assistance of Martin Sugden, Mirjana Misina, Hayley Salter and Helen Harvey.

Ole H. Petersen FRS
MRC Research Professor
The Physiological Laboratory
School of Biomedical Sciences
University of Liverpool, UK
2006

AC adenylyl cyclase
ACE angiotensin converting enzyme
ACh acetylcholine
ACTH adrenocorticotrophic hormone
ADH antidiuretic hormone
ADP adenosine diphosphate
Adr adrenaline
AEA arachydonoyl ethanolamide
2-AG 2-arachydonoylglycerol
AIDS acquired immunodeficiency syndrome
δ-ALA δ-aminolaevulinic acid
AMP adenosine monophosphate
AMPA α-amino-3-hydroxy-5-methyl-isoxazolepropionic acid
ANP atrial natriuretic peptide
AP action potential
APC *Adenomatous polyposis coli*
APUD amine precursor uptake and decarboxylation
ARP absolute refractory period
ASBT apical sodium-dependent bile transporter
ASIC acid-sensing ion channel
AT-I anti-thrombin I
ATP adenosine triphosphate
ATPS ambient temperature, pressure, saturated with water
a–v arterio-venous
AV atrioventricular
AVP arginine vasopressin
BAT brown adipose tissue
BC basket cell
BDNF brain-derived neurotrophic factor
BFGF basic fibroblast growth factor
BMI body mass index
BMR basal metabolic rate
BNP brain natriuretic peptide
Bötz C Bötzinger complex
2,3-BPG 2,3-bisphosphoglycerate
BTPS body temperature, pressure, saturated with water

c.a. carbonic anhydrase
$[Ca^{2+}]_i$ cytosolic free calcium concentration
CaM calmodulin
cAMP cyclic adenosine monophosphate
CBF cerebral blood flow
CCK cholecystokinin
CD Crohn's disease
cf climbing fibre
CFTR cystic fibrosis transmembrane conductance regulator
CFU colony-forming unit
CG chorionic gonadotrophin
cGMP cyclic guanosine monophosphate
CGRP calcitonin gene-related peptide
CHF congestive heart failure
CICR calcium-induced calcium release
CNS central nervous system
CO carbon monoxide
COMT catechol *O*-methyltransferase
COX cyclooxygenase
CP creatine phosphate
cPAG caudal periaqueductal grey
CPD citrate–phosphate–dextrose
CPG central pattern generator
CPK creatine phosphokinase
CREB cAMP response-element-binding protein
CRH corticotrophin-releasing hormone
CS chorionic somatomammotrophin
CSA central sleep apnoea
CSF cerebrospinal fluid
CSF colony-stimulating factor
CVLM caudal ventrolateral medulla
Cx connexin
DAG diacylglycerol
DH dorsal horn
1,25-DHCC 1,25-dihydroxycholecalciferol (calcitriol)
DHP dihydropyridine
DIT di-iodotyrosine
DMH dorsomedial hypothalamus

DMT1 divalent metal transporter type 1

DOC 11-deoxycorticosterone

L-DOPA L-dihydroxyphenylalanine

DRG dorsal respiratory group

DRG dorsal root ganglion

DTH delayed-type hypersensitivity

EC enterochromaffin

ECC excitation-contraction coupling

ECF extracellular fluid

ECG electrocardiogram

ECL enterochromaffin-like

ECT electroconvulsive shock therapy

EDHF endothelium-derived hyperpolarizing factor

EDRF endothelium-derived relaxing factor

EDTA ethylenediamine tetra-acetic acid

EEG electroencephalogram

EGF epidermal growth factor

EJP excitatory junction potential

ELISA enzyme-linked immunosorbent assay

EMG electromyogram

ENaC epithelial sodium channel

EOG electro-oculogram

EPSP excitatory postsynaptic potential

ER endoplasmic reticulum

ERV expiratory reserve volume

ET-1 endothelin 1

exp expiration

FAAH fatty acid amide hydrolase

FABP fatty acid-binding protein

FADH$_2$ flavin adenine dinucleotide (reduced)

FATP fatty-acid transporter protein

FEF forced expiratory flow (rate)

FEV$_1$ forced expiratory volume in 1 s

fMRI functional magnetic resonance imaging

FRC functional residual capacity

FSH follicle-stimulating hormone

FVC forced vital capacity

G protein GTP-regulatory protein

G17, G34 amino acid chain lengths of gastrin

GABA γ-aminobutyric acid

GAP GTPase-activating factor

GDP guanosine diphosphate

GEF GDP–GTP exchange factor

GEMM granulocyte, erythroid, monocyte and megakaryocyte

GFAP glial fibrillary acidic protein

GFR glomerular filtration rate

GH growth hormone

GHRH growth hormone-releasing hormone

GI gastrointestinal

GIP gastric inhibitory peptide

GIP glucose-dependent insulinotropic polypeptide

GL galanin

GLP glucagon-like peptide

GLP-1 glucagon-like peptide-1

GLUT2 glucose transporter type 2

GLUT5 glucose transporter type 5

GnRH gonadotrophin-releasing hormone

GoC Golgi cell

GORD gastro-oesophageal reflux disease

GPCR G-protein coupled receptor

GrC granule cell

GRP gastrin-releasing peptide

GTP guanosine triphosphate

H. pylori *Helicobacter pylori*

H$_2$O$_2$ hydrogen peroxide

Hb haemoglobin

HCG human chorionic gonadotrophin

HCl hydrochloric acid

HIV human immunodeficiency virus

HLA human leukocyte antigen

HMM heavy meromyosin

HMWK high molecular weight kininogen

11β-HSD-2 11β-hydroxy steroid dehydrogenase

5-HT 5-hydroxytryptamine, serotonin

$i_{b,Na}$ background sodium current

IBD inflammatory bowel disease

IBS inflammatory bowel syndrome

IC inspiratory capacity

$i_{Ca,L}$ L-type (long-lasting) calcium current

$i_{Ca,T}$ T-type (transient) calcium current

ICC interstitial cell of Cajal

ICF intracellular fluid

ICSI intracytoplasmic sperm injection

IDDM insulin-dependent diabetes mellitus

i_f 'funny' hyperpolarization-activated inward current

Ig immunoglobulin

IgA immunoglobulin A

IgD immunoglobulin D

IgE immunoglobulin E

IGF insulin-like growth factor

IgG immunoglobulin G
IgM immunoglobulin M
IJP inhibitory junction potential
i_K delayed rectifying potassium current
i_{K1} inward rectifying potassium current
IML intermediolateral cell column
i_{Na} fast sodium current
i_{NCX} sodium-calcium exchanger current
INR international normalized ratio
Ins-1 insulin substrate-1
insp inspiration
IP_3 inositol 1,4,5-trisphosphate
IPAN intrinsic primary afferent neurone
IPSP inhibitory postsynaptic potential
IRV inspiratory reserve volume
ISF interstitial fluid
IT inferior temporal
i.v. intravenous
IVF *in vitro* fertilization
αKG α ketoglutarate
LGN lateral geniculate nucleus
LH luteinizing hormone
LMM light meromyosin
LOS lower oesophageal sphincter
LTD long-term depression
LTP long-term potentiation
LV left ventricle
MABP mean arterial blood pressure
MAP microtubule-associated protein
MDP maximum diastolic potential
MEF mechano-electric feedback
MEG magnetoencephalogram
mf mossy fibre
MHC major histocompatibility complex
MI primary motor cortex
MIT monoiodotyrosine
MLCK myosine light chain kinase
MLCP myosine light chain phosphatase
MLR mesencephalic locomotor region
MMC migrating motor complex
MPQ McGill Pain Questionnaire
MSFP mean systemic filling pressure
MSH melanocyte-stimulating hormone
MT middle temporal
NA noradrenaline
NA nucleus ambiguus
NAD nicotinamide adenine dinucleotide

NADH nicotinamide adenine dinucleotide (reduced)
NADPH nicotinamide adenine dinucleotide phosphate (reduced)
NANC non-adrenergic non-cholinergic
NCC $Na^+–Cl^-$ co-transporter
NGF nerve growth factor
NIDDM non-insulin-dependent diabetes mellitus
NKA neurokinin A
NKCC2 $Na^+–K^+–2Cl^-$ co-transporter
NMDA *N*-methyl-D-aspartic acid
NO nitric oxide
NOS nitric oxide synthase
NPY neuropeptide Y
NSAID non-steroidal anti-inflammatory drug
NT neurotrophin
NTS nucleus of the tractus solitarius
OPG osteoprotegerin
OSA obstructive sleep apnoea
P_{50} Po_2 at which 50% saturation of the haemoglobin molecule occurs
PACAP pituitary anenylate cyclase-activating peptide
PAG periaqueductal grey
PAH para-aminohippurate
PAMP pathogen-associated molecular pattern
PC Purkinje cell
PCV packed cell volume
PDE cAMP phosphodiesterase
PEA palmitoylethanolamide
PEPT1 peptide transporter type 1
pf parallel fibre
PF3 platelet factor 3
PGE_2 prostaglandin E_2
PGG_2 prostaglandin G_2
PGH_2 prostaglandin H_2
PGI_2 prostaglandin I_2
PH posterior hypothalamus
PHI peptide histidine isoleucine
P_i inorganic phosphate
PI phosphatidylinositol
PIP phosphatidylinositol 4-phosphate
PIP_2 phosphatidylinositol 4,5-bisphosphate
PKA protein kinase A
PKC protein kinase C
PL (platelet) phospholipase
PLA_2 phospholipase A_2

PLC phospholipase C

PNS peripheral nervous system

POA preoptic anterior hypothalamus

POMC proopiomelanocortin

PP pancreatic polypeptide

PPI proton pump inhibitor

PPi pyrophosphate

PRG pontine respiratory group

PRL prolactin

PT prothrombin time

PTH parathyroid hormone

PTTK partial thromboplastin time with kaolin

PVB premature ventricular beat

PVN paraventricular nucleus

PYY peptide YY

$\dot{Q}$ cardiac output

R receptor

RANK receptor activator of nuclear factor κB

RANKL RANK ligand

RBF renal blood flow

REM rapid eye movement (sleep)

RF reticular formation

RMP resting membrane potential

ROC receptor-operated channel

RPA raphé/peripyramidal area

rPAG rostral periaqueductal grey

RPF renal plasma flow

RQ respiratory quotient

RRF retrorubral field

RRP relative refractory period

RV residual volume

RV right ventricle

RVLM rostral ventrolateral medulla

RVM rostroventral medulla

RyR ryanodine receptor

SA sino-atrial

SDA specific dynamic action

SERCA sarco-(endo-)plasmic reticulum calcium ATPase

SGLT1 sodium glucose-linked transporter type 1

SI primary somatosensory cortex

SII secondary somatosensory cortex

SMA (MII) supplementary motor area

SOM somatostatin

SP substance P

SR sarcoplasmic reticulum

STPD standard temperature and pressure, dry

SW slow-wave (sleep)

T_3 tri-iodothyronine

T_4 thyroxine

TA titratable acid

TBG thyroxine-binding globulin

TEA tetraethylammonium ion

TENS transcutaneous electrical nerve stimulation

TF trasferrin

TG thyroglobulin

TK tachykinin

TLC total lung capacity

T_m tubular maximum

TnC calcium-binding subunit of troponin

TnI inhibitory subunit of troponin

TnT tropomyosin-binding subunit of troponin

TNZ thermoneutral zone

TPR total peripheral resistance

TRH thyrotrophin-releasing hormone

TrK tyrosine kinase

TRP transient receptor potential

TRPV1 transient receptor potential vanilloid

TSH thyroid-stimulating hormone

TxA_2 thromboxane A_2

UC ulcerative colitis

UCP uncoupling protein(s)

UCP-1 uncoupling protein 1

$\dot{V}_{CO_2}$ carbon dioxide consumption

$\dot{V}_E$ pulmonary ventilation

$\dot{V}_{O_2}$ oxygen consumption

V1 primary visual cortex

V2 secondary visual cortex

VC vital capacity

VCG vector cardiogram

VH ventral horn

VIP vasoactive intestinal peptide

VMH ventromedial hypothalamus

VO_{2max} maximum rate of oxygen consumption

VOC voltage-operated channel

VRG ventral respiratory group

V_T tidal volume

VTA ventral tegmental area

Chapter 1

Cell Physiology

Physiology is the science of the functions and phenomena of living things. The aim of this book is to explain human physiology, but many of the underlying experimental data have been derived from animal experiments. Our bodies contain vast numbers of cells, which are the fundamental units of all living organisms.

1.1 Cells

Physiology is about how cells work and about how their environment is maintained so that the cells can function optimally.

Mammalian cells are very small, of the order of 10^{-5} m in diameter. This is about midway between people (of the order of 1 m) and atoms (10^{-10} m). A person has about as many cells—about 10^{14}—as a cell has molecules.

Although the detailed structure of cells is not revealed fully by light microscopy, due to its limited resolution ($0.2\,\mu m$), some of the major features can be observed in living cells by specifically staining individual components (Fig. 1.1). The cellular ultrastructure in all its complexity can be observed in electron micrographs of fixed tissue (resolution approximately 1 nm (10^{-9} m)).

In order to power cellular functions, there is a need for a continuous supply of matter (for example, glucose or amino acids), which can be transformed to generate usable energy in the form of **adenosine triphosphate (ATP)**. The **mitochon-**dria (Fig. 1.1) are the principal powerhouses of the cell, and this is where the main synthesis of ATP takes place. The details of metabolism are the domain of biochemistry.

Every cell is surrounded by fluid (**extracellular fluid, ECF**) and for normal cell function the composition of this bathing fluid must be maintained constant. This ECF is the medium through which all exchanges between cells and the external environment occur. The constancy of the ECF, necessary for the well being of the cells, is maintained by **homeostatic mechanisms** that monitor and regulate its temperature, osmotic pressure, pH and composition. Much of physiology is the story of homeostasis.

1.2 Homeostatic mechanisms

The composition of the ECF, and therefore the cell environment, is maintained constant through homeostatic mechanisms that monitor and regulate the functions of the circulatory system, the alimentary system, the respiratory system and the renal system. This monitoring and regulation is coordinated through the nervous and endocrine systems and requires receptors, central integration and output to the effectors.

Homeostatic mechanisms are triggered by alteration in some physiological property or quantity and act to produce a compensating change in the opposite direction, so as to return the system as

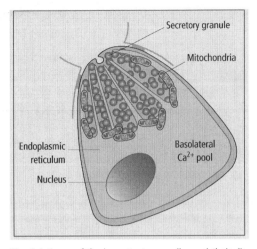

Fig. 1.1 Some of the important organelles and their distribution in a secretory cell (exocrine). The nucleus is surrounded by an extensive endoplasmic reticulum. The granules, containing material to be secreted (for example digestive enzymes in exocrine glands or hormones in endocrine glands) are clustered in one part of the cell, which is typical for exocrine cells. The mitochondria are predominantly localized on the border between the granules and the basolateral part of the cell containing the endoplasmic reticulum and the nucleus. (Modified from Petersen, O.H., Tepikin, A.V. & Park, M.K. (2001) *Trends Neurosci*, **24**, 271–76.)

close as possible to the normal situation (so-called negative feedback control). Minimum requirements are:

1 receptors, specialized to detect alterations in particular variables;

2 effectors, e.g. the circulatory system that carries nutrients and O_2 to the cells and removes metabolic waste products, including CO_2; the alimentary system that provides nutrients to the body; the respiratory system that carries out exchanges of gases with the external environment; the renal system that allows losses of unwanted solutes and water from the body; and the musculoskeletal system;

3 coordinating and integrating mechanisms, linking **1** to **2**. These are nervous and hormonal.

Nervous system

In essence this consists of **afferent nerve fibres** linking receptors to coordinating systems in the **brain** and **spinal cord**, and **efferent nerve fibres** that carry information from the coordinating systems to the effector organs. There are two major subdivisions of the efferent system: the **somatic nervous system** uses skeletal muscles as effectors for purposive behaviour and reflex actions; the **autonomic nervous system** sends its efferents to glands, the heart, and smooth muscle in hollow organs and blood vessels.

Endocrine system

This comprises cells, often arranged in groups called glands, which secrete **hormones** into the blood that affect the function of **target cells** throughout the body. Hormonal actions are generally slower and less sharply localized than those of the nervous system; they are, however, under the control of the nervous system through hormones produced in the brain (in the hypothalamus and the pituitary gland) that influence the other endocrine glands.

1.3 The importance of water in the body

About 60% of the body is water, the special properties of which are uniquely suited to life. Of this fluid, some 67% is in the cells (**intracellular fluid, ICF**) and 33% is extracellular (**ECF**). The ICF is high in K^+, the positive charge of which largely balances the negative charges of organic solutes. The ECF is high in Na^+ and Cl^-.

Distribution of water in the body

All substances exchanged between cells and their environment travel and react in solutions consisting of water, which is the main bulk constituent of all living systems. Water has a large dielectric constant, which reduces electrostatic forces 80 times and makes water a superb solvent for ionic compounds. Moreover, water dipoles are strongly attracted to dissolved ions and to charged surfaces, coating these with relatively immobile layers of water molecules that greatly modify the properties of ions in solution.

In a man about 60% of body weight is due to water. A 70-kg man therefore has about 42 L. In a woman, the relatively greater percentage of the body weight contributed by fat cells (which contain little water) means that about 55% of body weight is water. A 55-kg woman therefore has about 30 L of water.

This water is shared between the cells and the ECF that surround them. Difficulties in measuring the ECF volume have resulted in a variety of published values for cellular and extracellular water contents. Most commonly it is stated that two-thirds (67%) of the water is cellular and one-third (33%) extracellular. Using these ratios, it can be calculated that a 70-kg man would have 28 L of **intra-cellular water** and 14 L of **extracellular water**. In this man, 3 L of the extracellular water is in the **blood plasma**, most of the remaining 11 L constitutes the **interstitial fluid** (which includes lymph) that provides an aquatic habitat surrounding the cells. More accurately, about 1 L of the 11 L represents the **transcellular fluids** (cerebrospinal fluid, ocular, pleural, peritoneal and synovial fluids), but we usually ignore this in the simple calculations used to determine changes in body water and its distribution in health and disease.

Comparable approximate values for a 55-kg woman are intracellular water 20 L, extracellular water 10 L, plasma 2 L and interstitial fluid 8 L.

Clinically, the best guide to changes in body water is rapid alteration in body weight. When necessary, body water and water compartments are usually measured by methods that rely on the notion of 'volume of distribution'.

Dilution principle

A known amount of solute is injected intravenously. Then blood samples are obtained until a steady-state concentration of the injected substance is reached. Values have to be corrected for any urinary losses.

$$\text{Volume of space} = \frac{\text{amount given} - \text{amount lost}}{\text{conc. in plasma H}_2\text{O}}$$

The volumes of the compartments can be estimated from the volumes of distribution of substances thought to equilibrate in different compartments. For example, total body water has been estimated from the volume of distribution of urea and isotopes of water (deuterium oxide, tritiated water). Similarly, inulin, sucrose, mannitol and isotopes of Na^+ and Cl^- have been used to estimate extracellular water, and isotopically labelled albumin to estimate plasma water. Interstitial water cannot be measured directly but is (ignoring the transcellular volume) the difference between extracellular volume and plasma volume.

Intracellular and extracellular water have different solutes dissolved in them and so constitute two distinct fluids, the ICF and ECF. Skeletal muscle cell fluid and plasma are typical of ICF and ECF, respectively. The ICF has mainly **potassium** (K^+) with **organic anions**; ECF has mainly **sodium** (Na^+) and **chloride** (Cl^-), rather like diluted seawater. Their approximate compositions in $mmol\,L^{-1}$ are shown in Table 1.1.

1.4 Exchanges between capillaries and interstitial fluid

The heart and blood vessels comprise a transport system that carries water and solutes including hormones and gases (O_2 and CO_2) throughout the body. Circulating blood does not actually reach the cells. In the tissues, **capillaries** bring blood within 5–$10\,\mu m$ of most cells; but to get from blood to the interior of a cell, solutes like glucose and O_2 must:

1 cross the capillary wall;

2 cross a layer of interstitial fluid between the capillary and cell; and

3 cross the plasma membrane, which separates the ICF from the ECF.

The walls of most capillaries are relatively leaky. **Diffusion** is the dominant mechanism by which solutes and water cross the capillary wall as well as being the mechanism by which they move through the interstitial fluid. The roles of ultrafiltration and osmosis in capillary exchange are discussed in Chapter 16, Section 16.4.

Diffusion

Diffusion is a consequence of the thermal energies

Table 1.1 Blood plasma and skeletal muscle cell fluid as typical extracellular and intracellular fluids, respectively.

	Plasma (mmol L^{-1})	Muscle (mmol L^{-1})
Na$^+$	150	10
K$^+$	5	150
Ca^{2+}	2	10^{-4}
Mg^{2+}	1	10
Cl$^-$	110	5
HCO$_3^-$	27	10
Org$^-$ (e.g. lactate)	5	
Inorganic PO$_4^-$	2	
Org P$^-$		130
Prot^{17-}	1	2
pH	7.4	7.1
Osmolarity (mosmol L^{-1})	285	285

1 Plasma constituents are commonly expressed clinically per litre of plasma rather than per kilogram of water. Because protein occupies a finite volume, plasma values are somewhat lower than the values given in the table.

2 Cellular composition is not uniform; for example, some organelles (e.g. sarcoplasmic reticulum in skeletal muscle) contain ions at very different concentrations from those in the surrounding cytosol. Also, within the cytosol there exists a complex protein matrix contributed by microtubules, microfilaments and intermediate filaments and their associated proteins. Such large, relatively non-diffusible material contributes up to 30% of the cell volume.

3 Cell pH is not uniform and some organelles (e.g. lysosomes) may be much more acidic.

Table 1.2 Time taken to reach 99% equilibrium by diffusion of solute from a plane boundary in water at room temperature (Jacobs 1935). (From Robinson, J.R. (1981) *A Prelude to Physiology*, p. 26. Blackwell Scientific Publications, Oxford.)

Distance from boundary	Time
10 cm	53 days
1 cm	128 h
1 mm	76 min
100 μm	456 s
10 μm	0.0456 s
1 μm	0.000456 s
0.1 μm	0.00000456

dimensional representation with 67% cellular fluid and 33% ECF, most of which (80%) is interstitial fluid. In reality, however, because cells are three-dimensional and the interstitial fluid surrounds them, the thickness of the interstitial layer is much less than would appear from Fig. 1.2a. This is illustrated in Fig. 1.2b, which represents a cross-section through a spherical cell and its surrounding layer of interstitial fluid. With a cell radius of 10 μm, the thickness of the interstitial fluid layer is only approximately 1.2 μm. (In this representation, the plasma component is too small to be shown.) Thus the diffusional distances through the interstitial fluid are very small.

1.5 Movement across the cell plasma membrane

The cell (plasma) membrane

The plasma membrane is a lipid bilayer in which are embedded a variety of proteins.

A membrane (about 7.5 nm in thickness) separates the cell interior from the surrounding interstitial fluid. This is properly referred to as the plasma membrane to distinguish it from the membranes within the cells (e.g. mitochondrial membrane). It is composed of a mosaic of globular proteins embedded in a lipid bilayer with the hydrophilic ends of the lipid molecules oriented towards the outside of the membrane (Fig. 1.3). Both the protein and lipid molecules are free to move in the lateral plane of the membrane.

of the individual molecules. This results in Brownian (random) molecular movements. In the absence of concentration gradients this does not result in net transport, but if there is a difference in concentration of a particular solute between two regions, there will be more molecules leaving the high concentration region to move into the low concentration region than molecules moving in the opposite direction. Net flux of each species therefore occurs down its own gradient. Diffusion is very rapid over the relatively short distances within cells and between cells and capillaries, but very slow over longer distances (Table 1.2).

The major subdivisions of body water are often illustrated as shown in Fig. 1.2a, which is a two-

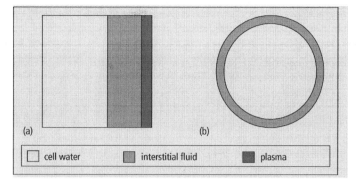

Fig. 1.2 (a) The major subdivisions of body water. (b) The relationship between cell water and the surrounding interstitial fluid for a spherical cell.

(a)   (b)

☐ cell water   ▨ interstitial fluid   ▩ plasma

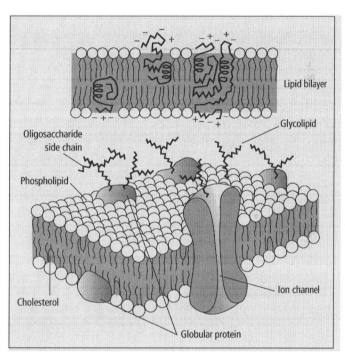

Fig. 1.3 The plasma membrane in cross-section (top) and in three dimensions (below). The globular proteins embedded in the lipid bilayer may be situated on one side of the membrane or extend through it. (Modified from Singer, S.J. & Nicolson, G.L. (1972) *Science* **175**, 720–31.)

Lipid bilayer

Glycolipid

Oligosaccharide side chain

Phospholipid

Cholesterol

Ion channel

Globular protein

Because of the nature of the lipid bilayer, the plasma membrane presents a formidable barrier to non-lipid-soluble solutes, for example, small ions (K^+, Na^+, Cl^-, HCO_3^-) and glucose. On the other hand, fatty acids and gases, for example, are much more permeable. The non-permeable molecules need special transmembrane transport proteins (**channels**, **carriers** and **pumps**) in order to be transferred across the plasma membrane.

Driving forces for solute movements

Net solute movement across the cell membrane

may be either passive (downhill, driven by the difference in chemical or electrochemical potential) or active (uphill, driven by the cell's metabolic energy).

The driving force for net movement of an uncharged solute from one solution to another is given by the difference in **chemical potential** ($\Delta\mu$) between the two solutions. This is formally expressed as:

$$\Delta\mu = RT \ln \frac{c_1}{c_2}$$

where R is the gas constant ($8.314\,\mathrm{J\,K^{-1}\,mol^{-1}}$), T is the absolute temperature (K), and c_1 and c_2 are the concentrations in $mol\,L^{-1}$ in solutions 1 and 2, respectively. Thus chemical work is expressed in $J\,mol^{-1}$.

If $c_1 > c_2$, then this represents the energy available to drive the net movement of 1 mol of c from compartment 1 to 2. This movement will occur spontaneously between a cell and its surrounding interstitial fluid if the membrane is permeable to the solute, and is called **passive transport** (also referred to as 'downhill' transport).

Conversely, if $c_1 < c_2$, net movement of 1 mol of c from compartment 1 to 2 can only occur if this amount of energy is expended by the system. In cell physiology, such energy expenditure results in **active transport** (also referred to as 'uphill' transport).

For **ions**, which are charged, there is an electrical potential difference (V) across the plasma membranes that needs to be considered, as well as a chemical concentration gradient, and it is the combined driving force, the **electrochemical potential** ($\Delta\tilde{\mu}$) that is important. The difference in $\Delta\tilde{\mu}$ for an ion of valency z between two solutions is:

$$\Delta\tilde{\mu} = RT\ln\frac{c_1}{c_2} \qquad + \quad zFV$$
$$\text{chemical energy} \;+\; \text{electrical energy}$$

Whereas chemical work is expressed in joule mol^{-1}, V is expressed in volts. Volts have the units joule coulomb^{-1} ($J\,C^{-1}$). Faraday's constant ($F = 96\,500\,C\,mol^{-1}$) in the equation allows the conversion of the electrical potential term into the same units as the chemical potential term, so that the two can be summed.

Mechanisms of membrane permeation

Lipid-soluble substances cross membranes passively by dissolving in, and diffusing through, the lipid bilayer. Water and water-soluble substances move through specific membrane proteins that may function as channels, carriers or pumps. Movement through channels is always passive; carrier-mediated movement may be passive or active. Movement via pumps is active.

These mechanisms may be classified as follows.

1 Permeation by dissolving and diffusing in the membrane lipid, e.g. O_2 and CO_2, steroid hormones. In so far as plasma membranes offer a fairly complete layer of lipid between the ICF and ECF, this mechanism should favour lipid-soluble substances of low molecular weight.

2 Permeation through specific membrane proteins. Protein molecules span the membrane lipid bilayer. Some of these can be permeated by ions and other solutes. Water also moves through specific protein molecules (aquaporins). The protein molecules that provide pathways for solute movements are classified into **channels** and **carriers**. A membrane channel may be open or shut. When open, it is accessible simultaneously from both sides of the membrane and contains one or more binding sites arranged in a transmembrane sequence. In contrast, membrane carriers have binding sites that are exposed sequentially to one side or other of the membrane (but never to both simultaneously). The rate of movement of ions through a single open channel can be some 10^6–$10^9\,s^{-1}$, a transport rate much greater than the highest known catalytic rates of enzymes, and comparable to the rates for free diffusion of ions in aqueous media. Movement mediated by a carrier is slower by orders of magnitude than that through a channel. The permeability of the membrane may be regulated by activation or inhibition of specific channels or carriers resident in the membrane and by the insertion into, or removal of, these proteins from the membrane.

Since movement of solutes through channels and carriers involves some interaction of the solute with the protein molecule, it is often possible to demonstrate **specificity**, **saturation kinetics**, **competition** between similar molecular species, and **inhibition**—properties similar to reactions catalysed by enzymes.

Modern techniques of molecular and structural biology allow identification of the amino acid sequences and three-dimensional structures of a variety of channels and carriers. Both channels and carriers consist of one or more protein subunits that span the membrane a number of times.

(a) **Membrane channels**, e.g. water, ions. The

properties of channels are rapidly becoming known through a variety of powerful techniques, particularly patch-clamping (Fig. 1.4) which permits the measurement of current passing through a single open channel in a fragment of membrane (Fig. 1.5). Ion channels allow specific ions, e.g. Na^+, K^+, Ca^{2+} or Cl^-, to move down their electrochemical gradients across the membrane, and are often named after the ions for which they show the greatest selectivity. A specific part of a channel (a 'gate') opens and closes; the processes that modulate this '**gating**' affect the probability of a channel being open or closed. Single-channel conductances range between 2 (close to the limit of detection) and 200 pS or more. There are three major types of gated channel. (i) **Voltage-gated channels**, sensitive to the voltage across the membrane in which they are inserted, e.g. the voltage-sensitive Na^+ channel involved in **action potential** generation. (ii) **Chemically-gated channels**, sensitive to a chemical (ligand) signal. Such signals may result from the binding of a ligand to a plasma membrane receptor. This may lead to direct activation of an ion channel, i.e. the receptor is an integral part of the ion channel (e.g. the acetylcholine receptor channel involved in neuromuscular transmission). This is referred to as a **receptor-operated** channel. More commonly, the interaction of the ligand with its receptor leads to the activation of a membrane-bound enzyme and the production of an intracellular chemical (**intracellular messenger**) which then opens or closes specific ion channels in the plasma or intracellular membranes. Some hormones or neurotransmitters are in this way able to release Ca^{2+} from intracellular stores, and this in turn increases the Ca^{2+} concentration in the cell water. This is important because many different channels can be activated by an increase in the intracellular Ca^{2+} concentration (Ca^{2+}-activated ion channels). In addition, changes in cell metabolism may alter channel activity (e.g. ATP inhibition of K^+ channels in some cell types). Receptor-operated channels allow more rapid transfer of information than can occur when channels are regulated via intracellular

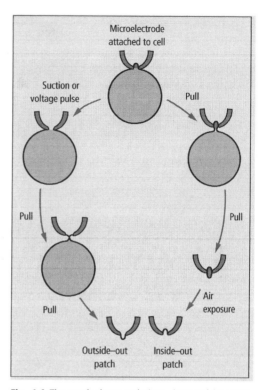

Fig. 1.4 The patch-clamp technique, invented by Erwin Neher and Bert Sakmann (jointly awarded the 1991 Nobel Prize for Physiology or Medicine, for their discoveries concerning the function of ion channels in cells), for measuring the very small currents flowing through individual ion channels in the plasma membrane. The first step is to attach a micropipette (electrode) to the cell surface. By suction, or a strong voltage pulse, the isolated plasma membrane covered by the pipette is broken and direct continuity between pipette interior and cell interior established. This configuration can be used to measure the total current flow across the whole of the plasma membrane. By pulling, bits of plasma membrane are excised, which reseal in the so-called outside-out configuration. In this configuration the outside of the excised patch of membrane is exposed to the outside solution and this configuration is therefore useful for investigating properties of ion channels normally activated by extracellular ligands (for example the neurotransmitter acetylcholine). Starting again from the initial cell-attached configuration, one can pull immediately and thereby isolate a plasma membrane vesicle excised from the cell. By exposing the vesicle—held at the tip of the micropipette—to air, the outer part of the vesicle is destroyed and an excised inside-out membrane patch has been created. This configuration is ideal for investigating the properties of ion channels normally activated by intracellular messengers, for example Ca^{2+} or cyclic nucleotides.

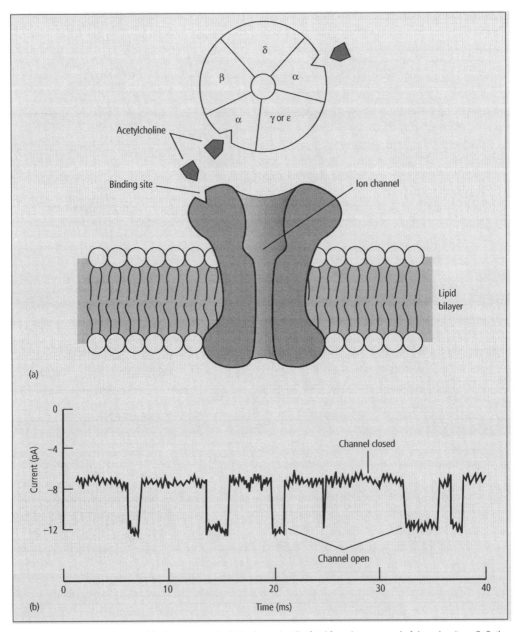

Fig. 1.5 (a) Structure of the acetylcholine receptor in skeletal muscle. The fetal form is composed of the subunits $\alpha_2\beta\gamma\delta$, the adult form $\alpha_2\beta\varepsilon\delta$. (b) Patch-clamp recording of current passing through an acetylcholine receptor channel (fetal form) of skeletal muscle.

messengers. (iii) **Mechanically-gated channels**, sensitive to mechanical deformation of the membrane, e.g. stretch-activated channels on sensory nerve terminals.

(b) **Carrier-mediated transport**. This can be subdivided into **facilitated diffusion**, where the net movement is passive and driven by the electrochemical potential gradient (e.g. glucose

exit into the blood from intestinal absorptive cells), and **primary** or **secondary active transport** (discussed below). As an example, consider how glucose, an important metabolic fuel for almost all types of cells, may be transported by facilitated diffusion. Glucose enters cells only very slowly by simple diffusion because of its size and water solubility. Its movement between interstitial fluid and cells therefore depends mainly on facilitated diffusion mediated by a family of glucose carriers (GLUT1, GLUT2, GLUT3 and GLUT4) whose occurrence differs from tissue to tissue. In most cells, the concentration gradient is such that glucose enters the cells via these carriers. In cells in some tissues (e.g. skeletal muscle and fat), glucose uptake (via GLUT4) is markedly stimulated by insulin. In these cells, insulin regulates the number of glucose transporters exposed to the extracellular surface by stimulating the fusion of cytosolic vesicles containing membrane-bound transporters with the plasma membrane. In some epithelial cells (e.g. small intestine and kidney) glucose is taken up from the lumen by secondary active transport which involves Na$^+$-dependent carriers located in the luminal membrane, the structure of which is quite distinct from that of the GLUT family of carriers. In these cells, glucose concentration rises above that in the interstitial fluid and glucose then moves from the cells to the interstitial fluid by facilitated diffusion via the GLUT2 carrier.

Energy-dependent transport across plasma membranes

In active transport, movement occurs against the electrochemical potential gradient. There are two types, primary and secondary. In primary active transport, the consumption of metabolic energy is coupled directly to the movement, which is independent of the downhill movement of any other species. In secondary active transport, the downhill movement of one species drives the uphill movement of another, and metabolic energy is not utilized directly. If the species move in the same direction across the membrane this is termed co-

transport; if the movements are in opposite tions, it is termed counter-transport.

Primary active transport

This has the following characteristics:
1 it is **coupled directly to a continuous suppl energy**;
2 it is **independent** of the downhill movemen any other solute or of water;
3 it can be shown to occur '**uphill**', i.e. to oc against the electrochemical potential gradie (For **uncharged molecules**, uphill is from lower higher concentration, i.e. against the chemic concentration gradient.)

Mechanism of primary active transport

At the molecular level primary active transport involves proteins which have their structure altered by reacting directly with, and hydrolysing, ATP. These proteins (enzymes) are called ATPases and there are three established categories: Na$^+$,K$^+$–ATPase (often referred to as the Na$^+$–K$^+$ pump or the Na$^+$ pump), Ca^{2+}–ATPases and a variety of H$^+$–ATPases (some of which also require K$^+$ and are called H$^+$,K$^+$–ATPases). As well as their presence in the plasma membrane, some of the Ca^{2+}–ATPases and H$^+$–ATPases are located on membranes lining cell organelles (e.g. Ca^{2+}–ATPase in the sarcoplasmic reticulum, H$^+$–ATPase in mitochondria).

As an example of active transport, consider the Na$^+$, K$^+$–ATPase. To maintain their steady state, high K$^+$, low Na$^+$ composition, cells need energy from metabolism to expel Na$^+$, which diffuses into the cell, and to take up K$^+$, which diffuses out of the cell. Poorly metabolizing cells gain Na$^+$ and lose K$^+$. If the cells recover, they take up K$^+$ and expel Na$^+$, both against electrochemical gradients. These movements of Na$^+$ and K$^+$ are coupled directly to the consumption of ATP. The protein that moves the ions across the membrane is itself an ATPase. To function, Na$^+$,K$^+$–ATPase requires Mg^{2+}; it is activated by cell Na$^+$ and extracellular K$^+$, and is inhibited by cardiac glycosides, such as ouabain. Three Na$^+$ are extruded from the cell and two K$^+$ are taken up with each cycle.

The Na$^+$,K$^+$–ATPase consists of two subunits—α

and β —in equal proportions. The unit responsible for the transport and ATPase activity is the α subunit; the β subunit is required for correct assembly and for the correct insertion of the protein into the plasma membrane. Different isoforms of both subunits are found in different cell types.

Secondary active transport

The cellular Na^+ concentration is much lower than that of the surrounding interstitial fluid and the membrane potential is negative on the inside. There is, therefore, a favourable electrochemical potential gradient for Na^+ entry to the cells. The energy in this gradient is used to drive the net movements of other solutes against their potential gradients by coupling their movement across the membrane to that of the passive downhill movement of Na^+. There is no direct coupling of metabolic energy to these movements. Instead, some of the energy inherent in the Na^+ gradient across the plasma membrane generated by the Na^+–K^+ pump is dissipated by the coupled flow of Na^+ with accompanying solute across the membrane.

If both the Na^+ and the other solute move in the same direction this is termed **co-transport**. Examples include the coupled entry of glucose with Na^+ and amino acids with Na^+ into small intestinal epithelial cells from the gut lumen, the movements of glucose and amino acids being uphill (i.e. against their own chemical or electrochemical potential gradients). If the Na^+ and the other solute move in opposite directions across the membrane this is termed **counter-transport** (sometimes also referred to as **exchange**). Examples include the coupling of Na^+ entry to cells to Ca^{2+} extrusion and to H^+ extrusion. The latter plays a central role in the regulation of cell pH (see below). Note that secondary active transport can involve ions other than Na^+ (e.g. Cl^-–HCO_3^- counter-transport).

Why is active transport important?

1 Active transport is important for maintaining normal ionic concentrations, in particular of Na^+, K^+, Ca^{2+} and H^+ which are essential for many intracellular activities.

2 Active transport is important for moving ions, water and other substances that accompany ions by sharing common carriers (i.e. co- and counter-transport) across plasma membranes, particularly in the kidney, stomach and intestine.

3 Active transport maintains the gradients of ionic concentration that are the basis of **resting membrane potentials** and **action potentials** used for signalling in nerves and for the activation of muscles.

4 The active extrusion of Na^+ is important for regulating cellular volume.

Examples of the types of membrane permeation through specific membrane proteins discussed in this section are illustrated in Fig. 1.6.

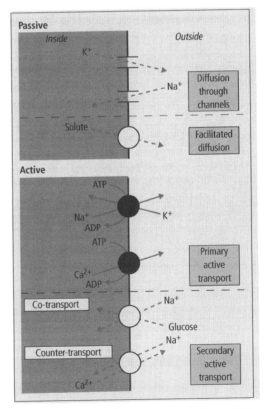

Fig. 1.6 Mechanisms of movement across plasma membranes. The solid lines and circles represent primary active transport; the dashed lines and open circles represent passive, facilitated or secondary active transport. ADP, adenosine diphosphate.

Regulation of intracellular Ca²⁺ and pH

The intracellular concentrations of free ionized Ca^{2+} and H^+ are in the nanomolar range and regulation of both is essential to normal cell function.

Intracellular Ca²⁺

Cellular membranes generally have a very low Ca^{2+} permeability and the concentration of free Ca^{2+} in the cytoplasm of inactive cells is regulated at around 10^{-7}–$10^{-8}\,mol\,L^{-1}$. As shown in Fig. 1.7, Ca^{2+} diffusing into the cell from the interstitial fluid down its electrochemical gradient may be expelled either by primary active transport (Ca^{2+}–ATPase), or by Na^+–Ca^{2+} counter-transport—an example of secondary active transport. Ca^{2+} can be transported into the endoplasmic reticulum and the nuclear envelope by a Ca^{2+}-ATPase and stored by binding to a number of binding proteins. The Ca^{2+} concentration inside the endoplasmic reticulum is much higher (~100–500 μmol L⁻¹) than in the cytoplasm. Therefore, when Ca^{2+} channels in the endoplasmic reticulum open in response to the generation of a special intracellular messenger, Ca^{2+} will be released into the cytoplasm. This is an important mechanism for the creation of cytosolic Ca^{2+} signals (see Chapter 2). The mitochondrial matrix is highly negative and Ca^{2+} can therefore move through a special channel, known as the Ca^{2+} uniporter, from the cytoplasm into the mitochondrial matrix. Ca^{2+} can move out of the mitochondria via a Na^+/Ca^{2+} exchanger. When the cytosolic Ca^{2+} concentration is increased, the mitochondria will rapidly accumulate the ion. Mitochondria can therefore restrict the movement of Ca^{2+} inside the cell. Uptake of Ca^{2+} into the mitochondria is crucial for the control of ATP production. Several enzymes in the metabolic cycle known as the Krebs cycle are Ca^{2+}-activated and an increase in the mitochondrial Ca^{2+} concentration is therefore an important signal for increasing ATP synthesis.

The level of free intracellular Ca^{2+} can rise as a result of either an increase in the permeability of the plasma membrane to Ca^{2+} or release from internal stores. Action potentials in muscle and nerve terminals increase intracellular Ca^{2+} primarily by opening voltage-dependent Ca^{2+} channels in the plasma membrane. In many cells opening of Ca^{2+} channels in the sarcoplasmic or endoplasmic reticulum membranes is also of great importance (see Chapters 2 and 5). Many neurotransmitters and hormones act by opening ligand-dependent Ca^{2+} channels (either directly or indirectly via

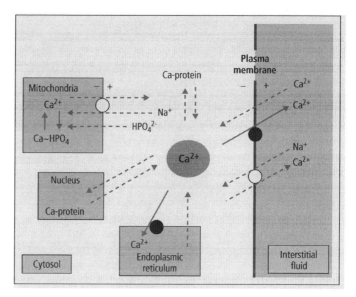

Fig. 1.7 Control of intracellular of intracellular Ca^{2+}. The solid blue lines and black circles represent primary active transport; the blue dashed lines and black open circles represent passive, facilitated or secondary active transport.

inositol 1,4,5-trisphosphate or cyclic adenosine monophosphate, cAMP; see Chapter 2).

Within cells, Ca^{2+} is an important regulator of many functions. It does this by influencing the activity of Ca^{2+}-binding proteins such as **troponin, calmodulin and synaptotagmin**. These proteins in turn control pathways that determine the activity of the cell (e.g. contraction, secretion). Thus Ca^{2+} is an important **intracellular messenger**.

Intracellular pH

Many cell functions (e.g. enzyme activities, growth) are also influenced by cell pH, and changes in H^+ activity can influence both the activity of cytosolic Ca^{2+} and the levels of cAMP. These in turn influence a variety of specific cellular functions. Since H^+ ions are formed continuously through cell metabolism, cells must be able to buffer H^+ ions and expel them to the interstitial fluid. In general, mammalian cell pH is approximately 7.0–7.2, i.e. slightly more acidic than the plasma pH of 7.4. This is considerably more alkaline than the pH of about 6.5 predicted from the Nernst equation (p. 14) if H^+ ions were distributed across the plasma membrane in electrochemical equilibrium. A major contribution to the removal of H^+ from the cell is Na^+–H^+ counter-transport. Also of importance in cell pH regulation is HCO_3^- transport for which a variety of pathways have been identified (e.g. Cl^-–HCO_3^- counter-transport and Na^+–HCO_3^- co-transport).

Endocytosis and exocytosis

Endocytosis and exocytosis represent energy-dependent processes by which molecules of large molecular weight are encapsulated in membrane as they enter or before they leave the cells.

These mechanisms allow energy-dependent transport of material between cells and the interstitial fluid. They differ from those discussed above in that bulk movements occur by processes that involve portions of membrane. These processes constantly add and delete membrane at the cell surface and are referred to as 'constitutive' in contrast to 'triggered' secretory events that release cellular material in response to an extracellular signal (Fig. 1.8).

In **endocytosis**, invaginations of the plasma membrane first enclose extracellular material and then seal, forming vacuoles or vesicles within the cell that may fuse with lysosomes where they and their contents are degraded. Alternatively, the vesicular membrane may be recycled. Endocytosis is of particular importance for uptake into cells of substances of large molecular weight, such as proteins, which do not otherwise cross plasma membranes.

Pinocytosis and **phagocytosis** are forms of endocytosis. Pinocytosis ('cell drinking') refers to the endocytotic uptake of solutions into cells, whereas phagocytosis ('cell eating') refers to the engulfing of particulate matter, e.g. bacteria and viruses, by neutrophils and macrophages.

Exocytosis is the reverse of endocytosis. Here substances are released from cells into the ECF by fusion of intracellular vesicles with the plasma membrane (Fig. 1.8). This results in an increase in the area of the plasma membrane that is then reduced by endocytosis. Important examples of exocytosis include the release of peptide hormones from endocrine glands, of enzyme precursors from exocrine glands in the gut, and of neurotransmitters from nerve terminals. These processes are triggered by an increase in the cytosolic Ca^{2+} concentration, for example due to influx of Ca^{2+} in response to specific stimuli.

Transcytosis is a combination of endocytosis occurring at one membrane of a cell (endothelial or epithelial) and exocytosis occurring at the other membrane. Thus a variety of macromolecules (e.g. plasma proteins) can be conveyed through the cell without degradation.

1.6 Resting membrane potential

The resting membrane potential (RMP) is largely a K^+ diffusion potential modified by the small finite permeability of the membrane to Na^+ or Cl^-. Its magnitude can be estimated using the Goldman equation or modifications thereof. Although ultimately responsible for generating the ionic gradients on which the membrane potential depends,

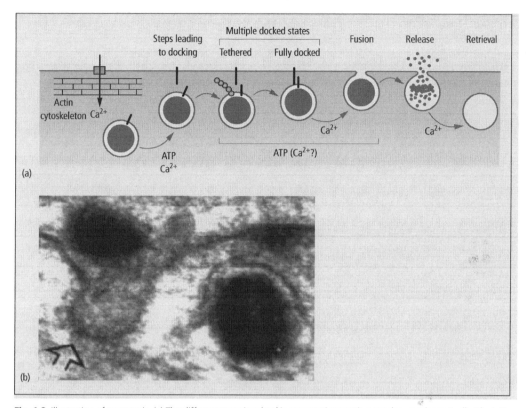

Fig. 1.8 Illustration of exocytosis. (a) The different steps involved in exocytotic secretion are shown schematically. The initi-ating step is Ca^{2+} influx across the plasma membrane, which increases the cytosolic Ca^{2+} concentration. In the presence of ATP this leads to docking—in several steps—of the granule at the plasma membrane. Thereafter fusion of the granule membrane with the plasma membrane (also Ca^{2+}-dependent) takes place. At the point of fusion, opening—i.e. direct continuity between the granule interior and the ECF—occurs, and the secretory material can move into the ECF (release of secretory material). The final stage is retrieval of the inserted granule membrane. (b) Electron microscopic image of an in-tact intracellular secretory granule and an exocytotic event (arrow). The image captures the moment just after the secreto-ry material has been released. The diameter of the secretory granule is approximately 100 nm. (From Burgoyne, R.D. & Morgan, A. (2003) *Physiol Rev,* **83**, 581–632.)

the Na⁺–K⁺ pump contributes only a few millivolts to the RMP as a consequence of its direct activity.

A difference of electrical potential is found across plasma membranes between the ICF and ECF. This difference, called the **RMP**, has a magnitude of up to −80 to −90 mV with the cell interior being nega-tive with respect to the interstitial fluid.

Diffusion potentials

The RMP is predominantly a **diffusion potential**. It arises because the plasma membrane is selective-ly permeable to ions. Consider a simple membrane

permeable only to K⁺, separating two solutions of different KCl concentrations (Fig. 1.9). Initially, there will be net K⁺ diffusion from side 1, the solu-tion with the higher K⁺ concentration, to side 2, driven by the chemical potential difference

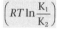

$$\left(RT \ln \frac{K_1}{K_2} \right)$$

(Fig. 1.9a). This will immediately create an electri-cal potential difference, with the side to which the K⁺ is moving being positive. This electrical poten-tial difference ($zF\Delta V$) will in turn increase the driv-ing force for K⁺ to move from side 2 to side 1. An

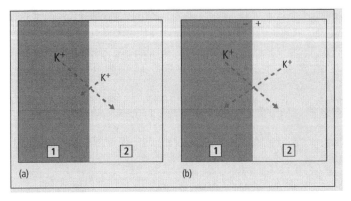

Fig. 1.9 Diffusion potential: (a) initially and (b) at equilibrium. The size of the K^+- symbols represent the relative magnitudes of the K^+ concentrations on sides 1 and 2.

equilibrium will be reached when the magnitudes of the two unidirectional fluxes of K^+ become equal (Fig. 1.9b). Now, the larger chemical gradient driving K^+ movement from side 1 to side 2 is balanced by the electrical gradient driving K^+ movement from side 2 to side 1.

It is essential to appreciate that very few ions actually move across the membrane during the establishment of the diffusion potential. For example, a change in potential difference of 100 mV would occur across 1 cm^2 of a membrane with properties similar to cell plasma membranes if only 10^{-12} mol of K^+ were to move. This charge separation would be confined to a distance of 10 nm across the membrane.

Recall that, for any ion c, the electrochemical potential gradient across the membrane is

$$\Delta\tilde{\mu} = RT\ln\frac{c_1}{c_2} + zFV$$

(p. 6). At equilibrium there is no electrochemical potential gradient across the membrane, i.e. $\Delta\tilde{\mu} = 0$. Therefore,

$$-zFV = RT\ln\frac{c_1}{c_2}$$

Nernst equation

The above equation can be rearranged by dividing both sides by zF.

$$-V = \frac{RT}{zF}\ln\frac{c_1}{c_2}$$

For a given ion, the electrical potential difference (V) across the membrane at equilibrium is called the **equilibrium potential** and is given the symbol E. Therefore,

$$E = \frac{RT}{zF}\ln\frac{c_2}{c_1}$$

(Note the inversion of the concentration ratio to allow for the removal of the negative sign from the potential difference term, E.)

This is the **Nernst equation** introduced by the German theoretical chemist W. Nernst (1864–1941). In effect it states either 'the maximum electromotive force that can be generated by a given ratio of concentrations of an ion, or the maximum ratio of concentration that can be sustained by a potential difference imposed from an external source'.

For use it is often convenient to put in actual values for the constants. This gives for monovalent ions at 37°C:

$$E = 27\ln\frac{c_2}{c_1} \quad or \quad E = 61\log_{10}\frac{c_2}{c_1}$$

where E has units of mV.

In the example illustrated in Fig. 1.9, with the membrane permeable only to K^+ (i.e. the only channel type present would be K^+-selective), the RMP would be the **equilibrium potential** for K^+ (E_K), with the magnitude given by the Nernst equation. Applying this and using values for K^+ concentrations in cells and ECF from Table 1.1, E_K is $27\ln 5/150 = 27 \times -3.33 = -90$ mV (inside negative). That is, if the plasma membrane was permeable only to K⁺, the RMP would be –90 mV. However, the measured RMP of most cells is significantly lower (–70 to –80 mV). The reason is that the plasma membrane is not totally impermeable to Na⁺, and Na⁺ ions diffusing down their concentration gradient (for example through Na⁺–amino acid co-transporters, Fig. 1.10) carry some positive charge into the cell and thus reduce the actual RMP to values less negative than E_K. In many cell types the distribution of Cl⁻, influenced by Na⁺-linked co-transport, also plays a role, since the plasma membrane can have a significant Cl⁻ permeability (i.e. contain Cl⁻ channels).

Equations for estimating RMP

The contribution of the diffusion of other ions to the RMP is expressed in the **Goldman equation**:

$$V = \frac{RT}{F} \ln \frac{P_K K_o + P_{Na} Na_o + P_{Cl} Cl_i}{P_K K_i + R_{Na} Na_i + P_{Cl} Cl_o}$$

where V is the membrane potential, P is the membrane permeability to the ion denoted by its subscript, o indicates the outside concentration and i the inside concentration. Note that because Cl⁻ is an anion the Cl⁻ concentrations are inverted in the Goldman equation.

A simpler version of the above equation, which assumes that Cl⁻ is passively distributed across the membrane and that, therefore, there is no net Cl⁻ diffusion, is the **Hodgkin–Katz equation**:

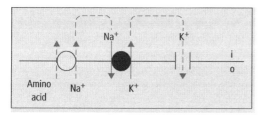

Fig. 1.10 A simple plasma membrane transport model. Recycling of Na⁺ and K⁺ through the Na⁺–K⁺ pump, Na⁺–amino acid co-transporter and K⁺ channel. In the steady state the only net transport is uptake of amino acid into the cell.

$$V = \frac{RT}{F} \ln \frac{K_o + bNa_o}{K_i + bNa_i}$$

where b is the ratio P_{Na}/P_K and is taken to be 0.01 for the resting axon. The equation predicts $V = 27$ ln(5 + 1.5)/(150 + 0.1) = 27 × –3.07 = –83 mV.

The good agreement of this predicted value with the measured RMP in some cell types supports the idea that the RMP in these cases is largely a K⁺ diffusion potential modified by the membrane's small permeability to Na⁺ ions.

What direct effect does the Na⁺–K⁺ pump have on RMP?

Since the Na⁺–K⁺ pump creates the unequal distributions of K⁺ and Na⁺ between cells and the ECF, its activity is indirectly responsible for the RMP. A pump that moved one K⁺ in for each Na⁺ out would carry no net charge and, therefore, no current across the membrane. However, the pump is not electrically neutral but transfers three Na⁺ out for every two K⁺ carried in. Thus current is generated directly by the pump, which is therefore termed **electrogenic**. However, provided that the membrane is much more permeable to K⁺ than to Na⁺, this electrogenic ion transport contributes relatively little (only a few millivolts) to the resting membrane potential, which is dominated by the K⁺ diffusion potential.

A simple membrane model

The simplest model of the electrophysiological properties of the plasma membrane must contain at least three transporters: K⁺ channels, the Na⁺–K⁺ pump and a Na⁺–amino acid co-transporter (Fig. 1.10). If the amino acid in question is neutral, then the RMP would be accounted for by the Hodgkin–Katz equation. In the steady state the only net transport would be uptake of amino acid, which is needed for protein synthesis.

1.7 Cell volume regulation

Cell volume reflects cell water content. Since plasma membranes are relatively permeable to water

(p. 6), water will be distributed between cells and interstitial fluid to maintain constant the **activity of water** in each compartment. Water activity is affected by solutes and by hydrostatic pressure. Water activity in a solution is decreased as the total concentration of solute particles is increased. It is increased when hydrostatic pressure is increased. A difference in water activity between compartments will result in a net movement of water across the membrane down its activity gradient—a process termed **osmosis**.

Osmosis and osmotic pressure

Osmosis is the net movement of water across a membrane driven by a gradient of water activity. Osmotic pressure is the hydrostatic pressure required to prevent osmosis. Osmolarity expresses the total number of osmotically active particles per litre of water.

An **ideal semi-permeable membrane** prevents diffusion of solutes but not solvent. Net movement of water across such a membrane (**osmosis**) will occur down the gradient of water activity and, therefore, from the more dilute to the more concentrated solution. It can be stopped by applying hydrostatic pressure to the more concentrated solution to raise its water activity. The hydrostatic pressure that just stops osmosis is the **osmotic pressure**, i.e. the pressure required to equalize water activities in the two compartments. A greater hydrostatic pressure in that compartment will raise water activity further and will cause water to leave the more concentrated solution. This is **ultrafiltration**.

The osmotic pressure ($\Delta\pi$) across an ideal semi-permeable membrane at equilibrium can be estimated by the **van't Hoff equation**:

$$\Delta\pi = RT\sum(c_1 - c_2)$$

where R is the gas constant, T is the absolute temperature (K) and $\sum(c_1 - c_2)$ is the sum of the difference in molar concentrations (mol L^{-1}) of all osmotically active solutes on sides 1 and 2 of the membrane.

Since osmotic pressure exists only when osmosis can occur, it is wrong to speak of the osmotic pressure of a solution. Instead, we use the term osmo-larity (osmol L^{-1}) to describe the effects of the total number of osmotically active particles per litre of solution. Mammalian fluids have an osmolarity of about 0.3 osmol L^{-1} and thus, when separated from pure water, would exert an osmotic pressure across an ideal semi-permeable membrane of about $RT \times 0.3 = 7.6$ atm or 5800 mmHg or 770 kPa at body temperature. However, when plasma is separated from interstitial fluid by the capillary wall, the difference in osmotic effect arises from the proteins and their associated counter-ions, which are largely restricted to the capillary lumen. Here, the protein concentration is about 1.5 mmol L^{-1} and the total osmotic pressure difference generated in this system approximates 25–30 mmHg.

The osmolarity of a solution can be estimated from the van't Hoff equation, by dividing the osmotic pressure in atmospheres by RT. An electrolyte like NaCl is dissociated in solution into two osmotically active ions, so its osmolar concentration will be approximately twice the molar concentration. The osmolarity of a solution can be measured in a commercial osmometer that relies on the fact that the osmotic pressure is related to the change in the freezing point or vapour pressure of the solution.

The term **osmolality** (osmol kg^{-1} solvent) is often used instead of osmolarity (osmol L^{-1} solution). However, since in dilute aqueous solutions molal concentrations (mol kg^{-1} water) closely approximate molar concentrations (mol L^{-1} solution), the terms osmolality and osmolarity are often used interchangeably.

Net flow of water across membranes

The net flow of water across a membrane per unit time (J_v) is given by

$$J_v = ALp(\Delta P - \Delta\pi)$$

where A is the area of the membrane available for flow, Lp is the hydraulic conductivity which is a measure of the ease with which water flows through the membrane, ($\Delta P - \Delta\pi$) is the driving force which is dependent on the differences in hydrostatic pressure (ΔP) and effective osmotic pressure ($\Delta\pi$) across the membrane.

Cell volume

Cell volume is determined by the cell content of osmoles and the extracellular osmolarity. Under physiological conditions, the colloid osmotic effect of impermeant cell solutes is offset by the Na^+–K^+ pump which effectively maintains Na^+ as an impermeant extracellular solute. Tonicity describes the behaviour of cells placed in a solution. If cells swell the solution is hypotonic, if cells shrink the solution is hypertonic, if cell volume is unchanged the solution is isotonic.

In the steady state, cell volume is constant and J_v = 0. Thus, $\Delta P = \Delta \pi$. Since animal plasma membranes cannot withstand appreciable gradients of hydrostatic pressure, both ΔP and $\Delta \pi$ between the ECF and ICF must be zero. This means that the osmolarities of both fluids must be identical. Since the plasma membrane is freely permeable to water, water will move rapidly between ECF and ICF in response to any tendency for alterations in water activities between these two compartments. The determinants of cell volume, therefore, are:

1 the total number of osmotically active particles within the cell; and

2 the osmolarity of the ECF.

The cell has a considerable quantity of impermeant solutes (e.g. proteins, organic phosphates) whereas the interstitial fluid is relatively devoid of these. There is, therefore, a colloid osmotic gradient that would draw fluid into the cells. Why then do cells not swell under physiological conditions? The Na^+–K^+ pump, by holding Na^+ extracellularly and preventing its accumulation in the cell, effectively offsets the colloid osmotic effect of cell macromolecules. If this pump ceases to expel Na^+ (e.g. when cells are chilled), Na^+ enters passively down its concentration gradient bringing Cl^- with it to preserve electroneutrality; to equalize its activity water then moves into the cells across the membrane and the cells swell.

Tonicity

The behaviour of cells in artificial bathing solutions cannot be predicted from the osmolarity of these solutions. It depends also on the permeability of the membrane to the solutes. For example, when cells are placed in $300\,mmol\,L^{-1}$ urea, which is approximately isosmotic with mammalian fluids, the cells will swell because urea enters and water follows. A new term is required to define the strength of a solution as it affects the volume of cells. This is **tonicity**, which is defined operationally thus:

1 if cells **shrink** in a solution, the solution is **hypertonic**,

2 if cells **swell** in a solution, the solution is **hypotonic**, and

3 if the cell volume is **unchanged**, the solution is **isotonic**.

Tonicity may also depend upon the functional activity and metabolism of the cells. Most cells swell grossly if their metabolism is inhibited, even in isosmotic NaCl solutions, because the cells gain NaCl. Consequently, isolated tissues need substrates and O_2 as well as the appropriate inorganic ions in bathing solutions designed to be isosmolar with normal ECF.

1.8 Movement of water and solutes across epithelia

Epithelia separate the internal from the external environment. Net movement of solutes and water may occur via the epithelial cells (cellular route) and between these cells (paracellular route). Net movement from lumen to interstitial fluid is termed absorption; net movement from interstitial fluid to lumen is termed secretion. On the basis of the properties of the paracellular route, epithelia can be classified as tight or leaky. The major solute absorbed by tight absorptive epithelia is Na^+. In the absence of hormonal stimulation, water permeability is low. Leaky absorptive epithelia transport a number of solutes and have a relatively high water permeability. Epithelial cells in a variety of organs can secrete an isosmotic NaCl solution. In such secretory epithelia, this involves activation of an apical membrane Cl^- conductance and movements of Na^+ from interstitial fluid to lumen via the paracellular route.

Epithelia separate the internal from the external environment and regulate movement of solutes and water to and from the body. Examples include the surface layers of the skin, lungs, wall of the alimentary canal and lining of the urogenital systems. The epithelial cells, which may be one or more layers thick, are separated by their basement membranes from supporting connective tissue containing blood vessels, nerves and smooth muscle fibres. It is believed that the transport functions reside only in the epithelial cell layer. All epithelial cells are separated from their neighbours by a space—the **lateral intercellular space**—whose size may vary (Fig. 1.11). They are held to each other at their luminal edges by junctions—**tight junctions** (Fig. 1.12).

Tight junctions were originally thought to be impermeable, but it is now appreciated that to a variable extent solutes and water may diffuse across them. There are thus two pathways by which solutes and water can cross epithelia, either through cells or between them. Substances passing between cells must cross tight junctions and pass through the lateral intercellular spaces—the so-called **paracellular** or **shunt pathway**. The amount passing through this shunt pathway differs between epithelia, depending on the difference in permeability characteristics of the tight junctions. Epithelia in which the paracellular pathway makes a significant contribution to total movements (e.g. proximal renal tubule, small in-

testine) are referred to as **leaky**, whereas those in which the cellular pathway predominates are referred to as **tight** (e.g. renal collecting duct, salivary gland ducts, amphibian skin and urinary bladder).

The importance of the concept of leaky and tight epithelia lies in the underlying physiological significance. In general, leaky epithelia are specialized for the bulk reabsorption of isosmotic solutions and lie more proximally, whereas tight epithelia lie more distally and are more selective in the manner in which they handle the load presented to them. Hormonal control of salt and water balance tends to be exerted on tight rather than on leaky epithelia.

Net flow of water across an epithelium per unit of time (J_v) is determined by $ALp(\Delta P - \Delta \pi)$ (p. 16) while net movements of solutes are determined by the following considerations. There are specific cellular transport pathways for a variety of solutes that allow unidirectional movement between lumen and interstitial fluid. In addition, solutes may diffuse in both directions through the paracellular pathway. The net solute flux (amount moved per unit time per unit area) is, therefore, the difference between two unidirectional fluxes. Net movement from lumen to interstitial fluid is termed **absorption**; net movement from interstitial fluid to lumen is called **secretion**. The net

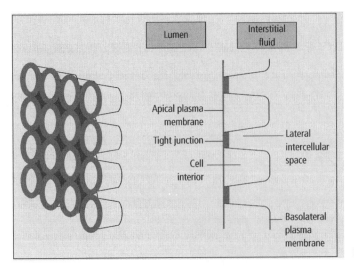

Fig. 1.11 Transporting epithelium.

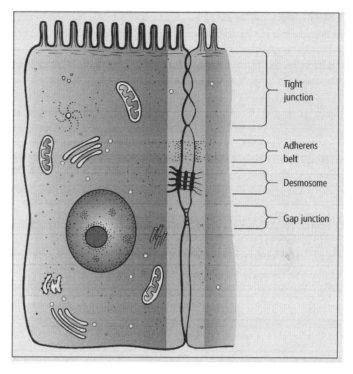

Fig. 1.12 Types of epithelial cell junctions. Tight junctions are formed by a series of connections between the outer surfaces of the plasma membranes of adjacent cells. They completely encircle the apical end of each cell, form an impermeable barrier for large molecules and are variably permeable to small solutes, ions and water. Cells are also held together by anchoring junctions, of which the adherens belt and the desmosomes are two examples. These junctions are connected to the cell cytoskeletal elements (adherens belt–actin filaments, desmosomes–intermediate filaments). Gap junctions provide a low resistance pathway between neighbouring cells through which small solutes, ions and water can pass (p. 25).

movement of any solute across an epithelium is determined by:

1 available surface area (since amount moved/unit time = area × flux);

2 time in contact with the available area;

3 electrochemical potential gradient, which will be influenced by blood and lymph flow;

4 properties of the epithelium, i.e. tight or leaky, together with the availability of specific transport mechanisms.

Absorptive epithelia

In general, epithelia that actively absorb ions primarily move Na^+. This transepithelial Na^+ transport generates a potential difference across the epithelial layer. The transepithelial potential difference in tight epithelia is high (>20 mV) whereas in leaky epithelia it is low (0–5 mV). Since electrical neutrality must be preserved, Cl^- follows passively, as does water when water permeability of the epithelium is sufficient. Mechanisms by which Na^+ crosses epithelia are summarized for a typical tight

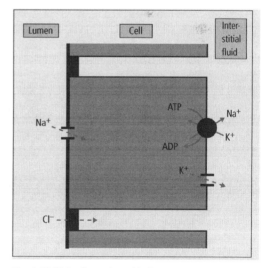

Fig. 1.13 Tight absorptive epithelium.

epithelium in Fig. 1.13. Unlike muscle, nerve and blood cells whose plasma membranes are symmetrical, the plasma membranes of epithelial cells are asymmetric. The apical portion, which faces the

19

lumen, has unusual permeability and transport characteristics. It has a high Na^+ and low K^+ permeability and no Na^+,K^+–ATPase. In contrast, the basolateral portion, consisting of the membrane beneath the tight junctions and adjacent to the capillaries, is similar in its permeability and transport properties to plasma membranes of non-epithelial cells. In general, in tight epithelia only Na^+ readily crosses the apical membrane (passively via aqueous channels) and, in the absence of hormonal stimulation, water permeability is low.

In leaky epithelia (Fig. 1.14), not only does Na^+ cross the apical membrane through channels, but entry of glucose, some amino acids and phosphate may be coupled to Na^+ entry. The electrochemical potential gradient for Na^+ entry is used to drive the accompanying solute into the cells from the lumen (i.e. co-transport). The active transport of Na^+ from cell to interstitial fluid is thought to involve the same Na^+–K^+ pump as described above (p. 9). The coupling of net water movement to net solute movement across leaky epithelia may involve the generation within the lateral intercellular spaces of a local region of Na^+ concentration, somewhat higher than that in interstitial fluid, reflecting the distribution and activity of the Na^+–K^+ pump. This provides an osmotic gradient moving water, either through the cells or tight junctions, from the lumen to the lateral intercellular space. This movement in turn creates a local hydrostatic pressure gradient so that fluid flows from the lateral intercellular spaces to the interstitium. However, the magnitude of any local osmotic gradient in the lateral intercellular spaces is now thought to be only a few milliosmoles per litre.

Counter-transport of Na^+ for cell H^+ is also often found. In addition, though often represented as coupled co-transport with Na^+ (Fig. 1.14), movement of Cl^- across the apical plasma membrane may be by counter-transport with cell HCO_3^- (or OH^-). In a cell with both Na^+–H^+ and Cl^-–HCO_3^- exchangers, the net effect will be Na^+ and Cl^- entry to the cell. H_2O and CO_2 are formed from the H^+ and HCO_3^- ions extruded from the cell. Loss of this Cl^- from the cell is shown as occurring through basolateral Cl^- channels, but this remains to be established. Alternatively, it has been suggested that a neutral K^+–Cl^- co-transporter may be responsible.

Secretory epithelia

A variety of inorganic and organic ions are secreted by epithelia and specific mechanisms are discussed in the appropriate chapters. These secretions result in the transfer of solutes and water to the surfaces of the body (internal or external) and are produced by exocrine glands. (This contrasts with secretions from cells that are carried in the plasma (hormones) which are produced by endocrine glands.)

Of particular interest because of its contribution to the production of many secretions (sweat, tears, saliva, pancreatic juice and some intestinal fluids) is the mechanism of isosmotic NaCl secretion, summarized in Fig. 1.15. The secretory cells comprise a relatively leaky epithelium. A Na^+–K^+–2 Cl^- co-transporter in the basolateral membrane is responsible for driving Cl^- into the cells against its electrochemical gradient. The accompanying Na^+ and K^+ are recycled back to the interstitial fluid via pumps and channels as shown in Fig. 1.15. In the quiescent state, the apical plasma membrane is relatively impermeable to Cl^-. Neurotransmitters or hormones stimulate secretion by increasing the cytosolic Ca^{2+} concentration and this opens Cl^- channels in the apical membrane and increases the

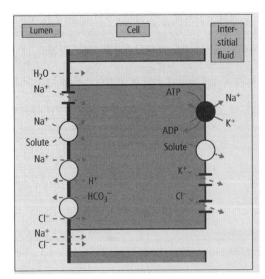

Fig. 1.14 Leaky absorptive epithelium.

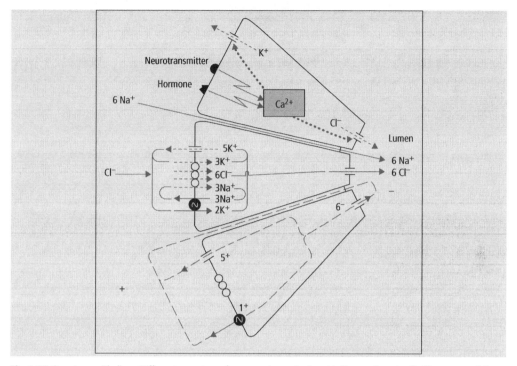

Fig. 1.15 Secretory epithelium. Different aspects are for convenience displayed in three adjacent cells. The upper cell shows the process of activating Ca^{2+}-dependent Cl^- channels in the apical, and Ca^{2+}-dependent K^+ channels in the basolateral plasma membrane, by increasing the cytosolic Ca^{2+} concentration in response to stimulation by either a neurotransmitter or a hormone. In the middle cell the ionic transport steps, mediated by various transport proteins are shown, highlighting the relative stoichiometries. In the steady-state the only net transport across the basolateral membrane is Cl^- uptake and the amount of Cl^- taken up per unit time must be equal to the amount of Cl^- leaving the cell per unit time through the Cl^- channels in the apical membrane. The lower cell illustrates the overall electrical circuit. The Na^+–K^+–$2Cl^-$ co-transport is electroneutral. The outward current through the K^+ channels and the Na^+–K^+ pump in the basal plasma membrane exactly matches the inward current (outward anion flux) through the apical Cl^- channels. (From Petersen, O.H. (1986) *Am J Physiol*, **251**, G1–G13.)

probability of K^+ channels being open in the basolateral membrane. The activation of basolateral K^+ channels counteracts the depolarizing tendency of the Cl^- channel opening and therefore preserves the electrochemical driving force for Cl^- exit into the lumen. Cl^-, therefore, moves from the cell to the lumen down its electrochemical gradient. As a

consequence of the increased luminal negativity, Na^+ passes from the interstitial fluid to the lumen through the leaky paracellular pathway to maintain electroneutrality. Water moves, both through the cells and through the paracellular pathway, down the osmotic gradient. Thus an isosmotic NaCl secretion is produced.

Chapter 2

Cellular Communication

Cells communicate with one another by chemical and electrical signals. There are also specialized sensory cells that respond to chemical, electrical, light, mechanical or heat stimuli that may come from external or internal sources. The cellular response to these signals may be simple and short-lived, such as depolarization, or it may be complex and long-lasting, such as the acquisition of memory. Nevertheless, the cellular mechanisms underlying these responses have much in common. Each of these signals is transduced into electrical or biochemical changes within the cell, which lead to a characteristic response. For example, the stimuli that give rise to the sensations of taste, smell, hearing and vision, and also certain neurotransmitters and hormones, can all control the opening and closing of ion channels and depolarize or hyperpolarize cells.

In this chapter we discuss how information is transmitted between cells, and how signals from the external and internal environment are received and transduced into electrical and biochemical changes within the cell.

2.1 How signals are transmitted between cells

Cells communicate with one another by chemical signals that either diffuse between cells (neurotransmitters, and paracrine and autocrine agents), or are disseminated in the blood (hormones).

These signals include small organic molecules (e.g. acetylcholine and adrenaline), and larger molecules such as proteins and steroids. Cells may also communicate with their immediate neighbours through gap junctions, which transmit both electrical and chemical signals.

Chemical signalling

The nervous and endocrine systems use chemical signals, neurotransmitters and hormones, respectively, for communication. **Neurotransmitters** are released from neurones, diffuse across a narrow synaptic space or cleft (<100 nm) and act on adjacent neurones, muscle cells or secretory cells in glands; **hormones** are transmitted in the circulation and act on cells of distant target organs. Hormones act at very low concentrations, typically 10^{-6} to $10^{-9}\,mol\,L^{-1}$ (but in some cases as low as $10^{-12}\,mol\,L^{-1}$), while the concentrations of neurotransmitters in synaptic clefts may reach $5 \times 10^{-4}\,mol\,L^{-1}$ (e.g. acetylcholine at the neuromuscular junction). In addition there are **paracrine agents** released locally by cells that act on neighbouring cells and **autocrine agents** that act on the cells that produced them. Therefore neurotransmitters, by definition, are paracrine agents, although they are not usually classified as such, and some hormones, e.g. gastrointestinal hormones, may also be classified as paracrine agents, because they may act locally as well as travelling in the blood stream to distant target organs. Secretions of neurones that are transported to distant target organs in the blood stream are referred to as **neurohormones**. Finally, certain cells secrete **growth factors** that are essential at critical stages in the development of their target cells.

Chemical signals may be ions or metabolites (e.g. Ca^{2+}, glucose or amino acids) which stimulate certain endocrine cells; they may be simple organic molecules (e.g. the neurotransmitters acetylcholine, noradrenaline and glutamate), or they may be more complex molecules (e.g. protein and steroid hormones). Even dissolved gases such as nitric oxide and carbon monoxide may act as chemical signals between cells. Many substances that were first identified as hormones produced in endocrine glands are also synthesized in the nervous system where they act as neurotransmitters or neuromodulators (see Chapter 3). Consequently, there is considerable overlap in the chemical messengers used by these two systems.

Synthesis and secretion

Neurotransmitters and many hormones that do not readily cross plasma membranes are packaged into **secretory vesicles** within the cell prior to their release by **exocytosis** (see Chapter 1). These include small polar organic molecules and large polypeptides. All cells can secrete proteins into the extracellular fluid (**constitutive secretion**), but only specialized cells do so in a regulated manner (**regulated secretion**). Regulated secretion occurs after an appropriate stimulus. Often a rise in the cytosolic Ca^{2+} concentration triggers exocytosis; the vesicles fuse with the plasma membrane and release their contents into the extracellular fluid (see Fig. 1.8).

Small polar organic molecules may be synthesized by enzymes in the cytosol, and then are actively accumulated within the vesicles by membrane-bound transporters. Alternatively, they may be synthesized, at least in part, by enzymes bound within the vesicles.

Polypeptide molecules, including proteins and glycoproteins that are destined for secretion, are first synthesized on the ribosomes of the rough (granular) endoplasmic reticulum as part of larger precursor polypeptides called **prepropolypeptides**. As they are synthesized, they are inserted into the intracisternal space of the endoplasmic reticulum and are subsequently modified by deletion of peptide sequences (Fig. 2.1). The 'pre' part of the prepropolypeptide is a **signal peptide**, which is involved in ribosomal attachment and transfer of the newly synthesized polypeptide across the membrane of the endoplasmic reticulum. After insertion the signal peptide is removed from the propolypeptide by a signal peptidase. Small vesicles containing the propolypeptide then bud off from the endoplasmic reticulum and transfer their contents to the Golgi apparatus by fusion with the Golgi membrane. In the Golgi apparatus the propolypeptide is packaged into secretory vesicles, and the 'pro' part is then split from the propolypeptide. Where the secretory product is a glycoprotein, carbohydrate groups are added by enzymes in the endoplasmic reticulum and these groups are further modified in the Golgi apparatus.

Lipophilic molecules are not packaged into vesicles for secretion. For instance, **steroid hormones** (e.g. cortisol, oestrogen and testosterone) are synthesized from cholesterol (Fig. 2.2) in steps that take place in the mitochondria, smooth endoplasmic reticulum and cytoplasm, and which require acetate, O_2, reduced nicotinamide adenine dinucleotide phosphate and other co-factors. They are not stored to any extent in the cells that synthesize them and they readily cross the plasma membrane of the cell. Therefore, their rate of release is directly related to their rate of synthesis.

Other signals

Thus far we have been discussing soluble chemical signals that pass from one cell to another. There are also proteins or glycoproteins attached to cell surfaces (e.g. adhesion molecules) or to the extracellular matrix (e.g. fibronectin, laminin, agrin) that provide signals for cell migration during development and for the localization of receptors, ion channels and enzymes to particular areas of the cell surface that best serve their function.

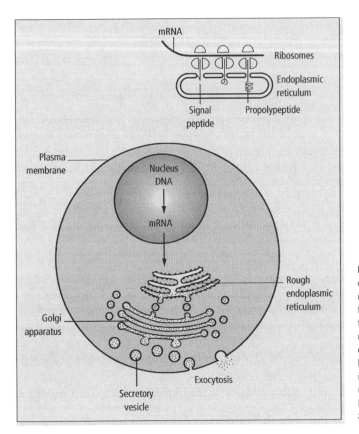

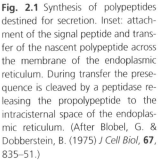

Fig. 2.1 Synthesis of polypeptides destined for secretion. Inset: attachment of the signal peptide and transfer of the nascent polypeptide across the membrane of the endoplasmic reticulum. During transfer the presequence is cleaved by a peptidase releasing the propolypeptide to the intracisternal space of the endoplasmic reticulum. (After Blobel, G. & Dobberstein, B. (1975) *J Cell Biol*, **67**, 835–51.)

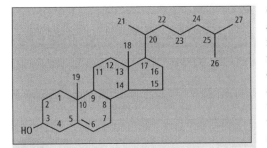

Fig. 2.2 Structure of cholesterol from which steroid hormones are synthesized.

Gap junctions

Membrane junctions that hold cells together (desmosomes and adherens belts), and those that impose a barrier to diffusion across layers of cells (tight junctions), have been mentioned previously (see Fig. 1.12). Another type, the **gap junction**, allows small organic molecules and ions to pass from cell to cell. In the regions of gap junctions, the plasma membranes of the two opposing cells come together to form a gap about 3 nm wide and small channels about 1.5 nm in diameter extend across the gap, linking the cytoplasm of the two cells (Fig. 2.3). The channels at gap junctions are formed from transmembrane protein assemblies called **connexons** (Fig. 2.3), of which there are several hundred at each gap junction. Two connexons from opposing membranes join together to form the aqueous pore or channel. Gap junctions are found in many tissues; in cardiac and smooth muscle cells they allow electrical signals to pass from one cell to another and thus synchronize their activity. In addition to ions, small molecules (<1500 M_r, e.g. sugars, amino acids and nucleotides) can also pass through the connecting

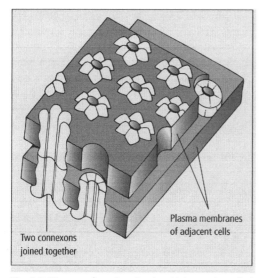

Two connexons
joined together

Plasma membranes
of adjacent cells

Fig. 2.3 Diagram of gap junction in which proteins called connexons form channels between adjacent cells. Each connexon is composed of six subunits and joins with a connexon in the opposing plasma membrane to form a channel that links the cytoplasm of adjoining cells.

2.2 How cells respond to external stimuli

Cells respond to a variety of external stimuli and transduce these signals into electrical and biochemical changes. In many instances this involves the interaction of a signal with a receptor in the plasma membrane. This may lead directly to activation of ion channels, but more commonly it induces the production of intracellular messengers that then regulate cell function. Guanosine triphosphate (GTP) regulatory proteins play a crucial role in coupling receptor occupancy to the generation of an intracellular biochemical cascade. Recognized intracellular pathways include the cAMP, the cyclic guanosine monophosphate (cGMP) and phosphoinositide systems. Ca^{2+} is a particularly important intracellular regulator; its cytosolic activity may be raised by influx across the plasma membrane or by release from intracellular stores controlled by the phosphoinositide system.

In some cases there is a direct link between a stimulus and activation of ion channels. Examples include stretch-activated channels in touch receptors and voltage-sensitive channels in excitable tissues (see Chapter 4). However, for chemical stimuli (e.g. gustatory, olfactory, neurotransmitters, hormones, growth factors, etc.) the first event leading to a cellular response is the interaction of the chemical signal (**ligand**) with its **receptor**.

Receptors

Receptors are molecular entities, either proteins or glycoproteins, which bind ligands with high affinity. (Note that cells, or components of cells, that respond to sensory stimuli are also referred to as 'receptors' but the two should not be confused.) Receptors for ligands that do not penetrate cells readily (e.g. most neurotransmitters, peptide hormones, etc.) are located in the plasma membrane, but some lipophilic ligands (e.g. steroid and thyroid hormones) have their receptors in the cytoplasm or nucleus.

Receptors usually have a high **affinity** for their ligands. They also exhibit **specificity** and only those cells that contain the appropriate receptors

channels. Cells connected by gap junctions are thus electrically and chemically coupled. The density of gap junctional channels varies enormously between different tissue types. Skeletal muscle cells have no gap junctions and are therefore completely isolated from each other. At the other end of the spectrum we find the extremely well coupled liver and pancreatic acinar cells, in which gap junctions are as densely packed as is physically possible.

The opening and closing of the gap junctional channels may be regulated by changes in voltage, cytosolic pH and intracellular messengers in much the same way that membrane ion channels are regulated (see below). For example, an increase in the intracellular cyclic adenosine monophosphate (cAMP) concentration can rapidly increase the permeability of gap junctions in certain tissues, whereas an increase in intracellular acidity can close the channels. This in turn will influence the rate of transfer of messengers between adjacent cells.

will recognize and respond to the ligand. It is necessary to use radioactively labelled ligands to study the kinetics of binding (Fig. 2.4). As the number of receptors is limited, the binding also shows **saturation** as the concentration of the ligand is increased.

The response of cells to signal molecules may vary with the intensity of stimulation. High concentrations of signal molecules can temporarily inactivate receptors (e.g. by phosphorylation of the receptor)—a process known as **desensitization**. The number of receptors in a cell may also vary with stimulation, leading to a decrease in the number of cell receptors (**down-regulation**), or to an increase (**up-regulation**). The number of receptors in the plasma membrane at any time represents a balance between their rate of insertion into the membrane and their rate of removal from the membrane. The ligand can enhance the rate of removal of receptor from the membrane by inducing receptor phosphorylation and the internalization of ligand–receptor complexes by endocytosis. These complexes are sequestered into clathrin-coated vesicles that are transported to endosomes from which they may be recycled back to the plasma membrane.

The distribution of receptors on a cell is not necessarily uniform. For example, in adult skeletal muscle fibres the acetylcholine receptors are clustered at the neuromuscular junction and there are few receptors in the extrajunctional regions. However, if the nerve is cut, there is a marked increase in the synthesis of receptors in the extrajunctional regions. Junctional acetylcholine receptors (composed of $\alpha_2\beta\epsilon\delta$ subunits) differ in one of their subunits from extrajunctional receptors (composed of $\alpha_2\beta\gamma\delta$ subunits) (see Fig. 1.5). These differences in the distribution and composition of the acetylcholine receptors are controlled by a number of factors, including muscle activity, the protein agrin in the extracellular matrix of the synaptic cleft and trophic factors released by the nerve terminals.

As discussed in Chapter 1, interaction of a ligand with its receptor may lead to direct activation of an ion channel, i.e. the receptor is an integral part of the ion channel. We call this a receptor-operated channel that allows very rapid transfer of information. A good example of a receptor-operated channel is the acetylcholine receptor in skeletal muscle. In other cases, the interaction of the ligand with its receptor leads to the activation of a membrane-bound enzyme and the production of an intracellular messenger—a slower process—that then regulates cell function.

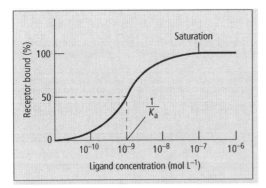

Fig. 2.4 Kinetics of binding of a radioactive ligand to its receptor. Specific binding is calculated by determining total binding of the radioactive ligand to its receptor and subtracting non-specific binding, which is measured in the presence of an excess of unlabelled ligand (agonist or antagonist). Note that binding becomes saturated as the concentration of radioactive ligand is increased and that the affinity constant (K_a) is given by the reciprocal of the ligand concentration at half maximal binding. Alternatively, it can be stated that the ligand concentration at half maximal binding is a measure of the equilibrium dissociation constant (K_d), which is the reciprocal of K_a.

Intracellular messengers

The first such intracellular messenger to be identified was **cAMP** (Fig. 2.5). Sutherland, who discovered the role of cAMP in the 1950s while studying the action of adrenaline on glycogenolysis in liver, called it a **second messenger**. It is synthesized from adenosine triphosphate (ATP) in a reaction catalysed by the enzyme **adenylyl cyclase**, which is stimulated or inhibited by many chemical signals. Ca^{2+} is now recognized as a particularly important intracellular messenger; stimuli may open channels allowing it to flow into the cell or be released from intracellular stores in the endoplasmic

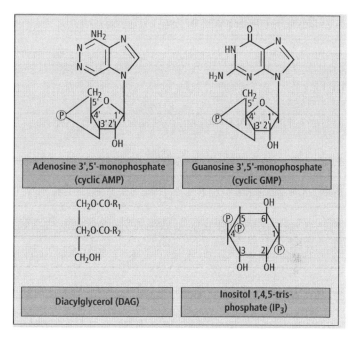

Fig. 2.5 Structure of some intracellular messengers.

reticulum. Other important intracellular messengers (e.g. cGMP, inositol 1,4,5-triphosphate and diacylglycerol) have since been identified (Fig. 2.5).

In many instances, but not all, these intracellular messengers affect **protein kinases** or **phosphatases**—enzymes that stimulate the phosphorylation or dephosphorylation, respectively, of other proteins. About one-third of eukaryotic proteins are phosphoproteins and **phosphorylation** is a major language of intracellular communication.

G proteins

In both the cAMP and the phosphoinositide systems that are described in detail later in this section, the step that follows the binding of the ligand to its receptor at the membrane surface, and that initiates the cell response, is the activation of a regulatory protein that binds GTP. Hence this protein is called a G protein. Many different ligand–receptor complexes are now known to activate G proteins, which have come to be known as **universal transducers**.

Large G proteins consist of α, β and γ subunits and so are referred to as **heterotrimers**. In the basal state, the α subunit of the G protein binds guanosine diphosphate (GDP) and the protein can be represented as βγα-GDP (Fig. 2.6). Following occupation of a surface receptor by its ligand, a conformational change in the G protein results in the exchange of GDP for cytoplasmic GTP, giving βγα-GTP. The α-GTP subunit then dissociates from the βγ subunits, and either the separated α-GTP subunit or the βγ-dimer interacts with an effector molecule. The effector may be an enzyme (e.g. adenylyl cyclase, phospholipase C-β, cGMP phosphodiesterase) or an ion channel (e.g. certain K$^+$ channels). Because the α subunit has GTPase activity, the GTP is subsequently converted to GDP and the inactive G protein is reconstituted as shown in Fig. 2.6.

A number of G proteins have been identified (Table 2.1). Some of these (G$_s$) stimulate adenylyl cyclase, others (G$_i$) inhibit this enzyme. Bacterial exotoxins have been particularly valuable in the identification of G proteins. **Cholera toxin**, which is produced by the bacterium that causes cholera, activates G$_s$ by catalysing adenosine diphosphate (ADP)-ribosylation of specific amino acid residues in the α subunit, so that it can no longer hydrolyse

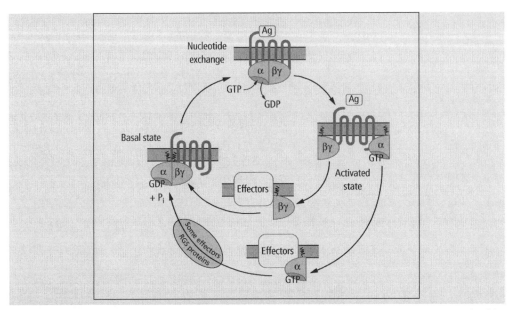

Fig. 2.6 Role of the G protein in signal transduction. The ligand (agonist; Ag) binds to the receptor on the outside of the plasma membrane and activates the G protein, which consists of $\alpha\beta\gamma$ subunits. In the basal (inactive) state, GDP is bound to the α-subunit. Activation involves a nucleotide exchange reaction in which GDP is replaced by GTP. The α-subunit then dissociates from the $\beta\gamma$-dimer, and either the α- or the $\beta\gamma$-subunit interacts with its specific effector. The spontaneous hydrolysis of GTP to GDP, catalysed by intrinsic GTPase activity, can be accelerated by various effectors, as well as by special regulators of G-protein signalling (the so-called RGS proteins). The GDP-bound α-subunit then reassociates with the $\beta\gamma$-subunit, reverting the G protein back to its inactive basal state. The GTPase activity of the α subunit breaks down GTP to GDP, causing the α-GDP subunit to dissociate from the effector and recombine with the $\beta\gamma$-dimer. P_i, inorganic phosphate. (From Wettschureck, N. & Offermanns, S. (2005) *Physiol Rev*, **85**, 1159–1204.)

Table 2.1 Heterotrimeric G proteins and their actions.

Type	Action	Comments
G_s	Stimulates adenylyl cyclase	Activated by cholera toxin
G_{olf}	Stimulates adenylyl cyclase in olfactory neurones	Activated by cholera toxin
G_{gus}	Stimulates adenylyl cyclase in gustatory cells	Activated by cholera toxin
G_i	Inhibits adenylyl cyclase	Activation blocked by pertussis toxin
	Activates Ca^{2+} channels	
G_o	Activates K channels	Occurs in high concentration in brain
	Inactivates Ca^{2+} channels	(approx. 1% of total protein);
		blocked by pertussis toxin
G_q	Stimulates phospholipase C-β	
G_t	Stimulates cGMP phosphodiesterase in photoreceptors	Known as transducin

its bound GTP. **Pertussis toxin**, which is produced by the bacterium that causes whooping cough, blocks the receptor-mediated activation of G_i and G_o, also by ADP-ribosylation of the α subunit, so that the complex remains bound to GDP.

The high concentration of G_o in the brain (Table 2.1) no doubt reflects the important role of this protein in the actions of the various neurotransmitters and neuromodulators. In some cases G_o may directly induce the opening of ion channels.

In addition to the heterotrimeric G protein family, there is another class of GTP-binding proteins of lower molecular mass, the Ras superfamily, also known as the 'small GTPases', which are discussed later in this chapter.

cAMP system

The enzyme adenylyl cyclase (formerly known as adenylate cyclase) converts ATP to cAMP plus pyrophosphate (PP_i). Depending on the G protein (G_s or G_i) that is activated by the interaction of the signal and its receptor, adenylyl cyclase activity may be either stimulated or inhibited.

Figure 2.7 summarizes the events that follow increased cAMP production. The raised level of cAMP within the cell stimulates **protein kinase A**, an enzyme that phosphorylates serine or threonine residues of other proteins. Protein kinase A is composed of two regulatory (R) subunits and two catalytic (C) subunits. cAMP binds to the R subunits, causing them to dissociate, and allows the free C subunits to phosphorylate cellular proteins. This may lead to specific changes in ion channel gating, enzyme activity, protein synthesis or gene activation, depending on the tissue involved. During this sequence of events, the initial signal is amplified many times. Eventually, the concentration of cAMP is restored to its basal level by degradation to adenosine monophosphate (AMP), this step being catalysed by the enzyme **cyclic nucleotide phosphodiesterase**. The phosphorylated proteins are deactivated by **phosphatases**.

In view of their specificity it may appear odd that the actions of so many hormones and neurotransmitters are mediated by cAMP. First, only certain tissues contain receptors that will react with a particular ligand to produce an increase in intracellular cAMP. Second, the responses of various tissues to raised levels of cAMP are different. For example, in response to an increase in cAMP, liver cells break down glycogen but heart cells increase their rate and strength of contraction.

In some cells an increase in cAMP activates the transcription of specific genes by stimulating the phosphorylation of a gene regulatory protein called the cAMP response element-binding protein (CREB), which in turn binds to a target DNA sequence that regulates gene transcription.

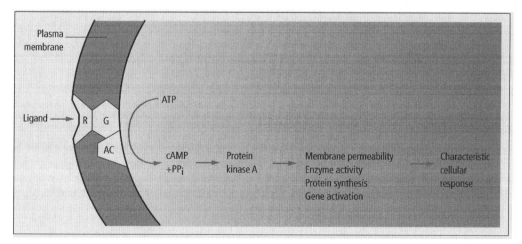

Fig. 2.7 Signals acting through cAMP. The ligand binds to its receptor (R) on the outer surface of the plasma membrane. At the inner surface are the GTP-regulatory protein (G) and the enzyme adenylyl cyclase (AC), which catalyses the conversion of ATP to cAMP. Binding of the ligand to the R–G complex allows the G unit to bind GTP and stimulate adenylyl cyclase activity. cAMP activates protein kinase A, which phosphorylates cellular proteins to produce the characteristic cellular response. PP_i, pyrophosphate.

cGMP system

The only other cyclic nucleotide found in animal tissues is **cGMP**, formed from GTP in a reaction catalysed by guanylyl cyclase. Some neurotransmitters and hormones operate by stimulating a membrane-bound guanylyl cyclase in a reaction that does not involve G proteins (e.g. atrial natriuretic peptide). There is also a cytoplasmic form of guanylyl cyclase; nitric oxide (NO) appears to be an important physiological activator of this form (p. 35).

In some cases a decreased level of cGMP mediates the actions of a signal. For instance, when light energy is absorbed by photoreceptor pigment in the retina, a G protein called transducin (G_t) is activated. This in turn stimulates a phosphodiesterase, leading to decreased cGMP concentration and closure of cationic channels (see Chapter 7).

Phosphoinositide system

Other chemical stimuli operate through the phosphoinositide system. Phosphoinositides (also known as inositol phospholipids) are a family of plasma membrane phospholipids containing inositol. Binding of a hormone to its receptor activates a different G protein or proteins (G_q) to those involved in the cAMP system. G_q then stimulates a phosphodiesterase (**phospholipase C-β**) in the plasma membrane (Fig. 2.8). This enzyme, on the inner face of the plasma membrane, cleaves phosphatidylinositol 4,5-bisphosphate (PIP_2) within the membrane to form **inositol trisphosphate** (IP_3) and **diacylglycerol** (DAG). IP_3 is water-soluble and diffuses throughout the cytosol. IP_3 binds to specific receptors (IP_3 receptors) in the endoplasmic reticulum membrane. The IP_3 receptors are cation channels permeable to Ca^{2+}, which open when IP_3 binds. Since the endoplasmic reticulum, as explained in Chapter 1, has a high Ca^{2+} concentration, this causes release of stored Ca^{2+} into the cytosol, thus increasing the cytosolic Ca^{2+} concentration.

In contrast to IP_3, DAG remains in the membrane and, in the presence of Ca^{2+} and phos-

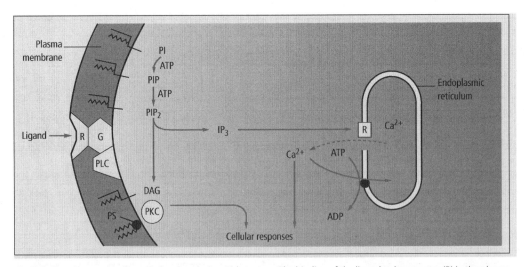

Fig. 2.8 Signals operating through the phosphoinositide system. The binding of the ligand to its receptor (R) in the plasma membrane activates the enzyme phospholipase C-β (PLC) via the GTP-regulatory protein (G_q). This enzyme cleaves PIP_2 in the plasma membrane to form the second messengers IP_3 and DAG. IP_3 mobilizes Ca^{2+} from the endoplasmic reticulum while DAG, in the presence of phosphatidyl serine (PS) and Ca^{2+}, activates the enzyme protein kinase C (PKC), and these actions lead to specific cellular responses. IP_3 and DAG are rapidly metabolized and their end-products recycled to form phosphatidyl inositol (PI), which is phosphorylated to form phosphatidylinositol 4-phosphate (PIP) and finally phosphatidylinositol 4,5-bisphosphate (PIP_2).

phatidylserine, activates **protein kinase C**. In its inactive state protein kinase C resides in the cytosol, but the binding of Ca^{2+} exposes its phospholipid binding site causing it to bind to the plasma membrane. Once activated by DAG this enzyme phosphorylates many intracellular proteins, including some that are also phosphorylated by protein kinase A. Phorbol esters, a group of chemicals that can induce tumours, are structurally related to DAG and also activate protein kinase C. This action may explain their cancer-inducing effects.

Finally, IP_3 and DAG are metabolized. The endproducts may be recycled to form phosphatidylinositol (PI), which is used to resynthesize PIP_2 as depicted in Fig. 2.8 or, in the case of DAG, a lipase may release arachidonic acid, the precursor of the eicosanoids, which include prostaglandins, thromboxanes and leukotrienes. When the intracellular IP_3 level goes down, the IP_3 receptor Ca^{2+}-release channels in the endoplasmic reticulum close, and Ca^{2+} is re-accumulated via the Ca^{2+} pump (Ca^{2+}–ATPase) in the endoplasmic reticulum, or pumped out of the cells via the Ca^{2+}–ATPase in the plasma membrane.

Thus, in this system, Ca^{2+} acts as a third messenger and events in both branches determine the appropriate cellular response. An increased cytosolic Ca^{2+} concentration may stimulate the activity of protein kinases or other regulatory enzymes in the cell either directly or through a Ca^{2+}-binding protein called **calmodulin**. Calmodulin, which binds up to four Ca^{2+} ions per molecule with high affinity, regulates the activity of many cellular enzymes, e.g. Ca^{2+}/calmodulin-dependent kinase II, phosphorylase kinase, adenylyl cyclase, cyclic nucleotide phosphodiesterase, Ca^{2+}–ATPase and myosin light-chain kinase.

Ca^{2+}-activation of calmodulin is usually associated with the translocation of this protein (Fig. 2.9). Since the normal, physiologically relevant Ca^{2+} signals occur in an oscillatory manner, this causes Ca^{2+}-dependent oscillations in local calmodulin concentrations (Fig. 2.9). For example, in the polarized secretory pancreatic acinar cells, the cytosolic Ca^{2+} release always starts in the apical secretory pole where the highest Ca^{2+} concentrations can be attained. The high local Ca^{2+} concentration in the

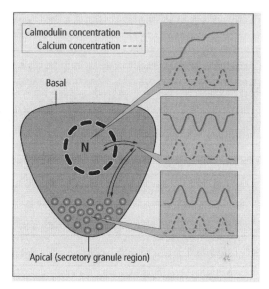

Fig. 2.9 Oscillations in the concentrations of Ca^{2+} and calmodulin in various regions of a polarized secretory cell in response to hormonal stimulation. (See text for further explanations.) N, nucleus. (From Craske, M., *et al.* (1999) *Proc Natl Acad Sci, USA* **96**, 4426–4431.)

apical pole causes translocation of calmodulin into the apical granular area and here the calmodulin concentration oscillates in synchrony with the Ca^{2+} concentration (Fig. 2.9). The movement of calmodulin from the basal part of the cell into the apical pole reduces the calmodulin concentration in the donor region, which therefore experiences calmodulin fluctuations that are exactly opposite to the Ca^{2+} oscillations (i.e. low calmodulin concentration when the Ca^{2+} concentration is high) (Fig. 2.9). After a delay, there can be a Ca^{2+}-dependent slower calmodulin translocation into the nucleus. Calmodulin binds in the nucleus and therefore only exits from this organelle very slowly. In this region, therefore, a gradual build-up of calmodulin occurs in response to regular cytosolic Ca^{2+} oscillations. The example shown in Fig. 2.9 illustrates that one intracellular signal (a cytosolic Ca^{2+} concentration rise) can cause different patterns of protein translocation changes in different regions of the cell, most likely serving different functions.

One should not necessarily think of the different

signalling systems as being entirely separate. For example, Ca²⁺ (via calmodulin) regulates enzymes involved in the synthesis and degradation of cAMP. In this way the Ca²⁺-signalling system has an important influence on the cAMP-signalling system.

Tyrosine kinase activation

Finally, there are a number of substances that do not appear to act through the recognized intracellular messenger systems discussed above. Some of these (e.g. insulin, epidermal growth factor, nerve growth factor) are known to interact with membrane-bound receptors that have intrinsic tyrosine kinase activity and can autophosphorylate their own tyrosine residues. This is in contrast to the protein kinases mentioned previously, which phosphorylate serine or threonine residues or other proteins.

Receptor tyrosine kinases are known to mediate growth, differentiation and survival responses to traditional growth factors. An example of their mode of action is that of the **insulin receptor**. The insulin receptor is composed of two α and two β subunits (Fig. 2.10). Insulin binds to the α subunit, which is in contact with the extracellular fluid, and activates the tyrosine kinase of the β subunit, which is located on the cytoplasmic side. This re-

sults in autophosphorylation of tyrosine residues on the β subunit. The insulin receptor is unique in that it has two transmembrane domains. Other tyrosine kinase receptors have only a single transmembrane domain and require ligand-induced receptor dimerization to function. In addition to receptor tyrosine kinases, there are **tyrosine-kinase associated receptors** that function in much the same way but are not covalently bound to the receptor, e.g. receptors for growth hormone, prolactin and cytokines.

Once autophosphorylation of the tyrosine residues has occurred, the activated receptor tyrosine kinase binds to and stimulates a variety of intracellular signalling proteins that result in phosphorylation and GDP–GTP exchange of other protein substrates as discussed below.

Small GTPases

Linked downstream of tyrosine kinase activation are small monomeric GTP-binding proteins (M_r ~ 21 000) belonging to the Ras superfamily, commonly referred to as the small GTPases. **Ras proteins** were first discovered as the hyperactive products of mutant genes that cause cancer (oncogenes). There are five major subfamilies: Ras, Rho, Rab, ARF and Ran, whose members are important regulators of many cellular functions,

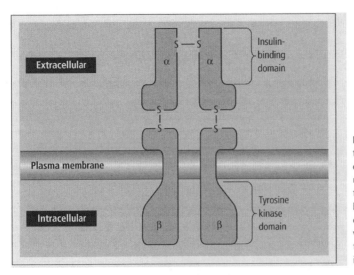

Fig. 2.10 Model of the insulin receptor. This comprises a glycoprotein composed of two α and two β subunits (M_r 13 0000 and 90 000, respectively) that are linked by disulphide bonds. Insulin binds to the α subunit on the extracellular surface and activates the tyrosine kinase domain of the β subunit, which is located on the intracellular surface.

such as cellular growth and differentiation, cell motility, intracellular transport, nuclear import, endocytosis and secretion. They regulate many intracellular signalling pathways, including serine/threonine kinase cascades and transcription factors. Like their heterotrimeric cousins (p. 27), they undergo GDP–GTP exchange and possess GTPase activity. Their activities are regulated by GDP–GTP exchange factors (GEF), which stimulate GDP–GTP exchange and by GTPase-activating proteins (GAP) which stimulate their intrinisic GTPase activity.

These GTPases respond to signals from plasma membrane receptors, such as tyrosine receptor kinases discussed above. The Ras family of GTPases are regulators of growth and differentiation. The Rho family proteins (including Rho, Cdc42 and Rac proteins) have profound effects on the actin cytoskeleton and are important in the regulation of cell shape and motility. For example, Rho plays an essential role in cytokinesis and regulates the formation of stress fibres and focal adhesions in cells; Rac is important in membrane ruffling associated with cell migration, together with Cdc42 which is involved in the formation of microspikes (filopodia) that protrude from migrating cells. In addition there are the Rab and ARF family proteins that regulate vesicular traffic in cells, and the Ran family proteins, which regulate the translocation of proteins through pores in the nuclear membrane.

Activation of nuclear receptors by lipophilic signals

In contrast to the signals involving hydrophilic ligands as discussed above, those involving lipophilic ligands that readily cross the plasma membrane (e.g. steroid and thyroid hormones) require intracellular receptors. Receptors for steroid and thyroid hormones are structurally related and belong to the **steroid–hormone receptor superfamily**. There are six classes of steroid receptors (i.e. glucocorticoid, mineralocorticoid, oestrogen, progesterone, androgen and calcitriol) and various isoforms of thyroid–hormone receptor. Steroid–hormone receptors are found in both the cytoplasm and nucleus while thyroid–hormone receptors are found exclusively in the nucleus. The classic view is that steroid hormones bind to specific cytoplasmic receptors and are then translocated to the nucleus (Fig. 2.11), but it is now considered that most steroid hormones, and also thyroid hormones, bind to receptors in the nucleus. The hormone–receptor complex undergoes dimerization and binds to **regulatory elements** on target DNA molecules, leading to the production (or suppression) of specific messenger RNA species. Consequently, the actions of steroid and thyroid hormones lead to changes in the concentrations of specific proteins that alter cell function.

2.3 Local mediators

There are many hormone-like substances released by cells that act locally, either on neighbouring cells (paracrine) or on the cells that secrete them (autocrine). Some, such as the eicosanoids and NO, are so ubiquitous that they are discussed below. Others, mainly polypeptides, such as growth factors, cytokines and kinins, are mentioned in the relevant sections of the book.

Eicosanoids

Eicosanoids are a group of substances derived from the polyunsaturated fatty acid **arachidonic acid**. This fatty acid, a 20-carbon moiety, can be formed from DAG produced by the phosphoinositide system or be released from membrane phospholipids through the action of the family of enzymes known as **phospholipase A_2** that require Ca^{2+} for their activity. Receptor-coupled G proteins may be involved in the regulation of phospholipase A_2, but their role is poorly understood. Metabolism of arachidonic acid leads to the formation of eicosanoids: **prostaglandins** and **thromboxanes** produced by the cyclo-oxygenase pathway and **leukotrienes** by the lipoxygenase pathway (Fig. 2.12). Prostaglandins (PG) occur in virtually all cells and are not restricted to the prostate gland after which they were named. They are subdivided alphabetically into various types (e.g. PGA, PGD, PGE etc.), which are further subdivided numerically

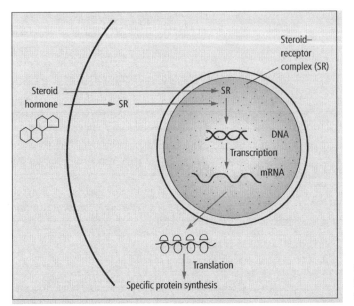

Fig. 2.11 Steroid hormone action at the cellular level. SR, steroid–receptor complex.

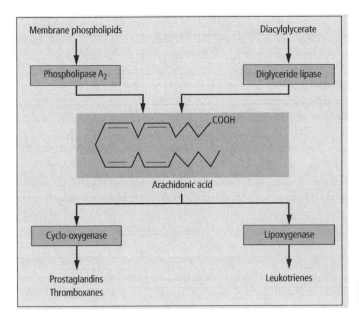

Fig. 2.12 Synthesis of prostaglandins, thromboxanes and leukotrienes.

(e.g. PGA_1, PGA_2 etc.). Together with the thromboxanes, they are referred to as **prostanoids**.

Not every cell produces the full range of eicosanoids and not all of the eicosanoids are second messengers, as defined above. Most have a very short half-life and are inactivated in the lung. Many leave the cells in which they are synthesized and diffuse locally to exert their effects on other cells, or on the cells that secreted them, by interacting with specific surface receptors coupled to G proteins. They are important in a great variety of cellular responses, including blood clotting, vasoconstriction, vasodilatation, bronchoconstriction, neuromodulation, pain, fever and inflammation.

The non-steroidal anti-inflammatory drug **aspirin** inhibits the enzyme cyclo-oxygenase and therefore blocks the synthesis of prostanoids.

Nitric oxide

NO is an important local mediator of communication between cells, acting as a paracrine agent and neurotransmitter. It is also a powerful activator of **cytoplasmic guanylyl cyclase**. NO is very labile and is formed in cells from the amino acid L-arginine in a reaction catalysed by a family of enzymes collectively named **NO synthase**. Neuronal and endothelial isoforms, expressed constitutively, are regulated by calmodulin and require elevation of the cystosolic Ca^{2+} concentration above the resting level. In response to immunological stimuli there is expression of a Ca^{2+}-insensitive isoform. Thus, there are both Ca^{2+}/calmodulin-dependent and Ca^{2+}-independent forms of NO synthase.

NO was first recognized to be a potent vasodilator released by endothelial cells that form a functional unit with the smooth muscle cells in blood vessels. In endothelial cells an increase in the cytosolic Ca^{2+} concentration stimulates NO synthase. The NO produced diffuses to the surrounding smooth muscle cells and activates a cytoplasmic guanylyl cyclase, thus increasing cGMP levels. This stimulates a cGMP-dependent protein kinase that phosphorylates proteins, either directly or by inhibiting protein phosphatases. One potential target appears to be K^+ channels, causing hyperpolarization and relaxation of smooth muscle.

2.4 Pathophysiological aspects

In view of the physiological significance of the cellular communication systems described in this chapter, it is unsurprising that abnormalities in these signalling pathways can cause serious problems. These will be dealt with when describing the various specific physiological systems in subsequent chapters. Here we shall focus on the important role of Ca^{2+} in cell death.

Ca^{2+} governs an enormous range of cell functions and is necessary for cell survival. As discussed above, physiological Ca^{2+} signals in the cytosol occur as repetitive spikes (Fig. 2.9) and are often highly localized in specific strategic sub-cellular regions. Cytosolic Ca^{2+} overload, often associated with mitochondrial Ca^{2+} overload and depletion of the Ca^{2+} store in the endoplasmic reticulum, can cause cell death. The two principal forms of cell death are apoptosis and necrosis. Apoptosis is a physiologically occurring phenomenon, which is important both in development, by removing cells that are not needed, and in the adult body by maintaining the size of organs in which cell division occurs. The balance between cell division and apoptosis is essential. If more cells are produced than die, this results in tumour formation; if more cells die than are newly produced, as a result of cell division, the result is atrophy. Apoptotic cell death, due to proteolysis or nucleolysis, can be triggered either by receptor-mediated or by mitochondria-mediated signalling pathways.

Necrosis is clearly a pathological process. There is irreversible cell swelling and loss of the integrity of the plasma membrane, with cell constituents being released into the interstitial fluid. This usually causes inflammation. Whether the result of an insult is apoptosis or necrosis is mainly dependent on the intracellular ATP concentration. Apoptosis requires ATP, so if the mitochondria are unable to synthesize ATP, necrosis is the only option. Cytosolic Ca^{2+} overload, due to excessive Ca^{2+} entry across the plasma membrane or excessive release from the endoplasmic reticulum, can cause mitochondrial Ca^{2+} overload, thus damaging their metabolic activity. Deficient disposal of Ca^{2+}, for example by reduced activity of the Na^+—Ca^{2+} exchanger in the plasma membrane, can contribute significantly to cellular Ca^{2+} overloading. Reduced mitochondrial ATP production will always contribute to further Ca^{2+} overloading. Lack of ATP will prevent Ca^{2+} extrusion across the plasma membrane via the Ca^{2+}–ATPase pump and also prevent Ca^{2+} pump-mediated uptake into the endoplasmic reticulum. A sustained elevated cytosolic Ca^{2+} concentration can activate proteases and endonucleases causing cell destruction.

The endoplasmic reticulum needs a high Ca^{2+} concentration in its lumen in order to be able to fold and process proteins normally. Although cytosolic Ca^{2+} signals can be generated physiologically by release of Ca^{2+} from the endoplasmic reticulum (Fig. 2.8), this does not normally empty the store. The release of relatively small amounts of Ca^{2+} into the cytosol is sufficient to generate substantial Ca^{2+} signals, due to the extremely low resting cytosolic Ca^{2+} level. Excessive (toxic) stimulation can cause complete depletion of the endoplasmic reticulum Ca^{2+} store, and this triggers, via a still poorly understood mechanism, excessive opening of Ca^{2+} entry pathways, contributing to further cytosolic Ca^{2+} overload.

Chapter 3

Introduction to the Nervous System

The nervous system comprises two closely interacting cellular networks, neuronal and neuroglial, specialized for the reception, integration and transmission of information. It is subdivided into the brain and spinal cord (the **central nervous system**; CNS), and the sensory and motor nerve fibres that enter and leave the CNS, or are wholly outside the CNS (the **peripheral nervous system**; PNS). The nervous system contains about 10^{11} neurones and 10^{12} glial cells, which occupy approximately equal brain volumes. Neuronal cell bodies tend to aggregate into compact groups (nuclei, ganglia), or into sheets (laminae) that lie within the grey matter of the CNS or are located in specialized ganglia in the PNS. Glial cells in the CNS are represented by astrocytes, oligodendrocytes and microglia, and by Schwann cells in the PNS. The nerve fibres (axons) course in the white matter of the CNS or along peripheral nerves. Groups of nerve fibres running in a common direction usually form a compact bundle (nerve, tract, peduncle, brachium, pathway). Many axons are surrounded by sheaths of lipid material called myelin, which is produced by either oligodendrocytes or Schwann cells.

3.1 Cells of the nervous system

Neurones are specialized for the rapid transmission of signals. Each neurone consists of a cell body, dendrites, an axon and synaptic terminals. The dendrites receive signals from other cells, the axon conducts signals from the cell body to distant targets, and the synaptic terminals transmit signals to other cells. Glial cells are integrated into a syncytium through numerous gap junctions; the latter are also instrumental for propagating Ca^{2+} waves, which serve as a means of inter-glial communications. Neurones and glia communicate via neurotransmitters released from both cell types. Glial cells nourish and protect the neurones. This includes providing them with various substances, maintaining extracellular ion homeostasis, participating in active uptake of many neurotransmitters, and forming the myelin sheath around axons. The glial cells are also involved in fighting brain damage in various pathological conditions.

Neurones

Neurones are more diverse in size and shape (Fig. 3.1) than cells in any other tissue of the body. Nevertheless they have certain features in common: they usually possess dendrites, a cell body, an axon and synaptic terminals (Fig. 3.2a).

Dendrites extend from the cell body and share with it the function of receiving information from synaptic connections with adjoining neurones. They are usually tapered and possess various protuberances, such as dendritic spines (Fig. 3.3), which are sites of contact with other cells.

The **cell body**, also known as the soma or perikaryon, contains the nucleus. In the cytoplasm

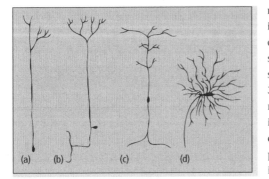

Fig. 3.1 Various types of neurones: (a) unipolar, e.g. invertebrate neurone; (b) pseudounipolar, e.g. dorsal root ganglion cell; (c) bipolar, e.g. retinal bipolar cell; and (d) multipolar, e.g. motor neurone.

surrounding the nucleus is an extensive array of rough and smooth endoplasmic reticulum (ER), represented by an internally continuous system of microtubules and cisterns, which extends from the nuclear envelope to axons and presynaptic terminals, as well as to dendrites and dendritic spines. The ER is responsible for protein synthesis and export to the neuronal processes. Large neurones replace as much as one-third of their protein content every day. In addition, the ER acts as a dynamic store of Ca^{2+} ions, which are released upon electrical or chemical stimulation.

The **axon** is a slender process ranging in length from a few hundred micrometres to more than a metre. The diameter of axons usually varies from 0.1 to 20 μm, although in some invertebrates it may be as much as 1 mm. The axon contains mitochondria, the ER, microtubules, neurofilaments, microfilaments and vesicles (Fig. 3.2b). The axon junction with the cell body is known as the **axon hillock**, which is an important site for the generation of action potentials. Axons are usually longer than dendrites, and at their ends they branch to form terminals that make contact with other cells at **synapses**. Axons stain more strongly than dendrites for a microtubule-associated protein, called tau, while dendrites immunostain specifically for another microtubule-associated protein (MAP) 2.

Synaptic terminals are the sites of release of

neurotransmitters and are usually in close proximity to another neurone or effector cell. A synapse consists of a presynaptic terminal containing synaptic vesicles packed with neurotransmitter, a synaptic cleft and a postsynaptic membrane (Fig. 3.3). The synaptic cleft between neurones is 20–30 nm wide and at skeletal neuromuscular junctions it is 50–100 nm. In electron micrographs, electron-dense areas on the cytoplasmic faces of pre- and postsynaptic membranes indicate sites of specialization for exocytosis of vesicle contents (**active zones**), and for the localization of postsynaptic receptors (**postsynaptic densities**). While most neurotransmitters are released close to effector cells, certain neurones release substances that act at some distance from their site of release, to modulate the activity of surrounding neurones. In the CNS, most of the synapses are closely enwrapped by the membrane of neighbouring astrocytes.

Rapid transmission of information by neurones relies on their ability to conduct action potentials, coupled with neurotransmitter release at synapses. These processes are discussed in more detail in the next chapter, as too is the ability of neurones to process and integrate information. Neurones also have a trophic ('nourishing') influence on the differentiation of sensory receptor cells (e.g. taste cells) and effector cells (e.g. skeletal muscle fibres). Their effect on taste cells is most likely due to the release of trophic factors, but their action on skeletal muscle fibres is also due to the electrical activity they induce in those cells.

In summary, neurones are specialized:
1 to receive information from the internal and external environment;
2 to transmit signals to other neurones and to effector organs;
3 to process information (integration); and
4 to determine or modify the differentiation of sensory receptor cells and effector cells (trophic functions).

Neuroglia

There are three types of neuroglial or glial cells in the CNS—astrocytes, oligodendrocytes and microglia (Fig. 3.4)—and one type in the PNS—

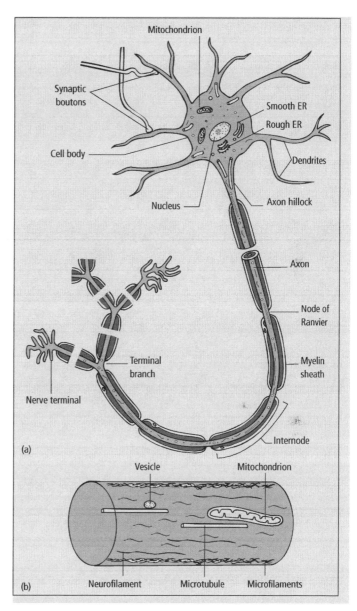

Fig. 3.2 (a) Diagram of a motor neurone. (b) Longitudinal view of an axon. ER, endoplasmic reticulum.

Schwann cells—that fill the spaces between neurones. Ependymal cells, which line the ventricles of the brain, may also be classified as glial cells.

Astrocytes are star-shaped cells with processes extending into the surrounding tangled network of unmyelinated nerve fibres (neuropil). These processes contain bundles of fibrils composed of **glial fibrillary acidic protein** (GFAP). (Note: Glial cell-derived tumours can be identified by GFAP immunostaining.) One role for astrocytes is to give structural support to neurones and their processes within the brain and spinal cord. Their processes form a framework or 'scaffolding' for neurones and some expand into end-feet on the pial surfaces of the brain or on capillaries. Astrocytes are internally connected into the syncytium by intercellular

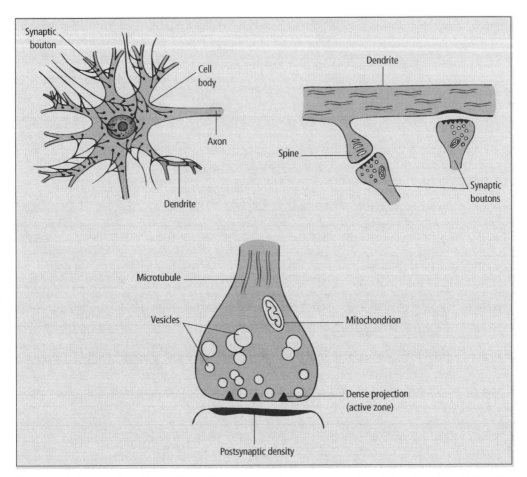

Fig. 3.3 Typical synapses found in the CNS. Left inset: numerous branches of axons from distant sites form synaptic terminals (boutons) on a cell body and dendrites of a neurone. Right inset: typical synapses on a dendrite.

channels or gap junctions formed by **connexons** (see Fig. 2.3). Astrocytes are able to express the same variety of neurotransmitter receptors as neurones, and astrocytic expression of these receptors matches the pattern expressed by their neuronal neighbours in every particular region of the brain. Thus, astrocytes and neurones are able to sense the same incoming information. In most cases astrocytes respond to the activation of neurotransmitter receptors by transient/oscillatory elevations in the intracellular Ca^{2+} concentration, which spread through the astrocytic syncytium in the form of **propagating Ca^{2+} waves**. Many astrocytes are able to release neurotransmitters (such as glutamate or

adenosine triphosphate), which in turn affect neuronal cells (Fig. 3.5). The astroglial plasmalemma has a high permeability to K^+, and resting membrane potentials are close to the potassium equilibrium potential (E_K), which helps to diminish increases in extracellular K^+ concentration in localized areas of the brain where there are high levels of activity. Astrocytes are able to remove excess K^+, which enters the glial cells through inwardly rectifying K^+ channels and then dissipates through the syncytium. Another function of astrocytes is to assist in the removal of certain neurotransmitters (e.g. glutamate, or γ-aminobutyric acid (GABA) after their release from neurones by virtue of

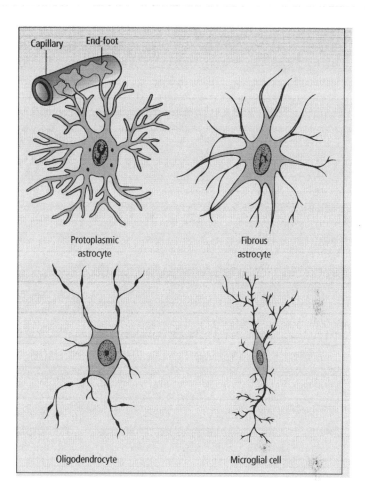

Fig. 3.4 Neuroglial cells.

Capillary

End-foot

Protoplasmic
astrocyte

Fibrous
astrocyte

Oligodendrocyte

Microglial cell

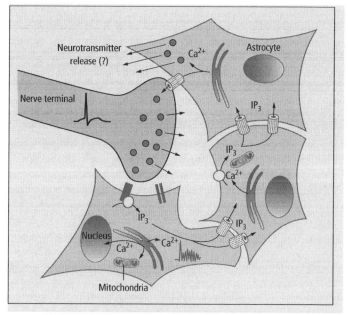

Fig. 3.5 Communication within neuronal–glial networks. Synaptically-released neurotransmitters activate glial receptors, which trigger synthesis of intracellular second messenger 1,4,5 inositol-trisphosphate (IP_3). The IP_3 induces Ca^{2+} release from the intracellular stores; IP_3 (and other second messengers and metabolites) can diffuse through gap junctions, interconnecting astrocytes into a syncytium, and thus produce propagating intercellular Ca^{2+} signals. Increases in astroglial Ca^{2+} can activate exocytotic release of 'glio' transmitters which signal back to neurones, thus integrating neuronal–glial circuits.

Neurotransmitter release (?)

Ca^{2+}

Astrocyte

Nerve terminal

IP_3

IP_3

Ca^{2+}

IP_3

IP_3

Nucleus

Ca^{2+}

Ca^{2+}

Mitochondria

specific transporters resident in the astroglial membrane.

Oligodendrocytes can be distinguished from astrocytes by having fewer and thinner processes. They form **myelin** sheaths around axons in the CNS, as do **Schwann cells** in peripheral nerves, by enveloping them with concentric layers of plasma membrane (Fig. 3.6). Myelin forms an insulating sheath around an axon, leaving small areas of axonal membrane exposed between successive myelin segments, known as the **nodes of Ranvier**. This organization is critical for **saltatory** (very rapid) propagation of action potential. Unmyelinated fibres in the CNS are not surrounded by oligodendrocytes, but in the PNS they are encircled by Schwann cells without the formation of concentric layers of myelin.

Microglia are smaller glial-type cells of non-neuronal origin that enter the brain shortly after birth. Microglial cells are then distributed throughout the brain and remain under resting conditions (characterized by a very small cell body and several fine processes). Injury to the brain activates microglial cells, which undergo proliferation and migrate to the point of injury where they differentiate into phagocytic cells and remove the debris. Brain injury also activates astrocytes (a process known as

reactive glyosis), which then proliferate and segregate the damaged area, forming a glial scar.

In summary, glial cells are specialized in:
1 maintaining structural integrity in the brain;
2 nourishing neurones;
3 controlling the ion composition of the extracellular space;
4 participating in the uptake of neurotransmitters;
5 integrating the information in the brain;
6 myelinating axons; and
7 defending the nervous system against damage and controlling brain repair.

3.2 General principles of intercellular communication in the nervous system

Cells in the nervous system communicate either through highly localized contacts (through chemical or electrical (gap junction) synapses), which is generally termed 'wiring transmission', or through more diffuse and global signalling that occurs via diffusion within the extracellular and intracellular spaces in syncytial cellular networks; the latter form of signalling is known as 'volume transmission'. There are fundamental functional differences between wiring and volume transmission. Wiring transmission is: rapid (milliseconds–seconds); extremely localized, exhibiting a one-to-one ratio (i.e signals occur only between two cells); unidirectional; and its effects are usually phasic. In contrast, volume transmission is: slow (seconds–minutes/hours/days); global, being one-to-many (i.e. the substance released by one cell may affect many receivers); sometimes bidirectional; and its effects are tonic. Extracellular volume transmission is involved in many well-documented cases of cell-to-cell signalling in the CNS; e.g. in signalling mediated by gaseous neurotransmitters such as nitric oxide (NO), in mediating the actions of neuropeptides released extrasynaptically, and in para-axonal transmission. The concept of intracellular volume transmission is relatively new, and to date it is believed to be confined mostly to the astroglial syncytium. These two principal pathways of signal transmission in the brain—working in concert—comprise CNS information processing by

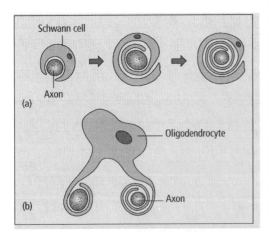

Fig. 3.6 Myelination of axons. (a) A Schwann cell in the PNS forms myelin around a portion of a single axon. (b) An oligodendrocyte in the CNS can form myelin around several axons.

integrating all neural cells, neurones and glia, into a highly effective information processing system.

3.3 Development, growth and regeneration of the nervous system

Cells of the nervous system are derived from embryonic ectoderm. Neurones and glial cells (except microglial) share the same precursor elements and are generated in the ventricular layer of the neural tube; they then migrate to their final position and send processes to their target regions. Structural components, which are synthesized in the cell body and carried by axonal transport, are incorporated at the growing tip of the axon, called the growth cone. The growth cone responds to environmental cues that help guide axons to their final destination. During development many neurones undergo a period of natural cell death, which reduces their numbers. Once development has occurred, neurones can no longer divide; regeneration of their axons can occur in the PNS, but is restricted in the CNS.

Early development of the nervous system

Cells of the very young embryo comprise three primordial types—ectoderm, endoderm and mesoderm. The nervous system develops from cells of ectodermal origin (Fig. 3.7). At an early stage, under the influence of the underlying notochord and mesoderm, the ectoderm becomes thickened to form the **neural plate**. At an intermediate stage, forces intrinsic and extrinsic to the neural plate drive the process of neurulation, in which **neural folds** are formed by ingression of surface ectoderm. At a late stage, the ingression of surface ectoderm is complete and the uplifted neural folds have joined in the midline to form the CNS primordium, the **neural tube**. Cells in the **neural crest**, which lies at the dorsal extreme of the neural tube, migrate along one of two major pathways and contribute to the generation of neural (e.g. dorsal root and autonomic ganglion cells, glial cells) and non-neural cells (e.g. endocrine cells) in many locations. The mesoderm becomes subdivided into

blocks (somites), which give rise to striated muscles and skeletal elements.

The innermost cells in the neural tube line the future ventricles of the brain, and are termed the ventricular layer. Neurones are generated by mitosis in the ventricular layer. Young postmitotic neurones migrate away from the ventricular layer, guided by radial glial cells, to settle in their final positions in the brain and spinal cord.

During early development the neurone sends out a number of neuronal processes, one of which develops into the axon; the others form the dendrites. Prior to differentiation these neuronal processes are referred to as **neurites**, which possess **growth cones** at their elongating tips. The growth cones react to various environmental cues (see below) that enable neural circuits to be established accurately without major trial and error.

Once initial contact has been established with the target region, the target cells may become hyperinnervated. Such is the case with the early motor input to developing skeletal muscles and sensory innervation of the skin. This **hyperinnervation** may represent an important trigger in the development and maturation of the target. Hyperinnervation of the target is not maintained to maturity, and there is a normal period during development, usually after the neural centre and target have established a functional relationship, when this hyperinnervation is lost by retraction of terminals from multiple innervated sites.

Neurotrophic factors

Substances derived from glial cells and target tissues promote the development and survival of neurones. The best characterized of such substances is **nerve growth factor** (NGF), a protein of M_r 135 000, which was first shown to stimulate the growth of neurites in dorsal root ganglia **in vitro**. A limited number of other neurotrophic factors that are essential for neuronal growth and survival, particularly during critical periods of development, have subsequently been isolated and classified as belonging to the **neurotrophin** family. In addition to NGF, this family includes brain-derived neurotrophic factor (BDNF), neurotrophin (NT) 3,

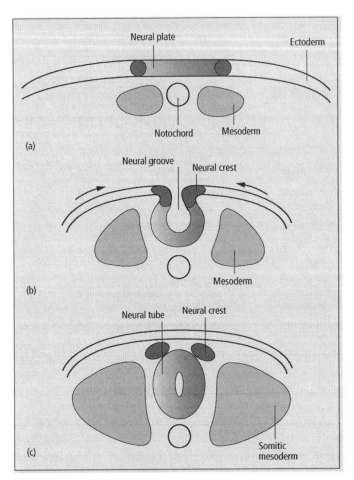

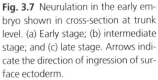

Fig. 3.7 Neurulation in the early embryo shown in cross-section at trunk level. (a) Early stage; (b) intermediate stage; and (c) late stage. Arrows indicate the direction of ingression of surface ectoderm.

NT4/5 and NT6. Different neurones respond to different neurotrophins. Sympathetic and sensory neurones have an absolute requirement for NGF during the early stages of their development, and die following the administration of antibodies to NGF at this time. Sympathetic neurones also require NGF for optimal maintenance at later stages. NGF is produced by target tissues and is specifically taken up into the nerve terminals of sympathetic and sensory neurones by receptor-mediated endocytosis and then transported to their cell bodies.

Axonal guidance

In the developing nervous system, outgrowing axons are guided to their distant targets by cues in the extracellular environment. Some extracellular matrix-bound molecules (e.g. laminin, fibronectin, collagen) promote axon outgrowth by interaction with specific receptors (integrins) in the growth cones of neurites. Other classes of guidance cues (e.g. semaphorins and netrins), either membrane-bound or diffusible, provide directionality by either attracting or repelling growth cones. Some guidance molecules, such as the netrins, may be simultaneously attractive to one neuronal subset and repulsive to another, depending on the nature of the interaction between the guidance molecule and the growth cone. The cellular mechanism involves binding of the guidance molecule to G protein-coupled receptors on the surface of the growth cone, which act through local fluctuations in intracellular calcium levels—involving

Ca^{2+} release from the ER—resulting in regional modification of the growth cone cytoskeleton and changes in direction of neurite outgrowth. Once axon pathways are established by these 'pioneer' axons, later outgrowing neurites may then grow along these axons to form bundles in which association is promoted by cell adhesion molecules.

Cell death

Many more neurones are produced during development than are actually required by the mature nervous system. There is a brief period of cell death when as many as 50% of neurones die, a phenomenon known as **apoptosis** (see also Chapter 2). This is a normal, genetically controlled response to specific developmental and environmental stimuli that is characterized by nuclear DNA fragmentation. The initial overproduction and subsequent death of neurones are thought to provide a mechanism that allows for optimal functional and numerical matching between the neural centre and its target cell population. Interactions between neurone and target are critical throughout the life of a neurone, since removal of the target tissue usually leads to its death.

Role of activity

There are certain critical periods in the development of young animals during which particular groups of neurones must be used if their synaptic connections are to be functionally maintained. For example, if one eye of a young kitten is covered during the second to the fourth month of age, the animal remains functionally blind in that eye for the rest of its life and there is a permanent deficit in the number of cortical synaptic connections relaying information from the deprived eye to the visual cortex. Strabismus (squint or 'lazy eye') in children has a similar result; the critical period here is from two to five years of age.

Growth, maintenance and axonal transport

In a large neurone the axon can occupy more than 99% of the volume of the cell. Since there are no ribosomes in axons and nerve terminals, proteins required for their growth and maintenance must be synthesized in the cell body and carried towards the nerve terminals by **axonal transport**. In mature axons substances carried by axonal transport exchange with existing structures, while in growing axons they are also incorporated into the growth cones of their elongating tips.

Axonal transport away from the cell body is referred to as 'anterograde' while that in the opposite direction is called 'retrograde'. Rates of anterograde transport have been determined by measuring the movement of radioactively labelled proteins after injection of labelled amino acids into regions containing cell bodies. This technique has revealed that there are several distinct rates of transport in axons—**one fast rate** of up to 400 mm day^{-1}, and **two slower rates** of 2–8 mm day^{-1} and approximately 1 mm day^{-1}.

Fast axonal transport involves the movement of organelles, such as synaptic vesicles and mitochondria, along the axon (Fig. 3.8). This movement can be best visualized in extruded squid axoplasm by video-enhanced contrast microscopy. Such studies show that the organelles travel along the outside of microtubules, and that such movement is powered by motor enzymes and adenosine triphosphate (ATP). The molecular motor for movement in the anterograde direction is **kinesin**, while that in the retrograde direction is **cytoplasmic dynein**. Recently, it has been shown that organelles also move along actin filaments (microfilaments), and that this movement is probably powered by a myosin-like protein.

Cytoskeletal proteins move at slow rates, although whether they move as monomers or filaments is not known. Tubulin and the neurofilament triplet proteins, which form the microtubules and neurofilaments respectively, move in the slowest component of slow transport. Other structural proteins—notably actin, which forms the microfilaments, and also a number of soluble proteins—move in the somewhat faster component of slow transport.

Retrograde transport can be elegantly demonstrated in histochemical studies in which a tracer

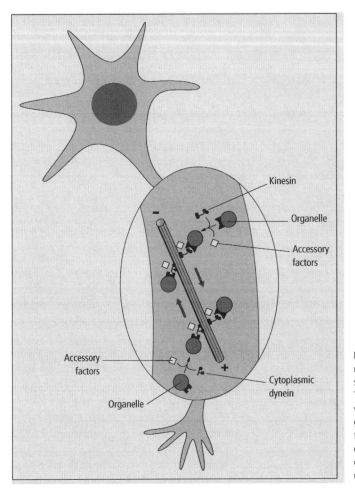

Fig. 3.8 Fast axonal transport of membranous organelles such as synaptic vesicles and mitochondria. The microtubules are polar structures with fast-growing (+) and slow-growing (−) ends. The molecular motors kinesin and cytoplasmic dynein drive organelle movement along microtubules towards the nerve terminals and the cell body, respectively.

substance, e.g. horseradish peroxidase, is injected into a region containing nerve terminals. The tracer is taken up into the nerve terminals by endocytosis, transported along the axon in vesicles, and subsequently appears in the cell body. This technique has proved to be of considerable value for tracing neural pathways in the brain. The rate of retrograde transport, via cytoplasmic dynein, approaches that of fast anterograde transport. Substances of physiological and pathological importance that are taken up at the nerve terminal and transported retrogradely include NGF, tetanus toxin and poliomyelitis virus.

Neural regeneration

PNS

If a peripheral nerve fibre is severed, the distal portion of the axon dies. Thereupon, Schwann cells surrounding the axon dedifferentiate and undergo mitosis, fill the nerve sheath distal to the cut and phagocytose the degenerating myelin (this process is generally known as **Waller degeneration**). Cell bodies of cut neurones undergo chromatolysis, a process involving dispersion of RNA-staining material (Nissl substance) and synthesis of new RNA. Thus, RNA coding for proteins involved in synaptic functions is lost and replaced by newly synthesized RNA, which codes for proteins necessary for regrowth of the axon. The proximal ends of cut axons sprout and will grow within the old nerve sheath, provided that they can make contact with it. This applies to both motor and sensory neurones. If, however, the more central portion (dorsal root) of a sensory nerve is damaged, regeneration into the spinal cord usually does not occur. There is little specificity in the regrowth of the peripheral axons, so that normal relations between particular motor neurones and muscles, and particular sensory neurones and their peripheral fields of innervation, are not accurately restored. The success of reinnervation of the original target area depends on the re-establishment of the original pathway. Hence, in attempting to restore function, it is helpful to suture the cut ends of the corresponding bundles (fascicles) together again.

Although there is little specificity in the regrowth of mammalian peripheral axons, it is noteworthy that motor axons grow back to form terminals at the original endplate sites on skeletal muscle fibres. It appears that they are directed by cues in the form of marker molecules present on the synaptic basal lamina that has been left behind. The marker molecule has been isolated and identified as a protein called **agrin**.

CNS

Damaged neurones in the CNS of higher vertebrates have a very limited capacity for regeneration. Axotomy often results in the death of the injured neurone, possibly because cells must be nourished by the retrograde transport of trophic factors. Cells surviving axotomy do produce axonal sprouts, but these fail to grow along their original pathway and form a tangled mass (neuroma) near the point of section. Recently it has been demonstrated that two proteins in the myelin produced by oligodendrocytes (but not Schwann cells) inhibit neurite regeneration. While this may appear to be a disadvantage, these neurite growth inhibitors could play an important role in restricting the growth of nerve fibres to specific pathways during CNS development and in preventing the establishment of aberrant pathways in the mature nervous system.

3.4 Divisions of the PNS

The PNS is that portion of the nervous system that lies outside the spinal cord and brain; it comprises both the somatic and the autonomic divisions. The somatic division contains all the peripheral pathways responsible for communication with the environment and the control of skeletal muscle. The autonomic nervous system comprises all the efferent pathways from controlling centres in the brain and spinal cord to effector organs other than skeletal muscle.

Somatic nervous system

This division includes all sensory (**primary afferent**) fibres from tissues such as eyes, ears, skin, joints and skeletal muscles and also includes the motor (**efferent**) fibres to skeletal muscles. The sensory fibres have their cell bodies in the dorsal root ganglia (Fig. 3.9) or brain; the motor fibres have their cell bodies in the ventral horn of the spinal cord or in the brain. Fibres enter or leave the spinal cord via pairs of spinal nerve roots (dorsal and ventral) at more or less regular intervals along each side. Fibres from the cell bodies of sensory neurones in the dorsal root ganglia pass via the dorsal roots to the periphery and to the spinal cord. In the spinal cord they branch and usually make synaptic contact with interneurones in the grey matter. The neurotransmitters released at these synapses include **glutamate**, **substance P** and other unidentified substances. Fibres from the cell bodies of motor neurones in the ventral horn of the spinal cord leave via the ventral roots.

The sensory fibres and motor fibres are collected together to form **peripheral nerves** (Fig. 3.10), which are covered by a connective tissue sheath (**epineurium**). Within the nerve the fibres are arranged into bundles (**fascicles**); each fascicle is surrounded by a **perineurium**, and each fibre by an **endoneurium**. The somatic sensory fibres range in size from small unmyelinated (class C) to large myelinated (class A) axons; the motor nerves are all large and myelinated (class A); class C axons carry **nociceptive** (pain) information. The most distal portions of the somatic nerves are usually

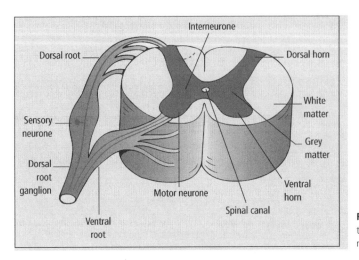
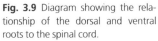

Fig. 3.9 Diagram showing the relationship of the dorsal and ventral roots to the spinal cord.

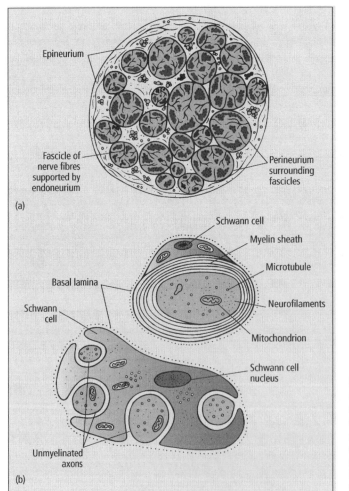

Fig. 3.10 (a) Cross-section of a peripheral nerve. (b) Enlargement of part of a fascicle showing myelinated and unmyelinated axons. Note that a number of unmyelinated axons are enclosed by a Schwann cell, while each myelinated axon is enveloped by layers of myelin from a single Schwann cell.

branched. The terminal regions of each sensory fibre go to adjacent receptors of the same type, while the intramuscular portions of each motor nerve innervate a number of similar muscle fibres. Somatic motor neurones release the neurotransmitter **acetylcholine**, which has an excitatory effect on skeletal muscle; there are no peripheral inhibitory actions exerted on skeletal muscle.

Autonomic nervous system

The actions of the peripheral autonomic nervous system are normally involuntary and are directed to the control of individual organ function and to homeostasis. Classically the autonomic nervous system is regarded as being solely motor in function, its fibres going to cardiac muscle, to smooth muscle and to glands. Sensory information comes from visceral and somatic afferent inputs. The peripheral autonomic nervous system (Fig. 3.11) is usually divided anatomically into the **sympathetic** and **parasympathetic systems**. Many tissues are innervated by both systems; when this occurs the two systems usually have opposing effects. In addition to these nerves there is a network of nerves that can act independently of the CNS. This network is often considered as another division of the autonomic nervous system and is referred to as the **enteric system**. Both the sympathetic and parasympathetic systems modulate the activity of this system.

The organization of the autonomic nervous system differs from the somatic division as all final motor (efferent) neurones lie completely outside the CNS (Fig. 3.11). The cell bodies of the peripheral neurones are grouped together to form **ganglia**. The efferent fibres passing from the CNS to the ganglia, the **preganglionic fibres**, are slow-conducting (class B and C) fibres which release acetylcholine (Fig. 3.12). The final motor neurones from the ganglia to the tissues, the **postganglionic fibres**, are mainly slow-conducting, unmyelinated class C fibres. These fibres and those from visceral sensory receptors run together as **visceral nerves**.

Sympathetic system

All preganglionic sympathetic neurones have their cell bodies in the thoracic and upper lumbar segments (T1–L3). The axons, along with somatic motor fibres, pass out of the spinal cord in the ventral roots (Fig. 3.13). On leaving the spinal column, the preganglionic fibres separate from the somatic nerves to form the **white rami communicantes** and join a distinct chain of sympathetic ganglia, the **vertebral** (paravertebral) **ganglia**. These ganglia are segmentally arranged and lie along each side of the spinal column. The preganglionic fibres either:

1 synapse with postganglionic neurones in one or more of the vertebral ganglia; or

2 leave the vertebral ganglia in visceral nerves and pass to **prevertebral ganglia** in the abdomen or to the **adrenal medullae**.

Many of the postganglionic fibres from vertebral ganglia leave the ganglia as the **grey rami communicantes** and join the spinal nerves that pass to peripheral tissue. Others, and also postganglionic fibres from prevertebral ganglia, join visceral nerves to particular organs.

The distribution of the postganglionic sympathetic fibres is not necessarily the same as the somatic motor fibres from the same segment and there is a lot of overlap between adjacent outflows. In brief, and very approximately, the T1 outflow passes to the head, T2 to the neck, T3–6 to the thorax, T7–11 to the abdomen and T12–13 to the legs (Fig. 3.11). Most of these postganglionic fibres release the neurotransmitter **noradrenaline** (norepinephrine) and are referred to as adrenergic fibres. The adrenal medullae can be thought of as modified ganglia that release the hormone **adrenaline** (epinephrine), and also some noradrenaline, into the blood stream rather than directly on to effector cells (Fig. 3.12). Some sympathetic nerves that innervate the blood vessels of muscles, sweat glands and hair follicles in the skin release acetylcholine instead of noradrenaline.

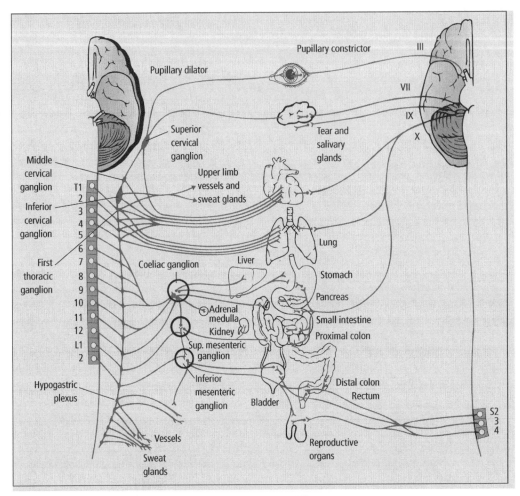

Fig. 3.11 Distribution of sympathetic (left) and parasympathetic (right) fibres.

Parasympathetic system

The preganglionic neurones of the parasympathetic system come from both the brainstem and sacral spinal cord (S2–4); the axons from the brainstem leave in cranial nerves III, VII, IX and X and the sacral axons leave in the ventral roots (Fig. 3.11). There are no vertebral (paravertebral) ganglia in this system; instead all ganglia are found adjacent to or within the effector organ. The postganglionic fibres from parasympathetic ganglia are relatively short and nearly all release **acetylcholine** as a neurotransmitter. In most cases the distribution of the parasympathetic outflow is more restricted than that of the sympathetic system. Thus, cranial nerve III supplies the smooth muscle of the eye (ciliary muscle and pupillary constrictor muscle), VII the lacrimal (tear) and submaxillary glands, and IX the parotid gland. The sacral parasympathetic outflow supplies the lower colon, rectum, bladder, the lower part of the ureters and the external genitalia. The major and most widely distributed parasympathetic outflow travels in cranial nerve X, the vagus. Approximately 70% of all parasympathetic preganglionic fibres leave the CNS in this nerve and supply all of the viscera in the thorax and most of the

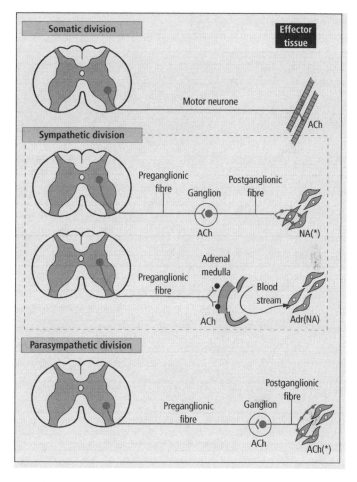

Fig. 3.12 Transmitters in the somatic, sympathetic and parasympathetic divisions of the PNS. ACh, acetylcholine; Adr, adrenaline; NA, noradrenaline. (*) Indicates that in addition to the classic transmitter, other co-transmitters may be released.

viscera in the abdomen. However, note that the vagus also carries many sensory fibres and a number of somatic motor nerves, e.g. to laryngeal and pharyngeal muscle.

It should be noted that there are many autonomically innervated tissues (e.g. in the cardiovascular, respiratory and urinary systems) where neurotransmitters other than noradrenaline and acetylcholine are released from postganglionic motor neurones to modify the activity of effector organs. At some sites these compounds (e.g. peptides, ATP, NO or opioids) are released along with the classical transmitter as a co-transmitter, while in others they may be the primary transmitter.

Enteric system

The autonomic nerves in the gastrointestinal tract differ from those in the other divisions as they form an extensive network in which many cells are not influenced by the CNS. The network is composed of ganglia and interconnecting bundles of axons that lie in the wall of the intestinal tract (from the oesophagus to the rectum) and form the myenteric and submucosal plexuses. A number of different neuronal types have been identified in the plexuses but a detailed knowledge of the relationships between ganglia and between cells is lacking. However, it is recognized that this system contains sensory neurones, interneurones (integrative) and excitatory and inhibitory motor

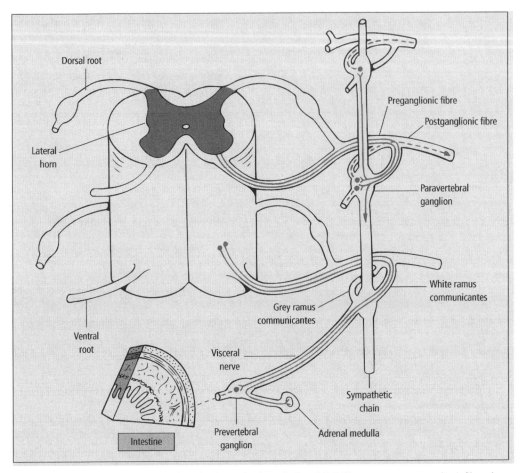

Fig. 3.13 Outflow of sympathetic fibres from the thoracolumbar spinal cord. Solid lines represent preganglionic fibres; broken lines represent postganglionic fibres.

neurones that can act together to generate coordinated patterns of activity. Many of the excitatory neurones (interneurones and motor neurones) release **acetylcholine** as a neurotransmitter, but others, particularly interneurones, may release **5-hydroxytryptamine** (5-HT, serotonin) or other compounds. The inhibitory neurones to smooth muscle do not release acetylcholine or noradrenaline as a transmitter and hence are referred to as **non-adrenergic, non-cholinergic nerves**. It has been suggested that they may be purinergic and release ATP, but more recent evidence suggests that a peptide (possibly **vasoactive intestinal polypeptide**; VIP) or NO may be involved.

3.5 Basic design of the CNS

The CNS comprises the brain lying within the skull and the spinal cord lying within the vertebral column. The brain consists of the brainstem, the cerebellum, the diencephalon and cerebrum. The brainstem, which links the spinal cord and the cerebrum, is composed of the medulla oblongata, the pons and the midbrain. The cerebellum is attached to the brainstem. The diencephalon comprises the thalamus, the subthalamus and the hypothalamus. The cerebrum consists of the right and left cerebral hemispheres, which are connected by the corpus callosum. The outer grey matter of the cerebral hemisphere constitutes the cortex. Within the white matter of each hemisphere are several collections of neuronal cell bodies, such as the basal ganglia.

During embryonic development the neural tube grows to form three longitudinal swellings at its anterior end. These swellings develop into the **fore-**, **mid-** and **hindbrain**. Their cavities form the **ventricles** and communicate with the canal in the **spinal cord**, which is formed from the remainder of the tube. The forebrain is divided into two regions, rostrally the **telencephalon** and caudally the **diencephalon**. The telencephalon is formed by a mid-portion and two lateral outpouchings, the primitive **cerebral hemispheres** or **cerebrum**, which grow first forwards and then backwards to cover most of the mid- and hindbrain (Fig. 3.14). The diencephalon gives rise to the **thalamus** and **hypothalamus**. The hindbrain gives rise to the **pons** and **medulla**, which together with the midbrain form the **brainstem**. Swellings of the hindbrain develop to form the **cerebellum**. The cerebellum and the cerebral hemispheres have two unique features:

1 their surfaces are extensively folded, forming depressions called **fissures** or **sulci** and raised portions called **gyri** in the cortex and **folia** in the cerebellum; and

2 unlike the brainstem and spinal cord, they have their grey matter on the outside and white matter on the inside.

Spinal cord

The spinal cord has a segmental structure with dorsal and ventral roots (see Fig. 3.9) arising on each side at more or less regular intervals. The **dorsal roots** carry information into the spinal cord from peripheral receptors; the **ventral roots** carry information out to effector organs, such as muscles. In cross-section each segment of the spinal cord shows a central butterfly-shaped area of grey matter and a peripheral zone of white matter (Fig. 3.9). The grey matter contains cell bodies of neurones. In the ventral horn of the grey matter lie the cell bodies of motor neurones whose axons leave in the ventral roots to innervate muscles; in the dorsal horn of the grey matter lie cell bodies of interneurones concerned with the processing of signals entering in the dorsal root axons.

The white matter of the spinal cord consists of tracts of ascending and descending axons (Fig. 3.15). In the dorsal quadrant of the white matter are the dorsal columns composed of axons that ascend to the brainstem conveying sensory information from skin, joints and muscles; in the lateral

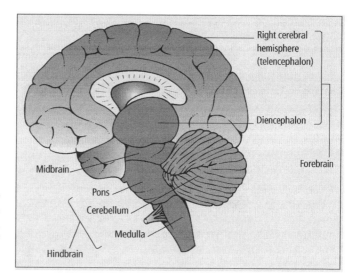

Fig. 3.14 A lateral view of brain after removal of the left cerebral hemisphere. (Adapted from Curtis, B.A., Jacobsen, S. & Marcus, E.M. (1972) *An Introduction to Neurosciences*, p. 13. Saunders, Philadelphia.)

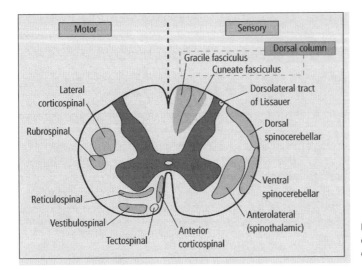

Fig. 3.15 Descending motor and ascending sensory tracts in the spinal cord.

quadrant there are both ascending tracts to the cerebellum and brainstem, and descending tracts from the cerebral cortex and brainstem. The spinal cord segments perform the initial processing of afferent information and contain the neural circuits for many reflexes, some of which are the basis of movement and posture.

Brain

The brain consists of three major subdivisions—the brainstem, the cerebellum, and the diencephalon and cerebrum.

Brainstem

This is an ancient part of the brain in an evolutionary sense. Although much smaller than the cerebellum, the brainstem is essential to life while the cerebellum may, with considerable residual but not life-threatening disability, be dispensed with. The brainstem links the spinal cord and cerebrum and is composed of three regions—the medulla oblongata, pons and midbrain (Fig. 3.14).

The **medulla oblongata** is continuous with the spinal cord and contains the same fibre tracts. The grey matter, however, is not organized in a continuous column but is broken into discrete nuclei, including motor and sensory nuclei for the throat,

mouth and neck, and nuclei involved in the control of the respiratory and cardiovascular systems and of movement and posture.

The **pons** may be recognized on the ventral surface (Fig. 3.16a) by the bulge of the brainstem formed by axons descending from the cerebrum and turning up into the cerebellum, which, in the intact brain, conceals the dorsal surface of the pons. The pons is continuous with the medulla and contains the same ascending and descending tracts in the reticular grey matter (**reticular formation**). It also contains nuclei that are involved in the control of the respiratory system and in motor and sensory functions of the face.

The **midbrain**, the smallest part of the brainstem, is continuous with the pons below and the diencephalon above. The ventral surface is characterized by the large **cerebral peduncles** (Fig. 3.16a) lying laterally and carrying axons from the cerebrum to the brainstem and cerebellum. The dorsal surface may be recognized by two pairs of protuberances, the **superior** and **inferior colliculi** (Fig. 3.16b). The superior collicular neurones are concerned with the processing of visual information and the inferior collicular neurones with auditory signals. The midbrain also contains nuclei concerned with the state of wakefulness of the brain and ascending tracts from the spinal cord on their way to the diencephalon.

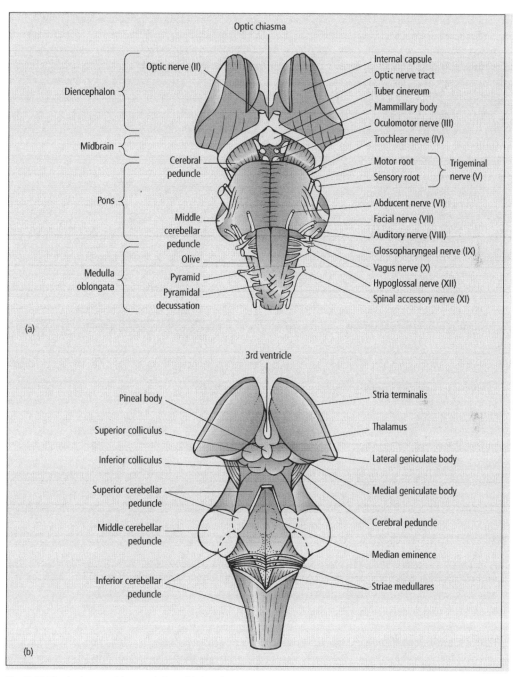

Fig. 3.16 The brainstem: (a) ventral view; (b) dorsal view. (Adapted from Truex, R.C. & Carpenter, M.B. (1969) *Human Neuroanatomy*, 6th edn, p. 31. Williams & Wilkins, Baltimore.)

The various **cranial nerves** have their superficial origins at different levels of the brainstem (Fig. 3.16a). There are 12 pairs of these and they innervate the skin and muscles of the face, structures in the head and neck and, in the case of the vagus (X) nerves, the thoracic and many of the abdominal viscera. Strictly speaking, the olfactory (I) nerves are connected to the forebrain, and not the brainstem. The optic (II) nerves are joined to the diencephalon via the optic chiasma. Cranial nerve pairs III and IV emerge from the midbrain, V–VIII from the pons and the remaining four pairs from the medulla.

The nuclei from which these cranial nerves have their origins may extend through a considerable length of the brainstem. Note that many of the nerves contain a mixture of fibres—motor and sensory, somatic and autonomic.

Cerebellum

This is a large organ overhanging the dorsal aspect of the brainstem to which it is attached to each side by three large bundles of white matter—the **superior**, **middle** and **inferior cerebellar peduncles**, which carry neural signals in and out of the cerebellum (Fig. 3.17a). Three cerebellar lobes can be recognized. On the superior aspect (Fig. 3.17b) the anterior lobe is separated from the larger middle lobe (sometimes called the posterior lobe) by the primary fissure. The anterior and middle lobes are further divided into a narrow median strip—the vermis—and two lateral **cerebellar hemispheres**. Rostrally, and seen only on the inferior aspect (Fig. 3.17c), are the **flocculus** and **nodule**, together forming the **flocculonodular lobe**. The anterior and middle lobes are transversely folded, the folds being termed **folia**. This folding vastly increases the surface area of the cerebellum.

All parts of the cerebellum have the same structure—a thin superficial layer of grey matter, the **cerebellar cortex**, covering a much larger expanse of white matter formed by axons entering and leaving the cortex. Deep in the white matter, close to the brainstem, lie the **intercerebellar nuclei**. A section at right angles to the long axis of a folium shows that it is much wider laterally than medially

and that subsidiary foldings of the folium, each with cortical grey matter and white matter, give the section the appearance of a tree, hence the name **arbor vitae** (Fig. 3.17a). The cerebellum has its major role in the control of the rate, range and direction of movement. The small, phylogenetically old, posterior lobe is connected to the organ of balance (labyrinth) and is concerned with the reflexes that ensure an upright posture.

Diencephalon and cerebrum

The **diencephalon** is covered by the cerebrum in the intact brain (Fig. 3.18a) and can only be seen if the brain is sectioned or if one hemisphere is removed (Fig. 3.14). Developmentally it represents that part of the forebrain from which the rudimentary cerebral hemispheres have budded off. Its walls have been thickened by the growth on either side of the mass of grey matter that constitutes the **thalamus**, and ventrally by the structures that make up the **hypothalamus**, so that the original cavity has become the narrow cleft of the **third ventricle** (Fig. 3.18b). The **thalamic nuclei** function in at least three ways. One group relays signals concerned with all types of afferent information, except olfaction, to the cerebral cortex on the same side. Another group relays signals to the motor cortex on the same side and receives information from the cerebellum and basal ganglia. A third group is concerned with sleep and wakefulness. The **hypothalamic nuclei** serve as regulating centres for autonomic functions (e.g. body temperature, heart rate and blood pressure). They control the release of hormones by the pituitary gland, and are involved in the expression of the emotions and the regulation of food and water intake.

The **cerebrum** consists of the right and left **cerebral hemispheres** (Fig. 3.18a). Connecting them in the midline is a large thick band of white matter known as the **corpus callosum** (Fig. 3.18b) made up of axons passing between the hemispheres. Each hemisphere comprises an outer layer, about 5 mm thick, of grey matter which is the **cerebral cortex**, covering a dense thick inner layer of white matter. The grey matter has a rich blood supply;

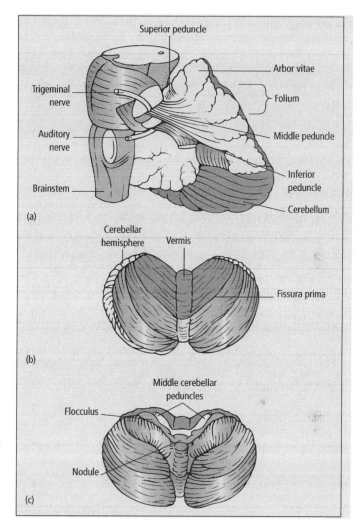

Fig. 3.17 The cerebellum: (a) lateral aspect; (b) superior aspect; (c) inferior aspect. (Redrawn from Johnson, T.B. & Willis, J. (eds) (1949) *Gray's Anatomy*, 30th edn, pp. 949, 954. Longmans, London.)

the white matter is less well-endowed. The white matter is composed of axons connecting different regions of the cortex with each other and connecting the cortex with the rest of the brain.

The cerebral cortex is folded into gyri and sulci, thereby increasing the surface area. The deepest sulci are called fissures. On the lateral surface of each hemisphere (Fig. 3.18a) the **lateral fissure** partially separates off the temporal lobe from the rest. This lobe contains the **primary auditory cortex**, which receives signals from the auditory receptors in the inner ear.

The **central sulcus** runs from the medial surface

to the lateral fissure (Fig. 3.18a). It is not as prominent as the lateral fissure but there are usually well-formed and continuous gyri on either side of the sulcus. The central sulcus forms the posterior boundary of the frontal lobe. The gyrus forming this posterior boundary and the anterior wall of the central sulcus is the **precentral gyrus**. This is the **primary motor cortex** containing neurones whose axons run down through the brainstem and spinal cord and synapse with motor neurones.

The **parietal lobe** lies behind the central sulcus. The posterior border of the sulcus is the **postcentral gyrus** of the parietal lobe—the **primary**

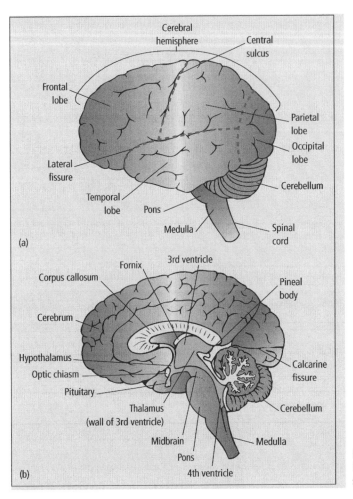

Fig. 3.18 The human brain: (a) lateral view; (b) view of a mid-sagittal section.

somatosensory cortex, which receives information from receptors in the skin, joints and muscle.

The **occipital lobe** is most posterior and little of it can be seen on the lateral surface (Fig. 3.18a). Examination of the medial surface (Fig. 3.18b), however, shows the **calcarine fissure** of the occipital lobe where the **primary visual cortex** is located. The occipital lobe is entirely concerned with the processing of visual information.

The **corpus callosum** (Fig. 3.18b) connects the two hemispheres and is surrounded by the **cingulate gyrus**, which is involved in the control of emotional behaviour.

Within the white matter of each hemisphere is a large collection of neuronal cell bodies, the **basal** ganglia. These consist of a group of nuclei that are concerned with the initiation and control of movement. They lie between the thalamus and cerebral cortex in each hemisphere and comprise the **claustrum**, the **putamen** and the **caudate nucleus**, and the **globus pallidus** (Fig. 3.19). Other smaller nuclei are for functional reasons usually considered along with the basal ganglia. The largest of these are the **subthalamic nucleus** and the **substantia nigra**, a darkly pigmented nucleus lying in the midbrain. The caudate nucleus and putamen are often referred to together as the **neostriatum**, while the putamen and globus pallidus are sometimes referred to together as the **lentiform nucleus** because of their combined shape. The term

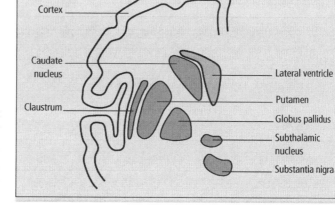

Fig. 3.19 Coronal section of the right cerebral hemisphere showing the location of the basal ganglia (claustrum, caudate nucleus, putamen and globus pallidus) and associated structures (subthalamic nucleus and substantia nigra).

corpus striatum includes all of these structures but not the claustrum.

Limbic system

This is a functionally related group of structures forming a fringe on the medial side of each hemisphere (Fig. 3.20). It is important in the regulation of behaviour and in memory. The structures concerned are many synapses away from the primary sensory or motor pathways and receive information from the overlying cortex, which, after processing, is directed back to the cortex. The limbic system comprises parts of the frontal and temporal lobe on either side, namely the **cingulate gyrus**, the **hippocampus**, the **septum**, the **amygdaloid nucleus** and the **anterior thalamic nucleus**. Some authors also include the hypothalamus. The cingulate gyrus lies above and around the corpus callosum (Fig. 3.20a). The hippocampus lies on the medial wall of the temporal lobe bordering the inferior horn of the lateral ventricle (Fig. 3.20b). It is a layered structure like the cerebral cortex but of simpler cellular pattern. The amygdala lies in the same region just in front of the hippocampus. The septum lies in the midline anterior to the hypothalamus between the lateral ventricles and ventral to the corpus callosum (Fig. 3.20). A large fibre bundle known as the fornix takes origin from the hippocampus and overlying cortex on each side (Fig. 3.20). This bundle arches forward underneath the corpus callosum accompanied by a similar but much smaller bundle of axons (stria terminalis) from the amygdaloid nucleus. The fornix and stria terminate in the septum and hypothalamus.

Meninges, ventricles and cerebrospinal fluid

The CNS is covered by three membranes or **meninges** (Fig. 3.21) comprising a tough outer layer, the **dura mater**, a middle layer, the **arachnoid**, in which lie the blood vessels, and an inner layer, the **pia mater**. Between the arachnoid and the pia mater is the **subarachnoid space**, which is in communication with the ventricles and contains **cerebrospinal fluid** (CSF), a specialized extracellular fluid. At the base of the brain, the subarachnoid space becomes enlarged to form cisterns, the largest being the **cisterna magna** (Fig. 3.21a).

The **ventricles** comprise the **lateral ventricles** in the cerebral hemispheres, the **third ventricle** in the diencephalon and the **fourth ventricle** in the hindbrain. The third and fourth ventricles are connected in the midbrain by a canal called the **cerebral aqueduct** (Fig. 3.21a).

Blood–brain barrier

Slow diffusion of many substances of low M_r between the blood and CSF and between the blood

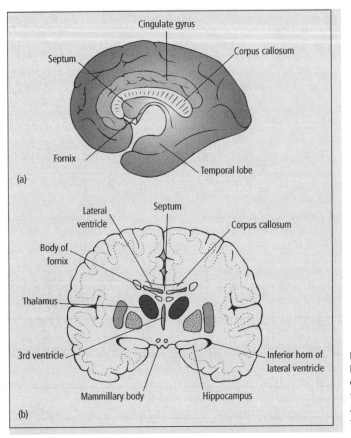

Fig. 3.20 The limbic system of the brain: (a) medial surface of the right cerebral hemisphere; (b) a frontal section through the junction of the third and lateral ventricles. See text for further information.

and brain suggests the existence of a **blood–CSF barrier** and a **blood–brain barrier**. These barriers are permeable to respiratory gases, to glucose and to lipid-soluble drugs like volatile anaesthetics. The endothelial cells of capillaries within the CNS are held together by **tight junctions**, and it is these which limit diffusional exchanges of water and water-soluble solutes. However, these cells are involved in the transport of solutes between blood and brain interstitial fluid. It should be noted that the blood–brain barrier is absent in certain structures called **circumventricular organs**, which abut on the third and fourth ventricles, e.g. the subfornical and pineal organs, the area postrema and the median eminence.

CSF

The CSF is formed predominantly by the **choroid plexuses** — rich networks of blood vessels covered with epithelial cells (**ependyma**) projecting into the ventricles (Fig. 3.21b). Fluid formed in the lateral ventricles passes to the third and fourth ventricles and to the central canal of the spinal cord. This movement is aided by the cilia on ependymal cells. The fluid escapes into the subarachnoid space through foramina in the ependymal lining of the fourth ventricle and circulates around the brain and spinal cord (Fig. 3.21a). Finally it is reabsorbed through the arachnoid villi into the sinuses of the venous system (Fig. 3.21c). In most regions of the brain, substances are free to diffuse between the ependymal cells and so there is a ready exchange of solutes between the CSF and the extracellular spaces of brain and spinal cord. The local environment of the neurones is further controlled by the activity of glial cells, which can adjust both K^+ and H^+ ion concentrations. Of the 700 ml of CSF

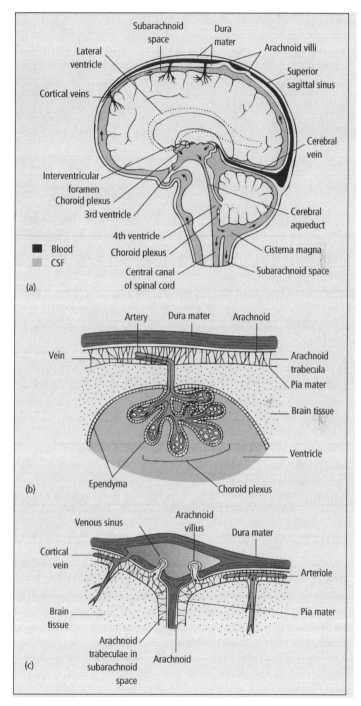

Fig. 3.21 Meninges, ventricles and CSF. (a) Flow of CSF. (After Rasmussen, A.T. (1937) *The Principal Nervous Pathways*, p. 4. Macmillan, New York.) (b) Choroid plexus. (c) Venous sinus.

Table 3.1 Composition of CSF compared with protein-free plasma, expressed as a ratio.*

Na+	1.0
K+	0.7
Ca2+	0.5
Cl−	1.1
HCO3−	0.9
Glucose	0.6

* Note that the protein content of CSF is $0.3\,g\,L^{-1}$ compared with $70\,g\,L^{-1}$ for plasma.

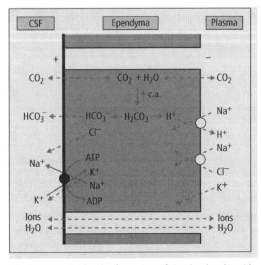

Fig. 3.22 Model for the formation of CSF by the choroid plexuses. c.a., carbonic anhydrase.

formed per day, about 70% is derived from the choroid plexuses and the other 30% comes from endothelial cells lining the brain capillaries. In adult humans the volume of CSF is about 140 ml (compared with about 250 ml for brain interstitial fluid), and when lying supine its pressure is about 10 mmHg, i.e. a little less than local venous pressure.

The composition of CSF differs from that expected if it were simply an ultrafiltrate of plasma (Table 3.1), indicating that it is actively secreted. One model for the formation of CSF by the choroid plexuses is illustrated in Fig. 3.22. One unusual feature of this is that the Na+,K+–ATPase is located in the apical plasma membrane. Note also that although CO_2 crosses the blood–brain barrier readily, HCO^-_3 does not. The HCO^-_3 in CSF is synthesized within the epithelial cells, in the reaction:

$$CO_2 + H_2O \rightleftharpoons H_2CO_3 \rightleftharpoons H^+ + HCO^-_3$$

The initial reaction is catalysed by carbonic anhydrase present in the epithelial cells. The primary secretion contains more HCO^-_3 than plasma (about $45\,mmol\,L^{-1}$), and it buffers H+ ions produced by neuronal and glial metabolism; this reduces $[HCO^-_3]$ to about $23\,mmol\,L^{-1}$. The decrease in $[HCO^-_3]$ may also reflect the mixing of choroidal CSF with fluid secreted by the capillary endothelial cells, which is thought to have a higher Cl− to HCO^-_3 ratio.

The functions of the CSF are as follows:

1 Conferring of buoyancy. The brain has little mechanical strength or rigidity. It weighs 50 g in CSF, compared with 1500 g in air, and so flotation in CSF protects it against deformation and damage from the innumerable accelerations imposed by movements of the head. Counter-pressure of CSF surrounding the blood vessels within the cranium and the spinal cord compensates for the gravitational effects of alterations in posture or external acceleration.

2 Maintenance of a constant ionic environment in the brain. This is important because the activity of neurones is highly sensitive to ionic changes.

3 Removal of waste substances. The CSF provides another route for removal of substances that have limited lipid solubility or are too large to move easily across capillary walls. In other tissues the lymphatic system, which is not found in the CNS, serves this function.

4 Intracerebral transport. Neuropeptides secreted into the CSF are carried from one region to another.

Chapter 4

Signalling in the Nervous System

4.1 Local potentials and action potentials

Electrical signals in neurones result from changes in their resting membrane potential. These changes in membrane potential can be divided into two types—local potentials and action potentials. In general, local potentials (also called graded potentials) occur at points where the neurones receive an input. Their amplitude is graded as a function of the intensity of the incoming stimulus. At the point of generation, the amplitude of the local potential is maximal; away from this point (within 0.2–2 mm) the amplitude falls rapidly. In contrast, for action potentials, the amplitude of the membrane potential change that takes place once the action potential is triggered is not affected by the intensity of the stimulus (termed an all-or-none response). In addition, the action potentials are conducted over longer distances, in some instances a metre or more, with little change in amplitude.

Neurones, like other cells, are electrically polarized so that their interior is negatively charged with respect to the outside of the cell (p. 13). Typical resting values for neurones are about −70 mV, compared to −90 mV for glial cells, −80 mV for skeletal muscle cells and −70 mV for smooth muscle cells.

The magnitude of the membrane potential can be estimated from the equilibrium potentials of the various ions and their conductances across the plasma membrane (p. 15). Ions move through channels that span the plasma membrane and that have the special property of being selectively permeable to particular ion species. At rest, the conductance through K^+-specific channels (g_K) is much greater than that through Na^+-specific channels (g_{Na}), and so the membrane potential approaches the equilibrium potential of the ion that is most permeable under these conditions; i.e. K^+ ($E_K \sim -90$ mV; calculated from the Nernst equation (p. 14)—applicable only in conditions of equilibrium when no net flux of ions takes place). When an excitable cell, such as a neurone, is stimulated, specific channels are activated (gated), and the current through them makes a greater contribution to the membrane potential. The potential developed will depend upon the equilibrium potential for each ion and on the relative contribution each makes to the total conductance (p. 15). In excitable membranes the major types of gated channels include: voltage-gated, chemically-gated (ligand-gated), and mechanically-gated channels (pp. 7–8).

Basic electrical properties of biological membranes

To understand the electrical changes that can take place within neuronal membranes, it is necessary to first consider some basic concepts of electricity, in the context of cellular membrane physiology. Small ions, which are electrically charged, can flow across biological membranes, and this current results in the separation of electrical charges. The intensity of the **current** (I, measured in amperes (amps; A)) passing through a membrane measures the rate of transfer of electrical charge (Q, measured in Coulombs (C)) from one side to the other in a unit of time (second) (thus, $1A = 1$ coulomb per second; Cs^{-1}). The **potential difference** (V, measured in volts; V) is a measure of the energy separated across the membrane per unit charge (joules per coulomb; JC^{-1}). For a given current, the potential difference generated increases proportionally with the **resistance** of the membrane, where resistance (R, measured in ohms; σ) is a measure of the difficulty with which charges can move through the membrane. This relationship is described by the classical formulation of Ohm's law:

$$V = IR$$

The reciprocal of resistance is called **conductance** (G, measured in siemens; S) and is a measure of the ease with which charge can move through the membrane. This parameter is used extensively when describing the basic properties of various ion channels.

Another important electrical parameter of the membranes is its **capacitance** (C). When a current is passed across, the membranes do not immediately change to a new, steady potential difference. Initially, some of the current passed simply changes the amount of charge (Q) stored on the membrane itself. The membrane, in separating charges across it, acts like a capacitor and the amount of charges separated per unit of driving force is the capacitance, such that $C = Q/V$, and its unit is the farad (F). The capacitance per unit area or **specific membrane capacitance** is similar for most biological membranes—about $1\,\mu F\,cm^{-2}$.

Local potentials

Whenever a net movement of electric charge takes place across the membrane a change in the potential difference results, which can go only in two directions: either the inside of the cell becomes more positive, with a concomitant decrease in the membrane potential difference—a process called **depo-**

larization; or the inside of the cell becomes more negative and the membrane potential difference is increased—termed **hyperpolarization**. A depolarization can result not only from the movement of positive charge into the cell, but also from an increased movement of negative charge away from the cell. The opposite movements of charge result in hyperpolarization: i.e. either a movement of negative charge into the cell, or positive charge away from the cell. In the nervous system, such local potentials are usually mediated by the opening or closing of various ion channels. This channel activity could result from either: the action of a chemical neurotransmitter—mainly at the synapse—generating a **synaptic potential** (or an **end-plate potential** at the neuromuscular junction; see below); or mechanical deformation of the membrane (inducing a **generator potential**) or activation of a specific sensory receptor (generating a **receptor potential**).

Local potentials have a number of important properties. First, the amplitude of the potential change that results from local electrical currents generated by ion channel activity is maximal at the site of generation. Like all electrical currents, their amplitude decreases exponentially with increasing distance travelled from the site of generation (**decrement**) (Fig. 4.1), such that local potentials are typically restricted to within 0.2–2 mm of their site of generation. Second, local potentials are **graded** (Fig. 4.2), i.e. the amplitude of the potential change is proportional to the magnitude of the stimulus (that is, a stronger stimulus will have a greater effect on ion channel activity, therefore inducing a greater movement of electric charge across the membrane). This also means that if a subsequent stimulus is generated prior to the complete disappearance of the first, it can elicit a larger response than it would have done alone (Fig. 4.3). This property is called **summation**, and summation takes place either **temporally** (stimuli arrive in quick succession; Fig. 4.3a) or **spatially** (two stimuli arrive at different, but relatively close, sites on the membrane; Fig. 4.3b). Summation of local potentials (either spatially or temporally) is particularly important as a basis for the initiation and propagation of action potentials.

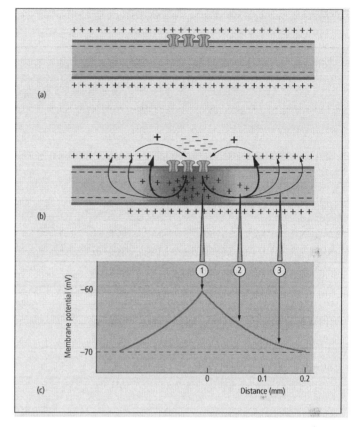

Fig. 4.1 Electrotonic spread of current along an axon following the generation of a local potential, and the resulting change in membrane potential. (a) The neuronal membrane at rest, with various ionic channels, closed. (b) Opening of the ionic channels in response to stimulation. The current flow is maximal at the site of generation, inducing the maximal change in membrane potential. The ionic charges diffuse away from the site of entry, and their density decreases with distance. (c) A plot of the decrease in the membrane potential with increasing distance away from the site of current injection.

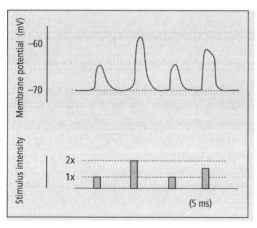

Fig. 4.2 Graded potentials. The amplitude of the local potentials is proportional to the strength of the stimulus applied.

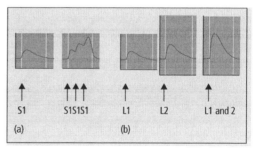

Fig. 4.3 The process of summation. (a) Temporal summation, with three stimuli of same intensity (S1) arriving in quick succession. (b) Spatial summation, with two stimuli, with different intensity (L1 and L2), arriving at the neurone at the same time but at different locations, separated by a few tens of micrometres.

Action potentials

The depolarizing local potentials discussed above result from small, inward, depolarizing currents. If such currents are sufficiently large, so that at various specific locations the neuronal membrane is depolarized to reach a certain potential, termed **threshold**, an **all-or-nothing** response—termed an **action potential**—ensues. Neurones and various types of muscle cells are called electrically excitable cells because their membrane properties and composition allow the generation and propagation of such action potentials. The action potential is probably the most important and fundamental neurophysiological process and, through its rapid and long-distance propagation, it mediates the integrative function of the nervous system.

Generation of the action potential

In simple terms, an action potential is generated by the sudden opening of specialized, fast Na$^+$ channels, which are voltage-dependent. The term 'voltage-dependent' means that these channels are sensitive to the membrane potential and are activated when membrane depolarization reaches a certain threshold level (for Na$^+$ channels in most membranes this threshold is $\sim$–55 mV) (Fig. 4.4). Termination of the action potential is caused by the activation of another set of voltage-sensitive channels, permeable to K$^+$. For a more detailed analysis of these events, the time-course of an action potential lasting under 5 ms can be divided into several stages (Fig. 4.4a). Following the resting state (**phase 1**), during the second phase, local potentials depolarize the membrane. Once the threshold is reached, fast, voltage-dependent Na$^+$ channels are activated and there is a sudden increase in Na$^+$ conductance (g_{Na}) (**phase 3**; see also Fig 4.4b). A powerful feed-forward, self-regenerating process is activated, during which Na$^+$ influx further depolarizes the membrane, activating additional Na$^+$ channels. At rest, the equilibrium potential of the membrane is dictated by the most permeable ion—K$^+$; however, during phase 3 of the action potential, Na$^+$ conductance is much larger

and therefore predominates. Accordingly, the membrane potential will move towards the equilibrium potential for Na$^+$, as dictated by the Nernst equation—E_{Na} ($\sim$+70 mV). This explains why, during the action potential, the polarity of the membrane can be completely reversed (positive charge inside), generating an **overshoot**. However, the membrane potential rarely reaches E_{Na}, and within less than a millisecond from the initiation of the action potential, a peak of depolarization is reached and the repolarization process (**phase 4**) takes over.

Repolarization is also controlled by ion channel activity, and results from two independent processes: a sudden, significant decrease in the Na$^+$ conductance and a slower, but continuous increase in the membrane conductance for K$^+$ (g_K). The decrease in g_{Na} is due to an intrinsic property of the fast Na$^+$ channels—**inactivation**, which occurs within milliseconds and is voltage-dependent, such that the more the membrane is depolarized, the stronger the inactivation (Fig. 4.5). The Na$^+$ channels have another important property—once the channels have been activated and then quickly inactivated during depolarization of the membrane, they will remain inactivated until the membrane potential returns to its resting level (Fig. 4.5). A second process, more directly and actively involved in repolarization, is the voltage-dependent activation of a set of K$^+$ channels. Following their opening, there is an efflux of K$^+$ along the electrochemical gradient from the cell into the extracellular fluid. This process is called **delayed rectification** due to its slower rate of activation and to the fact that it rectifies the anomalous situation of a membrane with a reversed polarity, as during the early phase of the action potential. In addition to delayed activation, these K$^+$ channels are also slow to close. As a consequence, when the Na$^+$ conductance is inactivated, they remain open, and the membrane is hence driven towards the K$^+$ equilibrium potential—E_K ($\sim$–90 mV). This explains the **after-hyperpolarization** that follows an action potential (**phase 5** in Fig. 4.4a).

Understanding the ionic basis of an action potential (Fig. 4.4b) helps to appreciate the various states of excitability of the neuronal membrane

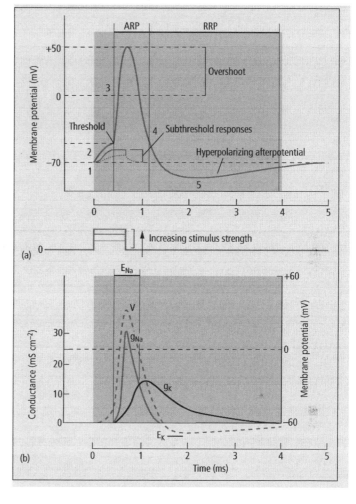

Fig. 4.4 Generation of an action potential. (a) (superimposed) The responses of a neurone to localized current pulses of different intensity. When threshold is reached, an action potential is generated. For description purposes, an action potential can be divided in various phases: absolute refractory period (ARP), during which the neurone cannot be activated; and the relative refractory period (RRP), during which the neurone can be activated only by stimuli larger than normal. (b) Time course of the changes in ionic conductances during an action potential in an axon; the sudden, rapid and large increase in Na$^+$ conductance (gNa) initiates the action potential. Later, a smaller increase in K$^+$ conductance (gK) terminates the action potential and leads to the hyperpolarization phase. E_{Na} and E_k illustrate the values of the electrochemical gradient for the two respective ions.

(Fig 4.4a). During an action potential the membrane is in an **absolute refractory period**, which means that no other action potential can be generated at that site, irrespective of the magnitude of the stimulus. (This is due to the fact that all fast Na$^+$ channels that mediate the upshot phase of the action potential are in a state of inactivation.) From when the Na$^+$ channels are beginning to be reactivated as the membrane is repolarized, until −50 mV or lower is reached—which occurs towards the end of the repolarization process—the neurone remains in a state termed the **relative refractory period** in which a new action potential can be generated, but only by stimuli of sufficiently large intensity (as the membrane is hyperpolarized and

thus a larger depolarization is required to reach the threshold).

Many of the functional properties of action potentials are explained by the characteristics of voltage-dependent Na$^+$ channels. The channels have two different ionic gates that regulate the flow of Na$^+$ ions. Accordingly, the channels can exist in three different states (Fig. 4.5). At rest, the **activation gate** is closed, while the other—**inactivation gate**—is opened (thus the channel is 'closed'). On reaching the threshold, the activation gate is opened, and Na$^+$ ions flow through unimpeded (the channel is therefore 'open'). Rapidly after activation the inactivation gate closes, while the activation gate remains open, and the channel is no

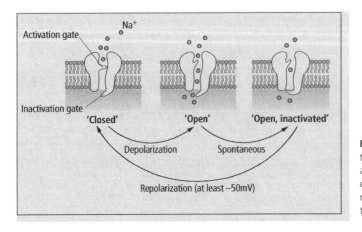

Fig. 4.5 Diagrammatic representation of the three configurations adopted by the voltage-sensitive Na$^+$ channel during the depolarizing and repolarizing phases of an action potential.

longer permeable to Na$^+$ (overall state 'open, inactive'). The channels are reactivated quickly, but only when the membrane potential falls to below −50 mV.

At the end of an action potential, the neurone recovers its resting membrane potential; however, the ionic composition is potentially altered since the action potential results in an influx of Na$^+$ during depolarization, and efflux of K$^+$ during repolarization. It can be calculated, taking into account the intracellular concentrations of both Na$^+$ and K$^+$, that less than 0.01% of the K$^+$ ions in a nerve fibre of 20 μm diameter is actually exchanged for Na$^+$ ions during the course of an action potential—an insignificant proportion. However, after several hundred impulses have passed in quick succession during periods of high activity, the total amount of K$^+$ ions lost may become significant, particularly for smaller diameter fibres; the ionic gradients must therefore be re-established via the Na$^+$–K$^+$ pump, using metabolic energy.

The existence of specific membrane channels and their role in the generation of action potentials is supported by the action of specific pharmacological blocking agents. For example: **tetrodotoxin** blocks voltage-dependent Na$^+$ channels and hence prevents the subsequent increase in g_{Na}; **scorpion venom** prevents Na$^+$ inactivation and so, after initiation of an action potential, the cell remains in a depolarized state; and **tetraethylammonium** blocks K$^+$ channels and leads to a delayed recovery of the action potential. **Local anaesthetics** prevent the generation of the action potential by inhibiting the voltage-dependent opening of Na$^+$ channels.

Propagation of the action potential

Most commonly, action potentials are generated only in specialized regions of neurones. For most neurones, the action potential is initiated at the **axon hillock**, representing the initial segment of the axon as it is formed from the cell body. This region contains a significantly higher density of fast, voltage-sensitive Na$^+$ channels, and therefore the cascade of ionic events generated by reaching the depolarization threshold is easier to trigger. In most instances, action potentials cannot be initiated in the dendrites or at other sites on the cell body because the density of Na$^+$ channels in these regions is lower. From the site of origin, an action potential propagates as a wave of excitation along the axon. At any one time, only a portion of the axon is depolarized. Although this local depolarization gives rise to a passive spread of current up and down the axon (Fig. 4.6), the propagation of the action potential is always **unidirectional**, since the regions behind the front end of propagation are in various stages of refractoriness. Thus, the local current is only effective at generating depolarization in the regions ahead of the action potential, by bringing resting Na$^+$ channels to threshold and hence generating subsequent action potentials.

Because the action potential mechanism involv-

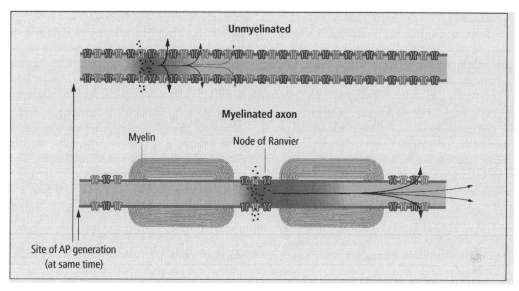

Fig. 4.6 Flow of current associated with the propagation of an action potential in axons—either unmyelinated (top) or myelinated (bottom). The figure also illustrates the differences in the speed of action potential conduction between the two types of axon.

ing membrane channels is relatively slow compared to the spread of an electric current, the further the local current can spread, the faster the action potential can travel. The **conduction velocity** can be enhanced by increasing the **diameter** of a fibre or by increasing its electrical insulation, through **myelination**. Increasing the diameter lowers intracellular resistance, because in large fibres more ions are available to carry the current and, as a consequence, depolarizing current spreads further along the fibre. For example, in squid giant nerve fibres, with diameters of up to 1 mm, the conduction velocity is approximately 25 $m s^{-1}$, compared to about $1 m s^{-1}$ for small (~1 μm) unmyelinated fibres. The wrapping of some axons with layers of myelin sheath increases the membrane resistance and decreases capacitance, both of which cause an increase in the conduction velocity. The conduction velocity of a myelinated nerve fibre of 20 μm diameter is approximately $100 m s^{-1}$ at 37°C. Most mammalian fibres of greater than 1 μm diameter are myelinated.

In addition to the effects on membrane resistance and capacitance, myelination restricts membrane current and the generation of action potentials to the **nodes of Ranvier** (Fig. 4.6). The nodes of Ranvier are characterized by a high concentration of voltage-sensitive Na^+ channels, which mediate the action potentials; the axonal membrane between the nodes is not excitable. The passing of an action potential from node to node is called **saltatory conduction**. However, it should be realized that at any instant an action potential travelling along a myelinated axon will cover several nodes and not simply a single one. For example, an action potential lasting 0.5 ms travelling at $100 m s^{-1}$ should cover a 50 mm length of the axon, and thus maybe up to 40 nodes. In summary, the benefits of myelination are:

1 higher conduction velocities for rapid signalling;

2 small diameters for conserving space; and

3 higher metabolic efficiency because of the reduced flux of ions and hence reduced expenditure of energy required to restore ionic concentrations.

Extracellular recording of nervous activity

For clinical neurology, measurement of peripheral nerve or muscle activity is of great diagnostic importance. Peripheral nerves contain axons, both sensory and motor, with a range of diameters—from large myelinated fibres with high conduction velocities to small unmyelinated slow-conducting fibres (see Table 4.1). The conduction of an action potential along these axons means a flow of electrical charge (i.e. an electrical current) into or away from the axons and into the tissue or medium surrounding the nerve. The resistance of the extracellular space is low in comparison with both the axonal membrane and intracellular longitudinal resistance, and thus the field potentials generated by one axon in the surrounding medium will be small. (Remember from above that $V_e = IR_e$, where V_e is the extracellular field potential and R_e is the small extracellular resistance.)

However, under experimental conditions, recording of single axon activity is possible if the axon is isolated electrically by immersion in mineral oil, which will minimize current dissipation. In this way, larger potentials can be recorded between two extracellular electrodes placed on the surface of the axon (Fig. 4.7). When an action potential reaches the first electrode, the underlying membrane reverses its polarity, because of the flow of positive charges (i.e. Na^+ ions) from the medium into the axon. Thus, the extracellular medium under the first electrode becomes negative compared to the medium under the second electrode, and by convention this is shown graphically as an upward deflection. When the action potential is propagating between the two electrodes, the potential difference falls to zero between the elec-

trodes. Later, as the electrical activity moves away from the first electrode to affect predominantly the area of the membrane under the second electrode, the potential difference is reversed. As such a recording shows both negative and positive components, it is referred to as a **di-** or **biphasic** action potential. If the action potential fails to reach the second electrode (e.g. due to the axon being damaged by crushing or a local anaesthetic is applied), only the first phase is recorded and the action potential appears as a single negative deflection—a **monophasic** action potential (Fig. 4.7b).

These mono- or biphasic action potentials, when recorded from a single axon, show the all-or-none and refractory characteristics of the intracellularly recorded action potential. In contrast, when the activity of a whole peripheral nerve, composed of hundreds to thousands of axons, is recorded, as in clinical measurements, the obtained record is a summed activity of action potentials being conducted along all the fibres. This is called a **compound action potential**. It is not all-or-none because of the different thresholds of various fibres. It increases in amplitude as the stimulus is increased until all fibres are excited. The compound action potential may also display a number of peaks (Fig. 4.8), each corresponding to groups of axons with different velocities of conduction. The separation of the peaks in one particular trace will depend also on the distance of the recording electrodes from the point of stimulation; the greater this distance, the greater the separation of the peaks (Fig. 4.8). In addition, the amplitude of these

Table 4.1 Classification of mammalian nerve fibres.

	Nerve fibre type		
	A	**B**	**C**
Fibre diameter (μm)	0.1–20	<4	0.3–1.5
Conduction speed (m s^{-1})	0.5–120	3–15	0.6–2.5
Spike duration (m s)	0.3–0.5	1.2	2.0
Absolute refractory period (m s)	0.4–1.0	1.2	2.0

The fibres in category A can be subdivided in a further 4 categories (α to δ). For specific comparison and similar classification of the sensory fibres, consult Table 6.1.

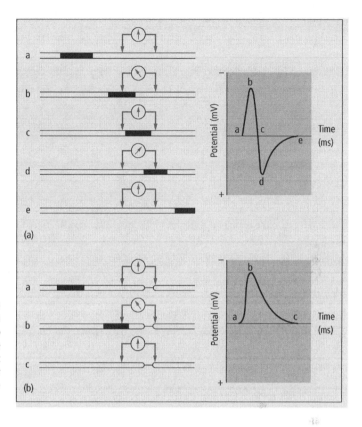

Fig. 4.7 Extracellular recording of an action potential conducted along an axon. The potentials corresponding to the positions of the conducted wave are indicated by a–e. (a) Biphasic record. (b) Monophasic record after crushing a portion of the axon between the recording electrodes.

peaks and their relationship to each other depend on the fibre composition of the nerve, with the larger fibres having the greatest amplitudes.

In clinical conditions, the **excitability** of a peripheral nerve is defined by either the voltage required to generate an action potential or by the length of time a stimulus is required for to achieve the firing of an action potential. The relationship between these two parameters, voltage and duration, generates a **strength-duration curve** (Fig. 4.9) that is characterized by two parameters of clinical importance: **rheobase** is the minimal voltage needed to produce an excitation with a long stimulus (normally 300 ms); and **chronaxie** is the time required to excite a nerve by a stimulus that is twice the rheobase.

Gasser (Nobel Prize, 1944) and his colleagues showed experimentally, in the 1930s, that the axons in peripheral nerves can be divided into three broad groups (A, B and C) according to their conduction velocities. The basic division is still valid, and the A fibres include all the peripheral myelinated fibres from 3 to 20 μm in diameter; the group is further subdivided into subgroups groups of decreasing size and conduction velocity, the α (12–20 μm, 70–120 ms⁻¹ velocity of transmission), β, γ and δ (2–5 μm, 10–30 ms⁻¹) fibres. The B group comprises the small myelinated fibres in visceral nerves (preganglionic autonomic), and the C group all small unmyelinated, afferent and efferent fibres. The conduction velocities and other properties of the fibres in the various groups can be seen in Table 4.1. A similar grouping, but using roman numerals (I–IV), is often applied to the sensory fibres (p. 123). The conduction velocity of a fibre is closely related to its fibre diameter, since this diameter determines the cross-sectional area and the intracellular resistance.

Conduction along fibres may be reduced or even blocked by cold, anoxia, compression and drugs.

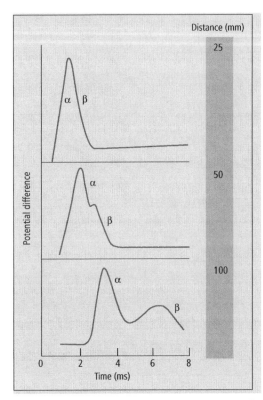

Fig. 4.8 Components of a compound action potential recorded at various distances from the recording electrodes. With increasing distance between the stimulation point and the recording electrode, the separation between the fast (α) and medium-fast fibres (β) becomes clearer. By 10 cm, the time taken by the axons of the slower fibres (about 6 ms) to depolarize is double that required by the fast fibres (3 ms).

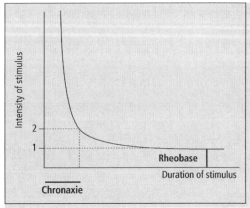

Fig. 4.9 Properties of action potentials. Rheobase defines the minimal intensity of a stimulus that is required to generate a response. Chronaxie defines the time required to generate a response that is two times larger than the response generated at rheobase level.

The conduction velocity decreases by approximately 3% of the maximal velocity for each 1°C fall. This is important in limbs or superficial tissues where the temperature may be well below the core temperature. Conduction block occurs in the large myelinated fibres at about 7°C and in the unmyelinated fibres at about 3°C. Compression and anoxia preferentially block large myelinated fibres. Thus, painful stimuli, which are transmitted in small unmyelinated fibres, can still be felt when other modes of sensation are lost. In contrast, local anaesthetics tend preferentially to block small fibres, the surface area to volume ratio of which is high.

As changes in the conduction velocity of peripheral nerves can also occur as a result of accident or disease states, such as **diabetes mellitus** or **Guillain-Barré syndrome**, studies of the compound action potential can be useful clinically. Neural degeneration and subsequent regrowth lead to the formation of thinner fibres with lower conduction velocities. Similarly, demyelinating diseases of the CNS, such as **multiple sclerosis**, may result in a reduction in thickness or a localized loss of myelin. Upon remyelination there is also a reduction in the distance between the nodes of Ranvier (internodal length), and this will affect negatively the conduction velocity. Similarly, with an extensive localized loss of myelin there may also be a conduction block.

Spontaneous action potentials

Some neurones spontaneously undergo fluctuations in their resting membrane potentials. These may generate action potentials even in the absence of external excitation. Such fluctuations in membrane potential have recently been shown to be generated by specific changes in membrane conductances, which may involve Na^+, Ca^{2+} and Ca^{2+}-dependent K^+ channels. Cells with these properties are important in the generation of rhythmic activity reflected in respiration and the electroencephalogram (EEG). They have also been shown to underlie the expression of some behavioural patterns in invertebrates.

4.2 Sensory receptors

The various sensory receptors form the interface between their surrounding environment and the nervous system. They usually detect a particular change in the environment, known as the adequate stimulus, and transduce this into electrical activity. Most receptors respond to a stimulus with a depolarizing receptor potential, which, if it exceeds threshold, will initiate action potentials in the sensory neurone. Some receptors respond to a continuous stimulus with a prolonged depolarization but others may adapt and respond only briefly. In most instances the frequency of action potentials in the sensory axons and the number of axons recruited are a reflection of the amplitude of the stimulus.

Sensory receptors are the link by which all information regarding the internal and external environment enters the nervous system. They are structures that convert different forms of stimulus energy into nerve impulses. However, they are limited in the range of stimuli that they can receive, and so restrict the information we perceive about our environment. Sensory receptors may be actual endings of sensory neurones or they may be specialized cells that initiate activity in some adjacent afferent (sensory) neurones.

Receptors are, to a large extent, **specific** or selective in their response, being sensitive primarily to one particular kind of energy. This energy, or change in energy, forms the **adequate stimulus** and a receptor transforms or **transduces** this particular kind of stimulus into a change in membrane potential. In some instances, the same receptor may also be able to transduce other forms of energy but with a much higher **threshold** of activation. Receptors are usually classified according to the kind of energy for which they are most specific, e.g. mechanoreceptors, thermoreceptors, chemoreceptors, photoreceptors and nociceptors (Table 4.2).

Transduction mechanisms

Activation of a sensory receptor by a specific stimulus can take place in several ways: a stimulus may act directly on the membrane of the nerve ending, e.g. free nerve endings in the skin; or alternatively, receptors may be highly specialized and the stimulus may act indirectly via either an **accessory structure**, e.g. a capsule or hair shaft, or via a **receptor cell**, e.g. rod and cone cells in the eye, taste buds in the tongue, hair cells in the ear (Fig. 4.10). Where an accessory structure is present, this usually plays an important role in transmission of the stimulus to the receptor, and is specifically adapted for the type of energy received.

A stimulus to a receptor cell induces a change in the membrane conductance leading to the generation of a localized receptor potential. This then evokes a local **generator potential** in the sensory nerve terminal, either by direct electrotonic spread or indirectly by the release of a chemical transmitter. If of sufficient strength, an individual generator potential initiates action potentials, which are then propagated along the sensory nerve to the CNS; alternatively this can occur through spatial and/or temporal summation of weaker generator potentials. The relationship between stimulus strength and amplitude of the receptor potential generated is linear and rather steep at lower stimulation strengths, but it saturates and flattens out at more intense levels of stimulation; therefore, very intense stimulation causes progressively smaller and smaller increments in action potential generation. This type of relationship allows the receptor to have a wide dynamic range of responses to stimuli that vary from very weak to very intense.

Adaptation

This is the term applied to the decline in the receptor potential shown by most receptors during the application of a constant or maintained stimulus. Receptor potentials in **slowly adapting** receptors, e.g. muscle spindles and Golgi tendon organs, are prolonged and decay slowly, while those in **rapidly adapting** receptors, e.g. hair receptors and

Table 4.2 Classification of receptors.

Receptor type	Adequate stimulus	Location	Examples of effective stimulus
Mechanoreceptors	Mechanical deformation	Skin	Touch, pressure, vibration
		Muscles and tendons	Changes in muscle length and tension
		Joints	Joint position and movement
		Viscera (e.g. blood vessels, lung, stomach, bladder)	Distension
		Cochlea	Sound vibrations, about 16 Hz to 20 kHz
		Vestibule (e.g. semicircular canals, utricle)	Linear acceleration, angular acceleration
Thermoreceptors	Heat changes	Skin	Warming or cooling
		Hypothalamus	Warming or cooling
Chemoreceptors	Certain chemicals	Carotid and aortic bodies	Changes in plasma P_{O_2}, P_{CO_2}, pH
		Medulla oblongata	Local changes in pH
		Tongue and gut	Acids, salts, sugars
		Nose	Odorous chemicals
		Hypothalamus	Changes in plasma osmolality
Photoreceptors	Electromagnetic radiation of particular wavelengths (400–700 nm)	Eye	Light
Nociceptors	Mechanical, thermal or chemical but only at an intensity which threatens or causes tissue damage	Skin	Pinch, crush, sting, heat above 45–50°C
		Deep structures (muscle, joint and viscera)	Excessive stretch

Pacinian corpuscles, quickly repolarize to values below threshold. Changes in receptor or generator potential to below threshold are reflected as changes in the discharge frequency of action potentials in the afferent fibres. During a constant stimulus, the impulse frequency in sensory neurones with slowly adapting receptors may remain at a relatively constant level for long periods of time (minutes to hours), hence they are also known as 'tonic' receptors. In sensory neurones with rapidly adapting receptors, the generation of action potentials may decline rapidly and cease altogether within seconds (Fig. 4.11). These types of receptors are best suited to detecting changes in the rates of activity; they are therefore also called 'rate' or 'phasic' receptors.

Coding of sensory information

The general view is that one sensory axon will carry only one type of information, but that the same axon will serve several receptors of the same kind. The afferent nerve fibre of a single sensory neurone, all its peripheral branches and central terminals, and any non-neural transducer cells associated with it, form together the **sensory unit** (Fig. 4.12). The area or part of the body covered by a sensory unit forms the **receptor field** of an individual neurone, and its size varies with the type of sensory information and anatomical location. Certain regions, e.g. fingertips and lips, are more densely innervated, with individual units having smaller receptive fields than other regions, e.g. trunk or

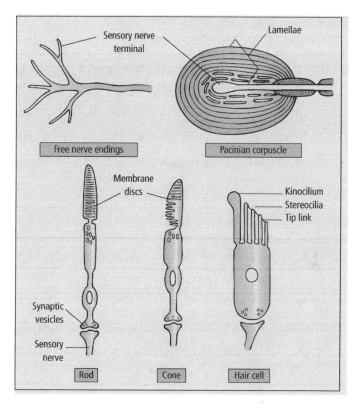

Fig. 4.10 Structure of various sensory receptors.

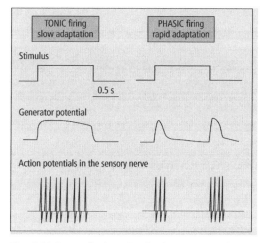

Fig. 4.11 Types of adaptation in the sensory pathway. Axons with tonic firing have slow adaptation, and fire action potentials for most of the time that the stimulus is present. Rapid adaptation is due to a phasic pattern of activity, in which generator potentials and resulting action potentials are fired only for a short time after the initiation and/or termination of the stimulus.

thigh. The number of receptors is larger in the centre of the field and diminishes towards the periphery, where it overlaps with neighbouring receptor fields. The size of the receptor field and the density of the receptors are important in allowing two-point discrimination, the capacity to differentiate clearly between two nearby stimuli.

An effective discriminatory power is also enhanced by the process of **lateral inhibition** in effect a biological contrast-enhancing mechanism, through which an active region (one sensory neurone firing action potentials) inhibits the activity in the surrounding area.

4.3 Synaptic transmission

Neural synaptic transmission

Neurones communicate with one another at synapses. At the majority of synapses the arrival of an action potential in the presynaptic region is followed by the release of chemical transmitters,

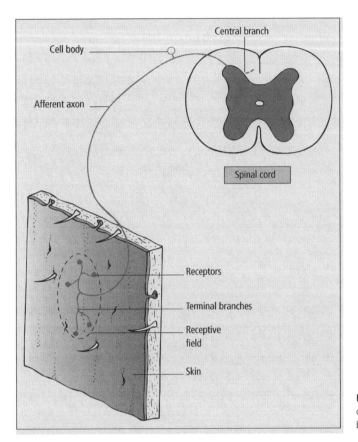

Cell body

Central branch

Afferent axon

Spinal cord

Receptors

Terminal branches

Receptive field

Skin

Fig. 4.12 A sensory unit and the receptive field supplied by its terminal branches.

which diffuse across the synaptic cleft. Transmitters interact transiently with receptors on the postsynaptic membrane and produce a change in membrane conductance and, consequently, membrane potential. Depending on the type of conductance change, the postsynaptic membrane may be either depolarized (excitatory postsynaptic potential, EPSP) or hyperpolarized (inhibitory postsynaptic potential, IPSP). Synaptic potentials can summate: if the final potential change is excitatory, action potentials may be initiated in the postsynaptic cell but if inhibitory, action potential generation will be suppressed.

The term **synapse** (from Greek **syn**, 'together' and **haptein**, 'to clasp') has been introduced by Sherrington (Nobel prize, 1932) to describe the point of contact between neurones. A typical neurone in the CNS receives inputs from many other neurones (**convergence**) and makes synaptic contact with many more (**divergence**; Fig. 4.13). For example, a motor neurone in the ventral horn of the spinal cord may receive some 20 000–50 000 synaptic contacts, called **synaptic boutons** (see Fig. 3.3), while a cerebellar Purkinje neurone can receive up to 200 000 inputs. The synapses are formed mainly between incoming axons and receiving dendrites (axodendritic synapses), although some of the axons reach the cell body of the next neurone (axosomatic synapses). In some cases, axoaxonal synapses are also formed, between two axons, and these type of synapses can play important modulatory roles (see Presynaptic inhibition). In addition to the normal intracellular organelles that are present in all cells, such as mitochondria and endoplasmic reticulum, the synaptic boutons also contain the **neurosecretory**

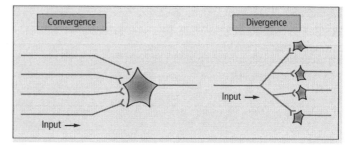

Fig. 4.13 Convergence and divergence of neural inputs.

vesicles, which store the neurotransmitters that are to be released by that neurone. For many of the neurotransmitters, the various sets of enzymes required for their synthesis and processing are present in the cytosol of the axonal terminal. (However it should be noted that peptide neurotransmitters (see below) are synthesized in the cell body and carried by axonal transport to the boutons.)

When an action potential arrives at a nerve terminal, depolarization of the membrane causes the opening of a set of **voltage-sensitive Ca^{2+} channels**. This generates an **influx of Ca^{2+}** and the subsequent increase in cytosolic Ca^{2+} ions triggers the **exocytosis** of neurosecretory vesicles, and hence the release of neurotransmitters into the synapse (the content of one vesicle, estimated experimentally to be a few thousand (5000–10000) molecules, is considered to be the unit of **transmission of information** between neurones—a **quantum** (plural: **quanta**) (Fig. 4.14). The neurotransmitter diffuses across the **synaptic cleft** (width of 50–60 nm) and binds to specific receptor molecules on a specialized part of the postsynaptic membrane—the **postsynaptic density**. Some of these receptors directly mediate a flow of ions through the membrane as, in the same protein complex, the receptor co-exists with a channel complex. Thus, binding of an agonist to the receptor induces a conformational change in another part of the protein complex, which changes the gating properties of the pore-forming part of the complex and allows the flow of ions; these types of receptors are called **ionotropic receptors**. Other receptors generate, through activation of different G proteins, an intracellular signalling response (see Chapter 2). Because these receptors involve a 'metabolic' response rather

than an ionic flux, the generic name for these is **metabotropic receptors**. The pathways activated by metabotropic receptors will trigger some specific intracellular responses, some of which modulate ionic channel activity.

The same neurotransmitter can activate various receptors with rather different functional properties. Consequently, the type of postsynaptic receptor involved will determine the speed of transmission of information; we can differentiate between **fast** and **slow synapses** on the basis of the **synaptic delay**, which defines the time elapsed between the excitation of the presynaptic nerve terminal and the permeability change in the postsynaptic membrane. In a fast synapse, the delay could be as little as 0.5 ms, increasing to more than 1 s in the slow synapses that use G proteins and other second messengers. Diffusion across the synaptic cleft is very rapid and, even for a fast synapse, most of the delay can be attributed to the time taken for presynaptic release of the transmitter (exocytosis). In the slow synapses, the delay is largely a result of the postsynaptic metabolic processes.

Within a presynaptic terminal, vesicles are docked at the active zone in preparation for release (Fig. 4.14) or are stored in a reserve pool bound to actin filaments by the protein **synapsin I**. At the active zone, Ca^{2+} influx through nearby voltage-sensitive channels activates, within microseconds, **synaptogamin**, a protein initiator of the fusion of vesicles with the presynaptic plasma membrane. The fusion process is then completed by other exocytotic proteins, such as syntaxin or SNAP-25. The rise in Ca^{2+} concentration also dissociates vesicles from the actin filaments, via a $Ca^{2+}/$

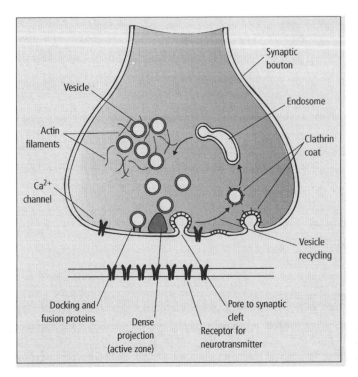

Vesicle

Actin
filaments

Ca²⁺
channel

Synaptic
bouton

Endosome

Clathrin
coat

Vesicle
recycling

Docking and
fusion proteins

Dense
projection
(active zone)

Pore to synaptic
cleft

Receptor for
neurotransmitter

Fig. 4.14 Release of neurotransmitter from a presynaptic nerve terminal and the recycling of vesicular membrane (see text for further explanation).

calmodulin-dependent protein kinase II, by inducing phosphorylation of synapsin I, thus mobilizing the reserve pool. Transmitter release is inhibited by **tetanus** and **botulinum** toxins, which enzymatically cleave specific proteins involved in docking or fusion. After release of neurotransmitter, the vesicular membrane is recycled by endocytosis, during which **clathrin**-coated pits form intracellular vesicles that fuse with endosomes and eventually produce new synaptic vesicles.

Once a neurotransmitter activates an ionic conductance on the postsynaptic membrane, a small localized change in membrane potential is produced (**postsynaptic potential**; effectively a local potential, as discussed above) that will result in either a depolarization (**EPSP**) or a hyperpolarization (**IPSP**) (Fig. 4.15a,b). Synaptic potentials of both kinds are generated at active synaptic sites across the whole neurone, depending on the incoming stream of information (i.e. action potentials). Note that not all the hundreds to thousands of synapses on a particular neurone need to be, or are, active at the same time, since in many instances they will

represent various independent neuronal pathways. As for any local potentials, the effects of the synaptic potentials can be summated, not only temporally or spatially (see above and Fig. 4.3), but also in respect to their electrotonic effect (depolarization or hyperpolarization). If the net result, after integration of all the various synaptic inputs, is a depolarization of sufficient magnitude at the axon hillock, then an 'all-or-none' action potential is triggered (Fig. 4.15c). This process of summation illustrates the complex nature of the neuronal computational capacity, which **integrates** signals from other neurones.

In addition to the **chemical synapses** described above, in which the transmission of information is mediated by chemical messengers (i.e. neurotransmitters), **electrical synapses** have also been described in the mammalian CNS. At these synapses, the adjacent cells are joined by gap junctions formed by grouping of specific proteins—**connexins** (see Chapter 2, p. 24), and the current from the presynaptic neurone passes directly to the postsynaptic neurone, where it changes the mem-

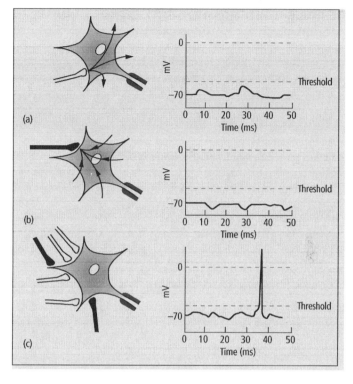

Fig. 4.15 Synaptic transmission in the CNS, as measured by an electrode placed on the axon. (a) Excitatory postsynaptic potentials (same single excitatory input (in white) being active at two time points, 7 and 25 ms, generating a flow of current into the postsynaptic neurone and generating the postsynaptic potential change—a slight depolarization). (b) Inhibitory postsynaptic potentials (an inhibitory input (in black) is activated 3 times, generating an outflow of current from the postsynaptic neurone and a resulting hyperpolarization). (c) Several excitatory and inhibitory inputs, firing at different rates. At one particular time point (35 ms), the summation of their independent activities was sufficient to bring the membrane potential of the postsynaptic neurone to the threshold for generation of an action potential.

brane potential. Such intercellular connections are common in some tissues (e.g. cardiac muscle and intestinal smooth muscle) or between certain types of cells (e.g. glia).

Ionic basis of synaptic potentials

During synaptic transmission the fast neurotransmitters activate various types of ionic channels. By altering the relative conductances to Na^+, K^+, Ca^{2+} and Cl^- ions, the membrane potential can be set to any value between the lowest (i.e. the equilibrium potential for K^+, $E_K \sim -90\,mV$) and highest (i.e. the equilibrium potential for Na^+, $E_{Na} \sim +70\,mV$) possible values. An EPSP is a depolarization of a few millivolts (Fig. 4.15a) that results from an overall increase in Na^+ conductance (g_{Na}). The channels with Na^+ permeability that are activated by neurotransmitters are significantly different from voltage-sensitive Na^+ channels that are activated during the action potential. In some cases, neurotransmitters can also activate a smaller K^+

conductance, so that the movement of positively charged Na^+ into the cell may, in part, be counteracted by the outward movement of K^+; however, the overall net influx of positive charges partially depolarizes the postsynaptic region. These potentials are called 'excitatory' because they bring the membrane closer to potential threshold and thus increase the likelihood that an action potential will be triggered.

Some inhibitory transmitters activate only K^+ conductances (g_K) so that a slight hyperpolarization, i.e. an IPSP, occurs (Fig. 4.15b), moving the membrane further away from threshold. More commonly, there is a simultaneous increase in the conductances for both K^+ and Cl^- (g_K and g_{Cl}). As E_{Cl} is usually close to the membrane potential ($E_{Cl} \sim -80\,mV$), an increase in g_{Cl} alone would not change the membrane potential, but more excitatory current would then be required to depolarize the cell as the membrane resistance is lowered; in addition, any depolarization will be opposed by Cl^- moving into the cell.

From the above, it would seem that synaptic transmission is a relatively straightforward sequence of action potential invasion of the presynaptic terminal bouton followed by transmitter release, diffusion across the synaptic cleft, interaction with a postsynaptic receptor and a resultant conductance change. But in addition to these events there are subtler interactions occurring within synapses. For instance, many neurotransmitters provide a rapid, self-limiting feedback that inhibits transmitter release. This autoinhibition is the result of neurotransmitter in the synaptic cleft acting also on presynaptic receptors (autoreceptors), to modify the rate of its release. Some neurotransmitters also exert slow modulatory influences on synaptic transmission. Such actions are more aptly called **neuromodulation** and may have their action at either pre- or postsynaptic sites.

Neurotransmitters

Many transmitter substances have been discovered in brain, spinal cord and peripheral tissues, and a list of established and putative neurotransmitters and neuromodulators is given in Table 4.3. Some of these substances are excitatory in their effects, others are inhibitory, and some have both actions. In many cases, the dual action of a single transmitter is due to their capacity to activate different subgroups of receptors, with different properties. The receptors are usually classified according to their affinity for particular pharmacological agents and/or to the type of physiological effect elicited. Amongst the neurotransmitters, nitric oxide (NO) appears to be unusual. Whereas 'conventional' neurotransmitters are synthesized, stored in vesicles and then released to act on surface receptors, NO, a gas, is synthesized when action potentials cause an elevation in the intracellular concentration of Ca^{2+} in the presynaptic terminal. A Ca^{2+}-activated specific enzyme, NO synthase (NOS), generates NO via the metabolism of an amino acid (L-arginine) (Fig. 4.16). Once produced, NO diffuses across the pre- and postsynaptic membranes, to act directly on the cytoplasmic guanylate cyclase in the postsynaptic cell (p. 35).

Of the compounds listed in Table 4.3, glutamate,

Table 4.3 Some of the substances that act, or are thought to act, as neurotransmitters or neuromodulators in the brain, spinal cord and peripheral nervous system.

Classical transmitters
Acetylcholine
Monoamines: adrenaline, noradrenaline, dopamine, histamine, 5-hydroxytryptamine (serotonin)
Amino acids: aspartate, glutamate, glycine, γ-aminobutyric acid
Other small-molecule neurotransmitters:
Purine derivatives: adenosine, adenosine triphosphate
Gases: Nitric oxide, carbon monoxide
Peptides:
adrenocorticotrophic hormone (ACTH)
angiotensin II
antidiuretic hormone (ADH)
calcitonin gene-related peptide (CGRP)
cholecystokinin (CCK)
β-endorphin
enkephalines: leu-enkephalin, met-enkephalin
gastrin
glucagon
gonadotrophin-releasing hormone (GRH)
neuropeptide Y (NPY)
neurotensin
oxytocin
somatostatin
substance P
thyrotrophin-releasing hormone (TRH)
vasoactive intestinal polypeptide (VIP)

γ-aminobutyric acid (GABA) and glycine play major roles in synaptic transmission in the CNS of vertebrates, and may be used to illustrate the complexity of synaptic transmission. Glutamate is the principal excitatory transmitter in most regions of the CNS. It acts through multiple subtypes of ionotropic and metabotropic receptors. The ionotropic glutamate receptors have been classified according to the pharmacological agents that selectively activate them, i.e. NMDA receptors (activated selectively by *N*-methyl-D-aspartic acid), AMPA receptors (activated by α-amino-3-hydroxy-5-methyl-4-isoxazolepropionic acid) or kainate receptors. Protein and sequence analysis of the

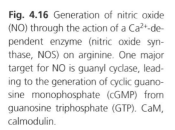

Fig. 4.16 Generation of nitric oxide (NO) through the action of a Ca^{2+}-dependent enzyme (nitric oxide synthase, NOS) on arginine. One major target for NO is guanyl cyclase, leading to the generation of cyclic guanosine monophosphate (cGMP) from guanosine triphosphate (GTP). CaM, calmodulin.

receptor/channel complexes has revealed further diversity within these subtypes, mainly stemming from the fact that each receptor is formed by various subunits that can combine in different ratios.

The AMPA and kainate (glutamate) receptors, when activated, allow the flow of Na^+ and K^+ ions through their associated channels. At membrane potentials negative to the reversal potential (around 0 mV for these channels), Na^+ influx predominates over K^+ efflux, so the net result is an inward current which depolarizes the neurone. This is the basis of fast glutamatergic EPSP.

The NMDA receptor/channel has special properties, which distinguish it from the other ionotropic glutamate receptors. Near the resting potential, the channel is blocked on the extracellular side by Mg^{2+} ions, which inhibits the flow of current even when glutamate is bound to the receptor. The block is relieved by depolarization, and this allows the conduction of Na^+, K^+ and Ca^{2+} ions (Fig. 4.17). The influx of Ca^{2+} at depolarized potentials is of particular importance because changes in the intracellular concentration of this ion can influence many processes within the postsynaptic neurone, e.g. long-term potentiation (see below).

The metabotropic glutamate receptors are linked via G proteins to ion channels and second messenger systems. At least eight subtypes have been identified and they have various actions, for example, some cause depolarization by inhibition of postsynaptic K^+ channels, while others are involved in presynaptic autoinhibition (see above).

In contrast to glutamate, GABA and glycine have largely inhibitory functions within the vertebrate CNS; GABA predominates in higher centres and glycine predominates in the brainstem and spinal cord. When released into the synaptic cleft, GABA can activate two types of receptors, $GABA_A$ and $GABA_B$, both of which inhibit the initiation of action potentials in neurones. $GABA_A$ receptors act through directly coupled channels that have a high conductance to Cl^-, while $GABA_B$ receptors act through G proteins that activate K^+ channels or inhibit Ca^{2+} channels. Glycine receptors, like $GABA_A$ receptors, are directly linked to Cl^- channels; as discussed above, an increase in Cl^- conductance stabilizes the membrane potential around E_{Cl}.

Synaptic plasticity

For many synapses, the effectiveness (or strength) of information transmission can change in response to various patterns of activity and a number of short- and long-lasting forms of synaptic plasticity have been described.

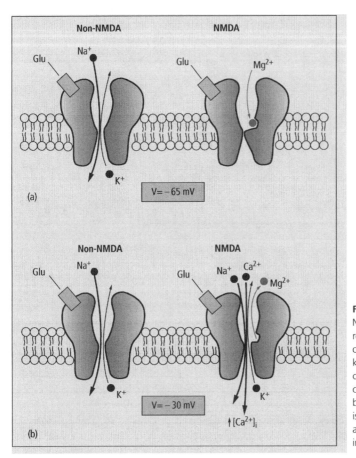

(a)

(b)

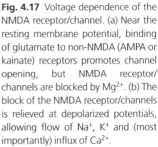

Fig. 4.17 Voltage dependence of the NMDA receptor/channel. (a) Near the resting membrane potential, binding of glutamate to non-NMDA (AMPA or kainate) receptors promotes channel opening, but NMDA receptor/channels are blocked by Mg^{2+}. (b) The block of the NMDA receptor/channels is relieved at depolarized potentials, allowing flow of Na^+, K^+ and (most importantly) influx of Ca^{2+}.

One relatively simple form of short-term plasticity is **facilitation**, an increase in synaptic efficacy observed at many excitatory synapses when a presynaptic action potential occurs shortly after a previous one (Fig. 4.18). The enhancement typically lasts less than 1 s, although it may be prolonged after a burst of high-frequency action potentials. The opposite process is called synaptic **depression**, and the mechanisms underlying both processes are believed to be purely presynaptic, resulting from changes in the amount of neurotransmitter being released as a consequence of residual elevations of $[Ca^{2+}]$ in the presynaptic terminal. In the case of facilitation, the increased presynaptic **residual Ca^{2+}** (i.e. Ca^{2+} that remains in the presynaptic cytosol following a previous stimulus) facilitates a Ca^{2+}-dependent process of exocytosis,

resulting in an increased number of neurotransmitter vesicles being released. In the case of the depression, the same residual increase in presynaptic $[Ca^{2+}]$ has a larger effect on a number of Ca^{2+}-dependent hyperpolarizing processes (e.g. activation of K^+ currents), so that the invading action potentials are less effective at releasing neurotransmitter. The difference between one effect and the other is entirely due to the balance of mechanisms that are present in each individual presynaptic bouton.

Longer-lasting forms of synaptic plasticity are interesting because, at the cellular level, they may represent a basis for learning and memory. These forms of plasticity, which include **long-term potentiation** (LTP) and **long-term depression** (LTD), are especially prominent in the hippocampal formation, neocortex, basal ganglia and (for LTD

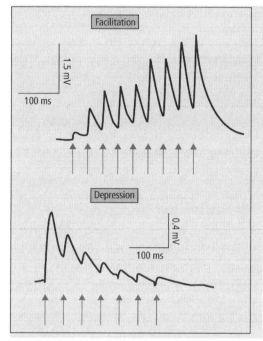

Fig. 4.18 Short-term synaptic plasticity. The activity of one particular synapse can be enhanced in certain stimulation protocols (facilitation), whereas others could be inhibited (depression). The differences are mainly due to the events and types of receptors present in the presynaptic bouton.

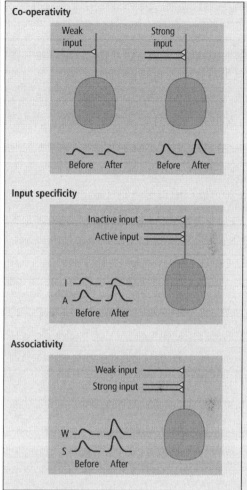

Fig. 4.19 Properties of the long-term potentiation process including cooperativity, input specificity and associativity (see text for more detailed explanations).

only) the cerebellum. LTP is experimentally activated by a brief period of high-frequency stimulation and the resulting enhancement of synaptic transmission lasts for hours or even days. LTD, at least as expressed in the hippocampus and neocortex, appears to be a reversal of the same process by repetitive low-frequency stimulation. A distinctive form of LTD occurs at specialized synapses in the cerebellum.

The form of LTP that has been studied most extensively occurs in the hippocampal formation and has a number of important and specific properties (Fig.4.19). This potentiation is initiated only if the input reaches a certain level; weak signals are not able to induce it, whereas a larger number of presynaptic fibres activated simultaneously are able to 'cooperate' in inducing the change in synaptic strength—a property called **cooperativity**. The second property of LTP is that of **input specificity**, which refers to the fact that synaptic transmission is strengthened only at the synapses that were originally active, and does not spread to other neighbouring synapses. Another property of LTP is its **associativity**, i.e. transmission is enhanced only at the synapses that are active at the same time, in association, even if their single input was of lower intensity. This process of synaptic transmission strengthening comes about because glutamatergic synapses on these neurones have postsynaptic AMPA and NMDA receptors. At lower levels of stimulation, or when only one synaptic input is activated, the release of glutamate will not be able to activate the NMDA receptor, due to its normal Mg^{2+} block. When two synapses are activated in quick succession on the same neurone, the role of the first one is to activate the more rapidly responding AMPA receptors. If this stimulation is strong enough, the postsynaptic potential depolarization will be large enough to relieve the Mg^{2+} block of the NMDA receptor/channels, so that the subsequent stimulation will be able to open the NMDA receptor and allow Ca^{2+} to enter the postsynaptic neurone. This postsynaptic Ca^{2+} influx, through a chain of events not yet entirely understood, leads to a long-term potentiation of the synapse at the site of Ca^{2+} entry.

Presynaptic inhibition

In presynaptic inhibition the excitation of a neurone (A), through the synaptic release of an excitatory transmitter by another neurone (B), is suppressed due to the action of another, inhibitory neurone (C) (Fig. 4.20). In practice, this modulatory activity by neurone C is achieved by controlling the amount of excitatory transmitter released from neurone B, and hence the level of stimulation of neurone A. Several processes may mediate these inhibitory effects. For example, control may be exerted by the release by neurone C of a transmitter, which causes some depolarization and partial inactivation of the voltage-dependent Na$^+$ mechanism in neurone B. In turn, this will reduce the effectiveness of action potentials that arrive at the axon terminal and reduce the influx of Ca^{2+} and the amount of transmitter released by neurone B, thus generating a smaller postsynaptic potential in neurone A. In this process, it is clear that only the specific input from neurone B is inhibited, while the general excitability of neurone A is not affected. Inputs arriving at neurone A through different pathways will proceed unimpeded.

Neuromuscular transmission in skeletal muscle

Synaptic transmission at skeletal neuromuscular junctions has a high safety margin, i.e. the invasion of the nerve terminal by an action potential always causes contraction of the muscle fibre. The action potential triggers an influx of Ca^{2+} followed by the release of acetylcholine from several hundred vesicles. Acetylcholine diffusing to the postsynaptic membrane activates ~100 000 nicotinic receptors that are also channels with high Na$^+$ permeability. The depolarization (endplate potential) induced by this change in conductance in turn activates voltage-sensitive channels, generating action potentials in the muscle fibres, which then transmit excitation to the remainder of the muscle fibres. Rapid degradation of the acetylcholine ensures that uncontrolled repetitive activation is avoided and that high frequencies of

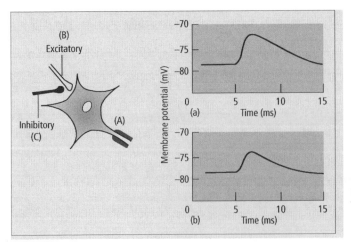

Fig. 4.20 An excitatory postsynaptic potential (a) before, and (b) during presynaptic inhibition. A, the neurone from which the membrane potential is measured; B, the excitatory input neurone; C, the inhibitory neurone.

neural activation are faithfully transmitted to the muscle.

Myelinated motor fibres branch into unmyelinated terminals which then form synapses (**neuromuscular junctions**) with skeletal muscle fibres. In adult mammalian skeletal muscles there is only one neuromuscular junction in the middle of each skeletal muscle fibre. At the junction the terminal branch of the axon lies in a shallow depression of the muscle fibre surface (Fig. 4.21). The pre- and postjunctional membranes are separated by the junctional cleft, which is about 100 nm wide and contains an extracellular matrix (**basal lamina**). The postjunctional membrane is thrown into a series of folds, which, together with the prejunctional membrane and junctional cleft, is called the **endplate**. The neurotransmitter released at the neuromuscular junction is **acetylcholine**. It is synthesized in the cytoplasm of the neurone in the reaction:

$$CH_3COCoA \quad + HOCH_2CH_2N^+(CH_3)_3$$
acetyl coenzyme A   choline

$$\rightarrow CH_3COOCH_2CH_2N^+(CH_3)_3 + HCoA$$
acetylcholine   coenzyme A

which is catalysed by the enzyme **choline acetyltransferase**. Acetylcholine is then packaged, together with adenosine triphosphate (ATP) and proteins into vesicles of about 50 nm in diameter.

The mechanism of release of acetylcholine is similar to that of other transmitters (see above). Briefly, when a nerve fibre is stimulated, an action potential invades the nerve terminal, causing the influx of Ca^{2+}. As a consequence, acetylcholine is released into the junctional cleft by exocytosis (Fig. 4.21), together with ATP, and most likely

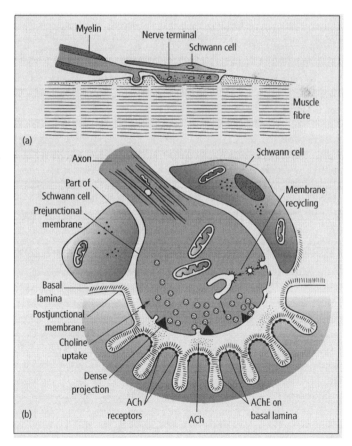

Fig. 4.21 Fine structure of a mammalian neuromuscular junction (endplate) in (a) longitudinal section, and (b) cross-section. ACh, acetylcholine.

other soluble proteins contained within the vesicles. The role of the ATP and proteins is not known. Exocytosis of acetylcholine is blocked by **botulinum toxin** produced by the bacterium *Clostridium botulinum* and by high $[Mg^{2+}]$. The vesicular membrane, which fused with the prejunctional membrane during exocytosis, is subsequently removed by endocytosis and re-utilized. Whereas in the CNS synapses only a few vesicles are released by each nerve impulse, the invasion of the motor neurone terminal by an action potential is followed by the release of several hundred **quanta**, each quantum comprising approximately 10 000 molecules of acetylcholine. A consequence of the release of such a large number of transmitter molecules, is that more than sufficient molecules are available during each nerve impulse to ensure the generation of an action potential in the skeletal muscle fibre that it innervates. For this reason neuromuscular transmission is said to have a high safety margin, with no transmission failures.

The acetylcholine diffuses across the cleft and binds to receptor sites on channels that are localized on the crests of the postjunctional folds (Fig. 4.21b). The binding of acetylcholine at two separate sites on the receptor induces a rapid conformational change that opens the channel pore that is inbuilt in the receptor and increases g_{Na} and g_K. Patch-clamp experiments, using the methodology described in Chapter 1 indicate that the channel may open (for about 1 ms) and close several times before the acetylcholine dissociates. The conductance change that results from the opening of a large number (10^4–10^5) of these channels results in a net influx of positive ions and a localized depolarization of the endplate, called the **endplate potential** (Fig. 4.22a). It has been calculated that opening of these channels by acetylcholine increases g_{Na} and g_K in the ratio of 1.3 : 1. Under normal circumstances, the endplate potential exceeds the threshold and an action potential is generated; but in the presence of receptor-blocking compounds, e.g. curare, subthreshold endplate potentials can be observed. During transmission there is a synaptic delay of 0.2–0.3 ms, much of which is attributed to the release of acetylcholine rather than to its subsequent diffusion across the cleft and the conductance changes that it provokes. There is a spontaneous release of acetylcholine from the nerve terminal; this is either **non-quantal**, presumably the result of some form of continuous leakage, or quantal, due to the exocytosis of individual vesicles. The quantal release gives rise to small transient fluctuations in membrane poten-

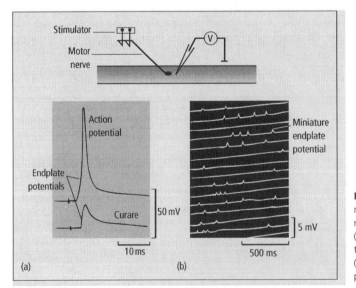

(a)   (b)

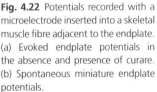

Fig. 4.22 Potentials recorded with a microelectrode inserted into a skeletal muscle fibre adjacent to the endplate. (a) Evoked endplate potentials in the absence and presence of curare. (b) Spontaneous miniature endplate potentials.

tial in the postsynaptic region called **miniature endplate potentials** (Fig. 4.22b).

The postsynaptic receptors at the skeletal neuromuscular junction are referred to as **nicotinic** because nicotine mimics the effects of acetylcholine at these junctions. Interaction of acetylcholine with its receptors is blocked reversibly by *D*-**tubocurarine** (curare), and almost irreversibly by α-**neurotoxins**. These neurotoxins (e.g. α-bungarotoxin, α-cobratoxin) are small proteins (M_r 8000) obtained from snake venoms which, when labelled with radioactive iodine, have been used to estimate the number of acetylcholine receptors (10^7) at the neuromuscular junction.

The acetylcholine released by each impulse is rapidly hydrolysed to choline and acetate by the enzyme **acetylcholinesterase** which is located in the basal lamina of the postjunctional membrane (Fig. 4.21b). Some 60% of the acetylcholine released by an action potential is hydrolysed before it crosses the synaptic cleft and the remainder is degraded within a few milliseconds. The choline produced by hydrolysis is taken up by a specific transport mechanism in the nerve terminal and re-utilized in the synthesis of acetylcholine. Any acetylcholine that diffuses away from the endplate into the blood stream is destroyed by **pseudocholinesterase** in blood and other tissues. The hydrolysis of acetylcholine is blocked by **organophosphates**, such as di-isofluorophosphate, which bind to the active site of the acetylcholinesterase and cause accumulation of transmitter in the synaptic cleft and prolonged activation of receptors.

Myasthenia gravis

This disease affects about 0.01% of the population and is characterized by a failure in neuromuscular transmission with repetitive nerve stimulation. The symptoms are weakness and fatigue—particularly of extraocular muscles—difficulty in swallowing and speech and, in advanced stages, respiratory failure. Hyperplasia of the thymus gland is frequently associated with this disease. Biopsy samples of intercostal muscles of myasthenic patients show a reduction in the amplitude of the endplate potentials and miniature endplate potentials. Consistent with these findings, a decrease in endplate acetylcholine receptors (up to 90%) has been found in binding studies with ^{125}I-labelled α neurotoxin. The symptoms of this disease therefore appear to reflect a deficiency in the number of acetylcholine receptors at the neuromuscular junction. Removal of the thymus gland often has a beneficial effect, and it has long been suspected that myasthenia gravis is an autoimmune disease. This has been confirmed by the demonstration of antibodies to acetylcholine receptors in these patients.

4.4 Transmission in the autonomic nervous system

Tissues innervated by the sympathetic, parasympathetic and enteric divisions of the autonomic nervous system receive either an excitatory, or both an excitatory and inhibitory, neural input. The neural input to these tissues first passes through ganglia, which have both a distributing and integrating function. The postganglionic fibres are largely unmyelinated and terminate in a densely branching network of varicose fibres in the effector tissue. Vesicle-bound transmitter substances such as acetylcholine, noradrenaline and other compounds are released from the varicosities into the neuroeffector junction and either excite or inhibit the effector cells by interacting with specific postjunctional receptors. Many of the autonomically innervated tissues are also affected by secretion of adrenaline and noradrenaline from the adrenal medullae.

The overall pattern of activity in the preganglionic autonomic nerves is controlled by the **hypothalamus**, and by centres in the **brainstem** and **spinal cord**. The output to some tissues is phasic; to others it is continuous (tonic) and of low frequency (e.g. 1–2 Hz to blood vessels). The activity in all these pathways is either initiated or modified by sensory input from visceral or somatic receptors (peripheral modulation), or by changes in emotional state (central modulation). When the change in activity occurs as a result of visceral input it is often referred to as an **autonomic reflex**.

Synaptic transmission in the autonomic nervous system

The activity in many postganglionic fibres is wholly dependent on preganglionic input. However, the ganglia are not simply relay stations, as significant levels of convergence, divergence and also synaptic integration occurs here.

Preganglionic transmission

In both sympathetic and parasympathetic divisions, the synaptic transmission between the preganglionic fibres and postganglionic neurones (the 'ganglionic synapse') is mediated by acetylcholine acting on nicotinic receptors. The nicotinic receptors on the postganglionic neurones are of a different molecular subtype (N_2) to the ones present at the neuromuscular junction (N_1). For both receptor types, activation induces a conformational change that opens an ionic channel (ionotropic receptors) permeable to both Na^+ and K^+; however, the N_2 subtype present on the postganglionic membranes has a higher Na^+ permeability, so that the activation of this receptor type leads to a depolarizing response in the postganglionic neurone. Another major difference between the N_1 and N_2 nicotinic receptors is their sensitivity to *D*-tubocurarine (curare); N_1 are inhibited (see Fig. 4.22) while N_2 are not—a block of muscular activity is not associated with a block of autonomic nervous transmission.

Postganglionic parasympathetic transmission

Parasympathetic postganglionic fibres are short and are usually confined to the walls of organs that are innervated. All of these fibres use **acetylcholine** as their neurotransmitter, which interacts with **muscarinic receptors** on the target cell. Depending on their particular type, activation of these receptors can induce either inhibitory or excitatory responses, partly due to the signalling pathways activated in the target cell. There are five different pharmacological subtypes of muscarinic receptors (M_1–M_5), encoded by five different genes, all of which interact with plasma membrane G proteins (Table 4.4). Three of these types (M_1, M_3 and M_5) stimulate the hydrolysis of phosphoinositides, with generation of IP_3 and a subsequent Ca^{2+} signal; subtypes M_2 and M_4 activate an inhibitory G protein that reduces the levels of cAMP (cyclic adenosine monophosphate) (for intracellular signalling pathways see Chapter 2).

The termination of the action of acetylcholine appears to be essentially the same as in skeletal muscle (see above, p. 87), although for this particular type of synapse, diffusion of neurotransmitter

Table 4.4 Classification of receptors (a) muscarinic, (b) adrenoceptors. (Adapted from Alexander, S., Peters, J.A., Mead, A. & Lewis, S. (1999) *Trends in Pharmacological Sciences*, **19**: Receptor & Ion Channel Nomenclature Supplement).

(a)

Type (tissue)	M_1 (neural)	M_2 (cardiac)	M_3 (small muscular and glandular)	M_4 (?)	M_5 (?)
Second messenger	IP_3/DAG	⇓ cAMP	IP_3/DAG	⇓ cAMP	IP_3/DAG

(b)

Type	α_1	α_2	β_1	β_2	β_3
Agonist potency	NA ≥ Adr	Adr ≥ NA	NA ≥ Adr	Adr > NA	Adr = NA
Second messenger	IP_3/DAG	⇓ cAMP	⇑ cAMP	⇑ cAMP	⇑ cAMP

Adr, adrenaline; cAMP, cyclic adenosine monophosphate; IP_3, inositol trisphosphate; NA, noradrenaline.

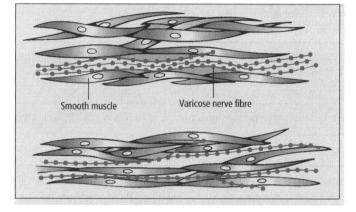

Fig. 4.23 Terminal branches of autonomic neurones. In some effector tissues they remain grouped together in bundles (top) but in others single fibres branch off from the bundle and the terminal branches make close contact with the effector cells (bottom).

Smooth muscle   Varicose nerve fibre

out of the junction may also be an important termination mechanism.

Postganglionic sympathetic transmission

Sympathetic postganglionic fibres are long and unmyelinated, with extensive branching in the terminal regions of contact with the target cells. In some tissues, the fibres remain in bundles with only an occasional terminal branch evident; whilst in others, many terminal branches are present (Fig. 4.23). Irrespective of their type of branching, the regions involved in neuronal transmission in these terminal branches appear as small swellings (approximately 1 μm in cross-section) and are called **varicosities**. Each neurone may have thousands of varicosities and each is responsible for the storage (except for NO) and release of transmitter.

The neurotransmitter released by these fibres is **noradrenaline**, which is synthesized from tyrosine in reactions catalysed by the enzymes outlined in Fig. 4.24. All of the reactions apart from the final one take place in the cytoplasm; the last step, from dopamine to noradrenaline, occurs in the storage vesicles. In addition to containing the transmitter and the enzyme dopamine β-oxidase, vesicles also contain chromogranins (proteins that have a role in the regulation of the secretory process and in mediating autocrine signalling) and ATP, which can also play a role in signalling, albeit less well defined. The rate-limiting step in noradrenaline synthesis is the conversion of tyrosine to dihydroxyphenylalanine. This process is regulated by a small quantity of noradrenaline that leaks from the vesicles and inhibits the activity of the enzyme tyrosine hydroxylase (i.e. end-product inhibition).

Once released, following the arrival of an action potential at the terminal branches, noradrenaline exerts its effects by interacting with α- or β-adrenoceptors, first classified by Ahlquist in 1948. These receptors are now relatively well characterized by a variety of pharmacological and molecular biology techniques, and are classified based on a number of criteria, including the type of intracellular signalling pathway used (Table 4.4). However, to understand the sympathetic effects on various tissues it is important to consider the heterogeneity of receptor distribution: on blood vessels, α_1 receptors predominate, while α_2 are in presynaptic terminals; β_1 receptors are predominant in the heart, whereas β_2 are predominant in the bronchial muscle in the lungs. Furthermore, some tissues have mixed populations of receptors and the response depends on the agent, the receptors, and their location. In a gross generalization, it could be said that activation of α_1 and β_1 receptors leads to excitatory responses (e.g. vasoconstriction or bronchial constriction (α_1) or increase heart rate and force of contraction (β_1)), whereas activation of β_2 receptors leads to an inhibitory response (e.g. vasodilation of smooth muscle in blood vessels, bronchi or intestinal wall).

Once released from the neurone, the action of

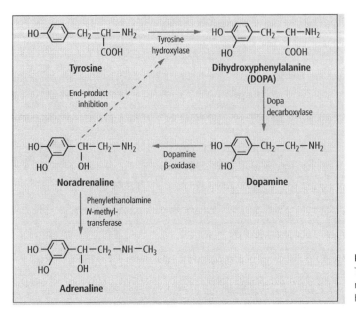

Fig. 4.24 Synthesis of noradrenaline. The broken line indicates the inhibitory effect of noradrenaline on tyrosine hydroxylase.

noradrenaline is not terminated by degradation, but is **inactivated** either by **uptake** or by **diffusion** away from the junction region. The uptake processes transport the intact amine across plasma membranes, either into the neurone (in which case it is called reuptake, or **neuronal uptake**) or into the effector cell (**extraneuronal uptake**; Fig. 4.25b). Estimates of the relative contributions of these two processes vary greatly but it would appear that in densely innervated tissues some 70% of the amine released is removed by neuronal uptake, 25% by extraneuronal uptake and 5% by diffusion. Extraneuronal uptake and diffusion may be more important in tissues that are innervated diffusely. A major portion of the amine accumulated by the neurone is transported into vesicles for reuse as a transmitter, with obvious benefit to the neurone. The portion of the transmitter taken up by the nerve and not recycled is degraded by **monoamine oxidase**, whilst the amines taken up by the extraneuronal tissue are degraded largely by **catechol-*O*-methyltransferase** (COMT). As the effects of catecholamines are not potentiated immediately by inhibition of either of these enzymes, it is believed that they are not involved in the termination of transmitter action. Rather, enhanced re-

sponses may be seen in the presence of inhibitors of neuronal uptake (e.g. cocaine and desipramine), or of inhibitors of extraneuronal uptake (e.g. corticosteroids).

Other types of synaptic transmission

In addition to the 'classical' transmitter substances, acetylcholine and noradrenaline, some neurones in the autonomic nervous system, particularly in the enteric nervous system, use either neuropeptides (e.g. neuropeptide Y, somatostatin, vasoactive intestinal polypeptide or enkephalin), ATP or NO as neurotransmitters (see also Table 4.3). Since pharmacological agents that block the action of acetylcholine and noradrenaline fail to inhibit the actions of these nerves, they are collectively known as **non-adrenergic non-cholinergic** (NANC) neurones. At present, there is evidence that these NANC substances may function, at different sites outside the CNS, as either primary transmitters or co-transmitters, or as neuromodulators.

For all the neurotransmitters active in the autonomic nervous system, their excitatory and inhibitory effects are the result of the receptor-mediated activation of G proteins and of

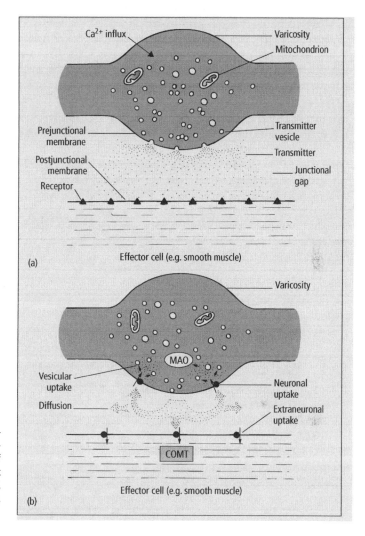

Fig. 4.25 (a) Chemical transmission at the sympathetic neuroeffector junction. (b) Inactivation of noradrenaline at the sympathetic neuroeffector junction. COMT, catechol-O-methyltransferase; MAO, monoamine oxidase.

changes in the levels of intracellular messengers. Excitatory effects are associated with an increase in intracellular Ca^{2+} that may arise through: depolarization of the plasma membrane of the target cells, due to an increase in conductance to Na^+ and Ca^{2+}, and action potentials (both of which promote the opening of voltage-sensitive Ca^{2+} channels in the cell membrane); and the release of Ca^{2+} from intracellular stores. For example, in the heart, noradrenaline acts via β_1 receptors to elevate cyclic adenosine monophosphate (cAMP); this, in turn, promotes the opening of voltage-sensitive Ca^{2+} channels in the cell membrane and Ca^{2+} release

channels in the sarcoplasmic reticulum, thus increasing the force of contraction. Other tissues are activated by the intracellular formation of IP_3 and diacylglycerol (DAG), which release Ca^{2+} from intracellular stores and stimulate protein kinase C, respectively. Inhibitory actions of transmitters can be accounted for in a similar manner, in that activation of G proteins may be accompanied by changes in the level of intracellular messengers, which increase conductance, mainly to K^+ or Cl^-, and hyperpolarize or stabilize the membrane; they may also be able to induce a sequestration of Ca^{2+}. In some tissues, inhibition is associated with an increase in the intracellular concentration of cyclic guanosine monophosphate (cGMP) that results from the actions of NO (see Fig. 4.16). ATP is a common constituent of vesicles and is another agent that acts as a co-transmitter. For instance, in vesicles derived from sympathetic neurones, there is a 4 : 1 molar ratio of noradrenaline to ATP. In the vas deferens of some animals the membrane potential of the smooth muscle responds to nerve stimulation with a biphasic, fast and then slow wave of depolarization. In this tissue it appears that the transmitter responsible for the fast component is ATP, which acts on directly coupled purinergic receptors, while the slow component is due to noradrenaline, which acts through α-adrenoceptors and G proteins.

Opposing actions of the parasympathetic and sympathetic systems

Many tissues have a dual autonomic innervation, and stimulation of one component usually results in effects opposite to those produced by stimulation of the other (Table 4.5). Further, it is clear that the effect of stimulating any one component may vary from tissue to tissue, being excitatory in some and inhibitory in others. Nevertheless, a closer study of Table 4.5 reveals that the **parasympathetic** effects are largely directed towards **maintenance** and **conservation** of bodily function. Thus, responses to parasympathetic stimulation include slowing of the heart, constriction of the pupils, contraction of the bladder (detrusor muscle) and increased secretion and motility in the digestive tract. In contrast, the effects of **sympathetic** stimulation, if examined together, are directed towards coping with stress and comprise the '**fight or flight**' response, described by W. Cannon in 1939. These changes include increased heart rate and contractility (inotropism), bronchodilation, pupillary dilation, inhibition of intestinal motility, constriction of the splanchnic vascular bed, decreased muscle fatigue, and elevated blood glucose and free fatty acids. However, this is not to say that the sympathetic system always acts *en masse* or that it is active only in stress. Indeed, most of the activity in the sympathetic nervous system is associated with normal homeostatic activity and its actions are localized (e.g. pupillary dilation and regional changes in blood flow).

The activity of tissues with dual innervation depends on the balance between parasympathetic and sympathetic discharge. Often one of the systems is dominant; for example, pupil diameter and resting heart rate are largely determined by the level of activity (tone) in their parasympathetic nerve supplies. Changes in effector activity are usually the result of reciprocal changes in both parasympathetic and sympathetic activity. Mutual antagonism in the periphery can occur either as a result of opposing actions of dual innervation of effector cells (e.g. as occurs in heart, bronchial smooth muscle and detrusor smooth muscle), or from suppression of synaptic transmission in ganglia.

Circulating catecholamines

The activity of some autonomically innervated tissues is influenced by both noradrenaline, released from nerves, and by catecholamines, released into the blood stream from the adrenal medullae. In humans, adrenaline comprises some 80% of the catecholamines released from the gland, the remainder being noradrenaline. The adrenaline and noradrenaline are synthesized and stored in different cells. An additional step in the synthetic chain (see Fig. 4.22) produces adrenaline by N-methylation of noradrenaline. The activity of the enzyme responsible for this step, **phenylethanolamine-N-methyltransferase**, is increased by steroids from the adrenal cortex.

The free plasma concentrations of these amines are low at rest, being 1–2 nmol L^{-1} (or 130–310 pg mL^{-1}) for noradrenaline, and 0.2–0.8 nmol L^{-1} (or 20–97 pg mL^{-1}) for adrenaline. All of the adrenaline comes from the adrenal medullae, but the noradrenaline originates both in the adrenal medullae and sympathetic nerves. Low levels are maintained at rest because the rate of release from the adrenal medullae is normally low and the half-life of the circulatory catecholamines is relatively short (less than 1 min in experimental animals). During

Table 4.5 Effects of parasympathetic (cholinergic) and sympathetic (adrenergic) stimulation.

Effector	Parasympathetic stimulation	Sympathetic stimulation
Heart		
Rate	Decreases	Increases (β_1)
Atrioventricular conduction	Decreases	Increases
Contractility	Decreases (atria only)	Increases (β_1)
Blood vessels		
Arterioles		
skin and mucosa		Constricts (α_1)
abdominal, mesenteric		Constricts (α_1)
skeletal		Constricts (α_1)
		Dilates (circulating Adrenaline; β_2 & cholinergic)
coronary	Dilates	Dilates (β_2)
		Constricts (α_1)
pulmonary	Dilates	Constricts (α_1)
brain	Dilates	Constricts (α_1)
penis, clitoris	Dilates (NO)	
Veins		Constricts (α_1)
Tracheal–bronchial smooth muscle	Contracts	Relaxes (β_2)
Gastrointestinal smooth muscle		
Longitudinal and circular	Increases motility	Decreases motility (α_1, β)
Sphincters	Relaxes (enteric NANC)	Contracts (α)
Urinary bladder		
Detrusor	Contracts	Relaxes (β_2)
Trigone (internal sphincter)		Contracts (α_1)
Genital organs		
General	Erection	Ejaculation
Seminal vesicle		Contracts (α)
Vas deferens		Contracts (α_1)
Uterus		Relaxes (depends on hormonal status) (β_2)
Eye		
Pupil	Contraction (sphincter)	Dilates (α)
Ciliary	Contracts	Slightly relaxes (β_2)
Pilo-erector		Contracts (α)
Skeletal		Increases glycogenolysis (β_2)
		Increases contractile force (β_2)
Salivary glands	Increases voluminous serous secretion	Decreases mucous secretion (submaxillary) (α)
Exocrine pancreas	Increases secretion	Decreases secretion (α)
Bronchial epithelium	Increases secretion	Increases secretion (α)
		Decreases secretion (β)
Sweat gland		Increases secretion (cholinergic)
Liver		Increases glycogenolysis (α_1, β_2)
		Increases gluconeogenesis (α_1, β_2)
Adipose cells		Increases lipolysis (β_3)
Insulin-secreting cells		Decreases secretion (α_2)

periods of stress—physical or emotional—the rate of release of adrenaline can increase about 10-fold.

Adrenaline has many actions similar to noradrenaline but, because it is a more potent β_2-agonist, it has more pronounced metabolic actions (see Chapter 11). These include elevation of blood glucose and an increase in metabolic rate. Adrenaline also produces vasodilation in those vascular beds in which the β to α receptor ratio is high, e.g. in skeletal and heart muscle.

Chapter 5

Muscle

Our bodies contain three kinds of muscle—skeletal, smooth and cardiac—classified according to their structure and function. Muscle cells are excitable and contain the proteins necessary for contraction. Muscles convert chemical energy into mechanical energy—movement. **Skeletal muscles** are characterized by the presence of thin, light and dark bands (striations) that are seen to lie across fibres when viewed through a microscope. These muscles form some 40% of the fat-free body weight. They are under voluntary control and are the only tissue through which we can directly influence our environment. In contrast to skeletal muscles, **smooth muscles** (which are also called involuntary or visceral muscles) lack transverse striations and are not under conscious control; they are found in viscera and blood vessels. **Cardiac muscle**, like skeletal muscle, is striated and like smooth muscle is not under conscious control; it generates the pressures required to drive blood around the vascular system and is described in Chapter 15.

5.1 Skeletal muscle

Skeletal muscle cells, known as fibres, are large and multinucleate, and are characterized by transverse striations and the ability to contract rapidly. The two functions of contraction of skeletal muscle are to maintain or move one component of the skeleton relative to its neighbour, and to produce heat. The force necessary to do this is generated by a regular array of actin and myosin filaments, the contractile proteins, and is fuelled by adenosine triphosphate (ATP) hydrolysis. The contraction of each muscle fibre is preceded by the generation, near the motor end-plate, of an action potential which travels along the muscle membrane and down the transverse (T) tubules. The action potential synchronizes and initiates each contraction by promoting the release of Ca^{2+} from the sarcoplasmic reticulum (SR). The elevation of intracellular Ca^{2+} stimulates the binding of myosin cross-bridges to actin; the subsequent flexing of the cross-bridges generates force. The force generated by a muscle is dependent on both the frequency of the action potentials in the muscle fibres and the number of muscle fibres activated by motor neurones. Each motor neurone innervates a number of muscle fibres that together form the basic functional contractile unit called the motor unit. The tension developed by muscles is used to move limbs or to resist their movement, to close sphincters that control the emptying of hollow organs, to move the tongue and regulate the vocal cords, and to perform other specialized functions. The heat produced by muscles is used to maintain body temperature, either by non-shivering mechanisms regulated by hormones or by shivering which is under direct neural control. The needs of the body for a range of contractions, from slow and sustained to fast and brief, are satisfied by the presence of muscles having different fibre types.

Basic biomechanics and contractions

Skeletal muscles are attached to bones via tendons. At the joints between bones, muscle contraction causes movement of the skeleton. If this movement takes the bones away from each other then the muscle is an extensor, e.g. triceps, and if the bones are brought closer together by the muscle contracting, it is a flexor, e.g. biceps. Many muscles exist as flexor–extensor antagonistic pairs. Muscles vary enormously in their capacity to generate force (tension) and in the rate at which this force can be developed. The maximal force that muscles develop is proportional to their cross-sectional area (up to $40 \, \text{N cm}^{-2}$); thus, the 'strength' of a muscle is dependent on the number of muscle fibres and on their diameters, as well as the orientation of the fibre bundles. Under the influence of testosterone the cross-sectional area of muscles increases, leading to greater muscular strength in the average man compared to the average woman. As the contractions of muscles depend on the shortening of a large number of subcellular units (sarcomeres) arranged in series, the speed with which a muscle changes length depends on the number of units in the series, on the rate of their change in length, and on the magnitude of any external applied force opposing the shortening of the muscle. Muscles contain varying amounts of fibrous and connective tissue that also contribute to their mechanical properties (see also tetanic contraction).

Muscles are said to be contracting when the contractile machinery is active and energy is being consumed. The term contraction applies whether the muscle is shortening, remaining at constant length or lengthening. In the latter case, the contractile process may be activated but the muscle as a whole may be forced to lengthen by the imposition of external force. Such **eccentric** contractions are a feature of normal muscle function, and are essential to our ability to move ourselves about while opposing the force of gravity. All types of contraction are employed in everyday use, but it is convenient to study muscle contraction when either the length of the muscle or its load is constant. When the length remains constant (**isometric** contraction), we measure the force (tension) generated by the contractile machinery. When the load remains constant (**isotonic** contraction), we measure the rate of shortening of the muscle. These forms of contraction are used in everyday activities, e.g. isometric contractions are involved in the maintenance of posture and isotonic contractions in the lifting of limbs.

Cellular structure of skeletal muscle

Skeletal muscles cells are known as muscle fibres and are some of the longest cells in the body. They are formed from the fusing of several cells during embryogenesis, and hence are multinucleate, and range in length from a few mm to up to 5 cm, with a diameter of 50–70 μm. To help maintain synchronous activity individual fibres retain only a single neural contact near their midpoint.

Muscle fibre force is generated by intracellular contractile proteins arranged into **myofilaments** (Fig. 5.1). The myofilaments are in bundles, called **myofibrils**, which run the whole length of the fibre. Each myofibril is surrounded by the **sarcoplasmic reticulum (SR)** (Fig. 5.2), and between the lateral cisternae of the SR are fine **T tubules** opening out on the surface membrane (the **sarcolemma**). The complex of a T tubule and the two adjacent SR cisternae is known as a **triad** (Fig. 5.2), and in human muscles these are located at the junction of the A and I bands, see below and Fig 5.1.

Sarcomeres and contractile proteins

Myofilaments are arranged into **sarcomeres**, which are considered to be the basic contractile units of muscle fibres. Each sarcomere is approximately 2 μm in length and its limits are defined by a Z disc (line) at each end. From the Z line, **thin actin** myofilaments (approximately 5 nm wide and 1000 nm long) project towards the middle of each sarcomere (Fig. 5.3 and 5.4), and in the central region of each sarcomere the filaments inter-

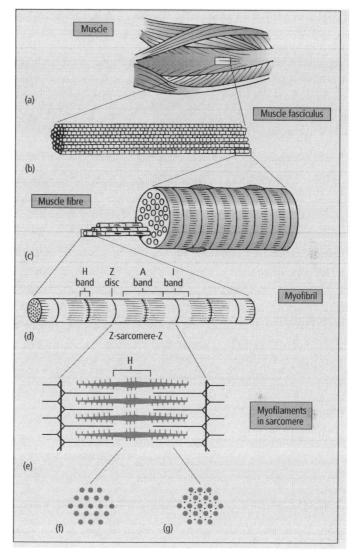

Fig. 5.1 Organization of muscle structure from whole muscle to myofilament (a–e) and transverse sections (f, g) showing the pattern of myofilaments. (Adapted from Bloom, W. & Fawcett, D.W. (1975) *A Textbook of Histology*, 10th edn, p. 306. Saunders, Philadelphia.)

digitate with **thick myosin** filaments (approximately 12 nm wide and 1600 nm long); each thick filament is surrounded by a hexagonal array of thin filaments (Fig. 5.1f,g).

Each thin filament is composed of two chains of globular actin molecules in a helical arrangement with two other proteins, tropomyosin and troponin lying in the grooves between the actin chains (Fig. 5.3a). Each thick filament is composed of myosin molecules (Fig. 5.3b) aligned with their tails parallel and pointing towards the middle of

the filament (Fig. 5.3c). Their heads are helically arranged along the filament and form **crossbridges** with the actin filaments.

The striated appearance of skeletal (and cardiac) muscle fibres is a result of the serial and parallel repetition of the myofilaments and the differing abilities of the actin- and myosin-containing regions to transmit light. As polarized light is not transmitted through the myosin-containing region (i.e. it is anisotropic), this region is called the A band (Fig. 5.1c). Light is transmitted through the

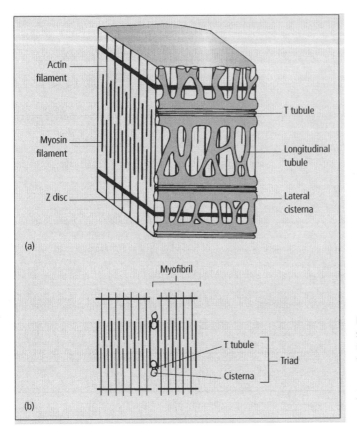

Actin filament

Myosin filament

Z disc

T tubule

Longitudinal tubule

Lateral cisterna

(a)

Myofibril

T tubule

Cisterna

Triad

(b)

Fig. 5.2 (a) Diagram illustrating the sarcoplasmic reticulum and T tubules in mammalian skeletal muscle. (b) A transverse section through sarcoplasmic reticulum and T tubules illustrating the relationship between a T tubule and two adjacent lateral cisternae (a triad).

actin-containing region (i.e. it is isotropic) and so it is referred to as the I band. In the middle of the A band where the myosin and actin filaments do not overlap, there is a lighter H band which marks the region devoid of cross-bridges, and in the middle of this is a finer dark M line. The Z disc lies in the middle of each I band.

Cytoskeletal proteins, extracellular matrix and muscular dystrophies

The repeated cell shortenings associated with muscle contraction requires that both the regular array of the myofilaments be maintained, and that the cell membrane and associated structures withstand the deformations that occur. These important requirements are met by a large group of proteins—some of which have only been identified in the last decade—contributing to the alignment and stabi-

lizing of myofibrils, maintaining anchorage to the surface membrane and extracellular matrix (basement membrane), and transmitting force laterally across the sarcolemma. The term **costamere** is used to encompass the subsarcolemmal structures that perform this function, arranged circumferentially in register with the Z discs.

The regular structure of skeletal muscles is maintained at rest and during changes in length by a network of stable filaments formed from such proteins as **titin** and **nebulin**. To date, titin is the largest protein in our bodies and a single molecule of it can stretch from the Z disc to the M line. In addition to stabilizing the sarcomeric structure by linking myosin filaments to the Z lines, titin is also responsible for the passive visco-elasticity of the myofibre. Nebulin, another huge protein, is a more rigid molecule linking Z discs to actin filaments. Several other proteins have been identified includ-

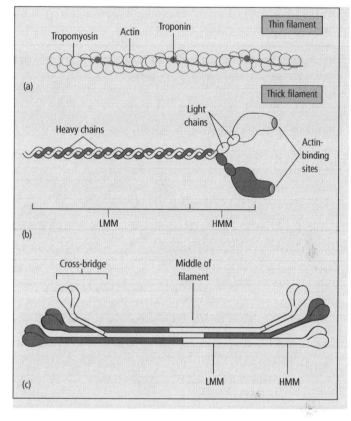

Fig. 5.3 (a) Actin filament composed of two chains of actin monomers arranged in a helix. In the grooves between these chains lie strands of tropomyosin and at regular intervals of about 40 nm are troponin molecules. (b) Myosin molecule composed of two filamentous heavy chains with globular heads bound to two pairs of light chains. The molecule can be cleaved by enzymes to produce a light meromyosin (LMM) fragment and a heavy meromyosin (HMM) fragment; the point of enzymatic cleavage is thought to be a region with some degree of flexibility. (c) The arrangement of myosin molecules in a filament. The LMM segment projects towards and forms the middle of the filament and forms the core, while the HMM segment extends to form cross-bridges.

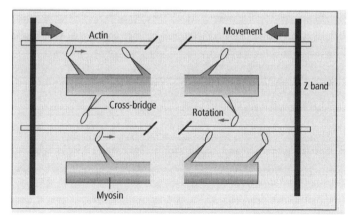

Fig. 5.4 Relative movement of actin and myosin filaments. This is accomplished by the rotation of the cross-bridge head, which contains the myosin ATPase. A second flexible point appears to exist where the cross-bridge joins the backbone of the filament.

ing **desmin**, a strong inelastic molecule that connects adjoining Z bands in a myofibril with adjacent myofibrils, and **skelemin** and **talin**, also with suspected roles in stabilization and linkage to the cell membrane.

A number of inherited diseases of muscle have been shown to be due to mutations in the molecules associated with costameres, including notably, some forms of dystrophy. The X-linked muscle wasting Duchene dystrophy for example, is caused by mutations in the gene encoding dystrophin. This protein forms a complex, which acts to connect the cytoskeleton to the basement membrane. The sarcolemma of dystrophic fibres is easily damaged during contraction, leading to excessive Ca^{2+} entry and a cycle of fibre degeneration and regeneration, until the regenerative potential is exhausted.

Resting membrane potential and action potentials

The resting membrane potential of skeletal muscle fibres is –75 to –85 mV. The basis of this membrane potential is similar to that found in other excitable cells; that is, a high intracellular concentration of K^+ and a selective permeability that favours potassium (see Chapter 1). The membrane potential of healthy skeletal muscles is stable and thus contractions have to be initiated by stimuli triggering action potentials. These triggers are the transmission of action potentials from the motor nerves to the muscle. The local depolarization (end-plate potential) generated by the interaction of neurally-released acetylcholine with the acetylcholine (nicotinic) receptors (see Chapter 1), is more than sufficient to initiate an action potential at the sarcolemma surrounding the end-plate. The ionic basis of the action potential in muscle is similar to that in nerves, i.e. the depolarizing phase is caused by a rapid increase in conductance to Na^+. However, in mammalian muscle the major contributor to repolarization is Cl^- influx, rather than K^+ efflux. Having many Cl^- channels and few K^+ channels in the muscle fibre membrane is an advantage during repetitive activity (e.g. during exercise); it minimizes K^+ accumulation in the T tubules, which could cause prolonged depolarization of the muscle fibre, and minimizes rises in K^+ concentration in the plasma, which could disrupt the rhythmic activity of the heart. The total duration of a muscle action potential may be several milliseconds longer than that of an axonal action potential. Once initiated in the middle of each muscle fibre, the action potentials are conducted at about 4–5 m s^{-1} towards both ends of the fibre by local current flow, as in unmyelinated axons (Chapter 4). Thus in a 3 cm long muscle fibre an action potential with a velocity of 5 m s^{-1} will activate a 15 mm length of fibre (from endplate-to-end) in 3 ms, so that activation is essentially instantaneous with respect to the timing of the changes in $[Ca^{2+}]$ elicited by this activation, as discussed below.

Contractile process: the sliding filament theory

If a muscle changes its length, the sarcomeres also change in length. However, the length of the thin and thick filaments remains the same, with the change in muscle length resulting from the filaments sliding over each other. This is the basis of the **sliding filament theory** developed by Hansen and Huxley in the 1950s; the muscle shortens but the myofilaments remain the same length. The forces generated during contractile activity arise in the regions where actin filaments overlap the cross-bridges, i.e. myosin heads. During contractions the myosin cross-bridges attach to adjacent actin filaments and flex towards the centre of the sarcomere (Fig 5.4 and 5.5), thereby generating a tension. The muscle shortens when the active tension generated between actin and myosin exceeds any passive tension applied to the muscle externally. As activation occurs at both ends of the myosin filament, the opposing actin filaments are drawn in towards the centre, the Z bands are pulled closer and the muscle fibre shortens.

Muscle contraction has at least three requirements:

1 that the actin and myosin must interact;

2 that the myosin cross-bridges must flex; and

3 that the system must be able to convert chemical energy into mechanical energy.

Of these, number two still engages muscle physiologists in vigorous debate; for example how far can a myosin head flex? Early X-ray diffraction studies of muscles at rest and in *rigor mortis* (see below) showed that the cross-bridges could have two stable positions—the resting position and the flexed position. More recent pulsed irradiation–diffraction (synchrotron) studies of muscles have demonstrated movements of the cross-bridges during contractions; but as with X-ray diffraction, critics would point to the large degree of interpretation needed when applying these techniques to living

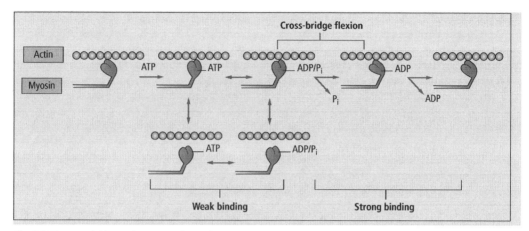

Fig. 5.5 The cross-bridge cycle. See text for explanation.

biological systems. Unravelling the mechanism involved in the transformation of chemical energy to mechanical energy has also proved elusive.

There is overwhelming evidence that ATP is the fuel used to operate the contractile machinery, and the myosin cross-bridges contain an ATPase. The rate of contraction of the sarcomeres appears to depend on the speed with which this enzyme can hydrolyse ATP. The interaction between actin and myosin is a multi-step process in which they may bind either strongly or weakly (Fig. 5.5). When neither ATP nor the products of its hydrolysis, adenosine diphosphate (ADP) and inorganic phosphate (P_i), are bound to the myosin head, the two proteins remain strongly bound. Consequently, muscles in which ATP is severely depleted (e.g. following death) are stiff and inextensible, a state referred to as **rigor**. When ATP or ADP/P_i are bound, the myosin rapidly attaches to, and subsequently detaches from, actin, in a weak binding relationship. This ATP-induced dissociation of actin and myosin allows the 'recocking' of the myosin head from its strongly bound flexed position in readiness for the next working stroke. When P_i is released from the myosin head, myosin undergoes a conformational change that results in both its strong binding to actin and the flexing of the myosin head (the working stroke), which generates the force to drive contraction. The subsequent release of ADP from myosin ensures strong binding

of actin and myosin until the next cycle of ATP binding and hydrolysis.

As a single cycle of cross-bridge attachment and detachment produces only a movement equivalent to 1% of the length of a sarcomere, it requires repetitive cycling to achieve shortening of the sarcomere and hence, muscle. Thus in each cycle the cross-bridge attaches to the actin, flexes, and then dissociates before returning to its initial configuration and a new binding site on the actin filament. These repetitive cycles throughout the sarcomere must also be asynchronous from surrounding myosin filaments, to ensure that the force exerted on an actin filament is maintained during a contraction. This activity results in the actin filament being pulled between the myosin filaments. When the muscle is unable to shorten, the elastic properties of the muscle fibres allow the cross-bridge mechanism to operate and force to be generated. Consider for example, pushing on a wall; force is generated in the arms of your muscle but they do not shorten (and the wall does not move). Actively resisting extension (**eccentric contraction**) is an important part of muscle function, both dynamic and static.

Length–tension relationship

A testable hypothesis arising from the sliding filament theory is that force should be directly proportional to the amount of interaction between the thick and thin filaments, as the more they overlap the more cross-bridges will be formed. As shown in Fig. 5.6 this hypothesis has proved to be correct, most impressively, in experiments performed on single muscle fibres.

In a single living muscle fibre the force generated can be shown to be related to the degree of overlap of the actin and myosin filaments (Fig. 5.6). It can also be seen that at long lengths, when there is no overlap of the actin and myosin filaments, the fibre is incapable of generating a force. In the intermediate range, when overlap of filaments is optimal, the force generated is maximal; at shorter lengths, the actin filaments overlap and interfere with each other and the force decreases. Eventually, at very short lengths (60–70% of the normal resting length), the Z discs will be pulled against the myosin filaments and the external force will again fall to zero. At this point the contractile machinery may still be active but the energy is used to distort the myosin filaments.

These findings relating to the length–tension relationship at the cellular and molecular level also apply to an entire muscle in our body. Thus, maximal muscle tension is generated when the muscle is approximately at normal resting length in the body. The relationship between the length of a muscle and the contractile (active) force that it develops can be examined by measuring the forces generated by a muscle at different lengths. Two forces can be measured: the **passive** force and the **total** force. When a relaxed (unstimulated) muscle held between a movable clamp and a force transducer (Fig. 5.7) is progressively stretched, an increasing force (tension), derived from an increasing resistance to stretch, can be measured (Fig. 5.7b). As the contractile machinery is not active, this force is passive and is due to the resistance exerted by elastic elements in the muscle—both extracellular components and also the elongation of myofilaments.

The force generated by stretch is not directly proportional to increase in length, as the elastic modulus increases with lengthening of the muscle. Some muscles, for example the back muscles of humans and the hind-leg muscles of kangaroos, which contain large amounts of elastic extracellular matrix material, can strongly resist extension by using purely passive mechanisms.

In Fig. 5.7b we can see that the **active** force developed when the muscle is stimulated at various lengths shows a similar relationship with length to that of the single muscle fibre. Thus the maximal active force is seen to occur near the natural resting length, and to decrease with changes in length from this position, just as it did at the level of a single sarcomere. The curve of **total** tension (Fig. 5.7b) is the sum of both the **passive** force (as described above) and the **active** force. (The amplitude of the

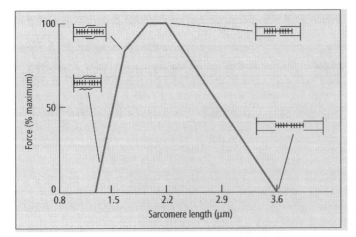

Fig. 5.6 The relationship between the contractile force and sarcomere length in a single muscle fibre. The insets illustrate the degree of overlap of the myofilaments at the sarcomere lengths indicated. (After Gordon, A.M., Huxley, A.F. & Julian, F.J. (1966) *J Physiol*, **184**, 170–92.)

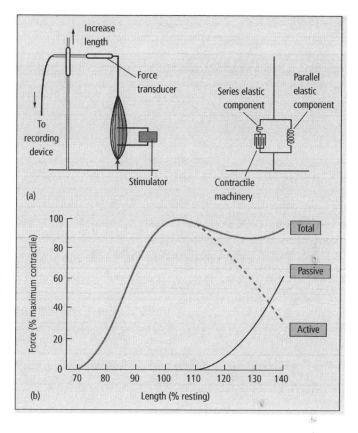

Fig. 5.7 (a) The experimental set-up used to study isometric contraction at different lengths (left) and a model of the contractile and elastic elements in muscle (right). (b) The relationship between force and muscle length. Note that the total force generated at each length is the sum of the active force generated by the contractile elements and the passive force due to extension of the elastic elements.

active force at any length is obtained by arithmetically subtracting the passive force from the experimentally measured total force.)

Excitation–contraction coupling

The term excitation–contraction coupling is used to discuss how events following the action potential at the sarcolemmal membrane lead to contraction. This coupling is accomplished via cytoplasmic Ca^{2+} and two regulatory proteins associated with the thin filament, tropomyosin and troponin. At rest this regulation is such that myosin ATPase activity is very low and thus the sliding of filaments cannot occur.

Myosin ATPase activity, and the contraction of muscle, depends on the interaction between the actin and myosin filaments, which is regulated by cytoplasmic Ca^{2+} (Mg^{2+} is also necessary for myosin ATPase activity but is in adequate supply).

At rest the free cytoplasmic Ca^{2+} concentration is so low ($10^{-8}\,mol\,L^{-1}$) that little interaction occurs. However, during activity the concentration rises sharply ($\sim 10^{-5}\,mol\,L^{-1}$); thus the free cytoplasmic Ca^{2+} regulates the development of tension within a muscle fibre and its control is vital.

Tropomyosin and troponin regulate contraction at the molecular level

In resting muscle, the free cytoplasmic Ca^{2+} concentration is low because the SR contains a membrane-bound pump (a Ca^{2+}–ATPase) that actively binds Ca^{2+} and then transports it to the lateral cisternae. However, this Ca^{2+} can be released by depolarization of T tubule membranes that come into close apposition with the lateral cisternae (Fig. 5.8). The T tubule membrane contains receptors that are sensitive to voltage (dihydropyridine receptors; DHP) and are mechanically linked to the Ca^{2+}-release sites on the SR. An action potential

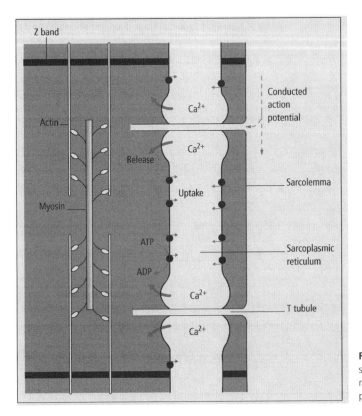

Z band

Actin

Ca²⁺

Conducted
action
potential

Ca²⁺

Release

Myosin

Uptake

Sarcolemma

ATP

ADP

Sarcoplasmic
reticulum

Ca²⁺

T tubule

Ca²⁺

Fig. 5.8 The release of Ca²⁺ from the sarcoplasmic reticulum and its reaccumulation by an active transport process.

propagating along the muscle and down the T tubules is sensed by the DHP receptors; this causes a conformational change at the SR, which opens the Ca²⁺ channels resulting in an elevation in the free intracellular Ca²⁺ concentration. The abundance of the SR and fast speed of action potential propagation ensures that the contractile activity in adjacent myofibrils is synchronized. The released Ca²⁺ binds to troponin.

At rest the interaction between actin and myosin (and the myosin ATPase activity) is inhibited by the **troponin–tropomyosin** complex (Fig. 5.3a). The troponin (Tn) component is a complex molecule spaced regularly along the actin filament, which has specific tropomyosin-binding (TnT), calcium-binding (TnC) and inhibitory (TnI) subunits. The inhibitory effect of the complex on actin–myosin binding is removed when Ca²⁺ binds to the TnC subunit. The change is associated with movement of the tropomyosin strands that lie in the grooves between the strands of actin mole-

cules. With this movement of the tropomyosin subtle changes in the conformation of actin occur, which unmask binding sites for the myosin cross-bridges and hence greatly enhances its interaction with myosin.

For **relaxation** to occur the central SR takes up the Ca²⁺ released from the lateral SR, using the Ca²⁺–ATPase pump. As the cytoplasmic [Ca²⁺] falls, Ca²⁺ is removed from TnC and this results in tropomyosin returning to its actin-blocking position. The myosin ATPase is then no longer activated, the filaments do not slide and therefore no further cross-bridges are formed. (Recall the role of ATP in this cycle—it is required for cross-bridge dissociation.)

In summary, for muscle to contract its motor neurone must produce an action potential and release ACh at the motor end-plate, which will depolarize the sarcolemmal membrane. This is sensed by DHP receptors and produces a conformational change in the lateral SR Ca²⁺-release channel, and thus Ca^{2+} rises and binds to TnC. This causes tropomyosin to move and reveal the myosin-binding sites on actin, and hence cross-bridges form. There will be many cycles of cross-bridges attaching and detaching, resulting in the filaments sliding and muscle contractions as ATP is hydrolysed by myosin ATPase.

The biochemistry of contraction

As mentioned above, ATP is the immediate source of energy for muscle contraction and is also required for Ca^{2+}-pumping back into the SR. However, very little ATP (~5 mM) is stored in a muscle—sufficient for only a few contractions. Thus ATP must constantly be supplied and renewed within the muscle cells. The short-term reserve for replacement is creatine phosphate (CP; also known as phosphocreatine), which forms a dynamic balance with free ATP; the enzyme creatine phosphokinase (CPK) ensures that this equilibrium is reached rapidly. Striated muscles have about 30 mM CP to buffer ATP, thus ATP is hydrolysed to ADP in the reaction:

$$ATP \rightarrow ADP + P_i$$

but the level of ATP is rapidly restored by the reaction:

$$ADP + CP \underset{}{\overset{CPK}{\rightleftharpoons}} ATP + C$$

As the last reaction is reversible, the CP is restored by the production of new ATP. How metabolism supplies the new ATP depends upon the individual's stored reserves and the availability of oxygen, and in addition, on the biochemical preference of different muscles. ATP may be derived from the metabolism of glucose and free fatty acids from blood, or from reserves of glycogen and lipid droplets in muscle fibres. The storage of glycogen is a characteristic of skeletal muscles.

Under anaerobic conditions, which may occur if the muscle is working hard, the breakdown of muscle glycogen proceeds via the glycolytic pathway to lactic acid. The end-product is lactic acid rather than pyruvic acid, and the oxidized nicotinamide adenine dinucleotide (NAD) generated by the conversion of pyruvic acid to lactic acid is used in an earlier step. As discussed below, some muscle will obtain a major portion of the ATP necessary for contraction from anaerobic metabolism. During aerobic conditions both fatty acids and pyruvate can enter the citric acid cycle via acetylcoenzyme A, and thus a far greater amount of ADP is converted to ATP. For example, anaerobic metabolism of 1 mol of glucose generates 2 mol of ATP, but aerobic metabolism in which pyruvate is further catabolized by the citric acid cycle generates 38 mol of ATP per mole of glucose.

The whole process, that is contraction and relaxation, operates with an efficiency of conversion of metabolic energy into external work of the order of 10–20%; the remainder is dissipated as heat.

Heat production

Our everyday experiences reveal that muscular work is accompanied by the liberation of heat and that the amount of heat generated by muscles is proportional to the effort. The rate at which muscles produce heat may increase during maximal contractile activity to 20–50-fold the resting level. To a large extent the amount of heat ($m W g^{-1}$ tissue) produced by a muscle depends on the physiological characteristics of the muscle; fast-contracting muscles produce about six times more heat that slow-contracting muscles. As these two types of muscles have similar abilities to develop force ($N cm^{-2}$ cross-sectional area), it is clear that fast-contracting muscles are less efficient than slow-contracting muscles. Shivering when exposed to cold results in an increase in the production of heat by muscles; with intense shivering it may rise to some eight times the resting level.

Precise measurements of the heat released from an isolated muscle contracting at a fixed length reveal that heat production is maximal at the *in vivo* length and diminishes with either increases or decreases in length.

Twitches and tetanus: the frequency–force relationship

Shortly after a muscle is stimulated by a single stimulus there is an increase in muscle tension, which then decays. The time course of an action potential and a contraction is shown in Fig. 5.9a. The time taken for the development of peak tension varies from 10 to 100 ms; its rate of decline also varies and both depend on the type of muscle being studied. A single contraction of this type is called a **twitch**. If the muscle is stimulated a second time, before it has had time to relax completely, the second response may add to the first and a greater peak tension is developed. This is referred to as **mechanical summation**. If the muscle is stimulated continuously, it fails to relax completely and during the period of stimulation the tension fluctuates (Fig. 5.9b). With increasing frequency of stimulation the maximum tension is increased, the oscillations become smaller and, eventually, at **fusion frequency** a smooth **tetanic**

contraction is produced. The tension produced in tetanus may be two to three times as great as that produced in a twitch. Note that while the twitch provides a useful experimental measure of the properties of the muscle fibres, it is not a behaviourally useful action since the time course of the twitch is usually too short for a behavioural response to occur. Skeletal muscles, therefore, are activated in normal behaviour by volleys of action potentials which produce fused contractions.

The substantial difference between the maximal tensions reached in a twitch and a tetanus has been attributed to the physical properties of the muscle and to changes in the cytoplasmic Ca^{2+} concentration. First, muscles are not rigid and the forces generated by the contractile machinery are transferred to limbs by elastic structures (the tendons and my-

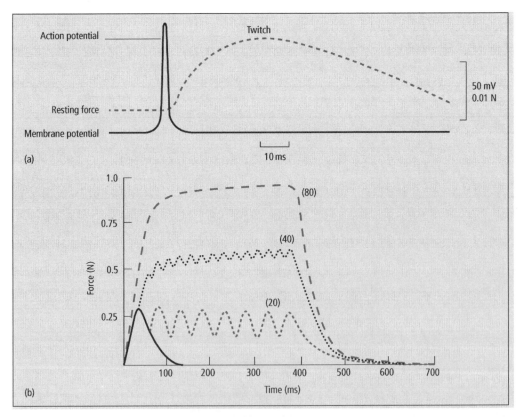

Fig. 5.9 (a) The time course of an action potential recorded intracellularly from a single fibre and the accompanying isometric twitch recorded from many fibres. (b) Isometric contractions from a rat extensor digitorum longus muscle showing the response to a single stimulus and to bursts of increasing frequencies (Hz), indicated in parentheses.

ofilaments). These are embedded in a viscoelastic medium (the cytoplasm, sarcolemma, sarcolemmal connective tissue and the connective tissue around fibre bundles), and many of these elements are arranged parallel to the contractile machinery. Thus much of the energy consumed in a twitch is used in overcoming the damping action of these elements. With continued activation, as in a tetanus, the elastic elements are already stretched and the maximum muscle tension is attained. Second, there is evidence that a higher level of cytoplasmic $[Ca^{2+}]$, and hence muscle activation, is reached during a tetanus.

Force–velocity relationship

The length–tension curve has described the ability of muscles to develop tension when the muscle is held at fixed lengths (isometric contractions). But, as mentioned earlier, the movement of limbs may be associated with the shortening of muscles under a constant load (isotonic contractions). It is an everyday experience that the lighter the load, the more rapidly it can be lifted. In fact, both the rate and the degree of muscle shortening depend on the load. The relationship between the rate of shortening, and the load carried, by a muscle is illustrated by the force (load)–velocity curve.

This relationship is determined by measuring the rate of shortening of a muscle as it lifts a variety of loads. The muscle is not initially subject to each load as this would alter the starting length of the muscle. However, before it can shorten the muscle must obviously first lift each load. Such an event is called an **after-loaded contraction**. When stimulated tetanically, an after-loaded muscle starts to contract. Initially, and until the tension exceeds the load, the contraction is isometric. After this, the muscle shortens isotonically and continues to shorten until it reaches the length at which (according to the length–tension curve) the maximal force it can develop is equal to the load. It is clear that with zero load the time required initially to shorten (the latency) will be minimal and the velocity of the contraction maximal (Fig. 5.10); as the load is increased the latency is increased and the

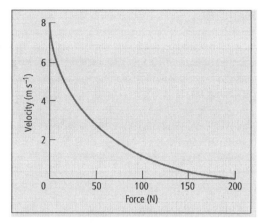

Fig. 5.10 The effect of force (load) on the velocity of shortening of human muscle. (Adapted from Wilkie, D.R. (1950) *J Physiol*, **110**, 249–80.)

velocity decreases. Finally, when the load is too heavy, the velocity of shortening is zero and the muscle is contracting isometrically. It can be seen from the force–velocity curve that the **power** (force × velocity) that a muscle develops is not constant. The power output of a muscle is in fact optimal when both the load and the velocity are moderate—hence the advantage of multiply-geared bicycles.

The reasons for the shape of the force–velocity curve are not known. One suggestion is that the myosin cross-bridges move continually as a result of thermal agitation and that there is only a limited space within which a cross-bridge and an actin site can interact. If this is correct and the actin filament is moving, the probability of successful union will decrease as the velocity of movement increases. Thus, at high velocities few cross-bridges are formed and the force is low because it is dependent upon the number of cross-bridges. Accordingly, the velocity of shortening will increase until the force generated by the muscle equals the load. If the force is either greater or less than the load, the velocity will either increase or decrease, respectively, which will in turn decrease or increase the number of bridges formed and the force generated. This idea is supported by the observation that the velocity of shortening in isotonic contractions is relatively constant.

Muscle fibre types

The diversity of muscular activity requires that muscles have different properties. Thus, some muscles are called upon to maintain a high level of tension for long periods without fatigue while others are required to produce intermittent rapid movements. These two extremes of activity are illustrated by the postural soleus muscle that reaches a peak tension in 80–200 ms (Fig. 5.11), and the extraocular eye muscles that develop their peak tension in 7–8 ms. The soleus muscle contains predominantly slow-contracting muscle fibres, and the extraocular muscles mainly fast-contracting muscle fibres. Muscles that have to perform both endurance and rapid actions have a more even mixture of these fibre types. When the properties of the slow (**type I**) and fast (**type II**) muscle

fibres are compared, pronounced differences are evident. The slow fibres have a low myosin ATPase activity and a high capacity to produce ATP by oxidative phosphorylation, which is aided by a well-developed blood capillary network and high levels of intracellular **myoglobin**. The latter is an O_2-binding protein (like haemoglobin; see Chapter 13), which both facilitates the diffusion of O_2 into these muscle cells and stores a small quantity of O_2 in the cells. The simultaneously high concentration of myoglobin and high capillary density in these muscles have led to the use of the term 'red muscle'.

There are two distinct groups of fast-contracting fibres. Both have a greater diameter and a higher myosin ATPase activity than the slow fibres, but their resistances to fatigue differ (Fig. 5.11b). The resistance to fatigue is correlated with a high ox-

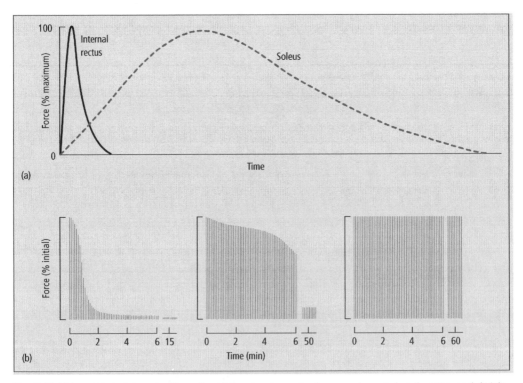

Fig. 5.11 (a) Isometric twitch contractions of cat internal rectus and soleus muscles scaled to the same peak height. (Adapted from Cooper, S. & Eccles, J.C. (1930) *J Physiol*, **69**, 377.) (b) Fatigue of fast (left), intermediate (middle) and slow (right) muscle fibres that were stimulated through their nerve supply at 40 Hz for 330 ms once each second. (From Burke, R.E., Levine, D.W., Tsairis, P. & Zajac, F.E. (1973) *J Physiol*, **234**, 723.)

idative capacity and those fibres with a high resistance are often referred to as **intermediate** fibres, required for example to perform marathon running. The largest and fastest contracting type II fibres (the so-called **fast** fibres) have a poorly developed oxidative metabolism and depend largely on glycolysis for the production of ATP; consider for example running the 100 m sprint. A summary of these and other properties of the different fibre types is given in Table 5.1. Thus differences at the molecular, biochemical and histological level underpin the broad physiological performance differences of our muscles.

Regulation of contraction at the gross level

The total force generated by a muscle depends on the number of active fibres and the level of activity in each fibre. Each motor axon entering a muscle makes contact with a number of muscle fibres; each of these fibres is innervated by a single terminal branch of that axon. Thus, groups of muscle fibres are activated synchronously.

Motor units

A **motor unit** comprises a motor neurone and the group of muscle fibres innervated by the branches of its axon (Fig. 5.12). Motor units vary greatly in size, ranging from one or two muscle fibres in the smallest units in muscles controlling the fine

movements of fingers or eyes, to more than 2000 in the largest units in limb muscles. All the muscle fibres in a motor unit tend to be very similar in their properties; so the terms type I and type II are used for both motor units and muscle fibres. In general, the type I units of slow muscles are rather similar in size and are not particularly large; in contrast, type II units of fast muscles range from very small to very large. The larger a motor unit is, the larger the axon and the nerve cell body of the motor neurone supplying it. This probably reflects the need for production by the cell of all the materials needed to keep every one of its nerve terminals functioning.

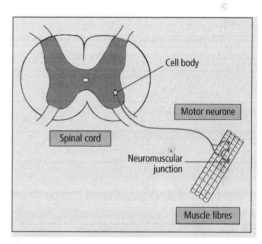

Fig. 5.12 A motor unit, consisting of a motor neurone and the muscle fibres that it innervates.

Table 5.1 Characteristics of type I and type II muscle fibres.

	Type I High oxidative	Type II High oxidative	Low oxidative
Rate of contraction	Slow	Fast	Fast
Myosin ATPase activity	Low	High	High
Main pathway for ATP production	Oxidative phosphorylation	Oxidative phosphorylation	Glycolysis
Number of mitochondria	Many	Many	Few
Myoglobin content (muscle colour)	High (red)	High (red)	Low (white)
Capillary density	High	High	Low
Glycogen reserves	Low	Intermediate	High
Rate of fatigue	Slow	Intermediate	Rapid
Fibre diameter	Small	Intermediate	Large

Gradation of tension

Increments in tension can result from an increase in the force generated by individual motor units or by bringing into action (**recruitment**) additional units. Extracellular recordings of the electrical activity of muscle fibres (electromyography) have shown that both these events occur, but not at the same rate. Thus, the initial development of muscle tension is thought to be due largely to recruitment of units. As explained below there is, in addition, an increase in firing frequency but the contribution of this to increments in tension is thought to be important mainly in the generation of larger forces.

The recruitment of motor units is not random but occurs in an orderly fashion from small to large. Low tensions are produced and precisely controlled by the selective activation of a number of small units. In fact, under most circumstances, a small proportion—paradoxically, the smallest ones—do most of the work. The largest units are activated only when a maximal effort is required and even then their activity is often brief.

Recruitment of motor neurones

The ordered recruitment from the **pool** of neurones supplying a muscle arises because the smallest cells are the most easily excited. The smaller surface area of the small motor neurones results in these cells having a higher input resistance. When similar excitatory synaptic currents are generated in the small and larger motor neurones, the small ones reach threshold first. As the intensity of excitatory synaptic activity in a motor neuronal pool increases, larger and larger motor units are recruited, and at the same time the frequency of discharges increases. However, there are also neural mechanisms that limit the discharge frequency of individual motor neurones to a frequency appropriate to the type of muscle fibres they innervate.

It should be noted that the contractions of skeletal muscles are not regulated solely by the motor units. These activities also make use of sensory information, including that from the muscles and limbs involved. The role of the muscle receptors

(the muscle spindles and Golgi tendon organs) in motor control is discussed in Chapter 8.

Development and maintenance of skeletal muscles

The speed with which muscles can contract and their ability to do work are not constant throughout life, but change as a person grows and ages; their performance is also influenced by exercise. The development, growth and maintenance of muscles are all dependent on the presence of an intact motor nerve supply.

Development of muscles

Skeletal muscle fibres are derived from cells of embryonic mesodermal origin. These myogenic precursors have their origin in the **somites**, the tissue blocks that are adjacent to the developing brain and spinal cord (Fig. 3.7). Myogenic precursors (myoblasts) migrate from the somites to the appropriate position in the body where, under the influence of unknown environmental signals, they may exit the mitotic cycle and fuse with one another to produce multinucleate embryonic muscle fibre myotubes. This process occurs in two stages: an early generation of primary myotubes defines the anatomy and fibre organization of the adult muscle, and acts as a scaffold to guide the formation of secondary myotubes. The number of fibres in skeletal muscles appears to be genetically determined, but the expression of their full genetic capacity is dependent on the normal development of the nerve supply to the muscles. If during early development the motor nerves fail to maintain contact, the muscles will be smaller than normal due to a decrease in the number of their fibres.

As well as influencing the number of fibres in a muscle, some property of the neural input also appears to influence fibre type. This has been demonstrated in a number of ways, but most obviously in that the muscle fibres within a motor unit are homogeneous with respect to such properties as contraction time, resistance to fatigue, enzymes of anaerobic and aerobic metabolism and myosin ATPase. These properties are determined early in development but they are not irreversible and changes can be seen in both developing and adult muscles, for example after denervation (see below). The ability of nerves to regulate the properties of muscles is referred to as a trophic influence but it is not known precisely how this influence is exerted. There is good evidence that nerve-induced muscle activity at the appropriate frequency (tonic low frequency for slow muscles and phasic high frequency for fast muscles) is important. Maintained low-frequency activation leads to a sustained rise in intracellular Ca^{2+}, which stimulates calcineurin, a Ca^{2+}-regulated phosphatase, leading to the activation of genes coding for slow-fibre specific contractile proteins. There is also evidence suggesting that specific messengers, **myogenic regulatory factors**, are released by motor nerves to influence the muscle fibres that they innervate. Experimentally, if the normal input to a muscle is cut and replaced with a nerve of a different type, the properties of the skeletal muscle will gradual transform to those of the muscle type previously innervated by the nerve. An exciting therapeutic use of this knowledge has been to transform the properties of skeletal muscle, e.g. latissimus dorsi *in vivo*, to become more like cardiac muscle in terms of non-fatigability, and to use it for cardiac assist in patients with failing hearts, by forming an additional ventricle.

Effects of training

Type I fibres make up about 30–40% of the cells in human muscles and they are about the same size in men and women (the mean diameter being ~60 µm). Type II fibres are larger in men (average diameter 69 µm) than in women (50 µm). The higher levels of testosterone are thought to underlie the larger size, and hence strength, of skeletal muscle in men, although female body builders show that musculature can be greatly increased in women by training. Two distinct responses to regularly performed strenuous exercise can be seen in muscle: hypertrophy of the fibres with an increase in strength (e.g. weight-lifters) and an increased capacity for aerobic metabolism (e.g. long-distance runners, cross-country skiers, swimmers).

Endurance exercise training gives rise to an increased capacity for oxidation of pyruvate and long-chain fatty acids. This is due to an increase in the density of mitochondria and hence in the amount of enzymes; for example, those of the tricarboxylic acid cycle and those involved in the activation, transport and oxidation of long-chain fatty acids. There is an increase in capillary density and myoglobin, which speeds the rate of diffusion of O_2 from cell membrane to mitochondria. Trained individuals have increased intramuscular stores of triglyceride and lowered concentrations of serum triglycerides, and their muscles can utilize lipids directly from blood.

The consequences of these changes are that during submaximal exercise, trained individuals derive more energy from fat and less from carbohydrate than do untrained individuals. Furthermore, in the trained individual, liver and muscle glycogen stores are better maintained during exercise and a greater proportion of oxygen is extracted from the blood supply to muscles.

Fatigue has two major causes: an inability to maintain an adequate motor drive from the central nervous system and a failure of excitation–contraction coupling. Fatigue resulting from voluntary exercise is normally evident before significant depletion of muscle energy reserves has occurred and, no matter how severe the exercise, muscle energy supplies are never depleted to the point of inducing rigor. (Recall that ATP is required for cross-bridges to detach). The process of fatigue is always reversible and training results in both its onset being delayed and its intensity reduced.

Effects of ageing

The ageing process results in a decrease in the size, speed and strength of skeletal muscles, and also a reduction in their fibre number. The age-related loss in skeletal muscle mass is referred to as **sarcopenia**. The death of type II motor neurones is an important factor, as it results in the denervation of type II muscle fibres, some of which will then die, while others will attract new input from nearby type I nerve terminals. This process results in an overall slowing of muscle contractile responses, a decrease in motor unit number, and an increase in motor unit size. In addition, motor unit fibres may become clumped within the muscle belly, in a way analogous to that of reinnervated muscles shown in Fig. 5.13. The potency of synaptic transmission also decreases with age due to structural changes at the neuromuscular junction.

Effects of damage to nerve or muscle

After the nerve to a muscle is sectioned, there are changes in both the muscle and the axons. Changes in the muscle fibres are particularly pronounced. Within a few days of denervation there is a small decrease in the resting membrane potential of the muscle fibres and an increase in their sensitivity to applied acetylcholine, due to the insertion of newly synthesized acetylcholine receptors throughout the sarcolemma (i.e. including the extrajunctional regions). A few days later the fibres develop spontaneous activity (**fibrillation**) due to instability of their membrane potential. Other changes, such as a pronounced decrease in the ability to develop tension, a change in enzymic composition and a decrease in fibre diameter (**atrophy**), may take longer to develop. In humans, the fibres may shrink down to some 10 µm unless they are reinnervated. If muscle fibres remain denervated for prolonged periods (months to years), they will gradually be replaced by connective tissue and fat.

When the nerve to a muscle is sectioned, some of the motor neurones die but others regenerate their axons. However, in higher vertebrates there is little or no specificity in the re-establishment of nerve–muscle connections. Regrowth of axons is aided and directed by the presence of the old nerve sheaths (hence the accurate suturing together of the cut ends of a nerve is important). Normally fibres belonging to a particular motor unit are well scattered across the muscle, but after regeneration they clump together (Fig. 5.13) as if the ingrowing nerve fibre made connections with all the muscle fibres in its immediate vicinity. Moreover they develop the characteristics of the motor neurone providing their input. However, reinnervation may not always be successful; when a whole limb is

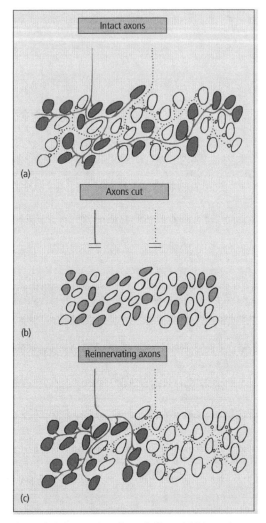

Fig. 5.13 Reinnervation of muscle fibres. (a) Prior to denervation the fibres innervated by each motor neurone are intermixed. (b) The muscle fibres atrophy following section of the nerve. (c) After reinnervation the muscle fibres of each motor unit tend to be grouped together.

denervated there is very little evidence of orderliness in nerve regeneration to muscles, and normal coordination of movement is never fully restored.

It is generally taken that damaged muscle fibres cannot divide and therefore lack the capacity for regeneration. They do however have endogenous stem cells—known as satellite cells because of their peripheral location—which are activated by damage and effectively repair the muscle. The small mononucleate satellite cells normally lie beneath the basal lamina of mature muscle fibres. These cells appear to be a special generation of myoblasts which migrate into the muscle region from the somite during development, but which do not then contribute immediately to the formation or growth of a muscle fibre. The appropriate stimulus triggers them to undergo mitosis, increase in number and ultimately fuse to repair the damaged fibres or to make new multinucleate muscle cells. It is actually possible to remove a muscle, mince it, pour the mince back into the appropriate place in the animal, sew up the skin, and produce a new but smaller functional muscle. Regeneration of the muscle in such cases is critically dependent on the presence of the nerve.

5.2 Smooth muscle

Smooth muscle has a wide range of functions including the regulation of gastrointestinal motility, the diameter of blood vessels and bronchioles, and uterine contractions. The characteristics and control of smooth muscle vary with location, enabling it to perform, in a tailored way, its tissue-specific functions. Smooth muscles control the movement of material through most hollow organs; for example, they propel material in the gastrointestinal tract, they restrict flow in arteriolar blood vessels and bronchi, and they expel material from the uterus, bladder and vas deferens. Smooth muscles also control piloerection and influence the dilator and constrictor muscles of the iris, thus affecting the amount of light reaching the retina. Smooth muscle cells usually exist in bundles or sheets. They are thin elongated cells, which may be connected to their neighbours electrically by low-resistance gap junctions that help coordinate contractile activity. Contraction is initiated by an increase in the concentration of intracellular Ca^{2+}, which acts through calmodulin, and phosphorylation of myosin light chain, i.e. regulation is thick-filament based. The contractions of smooth muscle are slower than those of skeletal muscle but more efficient. Smooth muscles vary in their level of activity from those that show more or less continuous activity, e.g. vascular tone, to those that

are quiescent for prolonged periods, e.g. urinary bladder. Activity in smooth muscles depends on a number of factors, including the character of the smooth muscle cells, their environment, neural input and hormones. All neural influences are exerted by the autonomic nervous system; some tissues are innervated by only one division, while others are innervated by both the parasympathetic and sympathetic divisions. Factors such as stretch, pH and oxygenation help to couple smooth muscle activity to the varying demands of the body.

Smooth muscle structure

A connective tissue sheath, the **epimysium**, surrounds the smooth muscle of each organ. Thin septa extend inwards from the epimysium to form the **perimysium**, which contains fibroblasts, capillaries, nerves and collagenous elastic fibres. The perimysium divides smooth muscle into discrete **bundles** (or sheets) of fibres. These bundles range from 20 to 200 μm in width, and anastomose with one another; these anastomoses can be seen at roughly 1 mm intervals along a fibre bundle (Fig. 5.14). An exception in which the smooth muscle is not organized into bundles is found in arteriolar walls, which may be only a couple of cell diameters in thickness.

The individual smooth muscle cells within a bundle are fusiform, or irregular elongated cells 2–10 μm in diameter, and vary in length from about 50 μm in arterioles to 400 μm in most other organs, and up to 600 μm in the pregnant uterus. They interweave and overlap with each other (Fig. 5.14) to form a network interlaced with collagen; smooth muscle cells may synthesize much of the collagen found in the extracellular space, i.e. they are both contractile and secretory cells. Damage to vascular smooth muscle cells can cause excessive matrix production and proliferation, causing a pathological narrowing of vessels.

Individual smooth muscle cells come into close contact with 10 or so neighbouring cells; at these points they may be connected by specialized intercellular junctions of relatively low electrical resistance called **gap junctions**. At these junctions the sarcolemma of the cells is separated by 3–5 nm and

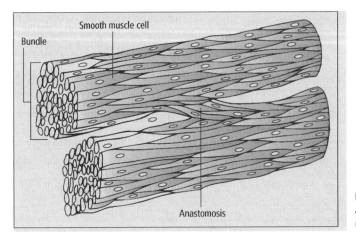

Fig. 5.14 Smooth muscle cells are arranged in bundles that are interconnected by an anastomosis.

the gap is bridged by structures that allow small ions to pass from cell-to-cell. The relatively low electrical resistance of these junctions allows current, which may have either an excitatory or an inhibitory effect, to pass from cell-to-cell. Alteration in gap junction permeability, e.g. by pH, provides a mechanism for changing the activity of smooth muscle. Where bundles exist, the direct coupling of cells within each bundle can result in the bundles being a functional (contractile) unit.

Pronounced differences between the structure of smooth muscles and striated muscles are seen at the ultrastructural level. Smooth muscle cells possess few mitochondria and a single nucleus—usually centrally located. The SR was originally considered to be poorly developed but recent confocal imaging techniques have shown it to be abundant in most smooth muscles, coming very close to the sarcolemma and encircling the nucleus (Fig. 5.15). The SR of most smooth muscles has both release channels gated by both Ca^{2+} and inositol triphosphate (IP_3). There is no specialization at the neuromuscular junction, and the myofilaments of actin and myosin are irregularly arranged. The actin filaments appear to be inserted into specialized structures in the sarcolemma—the dense bodies; costameres in skeletal muscle may be analogous to the better-known dense bodies. Long actin filaments radiate out in a longitudinal direction from dense bodies and there is a much higher ratio of actin to myosin compared with skeletal muscle. Smooth muscle cells lack troponin, and as detailed below, activity is regulated by another Ca^{2+}-binding protein, **calmodulin**, which is associated with the thick filaments. Various proteins have been identified in association with smooth muscle actin filaments, e.g. calponin and caldesmon, and appear to play a role in regulating contraction.

Contractile activity of smooth muscle: phasic and tonic

The variety of activity required by the different tissues containing smooth muscle leads to considerable variations in contractile activity and mechanisms of excitation. In some organs, only localized contractions occur (e.g. intestinal sphincters), while in others the whole organ may be involved (e.g. bladder). The contractions can be phasic with regular undulations of contraction and relaxation, or tonic with a steady level of force being produced over a long period of time (Fig. 5.16). The contractions of smooth muscle are slower than those of skeletal muscle. When excited by a single stimulus, there is often a long latency, a slow rise to peak tension (>1 s) and then a slow decline to the resting state. In many tissues, this single contraction may take several seconds and in some tissues last for minutes, e.g. uterine contractions in labour. Some smooth muscles, e.g. blood vessels, produce a more-or-less steady level of contraction

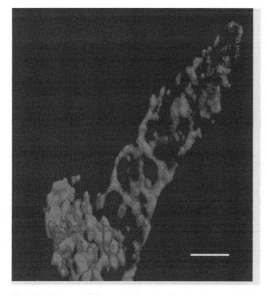

Force
(mN)   Phasic

(a)

Force
(mN)   Tonic

2 min

(b)

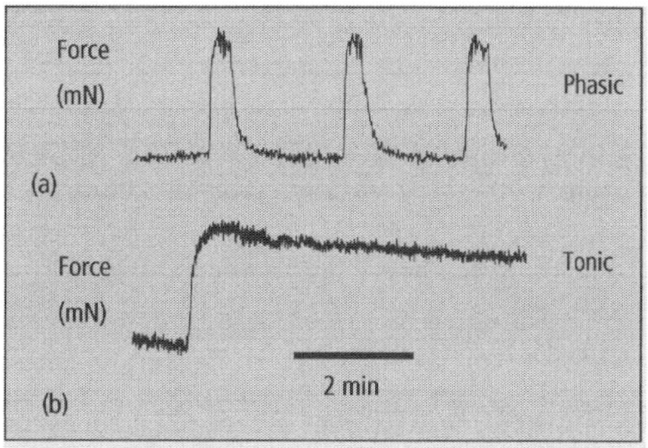

Fig. 5.16 The contractions of smooth muscle may be (a) phasic or (b) tonic.

Fig. 5.15 Image of the sarcoplasmic reticulum in a smooth muscle cell from the ureter, obtained using confocal microscopy. Scale bar, 5μm.

for many hours, referred to as tone or tonic activity. With trains of action potential or hormonal stimulation the forces generated by smooth muscles can reach levels similar to those found in skeletal muscles (30–$40\,N\,cm^{-1}$). However, unlike many skeletal muscles, smooth muscles can maintain their tension at a high level for long periods and over a wide range of muscle lengths. It seems probable that the low activity of the smooth muscle myosin ATPase may account for both the slow development of force and the relatively low O_2 consumption during contractions (<1/100 that of skeletal muscle). The efficiency of smooth muscle contraction is low, i.e. ~25% work/ATP compared to skeletal muscle, but its economy, the product of force and time per ATP, is greater. As with striated muscle the rate-limiting step in the cross-bridge cycle is P_i release. In smooth muscle the cross-bridge life-time is longer than in skeletal, which will also contribute to its greater economy. The ability to contract over a wide range of lengths (up

to four times the resting length) may be a result of the irregular arrangement of the myofilaments, and is clearly advantageous to their physiological role in surrounding organs, such as the bladder, as they fill with their contents.

Regulation of contraction—role of myosin phosphorylation

As with skeletal muscle, the force generated by smooth muscle is controlled by the level of intracellular free Ca^{2+}. In smooth muscle during stimulation, this Ca^{2+} may come from the interstitial fluid as a result of a change in membrane permeability, or it may be released internally from the SR as occurs in skeletal muscle. The incoming Ca^{2+} contributes substantially to the rising phase of the smooth muscle action potential (see below), and visceral smooth muscles will stop contracting in the absence of external Ca^{2+}. As a result of these changes, the cytoplasmic concentration of Ca^{2+}

may rise from a resting level of 10^{-8} mol L^{-1} to 10^{-6} mol L^{-1} or higher.

With this rise in concentration, more Ca^{2+} combines with the regulatory protein calmodulin to activate a highly specific protein kinase that phosphorylates the light (small) chains in the head of each myosin molecule. This is a prerequisite for the activation of the smooth muscle actin–myosin complex. This kinase is myosin light chain kinase, MLCK, and it phosphorylates a sereine residue, and thereby greatly increases the actin-activated myosin ATPase activity. The activity of MLCK is a target for modulation by some hormonal second messengers. Inactivation of the contractile mechanism is accomplished by the lowering of the intracellular concentration of Ca^{2+} and the activity of a phosphatase (myosin light chain phosphatase; MLCP) that dephosphorylates myosin light chain (Fig 5.17). The activity of MLCP is a key target for many hormonal second messengers, and in particular by phosphorylation; MLCP activity is greatly reduced if it is phosphorylated. This inhibition of MLCP can therefore lead to an increase in force without a change in $[Ca^{2+}]$, a process termed Ca^{2+}-sensitization in which the normal sigmoidal relation between $[Ca^{2+}]$ and force is right- or leftward-shifted. Thus, force production in smooth muscle may be viewed as the balance between the activities of MLCK and MLCP (Fig. 5.17).

Thin filament based regulation

While myosin phosphorylation is the dominant regulatory mechanism, recent evidence has supported an additional, thin filament based regulatory system operating in smooth muscles. This mechanism appears to be based around removal of the inhibitory influences of caldesmon and calponin on myosin ATPase, by phosphorylating them. The kinases required for this phosphorylation are stimulated when agonists bind to their receptors on the smooth muscle membrane.

The Ca^{2+}-independent pathways, i.e. sensitization, and thin filament-based regulation, will augment the contractile process initiated by excitation and Ca^{2+} entry through voltage-gated Ca^{2+} channels. However it is now recognized that some agonists act to modulate smooth muscle force without changing membrane potential; a process referred to as pharmaco-mechanical coupling to distinguish it from the usual electro-mechanical coupling. These agonists bind to receptor-operated channels, ROC, as opposed to voltage-operated channels, VOC, and produce IP_3 and other second messengers. The IP_3 will stimulate the release of Ca^{2+} from the SR, and other second messengers will activate the kinases that modify the regulatory mechanisms described above.

During tissue relaxation the Ca^{2+} that entered the cell for contraction is transported to the extracellular fluid or re-sequestered into the SR. Expulsion of Ca^{2+} from the cell is energy-dependent and due to the activity either of a Na^+–Ca^{2+} exchange mechanism or a Ca^{2+}-dependent ATPase.

Finally, in muscles that contract for long periods, there may be a decrease in the level of phosphorylation of myosin light chain while tension is maintained. It appears that dephosphorylation of the

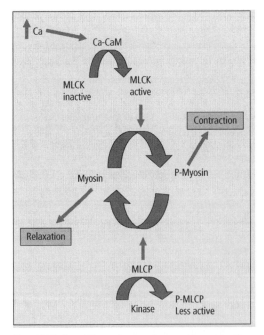

Fig. 5.17 Regulation of smooth muscle contraction occurs by altering the activity of myosin light chain kinase (MLCK) and myosin light chain phosphatase (MLCP). CaM, calmodulin.

cross-bridge while it is attached to actin may slow its dissociation. This 'latching' of cross-bridges may provide an energetically efficient means of maintaining tension.

In summary, the regulation of contraction in smooth muscles is more varied than in striated muscles and need not correlate with $[Ca^{2+}]$, membrane depolarization or myosin light chain phosphorylation.

Electrical activity is varied in smooth muscles

The resting membrane potential of many smooth muscles is in the range of -55 to -70 mV, and its basis is similar to that found in other excitable cells (see Chapter 1). There is, therefore, the same tendency for K^+ efflux leading to hyperpolarization, as the E_m for K^+ is -90 mV, and a strong inward driving force for Ca^{2+}, both electrically and chemically. One notable feature of smooth muscle cells is the relatively high $[Cl^-]$ and the modulation of excitability via Cl^- efflux, producing depolarization (as electrically it is equivalent to positive charge entering).

A description of electrical activity in smooth muscle cells is more complex than that of striated muscles because of their diversity. Not all smooth muscles exhibit action potentials, but in those that do they may be spike-like, but somewhat slower than in skeletal muscle, or plateau-type action potentials, as seen in cardiac cells (e.g. in the ureter; Fig. 5.18). A depolarization of some 20 mV is required to reach threshold and initiate an action potential, which reaches a peak of about 10 mV. If the stimulus is maintained, repetitive firing may occur, the frequency depending on the degree of depolarization.

In contrast to the action potential in nerves and skeletal muscles, in smooth muscles Ca^{2+}, not Na^+ ions are responsible for the inward current. The threshold depolarization is that required to open the voltage-sensitive Ca^{2+} channels. Thus the magnitude of the overshoot of the action potential is not directly proportional to E_{Na}, and removing Ca^{2+} ions from the bathing fluid abolishes action potentials, while increasing Ca^{2+} produces larger action potentials. Drugs that block these Ca^{2+} channels are used in the treatment of smooth muscle over-activity, for example hypertension.

Slow waves are a feature of some smooth muscles, e.g. gastrointestinal (GI). These are rolling changes in membrane potential of some 20 mV occurring over a timescale of many seconds and even minutes, rather than milliseconds. At the peak of the depolarization produced by the slow wave, trains of action potentials may be triggered. Thus contractile activity will map to the slow wave frequency. The ionic mechanism responsible for the generation of the slow waves is not fully understood at present.

As in cardiac muscle, some smooth muscles, e.g. ureter and GI tract, have pacemaker areas and/or specialized cells responsible for triggering electrical activity that can be transmitted rapidly to many cells via gap junction coupling. As discussed below, smooth muscles containing these pacemakers are spontaneously active. Other spontaneously active smooth muscles, e.g. uterine, have no anatomically defined pacemaker region but are suspected of having these cells distributed throughout them. However, this remains to be established. The mechanism underlying pacemaking activity is best understood for GI smooth muscle.

Types of smooth muscle

As mentioned above, the activity of smooth muscles may be phasic (rhythmical) and dependent on spontaneous mechanisms; other tissues are quiescent until stimulated by an incoming signal. The former have often been referred to as unitary (cells acting together) and the latter as multiunit (cells

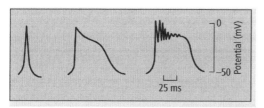

Fig. 5.18 Action potentials of smooth muscle may be spike-like (left), plateau-like (middle) or a mixture of these (right).

acting independently) smooth muscles, respectively, but these divisions are now of little use as they represent extremes, and smooth muscles may be considered to be a continuum, between these extremes. Smooth muscles may be conveniently divided into three groups according to their membrane properties; namely, spontaneously active, electrically inexcitable and intermediate.

Spontaneously active smooth muscle

Many visceral organs containing smooth muscle contract rhythmically (e.g. stomach, small intestine, ureter, uterus). As this coordinated activity is maintained without nerves and hormones, it must be initiated and coordinated by the smooth muscle cells, i.e. it is **myogenic** (as in the heart). Such activity usually depends on the spontaneous generation of action potentials, and the presence of a conducting system (the gap junctions). Two types of mechanism are responsible for the spontaneous generation of action potentials, **pacemaker** potentials and **slow waves**.

In some smooth muscles (e.g. ureter) there is a focal pacemaker region (in the case of the ureter this is in the renal pelvis) where groups of cells will depolarize to threshold; the subsequent action potentials are then conducted through the tissue. As mentioned earlier, in other smooth muscles, e.g. the uterus, the pacemaker regions are not constant in location, and it is thought that all regions within these tissues have the capacity to assume the role of pacemaker.

The rhythmic activity of the stomach and intestine results from the regular generation of depolarizing potentials (pacemaker potentials) in the highly specialized interstitial cells of Cajal (see Chapter 19). Thus the term myogenic can be misleading as it is not necessarily muscle cells that initiate the electrical activity, although it does occur in cells contained within the muscle. This initial depolarization spreads throughout the smooth muscle (Fig. 5.19). Not all activity in the GI tract can be attributed to slow waves triggering action potentials; for example in the fundus and body of the stomach the slow waves are larger but the spikes are smaller and occur only at the beginning

of the slow wave. In this area the contraction may be independent of action potentials and can be triggered by the slow wave exceeding the membrane potential for the initiation of contraction.

The spontaneous contractile activity of smooth muscles can be altered by nervous and hormonal activity, which may be either excitatory or inhibitory upon the underlying mechanisms, producing rhythmicity. For example, in the intestine acetylcholine, the transmitter released from parasympathetic nerves, causes the smooth muscle to depolarize. As a consequence, the number and frequency of action potentials on each slow wave are increased and the contractions are more forceful. In contrast, the inhibitory action of noradrenaline, the transmitter released from sympathetic neurones to the detrusor (bladder) muscle, and the inhibitory actions of non-adrenergic non-cholinergic autonomic neurones to the gut (see also Chapter 19) are due to hyperpolarization and movement of the membrane potential away from threshold. This may result in complete cessation of contractile activity while the spontaneous fluctuations in membrane potential continue at a subthreshold level. Hormones modify the activity of spontaneously active smooth muscles by a variety of mechanisms. Oxytocin for example can act on uterine smooth muscle cells to increase Ca^{2+} influx and the release of Ca^{2+} from the SR, as well as by decreasing Ca^{2+} efflux via the Ca^{2+}–ATPase of the plasma membrane. By affecting both the $[Ca^{2+}]$ within the cells, and the relationship between $[Ca^{2+}]$ and myofilaments force production (sensitivity), the normal phasic activity of uterine cells can be transformed into the strong and long-lasting contractions associated with labour.

Electrically inexcitable smooth muscle

This term applies to an extreme, but not unimportant, group of smooth muscles that do not generate action potentials (e.g. bronchial, tracheal and some arterial smooth muscles). In these tissues, the membrane potential remains stable until the tissue is stimulated. Stimulation may be the result of neurotransmitter release or the activity of paracrine or endocrine agents (e.g. histamine, bradykinin).

Stimulation is accompanied by depolarization and subsequent contractions. In tissues with a sparse innervation, excitation can spread because of the presence of gap junctions. The physiological advantage of these muscles may reside in their generally slow and sustained response to nerve stimulation.

Intermediate smooth muscle

This category includes smooth muscles in the iris, piloerector, blood vessels, vas deferens and seminal vesicles. Like electrically inexcitable smooth muscle they have a stable resting membrane potential and when stimulated they exhibit spike-like action potentials. The cells are linked by gap junctions, but conduction is decremental and so the contractions fail to spread throughout the tissue. The force of contraction is proportional to the frequency of the action potentials and is usually under neural control.

Activation of smooth muscle

Contraction of all smooth muscles is dependent on changes in the intracellular Ca^{2+} level. This can occur as a result of inherent myogenic mecha-

nisms, which regularly depolarize the muscle fibres, or as a result of neural or hormonal action. Contractions may also be induced by other means. For instance, some smooth muscles are relatively plastic when slowly stretched, but rapid stretching results in a depolarization and contraction. Such behaviour may be important in **myogenic autoregulation** of blood vessels (p. 387). In other tissues, local agents modify the force of contraction (e.g. the actions of O_2 and CO_2 on blood vessels of the lungs, and histamine on bronchial smooth muscle).

In tissues such as arterioles where the dominant influence is exerted by the nerves, irrespective of their type, excitation is usually the result of a depolarization (an **excitatory junction potential**; Fig. 5.20a). In the case of inhibition, hyperpolarization of the smooth muscle membrane occurs (an **inhibitory junction potential**; Fig. 5.20b). In nearly all cases, the increase in conductance arises as a result of the neurotransmitter interacting with specific surface receptors on the muscle fibres; one notable exception appears to be nitric oxide which is released as a neurotransmitter but acts directly on cytoplasmic guanylate cyclase in the smooth muscle to cause relaxation (p. 35). If the neuromuscular junction has a relatively small junctional

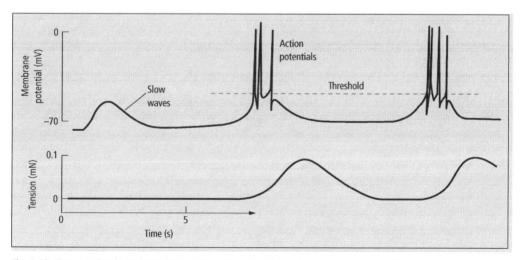

Fig. 5.19 Rhythmic depolarizations (slow waves), action potentials and contractions recorded from a strip of smooth muscle from the small intestine. The slow waves initiate action potentials on reaching threshold, and cause the muscle to contract. (In the stomach, the slow waves are usually larger in amplitude and may initiate contraction.)

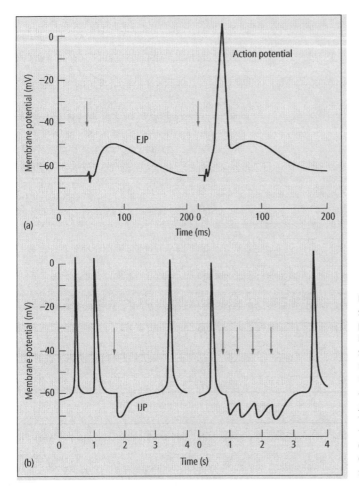

Fig. 5.20 Junction potentials in smooth muscle. (a) Excitatory junction potentials (EJP) recorded intracellularly from the vas deferens following stimulation (arrows) of its sympathetic nerve supply (left, subthreshold EJP; right, suprathreshold EJP leading to an action potential). (b) Inhibitory junction potentials (IJP) recorded intracellularly from longitudinal intestinal muscle following stimulation (arrows) of the intramural nerves (left, single stimulus; right, repetitive stimuli).

cleft (20 nm) then the junctional potential is distinct, with a fast rate of rise, lasting about 0.5 s; wider (400–500 nm) neuromuscular junctions appear to respond more slowly to nerve stimulation. In fact in some tissues (e.g. the tunica media of blood vessels), many of the muscle fibres may not be directly innervated; they may, however, be under some neural influence, as current will spread from neighbouring innervated regions (through gap junctions).

The contractile activity of many smooth muscles is influenced in a tissue specific manner by hormones and paracrines, which are discussed more in the relevant chapters, reflecting the highly specific nature of the receptors on the plasma membrane.

Some hormone receptors are expressed on many different smooth muscles and hence these hormones, e.g. adrenaline, will have widespread activities; for example, adrenaline can change the contractile activity of many tissues (e.g. blood vessels, bronchioles, the intestines). Similarly, the highly potent prostaglandins and thromboxanes have pronounced effects on a number of smooth muscles. For instance, prostaglandin F_2 is a potent stimulator of uterine contractility (and is used to induce labour at term), and of intestinal and bronchial smooth muscles.

Smooth muscle pathophysiology

It is clear from the widespread distribution of smooth muscle in the body that its control and correct functioning will be vital to our health. Many of the body's homeostatic mechanisms work via the autonomic nerve system affecting smooth muscle function. Consider for example what happens when blood pressure is elevated; its detection by baroreceptors alters autonomic activity and reduces the constriction of arterioles (as well as changing cardiac activity), to restore blood pressure. If a patient has elevated blood pressure then drugs to reduce the contraction of arterioles will be given; e.g. Ca^{2+}-channel blockers or drugs to reduce the effects of noradrenaline. Not all dysfunctions of smooth muscle can be so well controlled; for example, premature labour occurs when the mechanisms triggering the coordinated contractions of childbirth occur too early in pregnancy,

jeopardizing the fetus. The aetiology is usually unknown, and it is difficult to predict. It is almost impossible to stop the uterine contractions once labour has started, but Ca^{2+}-channel blockers, β mimetic drugs, or oxytocin antagonists may be effective for long enough (2 days) to administer steroids, which bring forward surfactant production in the baby's lungs and greatly increase its chances of survival. Many other common conditions such as asthma and bladder instability, also involve smooth muscle problems. The key to correcting the pathophysiological conditions affecting smooth muscles lies in obtaining a more complete understanding for each of the physiological processes and their modification.

Chapter 6

Sensory Systems

The term **sensory systems** applies to those parts of the nervous system concerned with the detection, transmission and analysis of information about stimuli from the internal and external environments. Some aspects of sensory stimuli are perceived, but much of the sensory information that is received by the body is outside the realm of consciousness. Sensory systems include the **receptors**, the **afferent nerve fibres** of sensory neurones and the **central pathways** activated by appropriate stimuli. This chapter considers the **somatosensory pathways** (signalling touch, mechanosensation, temperature and pain from the skin, muscles and joints) and **visceral pathways** (signalling the internal state, for example of blood vessels, gastrointestinal tract and heart). The following chapter deals with the pathways associated with the special senses, which arise in the eye, ear, nose and mouth.

6.1 Sensory neurones

Sensory neurones comprise the peripheral endings, afferent nerve fibres, cell bodies and their central processes through which changes in the environment are transmitted to the central nervous system (CNS). Here we consider the sensory neurones of two systems—somatic and visceral. The cell bodies of somatic neurones lie in the trigeminal and dorsal root ganglia; those of visceral neurones lie in various cranial and dorsal root ganglia. Sensory neurones vary in their sensitivity

to stimuli, in their axon diameter and in their electrical and chemical properties.

Like their receptors (see Table 4.2), sensory neurones may be classified as somatic or visceral. Their cell bodies are located outside the CNS in various ganglia. These cells are pseudounipolar (see Fig. 3.1) and their cell bodies do not receive synaptic inputs.

Somatic sensory neurones have their cell bodies either in the trigeminal or dorsal root ganglia. Their peripheral axons (somatic afferent fibres) travel in peripheral nerves carrying information from the skin, skeletal muscles, tendons, joints and bone; their central processes travel in the trigeminal or dorsal roots to the CNS.

Visceral sensory neurones have their cell bodies in various cranial nerve ganglia, such as the glossopharyngeal and vagal nerve ganglia, or in the dorsal root ganglia. Their peripheral axons (visceral afferent fibres) travel with sympathetic and parasympathetic nerves, or somatic peripheral nerves, and carry information from receptors in blood vessels and internal viscera, particularly the heart, lungs, bladder, rectum and genital organs. Their central axons either travel in the cranial VII, IX and X nerves to the nucleus of the tractus solitarius in the brainstem or, in the thoracic, lumbar and sacral regions, join the dorsal roots to enter the dorsal horn of the spinal cord with the somatic afferent fibres.

Within sensory ganglia, cell bodies differ in size,

staining properties and cytochemistry. There is some correlation between size and functional properties, with small diameter cells tending to be associated with high threshold, noxious or thermal stimuli. Many cells contain neuropeptides such as substance P and somatostatin, monoamines such as serotonin, or amino acids such as glutamate and aspartate. There is accumulating evidence that some of these act as transmitters in the dorsal horn; for example, substance P is thought to be one of the transmitters for nociceptive stimuli, whereas glutamate, acting on α-amino-3-hydroxy-5-methyl-isoxazolepropionic acid (AMPA) and N-methyl-D-aspartic acid (NMDA) receptors, underlies an important component of excitatory synaptic transmission in tactile sensation (p. 81).

The receptors for the somatic and visceral afferent fibres include: mechanoreceptors, which are sensitive, for instance, to skin indentation, muscle length or visceral stretch; thermoreceptors which detect changes in skin temperature; and nociceptors which detect potentially damaging stimuli (Tables 4.2 & 6.1).

As already discussed (p. 70), peripheral nerve fibres can be classified according to their diameter. In general, the greater their diameter, the greater their conduction velocity. Unfortunately, there are two overlapping classification systems for afferent fibres. It is common to use the alphabetical A–C system for cutaneous afferents and the Roman numeral I–IV system for muscle afferents (p. 70 and Table 6.1).

Associated with the differences in diameter, peripheral nerve fibres also show differences in the following functional properties:

1 Modality. Although there are no rigid correlations between diameter and modality, some general trends are clear, as shown in Table 6.1.

2 Conduction velocity. This increases with increasing fibre diameter and with myelination (p. 69).

3 Electrical threshold. When a nerve is stimulated by electrical pulses, the strength of the stimulus required to induce action potentials decreases with increasing fibre diameter. Consequently, small unmyelinated fibres require the greatest stimulation. This is a property of axons and does not reflect thresholds to physiological stimuli.

4 Refractory period. This decreases with increasing diameter; action potentials are of shorter duration and recovery is faster in large fibres. Thus, the frequency of firing in small unmyelinated fibres seldom exceeds 10 Hz, while short bursts of 500 Hz or more are occasionally seen in large myelinated fibres.

5 Sensitivity to local anaesthetics. Local anaesthetics, such as procaine and lidocaine, act on excitable membranes to reduce the voltage-dependent influx of Na^+ associated with the action potential, and hence to block activity. Small fibres are the most susceptible because of their high

Table 6.1 Characteristics of cutaneous sensory nerve fibres and their receptors.

Fibre type	Numerical equivalent	Diameter (μm)	Receptors	Modalities represented
Aβ	Smaller fibres of I and all II	4–16	Merkel cells, Pacinian corpuscles, Ruffini endings, Meissner's corpuscles, larger hairs	Touch, pressure, vibration, position sense
Aδ	III	1–4	Small hairs	Touch, pressure
			Specialized nerve endings	Cold
			Specialized nerve endings	Pricking pain
C	IV	0.5–2	Unknown mechanoreceptors*	Touch, pressure
			Unknown thermoreceptors	Cold, warmth
			Unknown nociceptors	Dull aching pain

* Not found in humans.

surface area to volume ratio. Thus, after application of local anaesthetic to a cutaneous nerve, sensations of temperature and pain are blocked before touch and pressure, which are associated with large fibres.

6 Sensitivity to ischaemia. A reduction in blood supply to a nerve, for example as a result of an embolism, a thrombosis or an occlusion due to a pressure cuff, blocks large fibres first, probably because of their greater volume and hence higher metabolic demands. Thus, in this type of block, vibration sensitivity and position sense are lost before the ability to appreciate pain or changes in skin temperature.

6.2 Somatosensory pathways

Inputs giving rise to sensation follow one of two routes within the CNS—the dorsal column pathway or the anterolateral pathway. The dorsal column pathway is more discriminative and precisely organized, while the anterolateral pathway is the only route for thermal or nociceptive inputs. Both pathways contain relay nuclei that act as synaptic stations where information can be modified by local and descending controls.

Afferent nerve fibres, except for those of the special sense organs, enter the CNS mainly via the spinal dorsal roots, and the trigeminal and vagal roots. The innervation areas of peripheral nerves to the skin show little overlap and hence section of a nerve gives a characteristic region of sensory loss.

However, fibres from one peripheral nerve enter the spinal cord over several dorsal roots, so that a particular innervation area is represented over a number of segments. The innervation area of the skin supplied by a single dorsal root is known as a **dermatome**. Dermatomes from adjacent dorsal roots overlap considerably so that section of a single root does not produce a region of complete anaesthesia.

After entering the spinal cord, fibres usually bifurcate to give ascending and descending branches, which mostly end in adjacent grey matter. Inputs giving rise to sensations usually follow one of two ascending pathways within the spinal cord—the **dorsal column pathway** and the **anterolateral pathway**.

Fibres destined for the dorsal column pathway are mainly large myelinated (Aβ) fibres, which enter the spinal cord via the more medially positioned dorsal rootlets. They bifurcate, giving one branch that enters the **dorsal horn** and a second branch that enters the ipsilateral **dorsal column** (Fig. 6.1).

The branches in the dorsal horn have a variety of destinations. Branches of the largest fibres from the annulospiral endings of the muscle spindles make direct synaptic contact with motor neurones in the ventral horn and can thus evoke a monosynaptic stretch reflex (Chapter 8). Branches from muscle, joint and skin mechanoreceptors synapse in the dorsal horn with the cells of origin of the **spinocerebellar tracts** which supply the cerebel-

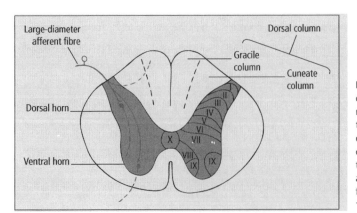

Fig. 6.1 Diagram showing the entry of a large-diameter (Aβ) afferent nerve fibre into the spinal cord and the passage of its branches into the dorsal horn, ventral horn and dorsal column. The roman numerals indicate the laminae of the spinal cord—10 anatomically defined layers. (Adapted from Rexed, B. (1964) *Prog Brain Res*, **11**, 58–90.)

lum with information used in the control of posture and movement. Other branches contact dorsal horn cells in different laminae (Fig. 6.1) depending on their modality, and are involved in local segmental activity.

Dorsal column pathway

The branches of the primary afferent fibres in the dorsal column ascend to the medulla without synapsing. There they synapse with neurones in a relay nucleus, the ipsilateral **dorsal column nucleus** (Fig. 6.2). These neurones send their axons to the opposite side of the medulla, forming a well-marked histological feature—the **sensory decussation**—where the fibres from the two sides cross. After crossing, the fibres ascend in a tract known as the **medial lemniscus**, which passes through the midbrain and terminates in a second relay nucleus, the **ventrobasal nuclear complex** of the thalamus. The thalamic neurones send their axons to layer IV in the postcentral gyrus of the cerebral cortex (**somatosensory cortex**) (see Fig. 6.7). Somatic inputs from the head enter the brainstem via the trigeminal root and first synapse in the trigeminal nucleus in the pons and medulla. From there, second-order fibres ascend to join the medial lemniscus, cross the midline and synapse in the medial part of the ventrobasal complex (Fig. 6.2); fibres from here project to the lateral part of the somatosensory cortex.

The dorsal column pathway carries information necessary for fine tactile discrimination, vibration sensitivity and position sense. Throughout the pathway the sensory modalities are preserved. Because the dorsal column pathway provides for these rather refined sensibilities, it is usually called the **discriminative** (specific) pathway. Since the medial lemniscus is a major component of this pathway it is also referred to as the **lemniscal system**.

Somatotopy

Receptive fields in this pathway remain fairly small and localized and, throughout the whole pathway

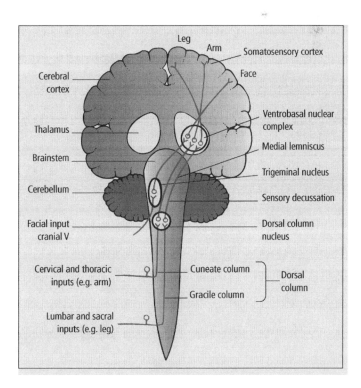

Fig. 6.2 Dorsal column pathway.

from the dorsal column to the somatosensory cortex, adjacent fibres or cells correspond to adjacent areas in the periphery. Thus, the body surface is represented in an orderly, topographic fashion known as **somatotopic organization**, which is more fully discussed on p. 129. Moreover, certain peripheral areas have higher innervation densities peripherally and therefore disproportionately larger central representations throughout the whole pathway.

Conduction properties

Activity in this pathway is relatively stable, showing little alteration with arousal and attention, and a lower susceptibility to blockage by general anaesthetics and hypoxia than that in the anterolateral pathway.

Anterolateral pathway

Fibres contributing to this pathway are the smaller myelinated (Aδ) and unmyelinated (C) fibres, which enter the spinal cord via the more lateral rootlets, together with some branches of larger fibres. Many bifurcate, sending branches rostrally or caudally in the dorsolateral tract (tract of Lissauer) before synapsing in the dorsal horn with second-order neurones most commonly found in laminae I and V. The axons of second- or third-order

neurones cross to the opposite side of the cord and ascend in the anterolateral tract (Fig. 6.3).

Axons in the anterolateral tract terminate in a number of regions (Fig. 6.4). Some axons travel directly to the thalamus (**spinothalamic tract**), terminating either laterally in the ventrobasal complex or in more medially located regions such as the intralaminar nuclei and posterior complex, and the nucleus submedius. These thalamic nuclei in turn provide inputs to various cortical regions, including the somatosensory cortex. Other axons of the anterolateral tract terminate in the reticular formation in the medulla, pons and midbrain (**spinoreticular** and **spinomesencephalic tracts**). These regions then relay to areas such as the thalamus and hypothalamus. For inputs from the face, the caudal part of the trigeminal nucleus in the medulla is considered to be analogous to the dorsal horn and sends projections to the thalamus as well as other brainstem regions.

Fibres entering the anterolateral pathway carry information about touch, pressure, cold, warm and noxious stimuli. While some cells remain modality-specific, others respond to both noxious and innocuous stimuli. At the thalamic level some cells can respond to somatic, auditory and visual inputs. Receptive fields in the anterolateral pathway also tend to be larger than in the dorsal column pathway and may include over half the body surface. Somatotopy in this pathway is therefore

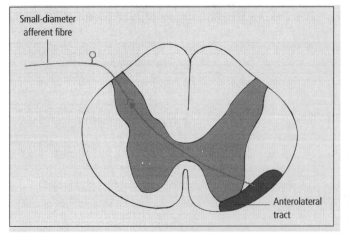

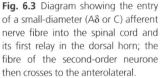

Fig. 6.3 Diagram showing the entry of a small-diameter (Aδ or C) afferent nerve fibre into the spinal cord and its first relay in the dorsal horn; the fibre of the second-order neurone then crosses to the anterolateral.

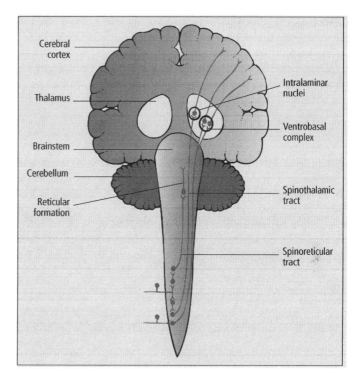

Fig. 6.4 Anterolateral pathway.

less precise than in the dorsal column pathway, with more overlap and less clear topography. In addition, responses can show marked alterations with attention, can habituate to repeated stimuli, and are less resistant to anaesthesia. For these reasons this pathway is often referred to as the **non-discriminative** (non-specific) pathway.

This is the principal pathway carrying impulses from nociceptive and thermal inputs, therefore damage to the anterolateral cord can produce analgesia in the opposite side of the body below the level of the lesion. Such damage can give rise to a dissociated sensory loss—touch to a particular region can still be felt (via the dorsal column pathway) but pain and temperature changes are not perceived.

Function of relay nuclei

On any sensory pathway, there are always several interruptions at synaptic regions known as **relay nuclei**; information can never travel via a single fibre from receptor to cortex. For somatosensory pathways, the relay nuclei consist of cells in the dorsal horns of the spinal cord, dorsal column nuclei, corresponding nuclei in the trigeminal system, and the ventrobasal nuclear complex of the thalamus. These nuclei are important in the functioning of the sensory pathways as they provide for interaction and modification of the input by excitatory and inhibitory mechanisms; such mechanisms are activated by ascending and descending pathways.

The mechanisms of excitation and inhibition at synapses have been dealt with in Chapter 4. Inhibition can be either presynaptic or postsynaptic. One situation in which both pre- and postsynaptic inhibition are thought to contribute to the functioning of sensory pathways is surround inhibition.

Surround inhibition

This is also called lateral or afferent inhibition. It is important in all sensory systems, particularly the visual and auditory systems, in the sharpening of contrasts, in the localization of stimuli and in spatial discriminative ability.

A sensory unit commonly has an excitatory receptive field surrounded by a region, the inhibitory surround, which when stimulated reduces the output of the unit (Fig. 6.5). The inhibitory surround of a unit is located in the excitatory fields of other adjacent sensory units which, when stimu-

lated, exert an inhibitory effect on that unit by way of interneurones. These interneurones may act either by pre- or post-synaptic inhibition. Thus, the unit with the greatest afferent input imposes the greatest inhibition on its neighbours.

At each central synapse, diverging connections may result in activity becoming widespread. Surround inhibition is important because it reduces the spread of activity. It occurs at synaptic relays at all levels of the sensory system, thus ensuring that the focus of activity is kept sharply localized, with weakly excited surround connections being inhibited by the strongly active centre. An example of how this works in two-point discrimination (p. 75) is shown in Fig. 6.6.

Descending control

Descending pathways originating in various regions of the brain exert control over the sensory, as well as motor, functions of the spinal cord. They act at every synaptic level to reduce irrelevant activity and to sharpen contrasts and improve discrimination. Pathways originating in the sensory cortex can influence transmission at all levels. For example, the removal of descending influences by the application of a cold block to the spinal cord alters the activity of dorsal horn cells caudal to

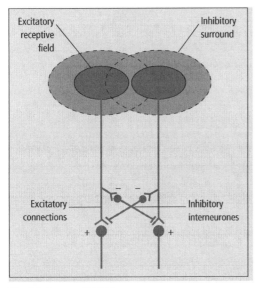

Fig. 6.5 Surround inhibition.

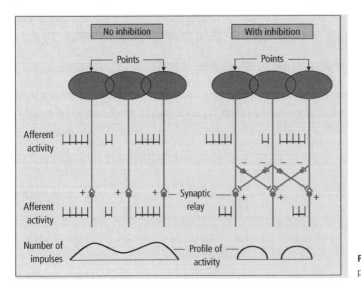

Fig. 6.6 Surround inhibition in two-point discrimination.

the block. Conversely, electrical stimulation in the midbrain around the periaqueductal grey matter produces analgesia in humans and animals. Such stimulation is thought to activate a descending inhibitory pathway from the raphe nuclei in the medulla. This pathway is serotonergic and exerts a powerful inhibitory effect on dorsal horn nociceptive cells.

These descending control pathways can be influenced by incoming activity in sensory pathways. In the control of pain for example, activity in spinoreticular pathways has been shown to influence descending inhibition. Nociceptive specific cells in lamina I of the spinal cord also project via a dorsolateral pathway to areas in the midbrain and medial thalamus and may modify the emotive aspects of pain and its control.

6.3 Somatosensory cortex

Inputs from somatosensory pathways end in a region of the cerebral cortex known as the somatosensory cortex. This is organized somatotopically with inputs from the legs ending medially, and those from the face laterally. Each body region has several representations, concerned with analysing different aspects of a stimulus. Stimulation of the periphery can elicit activity in the cortex, which can be recorded as evoked potentials in electroencephalogram (EEG) recordings or imaged by functional magnetic resonance imaging (fMRI).

The primary somatosensory cortex (SI) lies along the central sulcus in the postcentral gyrus (Fig. 6.7). The SI region is divided into three narrow strips, from anterior to posterior known as areas 3, 1 and 2. A second and smaller somatosensory area (secondary somatosensory cortex; SII) lies along the lateral fissure. For both SI and SII, inputs from the thalamus terminate mainly in layer IV, and from there activity spreads to more superficial and deep layers before passing to other cortical regions.

Organization of responses: somatotopy

Responses in the SI region result from stimulation on the opposite side of the body, except for some parts of the face, which are represented bilaterally. The responses in SI are somatotopically organized; for example, responses from the foot and leg are represented medially, responses from the face laterally and responses from the hand and arm in between (Fig. 6.8). The density of peripheral innervation determines the size of the corresponding cortical area. The particular area that is disproportionally enlarged varies in different species and reflects the behavioural use of different peripheral regions in discrimination. For instance, in the pig the snout representation is particularly large; in rats and mice it is the facial whiskers, and in humans the hands and lips. SII also shows somatotopic organization but this is less precise as cells generally have large receptive fields, which may be bilateral.

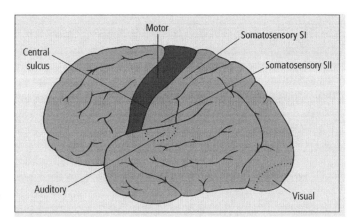

Fig. 6.7 Somatosensory cortex—primary (SI) and secondary (SII) areas.

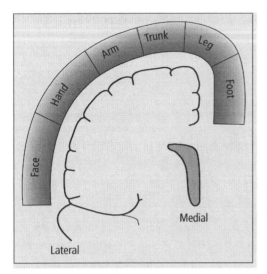

Fig. 6.8 Somatotopic organization. The sensory representations are indicated on a cross-section through the somatosensory cortex. (Adapted from Penfield, W. & Rasmussen, T. (1968) *The Cerebral Cortex of Man: a Clinical Study of Localization of Function*, p. 44. Hafner, New York.)

Response properties

In general the response properties of cortical neurones differ from those of the periphery with respect to their variability and receptive field size. Whereas the same stimulus delivered repetitively evokes highly precise activity in the sensory ganglion neurones, the responses in the somatosensory neocortex are highly variable. The high variability of cortical sensory responses likely reflects state and context dependent processing of the sensory information. Whereas receptive field size is small at the periphery, cortical neurones respond to larger areas. The broader receptive fields of cortical neurones is likely important to integrate sensory information and to form associations of sensory input with other information.

SI contains four representations of the body in narrow strips of cortex, which run parallel to the central sulcus. From anterior to posterior these representations lie in areas 3a, 3b, 1 and 2. Area 3 receives incoming signals, via the thalamus, from muscle stretch receptors (3a) or cutaneous receptors (3b), and contains cells that respond to simple joint movements or to punctate stimuli within localized receptive fields on the skin surface. All the cells within a 'vertical' column of cortex (i.e. from the pial surface to the white matter) have similar receptive fields, adaptation rates and respond to similar modalities (e.g. touch, pressure or joint movement). The characteristic of cells in one vertical region sharing similar response properties is known as **columnar organization**, as first described by Vernon Mountcastle; this is also a feature of other sensory cortices such as the visual area, as found by David Hubel and Torsten Wiesel (p. 152).

Response properties of cells in areas 1 and 2 are more complex than in area 3. Thus cells in area 3 have relatively localized receptive fields, e.g. corresponding to part of one finger, while those in areas 1 and 2 are larger, e.g. encompassing all fingers. This complexity is partly due to convergence of inputs, with area 1 receiving inputs from both the thalamus and from cells in area 3; area 2, in turn, receives inputs from area 1. Some cells in area 1, and many in area 2, show 'direction sensitivity' indicating that they respond preferentially to movement of an object in a particular direction within their receptive field. For area 1 the thalamic input is from rapidly adapting cutaneous receptors, so these cells are thought to be concerned with discrimination of texture—for instance, when we rub our fingers over a surface.

Area 2 contains some cells that are sensitive to the orientation of the edges of an object; cells may also respond to both tactile stimuli and joint movement—as occurs, for instance, when an object is grasped. These properties mean that cells in area 2 are probably involved in perception of the three-dimensional size and shape of objects (known as **stereognosis**). Cells in area 2 project to the motor cortex and are involved in fine manipulative skills. Lesions in the hand region of areas 1 and 2 cause severe impairment in both fine tactile discrimination and fine finger manipulations. Electrical stimulation of the somatosensory cortex can elicit sensations of numbness, tingling or normal tactile sensations attributed to the corresponding part of the periphery.

Sensory responses

Stimulation of the limbs or other parts of the periphery can elicit a mass response in the SI cortex, which consists of the inhibitory and excitatory postsynaptic potentials of many activated cells. This mass response is known as an evoked potential and can be recorded from the surface of the SI cortex, or even through the scalp (EEG) if averaging techniques are used to improve the signal-to-noise ratio. The potentials most commonly consist of a series of alternating positive and negative waves, the first wave being surface positive (Fig. 6.9). Evoked potentials can also be recorded in the visual and auditory systems.

In a similar way to EEG recording, the corresponding magnetic fields generated by brain electrical activity can also be recorded at high temporal resolution in the magnetoencephalogram (MEG). By simultaneously recording from many EEG or MEG sites, the spatial location of cortical activity can be estimated. Cortical activity evoked by tactile stimuli can be imaged at high spatial resolution using fMRI, revealing localized processing of information within the somatopic map. However, the fMRI technique has poor temporal resolution, and therefore complements the EEG and MEG recordings, which have low spatial resolution but high temporal resolution.

The **latency** of an evoked potential varies in different sensory systems and in different animals, but is very consistent under similar stimulating and recording conditions. This has proved valuable in the early diagnosis of certain diseases like **multiple sclerosis** in which the latency of the evoked potential is increased because of loss of myelin along the pathway. Evoked potentials can also be used to assess the integrity of a sensory path in infants or comatose patients.

6.4 Modalities of sensation

Stimulation of sensory receptors gives rise to a number of perceived sensations. Thus mechanoreception results in sensations such as touch, visceral distension and kinaesthesia or limb position. Thermoreception produces sensations of warmth or cold, and nociception may result in pain. Various anomalies in pain sensations, such as referred pains, are common.

Now that the nature of the receptors, sensory neurones and central pathways involved in sensation have been discussed, we can consider in more detail the various modalities of sensation.

Mechanoreception

The sensations usually associated with gentle mechanical stimulation of the skin are **touch** and **pressure**, although more complex sensations such as **vibration** and **tickle** are also recognized. Figure 6.10 illustrates the kinds of mechanoreceptors to be found in hairy and glabrous skin of mammals. Muscles and joints contain receptors, which contribute to **position sense** as well as responding to

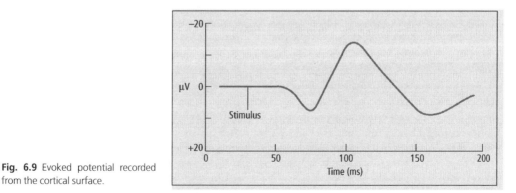

Fig. 6.9 Evoked potential recorded from the cortical surface.

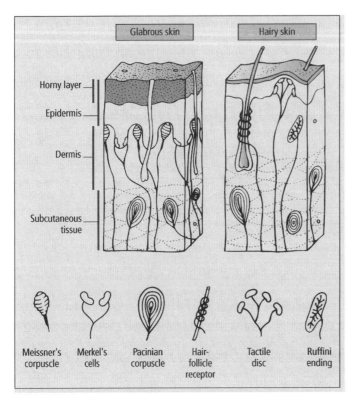

Meissner's corpuscle   Merkel's cells   Pacinian corpuscle   Hair-follicle receptor   Tactile disc   Ruffini ending

Fig. 6.10 Mechanoreceptors in glabrous and hairy skin. (From Schmidt, R.F. (1981) *Fundamentals of Sensory Physiology*, p. 86. Springer-Verlag, New York.)

pressure and stretch. Viscera have only a few mechanoreceptors.

Mechanoreceptors are specialized to detect particular properties of the stimulus such as its position, intensity, duration, velocity or acceleration. Mechanical stimuli can have both **static** and **dynamic** components. The static component refers to a constant force such as that exerted on a stationary joint (e.g. the hip joint when standing) or on the skin by steady pressure. For the dynamic component, the force changes with time, such as occurs on joints during limb movement or on the skin during the process of indentation. Receptors that respond when a stimulus is static are **position** or **length** detectors. The frequency of nerve impulses is proportional to the position (e.g. joint angle, skin position) or length (e.g. muscle length), and receptors maintain their response as long as the position or length is maintained. These receptors are described as **tonic** receptors, and the type of response is known as 'slowly adapting' (p. 74).

As well as location and modality, these receptors can provide information about the 'intensity' and 'duration' of the maintained force by the frequency and duration of their response. Examples are Merkel receptors and Ruffini endings in the skin (Fig. 6.10), and both are probably involved in the sensation of pressure on the skin.

Receptors detecting the dynamic component of a stimulus respond during a change in position and cease to respond after the movement finishes. Such receptors detect **velocity**, and their discharge frequency is dependent on the magnitude of the velocity change. Their response is described as **phasic** or rapidly adapting (p. 74). Examples of this type of receptor are Meissner's corpuscles in glabrous skin and hair follicle receptors in hairy skin. They are important for touch (e.g. in texture discrimination) when we move our fingers over a surface.

Some receptors show both a tonic and phasic pattern of response, giving impulses of higher frequency during a change in length (dynamic component), but continuing to respond during a maintained displacement or fixed length (static component). An example of such a receptor is the muscle spindle, found in skeletal muscles (p. 188), which contributes to our sense of limb position.

A third type of receptor responds to rapid transients in skin displacement, i.e. to **acceleration**. These receptors are very rapidly adapting and may discharge only one impulse for each stimulus. Two types are known—Pacinian corpuscles and certain hair receptors. Rapidly repeated stimulation of these receptors evokes a sensation of vibration. Pacinian corpuscles are extremely sensitive to vibration and detect very small amplitudes of the order of $1\,\mu$m, particularly between 150 and 300 Hz.

Touch

Tactile sensations can be produced by indenting the skin on the fingertips by as little as $10\,\mu$m. Localized regions or **touch points** occur which are more sensitive to touch or pressure than surrounding areas. In the fingertips the thresholds of the receptors are significantly lower than surrounding areas. The capacity for **spatial discrimination** also varies over different parts of the body. For example, two-point discrimination (Fig. 6.6), assessed with the pointed arms of a pair of calipers, is 1–3 mm over the tips of the fingers and tongue; in contrast, the minimum spatial discrimination is 20–50 mm over the forearm and back. Usually touch involves an active movement of the skin over an object. This movement greatly improves our ability to discriminate surface texture, as well as the size, shape and consistency of an object.

Kinaesthesia

In muscle and tendons there are mechanoreceptors providing information about muscle length and tension. These are usually associated with **muscle spindles** (p. 188) and **Golgi tendon organs** (p. 191). In joints there are mechanoreceptors that respond to bending of the limbs. These may be Ruffini endings in joint capsules, Golgi endings in

ligaments, or Pacinian corpuscules associated with joints and along bones and ligaments. All of these receptors (and mechanoreceptors in the skin) may be involved in the subconscious control of posture and movement, and also in the conscious awareness of position and movement, which is called **kinaesthesia**. All receptors signalling information about the position of the limbs and body are called **proprioceptors**. Our present understanding of the roles of the various proprioceptors in position sense is summarized below.

Recordings from joint receptors indicate that they respond mainly at the extremes of movement of a joint or to movements in more than one axis of rotation (e.g. flexion–extension and abduction–adduction). They are therefore unlikely to provide accurate information on mid-range positions. However, stimulation of single-joint afferents can be perceived as movement of the appropriate joints.

Muscle spindles and Golgi tendon organs also give information about the state of joints and can provide accurate information about position. Indeed, various lines of evidence suggest an important role for these receptors in kinaesthesia. Thus, vibration of muscles (a powerful stimulus for muscle spindles) can give rise to illusions of movement and inaccurate estimation of joint position. These illusions remain even if the joints and skin are anaesthetized. When the tongue, which has no joints or joint receptors, is anaesthetized so that information from mucous membranes is lost, its position can still be distinguished, presumably by signals from muscle spindles. However, activity of single muscle spindle afferents around a joint is not perceived as joint movement, so it is presumably the activity in the population of fibres that is important in kinaesthesia.

The contribution of cutaneous afferents to joint position is still uncertain. These afferents respond mainly at the limits of joint movement. They can facilitate detection of passive finger movement, but skin anaesthesia has little effect on kinaesthetic performance.

In conclusion, it appears that summed activity from muscle receptors may be the principal input for normal position sense. However, joint and skin receptors may play a role in situations where input from muscles is impaired, and at the extremes of movement.

Thermoreception

There are two types of cutaneous receptors associated with thermal sensation—**cold receptors** that respond to a decrease in skin temperature and **warm receptors** that respond to an increase. These receptors are active in detecting localized changes in temperature (e.g. when a cold object is touched) as well as in detecting changes in ambient temperature. Together with receptors in the hypothalamus and spinal cord, they are also involved in the regulation of body temperature (Chapter 23). The structure of cutaneous thermoreceptors is not well defined but they are probably free nerve endings endowed with temperature sensitive ion channels encoded by the transient receptor potential (TRP) gene family; they are supplied by small myelinated (Aδ) and unmyelinated (C) fibres.

The afferent fibres associated with temperature receptors usually show a basic discharge at the normal physiological skin temperature (32°C). As the skin temperature falls, activity in the afferent fibres from cold receptors increases and may peak at a skin temperature of 15–20°C; in those from warm receptors the activity increases with temperature until it reaches a peak at 40–45°C. At this temperature there may also be a transient paradoxical response from cold receptors, although they are normally silent above 40°C.

Our ability to detect actual skin temperature and temperature changes depends on factors like the area of skin affected, the initial skin temperature and the rate of temperature change. For steady temperatures, the body has a neutral zone from about 20 to 36°C (the actual range being variable) in which there is no persisting sensation of body temperature. For temperatures above or below this range, persisting sensations of cold or warmth are experienced. Above about 45°C, pain rather than warmth is usually reported. Changes in temperature of the order of 0.1–0.3°C can be detected if rapid; slower changes may require a shift of 5°C to be detected.

Pain

Pain can be described as the sensation resulting from stimuli that are intense enough to threaten or to cause tissue injury. Such stimuli may be mechanical (e.g. scratch), chemical (e.g. acid) or thermal (e.g. burn). The receptors that respond to these painful stimuli are known as **nociceptors** (Table 4.2). Unlike other sensations, pain sensations often show no simple correlation with the stimulus intensity or extent of tissue injury. Areas of apparently normal skin may show increased sensitivity (**hyperalgesia**), while massive tissue destruction may occur without pain. Thus the location and type of injury are important. Pain sensitivity also varies in different individuals, races and cultures. Even the same injury in the same individual can cause different degrees of pain, depending on the situation. For example, injuries in accident victims are often not remembered as painful at the time of the accident. Such variability suggests that the sensation of pain is complex and under the influence of powerful controls (see below).

It is usual to consider pain as having two components—the sensation *per se* and the emotional overtones of suffering and distress associated with it. The sensation itself depends on activity that travels in the anterolateral pathway to thalamic and cortical cells. In primates, neurones responsive to nociceptive stimuli have been recorded in the pre- and postcentral gyri. Some cells have localized contralateral receptive fields, and are thought to be involved in the discriminative aspects of pain. This is supported by reports in humans that epilepsy generated in this region has an aura of localized pricking pain. Other nociceptive postcentral cells have large receptive fields (sometimes the whole body) and may project to prefrontal cortex and limbic regions involved in the motivational and arousing aspects of pain. While the sensation and its emotive overtones usually occur together, certain procedures may leave one without the other. Thus pain sensations may occur without distress after frontal lobotomy operations, while damage to parts of the thalamus may lead to a particularly intractable sensation of pain known as the **thalamic syndrome**. Certain drugs may also have different effects on the two components; morphine, for instance, is especially effective on the emotive component.

Somatic pain

Nociceptors in skin, muscles and joints are free nerve endings supplied by either small myelinated (Aδ) fibres or unmyelinated (C) fibres. The endings of Aδ and C fibres signal high-intensity mechanical or thermal stimuli. Some C fibres are less selective (polymodal), responding to high-intensity mechanical, thermal and noxious chemical stimuli. Although these different receptor classes exist, neurologists commonly test pain sensitivity by a pinprick. When stimulated, nociceptors usually respond with a vigorous burst of activity. Sometimes the two groups of nerve fibres give rise to a double sensation, with the pain differing in latency and quality. These is a sharp initial pain, thought to be due to the faster conducting A fibres, then a longer-lasting, aching pain due to activity in C fibres. Nociceptive afferent fibres project to the dorsal horn and thence via the anterolateral tract to the thalamus (p. 228). **Substance P**, a peptide present in afferent terminals, is a likely transmitter for nociceptive afferents in the dorsal horn.

Many nociceptors show **sensitization**; that is, an increase in activity in response to repeated stimuli. Such sensitization at least partly underlies the hyperalgesia found in an injured area, although changes in central transmission also occur. Recent results from a study on the knee joint suggest there are normally 'silent' receptors, which become activated during arthritis. Various factors such as pH, histamine, adenosine triphosphate, serotonin, kinins and prostaglandins released in association with tissue damage have all been implicated in receptor activation. Macrophages and mast cells are also involved (via cytokines) in the hyperalgesia associated with inflammation. There is recent evidence that neurotrophins such as nerve growth factor (p. 43) play a key role in activating these immune cells and increasing the inflammatory hyperalgesia. Other factors, such as substance P released from peripheral nociceptor terminals,

may contribute to vasodilation and the inflammatory process. Cramping pains may occur with excessive use of skeletal muscles, as a result of stimulation of nociceptors by unknown factors.

Central changes in responsiveness in pain pathways include increased sensitivity of neurones in the dorsal horn. A steady input from nociceptors produces a progressive increase in response, a phenomenon known as 'windup'. This change can occur even in unconscious patients and some surgeons advocate the infiltration of local anaesthetic into regions prior to cutting in an attempt to prevent windup and hence reduce post-surgical pain.

Descending controls

The variability of pain sensations in different situations suggests powerful descending controls may be present. A region around the aqueduct in the midbrain, the periaqueductal grey matter, has been shown to be involved in the control of transmission in pain pathways. Thus stimulation of this region in both animals and humans produces a powerful analgesic effect. The periaqueductal grey matter has projections to the raphe nuclei and adjacent reticular formation in the rostroventral medulla (see Fig. 8.6). Serotonergic cells of nucleus raphe magnus project via the dorsolateral funiculus to dorsal horn cells at all spinal levels. This pathway provides both direct and indirect inhibition of dorsal horn cells, including nociceptive neurones in laminae I, II and V. Activation of the periaqueductal grey matter is thought to lead indirectly to analgesia by activating these descending inhibitory pathways from the raphe nuclei as well as possible noradrenergic pathways.

Visceral pain

Responses from visceral receptors, including nociceptors, have been studied in the vagus and other visceral nerves. As in the skin, visceral nociceptors are thought to be free nerve endings and occur in the walls of most hollow viscera, mesenteries and blood vessels. Like somatic nociceptors, they are supplied by small myelinated and unmyelinated afferent fibres.

It is unclear to what extent viscera contain specific nociceptors. Many afferents from the heart, lungs, intestine and bladder respond to innocuous mechanical stimuli as well as to damaging stimuli. However, specific responses have been reported from heart, ureter and gallbladder. Effective stimuli are either excessive stretch or ischaemia. In the heart, for example, afferents have been described which respond only to interruption of coronary blood flow, while in the ureter there are afferents responding specifically to overdistension. Nociceptors are not present at all in some tissues, for example the brain, so brain tissue can be cut without giving rise to pain. The dura, on the other hand, is extremely sensitive.

The sensations most commonly detected from viscera are either fullness or pain. Thus, stretch in the rectum or bladder gives rise to the sensation of fullness and triggers emptying reflexes. Excessive stretch or distension of many viscera gives pain, which is often colicky or intermittent, for example, biliary colic or ureteric colic. Alternatively, severe visceral pain can also occur with ischaemia, as for instance in angina pectoris. Visceral pains are commonly poorly localized and may be referred to other parts of the body.

Referred pain

Damage to an internal organ is commonly associated with pain or tenderness not in the organ but in some skin region sharing the same segmental innervation. A classic example of this is the referral of cardiac pain to the left shoulder and upper arm. The most likely explanation for referred pain is that some central cells receive both cutaneous and visceral inputs. Such cells have been described in lamina V of the dorsal horn. In the normal situation, lamina V cells are activated by skin inputs. When the visceral organ is injured, it activates the same cell in the dorsal horn and this is interpreted as injury to the skin. The skin, though uninjured, feels tender and local anaesthetics applied to the skin help to relieve pain by reducing the total sensory input to the central cells.

Phantom-limb pain

The amputation of a limb is often followed by the feeling that the limb is still present. The phantom area gradually shrinks and may completely disappear, but a small percentage (5–10%) of amputees are left with a persistent and severe pain apparently from the absent region. The pain is thought to arise centrally because sectioning of the contralateral anterolateral tracts may give only temporary analgesia, and the pain may return and be felt at the same site, as preoperatively. However, in some cases the pain may be relieved for long periods by a prolonged or severe stimulus to the stump, although in others the stump may be reamputated or anaesthetized without any relief. Recent work suggests that phantom-limb pain from an amputated hand might be relieved through a training procedure, which might induce somatosensory cortical reorganization. In the so-called mirror box therapy, the patient is asked to place his stump behind a mirror to reflect the image of the intact hand in the place where the stump would normally be seen. This can trick the brain into believing that the hand is intact and apparently pain can be relieved.

Itch

Itch is thought to be a distinct sensation with its own receptors, which, like nociceptors, are free nerve endings. Receptors are localized to the basal layer of the epidermis; itch is only felt in the skin, not in deep tissues. The receptors are sensitive to histamine, either applied directly or released indirectly by activation of mast cells. Itch receptors are connected to $A\delta$ and C fibres, with activity travelling centrally via the anterolateral pathway. Positron emission tomography studies have shown that itch sensations are associated with widespread activation of the prefrontal and premotor cortex, possibly related to planning of scratch movements. Like other nociceptive responses, itch sensations can be strongly influenced by descending controls.

Opioids

Opiates, such as morphine, heroin and codeine, are amongst the most powerful analgesics known. When administered intravenously they act centrally by combining with receptors in many regions, including those associated with pain perception and its control such as parts of the limbic system, the periaqueductal grey matter and the dorsal horn.

An increased understanding of the actions of these exogenous opiates has occurred with the discovery of endogenous **opioid peptides** (p. 235). There are three classes of these endogenous opioids—enkephalins, endorphins and dynorphins, which are all powerful analgesics when administered intracranially. (They are not effective when injected intravenously because they do not cross the blood–brain barrier and are rapidly degraded.) The **enkephalins** are pentapeptides (tyrosine–glycine–glycine–phenylalanine–methionine/leucine) produced within the brain in regions such as the periaqueductal grey matter, limbic system, thalamus and substantia gelatinosa of the spinal cord. The **endorphins** and **dynorphins** are larger molecules containing the met-enkephalin or leu-enkephalin sequence. Dynorphins have a widespread distribution similar to enkephalins, whereas the endorphins are mainly localized to the hypothalamus.

Although quite different in structure, both the opiates and opioid peptides act by binding to similar receptors. Three classes of opiate receptors have been described—μ, δ and κ. Morphine and other exogenous opiates are potent agonists of the μ receptor, enkephalins bind mainly to δ receptors, endorphins to both μ and δ receptors, and dynorphin activates κ receptors. The three receptor classes are widely distributed in the brain and are probably involved in other activities besides nociception. Descending pain control involves the opiate peptides and their receptors in the periaqueductal grey matter, raphe magnus and dorsal horn. It has been reported that levels of the peptides are decreased in chronic pain states. There is some evidence that μ receptors are particularly effective for inhibiting noxious thermal stimuli and κ for mechanical stimuli. In the dorsal horn, μ receptors are present on both nociceptive afferents and postsynaptic cells. Descending serotonergic fibres activate enkephalin-containing interneurones, which in turn inhibit transmission of nociceptive signals. The mechanisms of inhibition are both presynaptic (p. 84) by blocking release of substance P and glutamate from afferent endings, and postsynaptic by inhibiting dorsal horn cells.

In addition to being released from central afferent endings, substance P is also released from peripheral terminals and plays a role in vasodilation and inflammation. Opioid peptides act peripherally by reducing this release. These peptides may also play a role in **acupuncture** as some of the effects of acupuncture can be blocked by the opiate antagonist naloxone.

Chapter 7

Special Senses

7.1 Vision

Our brain derives knowledge of the world around us from visual stimuli. Vision is the process in which the brain uses information from light-sensitive receptors in the retina to create a representation of the external world; at least one-third of the human cortex (more than a billion nerve cells) is devoted to this task, indicating its importance in human perception. The eye is the receptor organ for vision. Light enters the eye through the pupil and is focused by the cornea and lens on to the retina at the back of the eyeball. When focusing on a close object (near response), the lens rounds up, the pupil constricts and the eyes converge. Six different muscles move each eyeball in its socket, allowing us to follow a moving object (smooth-pursuit movement) or switch our gaze from one spot to another (saccadic movement).

Functional anatomy of the eye

The eye is approximately spherical with three peripheral layers: a tough outer fibrous layer (the **sclera** and **cornea**); a middle layer comprising the vascular **choroid** and the muscular **ciliary body** and **iris**; and an inner neural layer, the **retina** (Fig. 7.1). Nerve fibres leave the eye at the **optic disc**. Blood vessels supplying the retina also enter and leave the eye at this site. Many blood vessels run over the inner surface of the retina. The two inner chambers of the eye contain the **aqueous** and **vitreous humours**; suspended between these is the **lens**. The shape of the eye is maintained by an intraocular pressure of approximately 15 mmHg; intraocular pressure is maintained by a balance between the formation and drainage of aqueous humour, which is secreted by the ciliary processes and flows from the posterior chamber to the anterior chamber, where it drains through the canal of Schlemm.

Light enters the eye through the cornea, passes through the aqueous humour and the pupil, then through the lens and vitreous humour and, finally, through the neural elements of the retina to reach the photoreceptors (**rods** and **cones**) on the posterior surface of the retina. Highest acuity (central) vision depends on focusing light rays on to the **fovea centralis** (Fig. 7.1). Vision in man involves the detection of a very narrow band of light ranging from about 400–750 nm in wavelength.

Physiological optics

When focused at infinity the eye has 60 **dioptres** (D) of refraction (power in dioptres = 1/focal length in metres). Most refraction (45 D) occurs at the air–cornea interface while the lens provides 15 D, which can be increased for focusing on objects close to the eye. Changing the point of fixation from an object at infinity to one nearby involves the **near response**, which has three components:

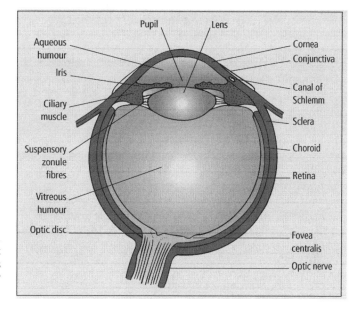

Pupil | Lens
Aqueous humour
Iris
Ciliary muscle
Suspensory zonule fibres
Vitreous humour
Optic disc

Cornea
Conjunctiva
Canal of Schlemm
Sclera
Choroid
Retina
Fovea centralis
Optic nerve

Fig. 7.1 The eye in horizontal section. To reach the photoreceptors, light must traverse the cornea, the aqueous humour, the lens, the vitreous humour and the inner layers of the retina.

1 Accommodation. The refractive power of the lens is made greater by increasing its surface curvature, particularly its anterior surface. In childhood, the power of accommodation is about 10 D, but this decreases with age (**presbyopia**). When focused at infinity, the lens is pulled flat by tension in the **zonule** (lens ligament). Accommodation is achieved by contracting the ciliary muscles, under the control of parasympathetic nerve fibres in cranial nerve III (oculomotor nerve). The ciliary muscles are orientated in a circular fashion so their contraction causes the zonule to move forwards and to slacken, releasing the lens from tension and allowing it to round up due to its inherent elasticity (Fig. 7.2).

2 Constriction of the pupil. This is referred to as **miosis** and results in a better depth of focus, since with constriction light rays pass only through the central part of the lens. Pupil size is controlled by both sympathetic and parasympathetic nerve fibre supply to the muscles of the iris. Sympathetic fibres (cervical) contract the dilator muscle, which is radial, and thereby dilate the pupil (**mydriasis**); parasympathetic fibres (cranial nerve III) contract the sphincter muscle, which is circular, and thereby constrict the pupil. Since diffraction errors can be associated with too small a

pupil, the optimal pupil size is approximately 2 mm diameter.

Constriction of the pupil reduces **spherical aberration** (light entering near the periphery of the lens being refracted more strongly than near the centre). **Chromatic aberration**, caused by the differing degrees of refraction of short (blue) and long (red) wavelengths of light, is also reduced, although never fully corrected. The perceptual consequences of this are minimized by the fovea having very few blue cones, and containing a yellow pigment, which strongly absorbs blue and violet light. Thus short-wavelength light does not affect the cones and the fovea responds only to longer wavelengths of light.

3 Convergence of the eyes. This ensures that the light rays from an object fall on corresponding parts of each retina to give a fused image. It is achieved by contraction of the left and right medial recti muscles (Fig. 7.3) controlled by cranial nerve III.

Light reflex

The light reflex induces constriction of the pupils (miosis) in response to light or when looking at near objects. This reflex has two components:

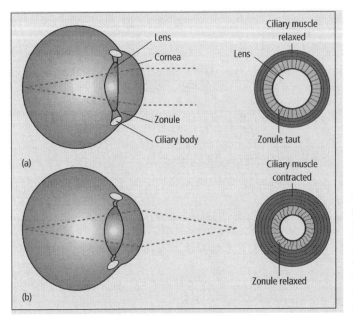

Fig. 7.2 Accommodation for near vision. (a) In distant vision the circular muscle of the ciliary body relaxes and the fibres of the zonule become taut, causing the lens to flatten. (b) In near vision the ciliary muscle contracts and the fibres of the zonule relax, allowing an increase in curvature of the lens, particularly its anterior surface.

when light is shone into one eye, the **direct** light reflex results in the pupil of that eye constricting; at the same time, the **consensual** light reflex causes the pupil of the other eye also to constrict. The afferent pathway for the light reflex is via the optic nerve to the pretectal region of the midbrain and the efferent pathway is along parasympathetic fibres of cranial nerve III.

Eye movements

Each eyeball is moved by four rectus muscles (superior, lateral, inferior and medial) and two oblique muscles (superior and inferior) (Fig. 7.3a). The lateral rectus is controlled by cranial nerve VI (abducens nerve), the superior oblique by cranial nerve IV (trochlear nerve) and all the others by cranial nerve III (oculomotor nerve). When looking straight ahead, these skeletal muscles have the actions shown in Fig. 7.3b. The two eyes may be moved in the same direction (conjugate movements or versions) or in opposite directions (disjunctive movements or vergences), as occurs, for instance, during accommodation. When altering fixation from one object to another, the eyes move in rapid jumps called **saccades**. Even at rest the

eyes are never still, but move in constant microsaccades, an activity that is essential for vision. The eyes can, however, move smoothly without making rapid jumps, as in **smooth-pursuit** movement when the eyes fixate on a moving object. A **squint** (strabismus) occurs when the visual axis of one eye is not fixed on the object being viewed by the other.

Transduction in photoreceptors

Light focused onto the retina is absorbed by visual pigments in the photoreceptors—rods for monochromatic and night vision, cones for colour and day vision. Rod photoreceptors contain the pigment rhodopsin; cones contain three colour pigments (red-, green- and blue-sensitive opsins). Each pigment also contains retinal, which is isomerized by photons and split from opsin in a process known as bleaching. Light induces a hyperpolarizing potential in the photoreceptors. On entering the dark, the pigment is regenerated, allowing dark adaption.

The photoreceptors, **cones** (used for colour and daylight vision) and **rods** (used for monochromatic and nocturnal vision) are arrayed along the

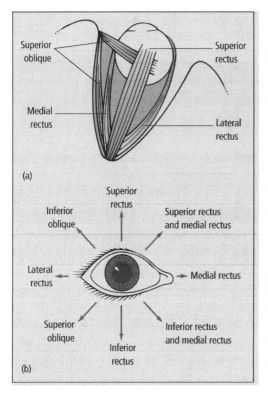

(a)

(b)

Fig. 7.3 (a) Extraocular muscles of the right eye as seen from above (inferior oblique and inferior rectus are situated below). (b) Directions of movement of the right eye, mediated by its extraocular muscles.

outer surface of the retina next to the pigment epithelium (see Fig. 7.8). The photoreceptors are supplied by blood vessels from the choroid, not by those on the inner retinal surface. This is why detachment of the retina from the choroid (**retinal detachment**) leads to extensive damage to rods and cones. Some of the differences between rods and cones are summarized in Table 7.1.

Photopigments

The transduction of light energy into a receptor membrane potential begins when photons are absorbed by photopigments located in the outer segments of the receptors. Each photopigment consists of a protein **opsin**, and a chromophore **retinal** (an abbreviation of retinaldehyde, the aldehyde of vitamin A). There are four forms of opsin giving four photopigments—the rod photopigment **rhodopsin**, and the three cone photopigments: **erythrolabe** (red-sensitive), **chlorolabe** (green-sensitive) and **cyanolabe** (blue-sensitive). Their absorption spectra are shown in Fig. 7.4. Perception of different colours depends on light of a particular wavelength causing different degrees of excitation of the three cone types.

The threshold sensitivity of the eye to dim light depends on the wavelength and on whether the eye is adapted for night vision (**scotopia**) or day

Table 7.1 Ways in which rods differ from cones.

Rods	Cones
120×10^6 per eye	8×10^6 per eye
Not found in the fovea, but fairly evenly distributed throughout the rest of the eye	Red- and green-sensitive cones highly concentrated in the fovea, and blue-sensitive cones near the fovea
High sensitivity to light; longer outer segments, relatively more photopigment	Lower sensitivity; shorter outer segments, relatively less photopigment
Used for night vision; pigment is fully bleached in bright light so that rods are inoperative in daytime	Used for daytime vision
Many rods linked to each retinal ganglion cell so that receptive fields are larger, hence relatively lower acuity	Smaller receptive fields, especially in fovea where limit is diameter of one cone (~2 μm)
Do not give colour sensation	Give colour sensation
Pigment (rhodopsin) is in membranous discs inside the rod outer segment	Pigment (red-, green- or blue-sensitive) is incorporated in folds of the cone outer segment membrane
Sensitive to light rays with wide angle of incidence, including those traversing the periphery of the lens	Greater directional sensitivity, less sensitive to light rays traversing the periphery of the lens

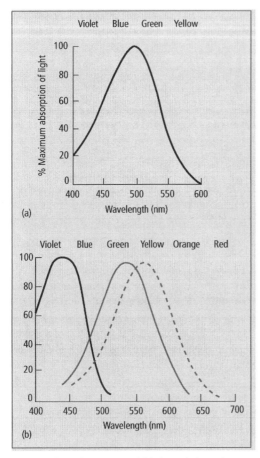

(a)

(b)

Fig. 7.4 Absorption spectra of (a) the rod photopigment and (b) the three cone photopigments.

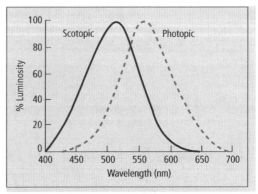

Fig. 7.5 Relative sensitivity to different wavelengths of light for eyes that are dark-adapted (scotopic vision) and light-adapted (photopic vision). The scotopic sensitivity is measured by adjusting the luminosity of light of different colours until the intensity matches that of a reference light. Photopic sensitivity is measured in a similar manner using a **flicker photometer** where the reference and test lights alternate at a frequency of 20 Hz so that differences in colours are not noticed.

foveal region, can act as waveguides, so that once a photon has entered the outer segment it will be internally reflected, maximizing its chances of being absorbed by photopigment. Absorption of a photon results in isomerization of the chromophore retinal from 11-*cis* (which binds to opsin) to all-*trans* (which does not bind to opsin). Isomerization starts a series of reactions ending in separation of retinal from opsin, a process known as **bleaching**. The all-*trans* retinal is transported to the pigment epithelium where it is regenerated to the 11-*cis* isomer.

Adaptation

The sensitivity of the eye depends on the ambient light intensity. When moving from a light environment into a darker one, there is a gradual increase in sensitivity, allowing dimmer lights to be seen, a mechanism known as **dark adaptation** (Fig. 7.6). This has four principal components:

1 pupil dilation, which can account for up to a 16-fold increase in sensitivity;

2 neural changes mediated by amacrine cells in the retina resulting in retinal neurones becoming

vision (**photopia**). The scotopic spectral luminosity curve (Fig. 7.5) shows maximum sensitivity to light of wavelength 507 nm, and is characteristic of the absorption spectrum of rhodopsin, while the photopic spectral luminosity curve (Fig. 7.5) has a peak at 555 nm and is characteristic of the combined absorption spectra of the three cone pigments. Thus, in scotopic vision the eye is most sensitive to green, while in photopic vision it is most sensitive to yellow. The shift from scotopic vision to photopic is called the **Purkinje shift**.

The outer segments of rods and cones are long narrow thread-like structures 2 μm in diameter. They sometimes, particularly in the cones in the

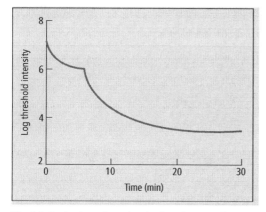

Fig. 7.6 Dark adaptation. The absolute threshold for perception of light, measured at different times after entering a dark room. The inflection in the biphasic curve reflects the time at which rod vision becomes more sensitive than cone vision. Note the logarithmic scale for the threshold; overall sensitivity increases by 5 orders of magnitude.

more excitable and the inhibitory components of receptive fields being suppressed;

3 an increase in **receptor sensitivity** due to regeneration of photopigments from their bleached forms, a process requiring less than 10 min in cones and about 30 min in rods; and

4 a decrease in **residual activation** of the cascade from bleached photopigments ('dark–light'). This can explain why dark adaptation can occur following flashes that bleach less than 3% of pigment.

Sensitivity is limited by the amount of pigment available; rods are fully bleached in daylight. On entering a dark environment, regeneration of photopigments starts, but since rods contain more photopigment than cones they take longer to regenerate fully. Therefore dark adaptation has two components, with an inflection in the curve at the time when rods become more sensitive than cones (Fig. 7.6). The overall change in sensitivity is by a factor of about 10^5 occurring over 30 min, of which a smaller fraction is due to dilation of the pupil and neural mechanisms within the retina, and most to regeneration of photopigment. A much faster (3–5 min) period of **light adaptation** occurs when going from a dark environment into a brighter one, resulting from pupil constriction and bleaching of photopigments.

After-images

Visual sensations outlast the stimulus, allowing us to perceive a series of images (e.g. a movie) as continuous smooth action. This reflects the bleaching of photopigment briefly outlasting the stimulus, and can be illustrated by applying a bright stimulus as a single brief flash. If you then regard a white or pale grey background you perceive first a positive and then a negative after-image, the positive due to photo-pigment bleaching and the negative due to neural mechanisms, fatigue and surround inhibition. Negative after-images are seen as complementary (opponent) colours; dark for a bright image, red for a green image, and so on. Movement and pattern after-images can also be demonstrated using appropriate stimuli, such as a rotating spiral.

The **critical fusion frequency**, the frequency at which a flickering stimulus appears to be continuous, depends on the frequency of action potentials fired by retinal ganglion cells. In dim light, when action potential frequency is relatively low, it may be less than 10 Hz, but in bright light it may range up to more than 60 Hz. This enables us to perceive the intermittently presented images in films and television as continuous.

Receptor potential

Photoreceptors are depolarized in the dark, and the bleaching of photopigment by light induces a **hyperpolarizing** receptor potential. The outer membrane of the outer segment contains cyclic guanosine monophosphate (cGMP)-gated ion channels (selective for Na^+ and Ca^{2+}) responsible for the receptor potential. In the dark, the cGMP-gated channels are open, allowing a steady current to enter (Fig. 7.7). This inward current keeps the cell depolarized, near –40 mV, and the transmitter (glutamate) is continually released from the synaptic terminal. Light closes the outer segment channels, the membrane hyperpolarizes and transmitter release decreases.

During normal photopic vision, light induces a hyperpolarizing receptor potential and dark a depolarizing receptor potential—a dark object on a lighter background can be considered an

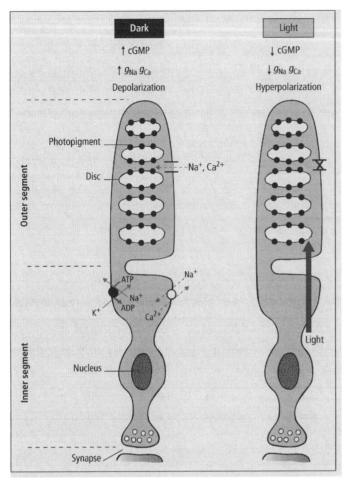

Fig. 7.7 Current flow in a rod photoreceptor cell in response to dark and light. The outer segment is packed with membrane discs containing photopigment while the inner segment contains the nucleus and bulk of the cytoplasm. In the dark the cGMP levels increase, Na^+/Ca^{2+} ion channels open and Na^+ and Ca^{2+} ions flow into the outer segment, depolarizing the cell. Na^+ and Ca^{2+} ions diffuse from the outer to the inner segment where they are removed by the Na^+,K^+–ATPase/sodium pump and by Na^+–Ca^{2+} exchange, respectively. In the light the cGMP levels decrease and Na^+/Ca^{2+} ion channels close, hyperpolarizing the cell.

excitatory visual stimulus—by way of a complex sequence of reactions.

Light-triggered cGMP cascade

The membranous discs in the outer segments of rods, and the equivalent membrane folds in cones, contain three major proteins: visual pigment (**retinal** plus **opsin**); a G protein called **transducin**; and **cGMP phosphodiesterase**. Upon absorbing a photon, 11-*cis* retinal isomerizes and triggers a series of conformational changes in the protein part of the visual pigment molecule. The isomerized molecule is free to diffuse laterally in the membrane and can activate a number of molecules of transducin. This catalyses the exchange of guanosine diphosphate (GDP) for guanosine triphosphate (GTP) on the α subunit of transducin. The binding of GTP causes liberation of an active α-GTP subunit, which in turn disinhibits cGMP phosphodiesterase leading to rapid hydrolysis of cGMP, with the result that a single photon hitting a rod can close about 300 outer-segment ion channels. The mechanisms by which the light response is terminated are not fully understood. They include phosphorylation of isomerized rhodopsin to inactivate it, and hydrolysis of the α-GTP subunit to α-GDP. For reasons that are as yet not fully understood, amplification in the cone cascade is much less, with more photons being required to give the same response.

In the dark, Na^+ and Ca^{2+} enter the outer segment through the cGMP-gated conductance channels (Fig. 7.7). Na^+ accumulating in the outer segment diffuses into the inner segment, where it is removed by the Na^+–K^+ pump (Na^+, K^+–ATPase); Ca^{2+} ions are removed by the Na^+–Ca^{2+} exchange carrier. In the dark, elevation of the concentration of cGMP increases the influx of Ca^{2+}. Increased concentrations of Ca^{2+} result in an inhibition of the enzyme controlling the synthesis of cGMP (guanylate cyclase), thus lowering cGMP; this therefore provides negative feedback control of cGMP levels. Conversely, in the light, as the cGMP-regulated channels close, Ca^{2+} continues to be removed and its concentration becomes reduced, allowing cGMP levels to increase. This system is involved in adaptation to light, and it stabilizes levels of cGMP in the dark so that only 1–2% of the cGMP-regulated channels are open, reducing the load on the photoreceptor cell metabolism.

The cGMP-regulated channel openings in the outer segment are unitary events with a mean duration of about 1 ms and a unit conductance of about 0.1 pS. This small effective conductance ensures that the amplitude of dark current noise (spontaneous channel openings due to random thermal motion) is small compared to the electrical signal resulting from reception of a photon, thereby allowing detection of single photons.

Electro-oculogram and electroretinogram

There is a steady potential difference of about 6 mV between the cornea (positive) and the posterior portion of the interior of the eye—the fundus (negative)—generated predominantly across the pigment epithelium. As a result of this potential difference, electrodes placed on the skin at each side of the eye detect a change in potential when the eye is moved in a horizontal direction. The record so obtained during eye movements is called an **electro-oculogram**.

Illumination of the eye causes a series of smaller changes detected between an electrode on the cornea and an indifferent electrode. This is known as an **electroretinogram** and its early part reflects electrical activity within the receptors.

Retina and visual pathways

Light has to pass through three layers of retinal neurones to reach the photoreceptors. A change in photoreceptor potential is transmitted to the ganglion cells, either directly via bipolar cells or indirectly via horizontal and amacrine cells. Action potentials are not generated until the ganglion cells are reached. Axons from the ganglion cells converge at the optic disc (blind spot) and travel in the optic nerve to the lateral geniculate nucleus; those from the nasal half of each retina cross over (decussate) at the optic chiasm, while those from the temporal halves stay on the same side. In primates, the vast majority of ganglion cell axons synapse with cells in the magnocellular and parvocellular layers of the lateral geniculate nucleus. These cells project to the visual cortex to give rise to the conscious sensation of vision. Other ganglion cells target different parts of the lateral geniculate nucleus, or other subcortical nuclei (e.g. superior colliculus) as part of various visual reflexes (e.g. for eye movements, pupillary dilation and lens accommodation). Different aspects of vision can be identified, such as movement, texture, stereoscopic vision, colour, high-acuity perception of form and contours. Different parts of the brain show different degrees of specialization for these aspects of vision. The old idea that they could be simply related to differences in the subcortical properties of the magnocellular and parvocellular systems has been challenged. It is now clear that there is considerable intermingling of the two systems in the cortex.

The retina

The retina is an outgrowth of the brain and, in addition to the photoreceptors (rods and cones), contains four other types of neurone: **bipolar** cells, **horizontal** cells, **amacrine** cells and **ganglion** cells. It is composed of three cellular layers with two synaptic (plexiform) layers interposed between them (Fig. 7.8). Light passes through the retina to reach the photoreceptors (rods and cones) at its outer surface; these are the only light-sensitive cells in the retina. Behind the neural layer

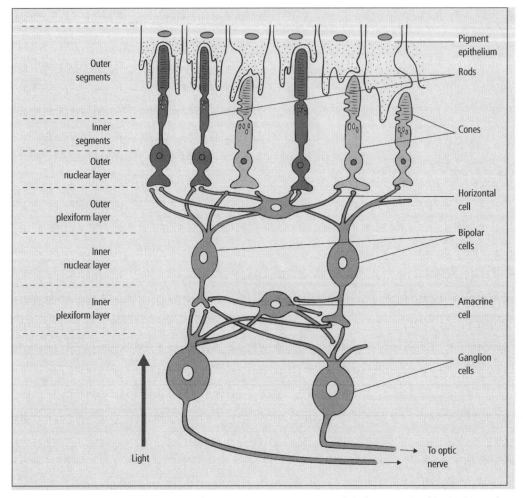

Fig. 7.8 Cellular layers of the retina. (Adapted from Dowling, J.E. & Boycott, B.B. (1966) *Proc Roy Soc (B)*, **166**, 80–111.)

of the retina lies the **pigment epithelium**. This absorbs stray light, preventing blurring of the image, and is involved in the metabolism of visual pigments (see p. 141). In patients with **retinitis pigmentosa**, pigment-containing cells migrate into the neural layer. This retinal degenerative disease has been linked to genetic defects in the metabolism of the chromophore component of visual pigments.

There are no photoreceptors overlying the optic disc and therefore light falling on it cannot be seen, hence the term **blind spot**. At the fovea, where visual acuity is greatest, the orderly layering of the retina is modified with neural elements—other than cones—displaced to the sides, and retinal blood vessels absent.

All signals originating in photoreceptors must pass to ganglion cells via bipolar cells, which are part of both **direct** (photoreceptor → bipolar → ganglion cell) and **indirect** (photoreceptor → horizontal or bipolar → amacrine → ganglion cell) pathways (Fig. 7.8). Horizontal cells contact photoreceptors over a relatively wide area, and are electrically coupled to one another via gap junctions; every photoreceptor is contacted by a horizontal cell. In primates, outputs from horizontal cells are not well known, and may be directed back to photoreceptors or bipolar cells, or to both. There are at least 20 types of amacrine cells, which link bipolar and ganglion cells, providing alternative, indirect routes between them. Amacrine cells are involved in a number of complex circuits, which give individual ganglion cells particular receptive field properties.

Bipolar cell receptive fields are circular, detecting differences in luminance between an inner circle and a surrounding annulus (see Fig. 7.13); they detect spatial **contrast** in the image. Those excited by light in the centre of their receptive field are named **ON-bipolar cells** and those excited by dark in the centre of their receptive field as **OFF-bipolar cells**. Direct connections from bipolars to ganglion cells are all excitatory, so ON-centre bipolars supply ON-centre ganglion cells, and OFF-centre bipolars supply OFF-centre ganglion cells. Photoreceptors, bipolars and horizontal cells do not fire action potentials (some amacrine cells may); the first action potential in the direct pathway occurs at the ganglion cell.

Ganglion cells

Ganglion cells are the only output cells from the retina; their axons (about 10^6) leave the eye at the optic disc to form the optic nerve. Ganglion cell axons are unmyelinated and hence transparent until they reach the optic nerve, where most become myelinated. They project in the optic nerve to two major subcortical visual centres, the **superior colliculus** and the **lateral geniculate nucleus** (LGN). The pathway to the superior colliculus is concerned with eye movements and orientation to visual stimuli; that to the LGN projects to the cortex and is concerned with the sensation of vision. There is partial crossover of the optic nerve fibres; those from the nasal halves of the retinas cross, while those from the temporal halves remain ipsilateral, so that visual stimuli in the left halves of the visual fields of both eyes excite the right visual cortex and *vice versa* (Fig. 7.9).

Ganglion cells respond to a variety of different properties of the stimulus. Some respond to objects brighter than the background, others to darker, generally with on–off circular-shaped fields (see Fig. 7.13). Some give sustained responses, some transient; some are colour-coded, some are not, and so on. They can be classified into three main groups: M, P and 'others'. The M cells (Fig. 7.10a), which comprise about 16% of the total ganglion cell population, are relatively large, with wide dendritic fields and fast-conducting myelinated axons in the optic nerve. They are most sensitive to

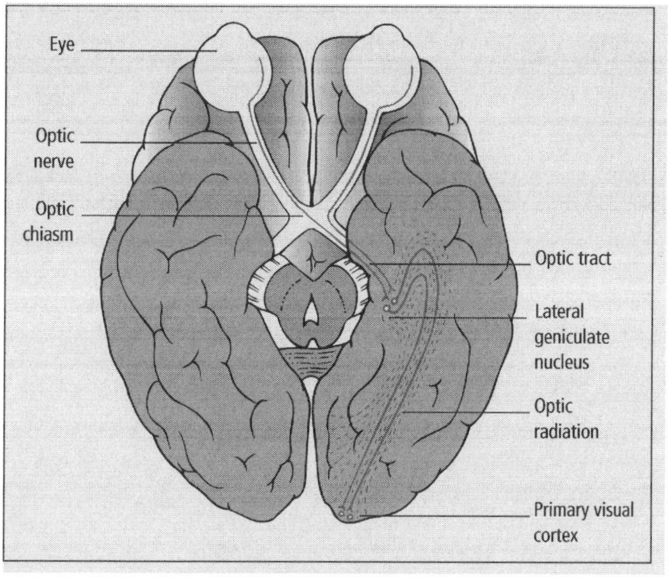

Fig. 7.9 The visual pathway and visual area 1, as viewed from below. Images from the right field of view fall on the left hemiretinas of the two eyes, and these project, via the optic nerve, optic chiasm (where axons from the nasal half of each eye cross over and those from the temporal half stay on the same side), lateral geniculate nucleus and optic radiation, to visual area 1 in the left cortical hemisphere.

Labels in figure: Eye, Optic nerve, Optic chiasm, Optic tract, Lateral geniculate nucleus, Optic radiation, Primary visual cortex

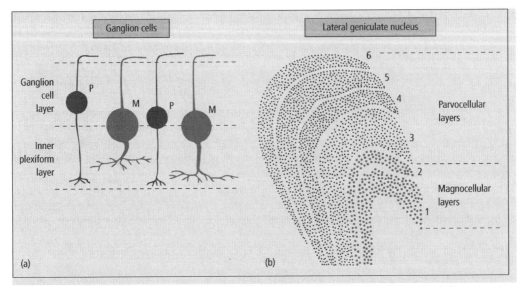

Fig. 7.10 (a) M and P ganglion cells in the retina and (b) the magnocellular and parvocellular layers of the left lateral geniculate nucleus cut in the frontal plane. (Adapted from Perry, V.H., Silveira, L. & Cowey, A. (1990) *Ciba Symp*, **155**, 5–14.)

relatively low spatial frequencies, have high contrast sensitivity, are very sensitive to movement and do not respond to colour contrasts. The P cells are smaller with relatively small dendritic fields and slower-conducting myelinated axons; they are most sensitive to high spatial frequencies, have poor contrast sensitivity, and show colour opponency. The 'others' have been classified on morphological grounds into at least 10 types but their functional properties are less well characterized.

The M ganglion cells project to the **magnocellular** layers of the LGN; the P ganglion cells project to the **parvocellular** layers of the LGN (Fig. 7.10b). Many of the 'others' also project to the LGN, including one type (blue-ON, yellow-OFF) that projects to the **koniocellular** layers of the LGN, which are thin layers interdigitated between the parvocellular and magnocellular layers. Ganglion cells project to a variety of nuclei, including the superior colliculus (reflexes involving attention to movement), the suprachiasmatic nuclei (involved in diurnal rhythms), ventral LGN (part of the reflex pathway regulating the size of the pupil), pretectal complex (concerned with the near response, i.e. vergence, miosis and accommodation), and the accessory optic system (projecting to the dorsal,

lateral and medial terminal nuclei in the midbrain and mediating eye movement reflexes).

Divisions of the visual system

The LGN has six major layers comprising two ventral magnocellular layers (1 and 2) and four dorsal parvocellular layers (3–6; Fig. 7.10b), which receive inputs from M and P ganglion cells, respectively. These layers receive inputs from either the ipsilateral eye (layers 2, 3 and 5) or contralateral eye (layers 1, 4 and 6). There are also six thin koniocellular layers interdigitated between the major layers.

The magnocellular and parvocellular divisions in the LGN perform different tasks in analysing visual information from the retina. The question remains—does this division persist in the rest of the visual pathway? It used to be thought that there were three processing streams leaving striate cortex; one fed by the magnocellular division, processing information pertaining to movement and stereoscopic vision and two fed by the parvocellular system, processing information pertaining either to colour, or to shape (form). The latter streams correspond to the so-called blob regions of the visual cortex that contain high levels of cytochrome oxidase (Figs 7.11 & 7.12), and to the interblob regions. It is now thought that there are just two streams; one associated with the blobs and one associated with interblobs. However, it is also clear that all three geniculate divisions (magno-, parvo- and koniocellular) project to both blobs and interblobs. Furthermore, the functional properties of the streams are much less categorical, particularly in the distinction between colour and form — cells selective for both colour and orientation are common in striate cortex.

Regions of cerebral cortex involved in vision

At least a third of the human cortex is thought to be involved in processing visual information, reflecting the profound influence of visual sensation in human perception. The **primary visual cortex** (V1; also known as the striate cortex), which is located in the occipital cortex on the walls of the calcarine fissure, receives inputs from LGN (Fig. 7.9). The entire contralateral visual field is represented, ending precisely at the vertical meridian. Other visual areas, V2–5, are located in the peristriate and

more anterior cortex and are concerned with different aspects of visual perception. Thus V4 appears to specialize for colour contrast and V5/MT for motion detection but both areas contain neurones selective for stereopsis. Many of these areas during visual activation can now be observed directly in human and non-human primates by magnetic resonance imaging.

Processing visual information

Retinal and lateral geniculate cells have centre-surround receptive fields, while most neurones in the visual cortex respond to more complex stimuli. Uniform illumination of the whole receptive field gives, on average, little excitation; neurones respond best to contrasts in illumination. Some neurones in the visual cortex are stimulated best by the bars or edges of a particular orientation or spatial frequency, or by specific colours, or by movement. Information about the disparity of images on the two retinas is used to give stereoscopic perception of depth and distance. Neurones of the visual cortex with closely related functions are arranged anatomically in radial columns with cells

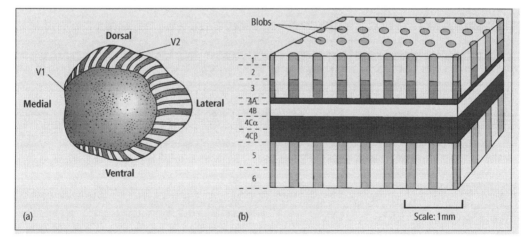

Fig. 7.11 Distribution of cytochrome oxidase-positive regions in visual areas 1 and 2 of the monkey visual cortex. (a) A section of monkey cortex cut parallel to the surface, showing blobs in V1 and thick and thin stripes and pale interstripes in V2. (b) Schematic representation of the three-dimensional distribution of cytochrome oxidase-rich cells in V1. The blobs are found in all layers except layer 4; they are most obvious in layer 3, as indicated by the gradation in the degree of stippling. (From Tootell, R.B.H. *et al.* (1988) *J Neurosci*, **8**, 1500–30.)

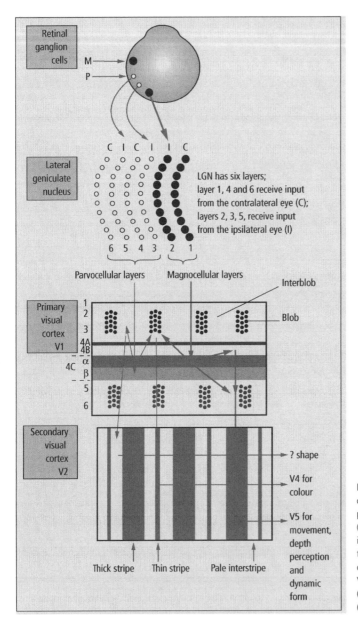

Retinal ganglion cells

M

P

Lateral geniculate nucleus

C I C I I C

LGN has six layers; layer 1, 4 and 6 receive input from the contralateral eye (C); layers 2, 3, 5, receive input from the ipsilateral eye (I)

6 5 4 3 2 1

Parvocellular layers   Magnocellular layers

Interblob

Primary visual cortex V1

1 2 3 4A 4B 4C α β 5 6

Blob

Secondary visual cortex V2

? shape

V4 for colour

V5 for movement, depth perception and dynamic form

Thick stripe   Thin stripe   Pale interstripe

FIG. 7.12 Diagrammatic illustration of the magnocellular and parvocellular pathways from retina to visual cortex (see text for explanation). The shading in the bottom half of the figure illustrates the distribution of cytochrome oxidase staining, showing blobs in V1 and thick and thin stripes in V2. (Adapted from Livingstone, M.S. (1988) *Sci Am*, **258**, 68–75.)

responding to the same region of the retina, dominated by the same eye and sharing the same orientation or colour preference. These columns are arranged in groups (hypercolumns) in such a way that a small region of the visual cortex receives inputs from all possible receptive fields belonging to a small region of visual space.

Parallel processing

Information processing is carried out in both a hierarchical and parallel manner. A hierarchically ordered series of ascending connections, from lower to higher centres (e.g. retina to thalamus to cortex), explains the responses of many cells to specific stimuli. At each stage the relatively simple properties of individual cells combine to form a picture of increasing complexity. In addition, information concerned with different aspects of visual perception, e.g. colour, high-acuity vision, movement, stereoscopic depth and periodic pattern detection, is carried along separate parallel paths.

Separation into parallel pathways carrying different components also starts in the retina (e.g. with different receptors and ganglion cells), is maintained in the LGN (magnocellular and parvocellular divisions) and is seen in the cerebral cortex where new divisions emerge (Fig. 7.12). The magnocellular pathway projects to layer 4Cα and the parvocellular division projects to layer 4Cβ. Both 4Cα and 4Cβ then project to layers 4B, 4A and 3/2, so mixing inputs from the magnocellular and parvoclluualr divisions in the blobs and interblobs of the upper cortical layers. The blob regions of the primary visual cortex (V1) to the thin stripes of the secondary visual cortex (V2), and the interblob regions project to both the thick stripes and interstripes of V2. Both thin stripes and interstripes project to V4 whereas the thick stripes project to V5/MT. Recent recording studies in V2 show that neurones selective for colour are relatively more common in the thin stripes, and neurones selective for orientation are more common in the thick stripes and interstripes; but on an individual neuroneal basis there is no correlation between colour selectivity and orientation selectivity. The relative distribution of directionally selective neurones is less clear cut. Although there is good evidence for parallel retino–geniculate pathways and the involvement of different cortical regions in the analysis of different aspects of visual sensation, there are also extensive interconnections between the different regions. This is considered important for providing overall integration, usually referred to as **binding**, of visual sensation and perception.

Receptive fields

A cell is defined as being part of the visual system if it responds to visual stimuli presented to the eye. 'Receptive field' is an abstract concept, being more than just an area of visual space within which a stimulus will affect the cell. 'Receptive field' in this context includes the pattern of the stimulus, which will alter the response of the cell: that is, the shape, colour, orientation, movement, direction and binocularity of the effective stimulus. For cells early in the visual pathway, the receptive field map can predict the optimal stimulus (e.g. the simple ON-centre, OFF-surround of ganglion cells; see below). For many cells, the receptive field map does not predict the optimal stimulus (e.g. cortical complex cells; see below).

Centre-surround receptive fields

Retinal ganglion cells and LGN neurones have centre-surround receptive fields. Many cells have action potentials even in the dark; small light or dark spots presented within the receptive area may increase or decrease the frequency of action potentials. Excitatory and inhibitory regions of the receptive field are arranged in the form of an annulus surrounding a central circle (Fig. 7.13). If a bright spot stimulates the central region (ON-centre unit), then light will inhibit the surround. Conversely, if a dark spot stimulates the central region (an OFF-centre unit), then dark will inhibit the surround. Units with centre-surround receptive fields give little or no response to uniform stimulation throughout their field; they respond only to **contrasts** in illumination. In consequence, signals in the optic nerves are primarily responses to **differences** in illumination within the visual fields, while constancies must be inferred by the visual centres in the brain. This allows a high degree of economy in the amount of information needed to form a visual perception. It also limits the size of a visual object within which differences in luminance can be detected.

The retina and LGN also possess colour-sensitive units, with centre-surround receptive fields to spectrally opponent colours, for example, red centre, green surround and *vice versa*.

Orientation sensitivity

Some neurones in layer 4 of V1 have centre-surround receptive fields, but the majority of cells in other layers respond to contours, or to contrasts in

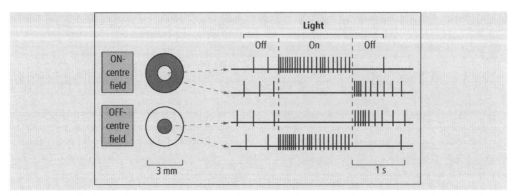

Fig. 7.13 Receptive fields of retinal ganglion cells and of neurones in the LGN. Most receptive fields at these levels have a centre-surround arrangement. Most cells, when impaled with a microelectrode, are observed to fire irregularly, even in complete darkness. ON-centre units are excited by a light spot in the central region of their receptive field and are inhibited when the light spot is moved to the surrounding annulus. When the light spot in the surrounding annulus is turned off, there is a brief period of excitation. OFF-centre units show the opposite pattern of responses. The centre and surround regions interact in an antagonistic way and so uniform illumination gives little or no response.

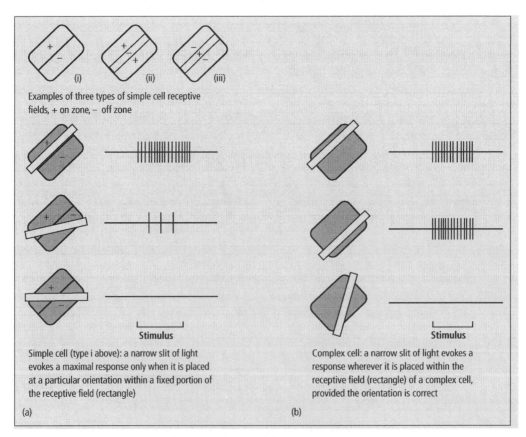

Fig. 7.14 Receptive fields of neurones in the visual cortex. (a) Simple cell responses to a bar of light. (b) Complex cell responses. (c) (*opposite*) Comparison of complex and end-stopped complex cell responses.

either colour or luminance, which have straight edges and usually lie at particular orientations. Receptive fields of characteristic neurones in the visual cortex are shown in Fig. 7.14.

Simple cells respond to bars or edges with a particular orientation and with a particular optimum width within a fixed portion of visual space (Fig. 7.14a).

Complex cells respond to bars or edges with particular orientations and with a particular optimum width, but placed anywhere within a larger region of visual space (Fig. 7.14b).

End-stopped cells may be simple or complex.

They have the particular property that they are inhibited if the contour to which they respond extends outside a certain limited region of their receptive field (Fig. 7.14c). This property means that these cells are stimulated by contours only if they end within their receptive field, or if they change in direction. End-stopped cells respond, therefore, to discontinuities in contour, such as corners, curves and ends of lines.

Colour sensitivity

Colour-sensitive cells have recently been shown also to be sensitive to orientation. Single opponent

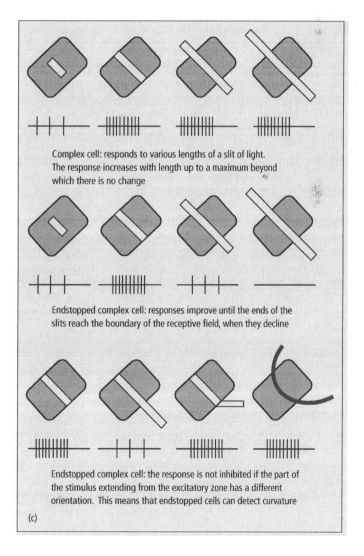

Complex cell: responds to various lengths of a slit of light. The response increases with length up to a maximum beyond which there is no change

Endstopped complex cell: responses improve until the ends of the slits reach the boundary of the receptive field, when they decline

Endstopped complex cell: the response is not inhibited if the part of the stimulus extending from the excitatory zone has a different orientation. This means that endstopped cells can detect curvature

(c)

Fig. 7.14 *Continued.*

cells, as seen at the level of retinal P ganglion cell or LGN, are excited by one colour in their centre and by the opponent colour in their surround (e.g. red centre/green surround or blue centre/yellow surround). Some cortical cells do not respond to luminance boundaries—they have cone-opponent receptive fields. Other cells can respond to both chromatic and luminance boundaries; these are double-opponent cells, which are excited by one colour and inhibited by its opponent in their receptive field centres, and inhibited by the colour and excited by its opponent in their surrounds. Some cortical cells respond only to luminance boundaries, they show no cone opponency.

Disparity

Disparity-sensitive neurones give their optimum response to stimuli presented at slightly disparate points on the two retinas, and are thought to have a role in stereoscopic perception of depth and distance. **Far** neurones are excited by disparate points past the fixation point and inhibited by those nearer, whereas **near** neurones behave in the opposite fashion. **Flat** neurones are not disparity-selective, and give similar responses to stimuli at varying distances within the disparity range of binocular interaction.

Columnar arrangement of visual cortex

Neurones in the visual cortex are arranged in radial columns, in which all cells have closely related functions. Within V1 several types of columns associated with different aspects of the visual response can be recognized.

Ocular dominance columns

The left half of each visual field projects to the right half of each retina, divided down the vertical meridian (Fig. 7.9). This in turn projects to V1 in the right hemisphere. The opposite is true for the right half of each visual field, which projects to the left hemisphere. Corresponding regions of each retina project to closely adjacent neurones in appropriate regions of V1, and these neurones are arranged in ocular dominance columns (Fig. 7.15); that is, cells in one column respond preferentially to inputs from one eye. Columns with the same ocular dominance are arranged in short lines or stripes approximately 400–500 μm wide. A microelectrode passing radially through the cortex might successively record signals from 50 different neurones, but all these neurones would have a dominant input from one eye. If the microelectrode was moved sideways by a millimetre, and the recording repeated, it might now register a series of neurones dominated by the other eye, all with receptive fields in the same small region of visual space.

Orientation columns

Neurones within a cortical orientation column (approximately 50–100 μm wide) share the same orientation preference, although they may be simple, complex or end-stopped. If the recording electrode is moved sideways a few tens of microns, the orientation preference would change by 15–30° in a progressive and orderly manner, coming full circle within a millimetre (Fig. 7.16). Both ocular dominance and orientation columns are arranged in orderly rows, but these are not congruent with one another, so that if you recorded along a row of cells with a common orientation preference, ocular dominance would shift alternatively from one eye to the next, and receptive fields would appear in adjacent regions of visual space.

Cytochrome oxidase blobs

Cells in the blobs form columns (Fig. 7.11) concerned with processing of colour; orientation columns lie in the interblob regions. Both blob and interblob cells form part of ocular dominance stripes.

Hypercolumns

The orderly arrangement of V1 into orientation or ocular dominance stripes or colour-sensitive blobs has the consequence that a small region of cortex, a square millimetre or so in area, will receive inputs from all possible receptive fields within a small

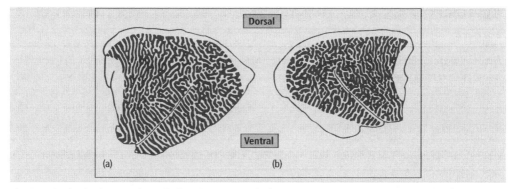

Fig. 7.15 Ocular dominance columns in the striate cortex (VI) of a monkey as revealed by autoradiography of sections tangential to the exposed surface of (a) the left and (b) the right occipital lobes. The dark stripes are metabolically active areas, as revealed by the radioactive 2-deoxyglucose technique, and correspond to input from one eye while the other eye is masked. Note the alternating pattern of inputs from each eye; each stripe corresponds to an ocular dominance column. (From Tootell, R.B.H. *et al.* (1988) *J Neurosci*, **8**, 1500–30.)

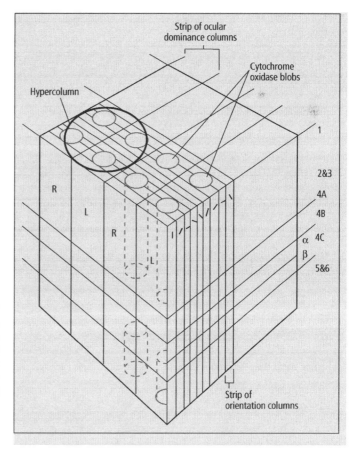

Fig. 7.16 Modular arrangement of cortex in visual area 1. A small region of cortex, constituting a hypercolumn, contains columns of cells of all possible orientation preferences, with left or right eye dominance, and cytochrome oxidase blobs containing cells devoted to analysis of colour. (From Livingston, M.S. & Hubel, D.H. (1984) *J Neurosci*, **4**, 309–56.)

region of visual space. This region is a hypercolumn, responsible for the primary processing of visual information from this space (Fig. 7.16). A hypercolumn contains cells with all possible orientation preferences from both eyes, and colour-sensitive neurones, receiving projections from a restricted region of visual space. An adjacent part on the retina (and hence of the visual space) is represented within an adjacent block of cortex. Thus the whole visual field is analysed in an orderly topographic arrangement.

Recent evidence indicates that this columnar organization is a feature of higher visual areas as well as V1.

High-acuity vision

High-acuity analysis of contour and form is a function of the parvocellular system. Acuity is not limited by optics, but by the resolving power of the retina. In the fovea the limit to visual acuity is set by the distance between two cones—about 2.5 μm or 0.5′ (~0.01°) of arc. Away from the fovea, receptive fields get larger, involving groups of cones, and acuity is correspondingly lower.

For routine clinical purposes, one measures acuity using a **Snellen chart** in which letters of the alphabet are arranged in lines and the size of the letters in each line is such that the details of the letters each subtend 1′ of arc at defined distances from the eye. The test is usually conducted at 6 m from the chart to exclude the effects of accommodation, and the line of smallest letters that the subject can correctly read is determined. Visual acuity is expressed as a fraction in which the numerator is the testing distance (6 m) and the denominator is the distance at which details of the smallest, correctly read letters subtend 1′ of arc. For a normal person this is 6/6. A myopic person could detect only larger letters, for example those subtending an angle of 1′ at a distance of 12 m (i.e. twice as big), giving a measure of acuity of 6/12.

Stereoscopic vision

When viewing an object with binocular vision, accommodation and convergence of our eyes causes the image to focus on corresponding portions of each retina. Any part of the object that is nearer or further from the fixation point will project an image that is at some distance in the horizontal direction from the point of focus (Fig. 7.17). However, the two eyes view the object from slightly different positions and the image of the object does not fall exactly on corresponding positions of the two retinas. This difference depends on the distance of the object from the fixation point and is referred to as **binocular disparity**. Stereoscopy

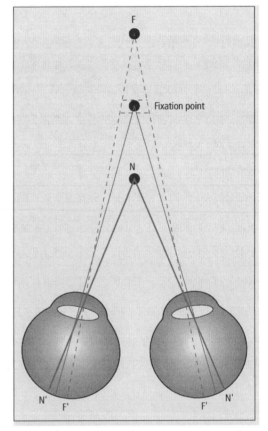

Fig. 7.17 Binocular vision—the image of an object is focused on corresponding points of the two retinas. When our eyes are fixed on one part of an object, images from more distant regions (F) will project to regions nasal to the corresponding points (F′); those from closer regions (N) will project to regions temporal to the corresponding points (N′).

involves the use of this binocular disparity to give rise to three-dimensional perception. With knowledge of disparity at the two retinas, an estimate of distance can be made from the geometry of the situation. Stereopsis is a basic function of vision, and does not require recognition of objects. There are also monocular cues for depth perception (as can be determined by closing one eye) including relative size of objects, occlusion/superposition, parallax, perspective, shadow casting (e.g. to distinguish pits and bumps), texture gradients, rotation and the relative movement of parts of an object, and awareness of the need to accommodate.

Colour vision

'Light' is defined as the spectrum of electromagnetic energy that we can see (wavelengths 400–700 nm). Light with a uniform mixture of wavelengths is seen as white (we may also see a mixture of two monochromatic lights as white). A pigment absorbs some light and reflects the rest and the pigment appears the colour of the reflected light. Green leaves, for example, absorb long- and short-wavelength light, and reflect the middle wavelengths.

Humans can discriminate about 100 variations of wavelength and 30–80 variations of spectral purity of each wavelength, even when stimuli have been equated for luminance. In other words, several-thousand colour combinations can be discriminated at a constant level of luminance, compared with about 30 discriminable variations in intensity contrast. We are colour-blind in dim light (scotopic vision).

Visual receptors

We have three types of cones, with peak absorptions at 420 ('blue', actually violet), 530 ('green', actually green) and 560 nm ('red', actually yellow–red; Fig. 7.4b). The rod pigment, rhodopsin, reflects blue and red and therefore looks purple, with peak absorption in the green. The three cone types have broad sensitivity curves with much overlap and the sensation of colour depends on the extent to which each is excited. When all three types of cone are stimulated equally, the light is perceived as white.

Inherited variation in human colour vision

Individuals with normal colour vision can match any spectral colour by using a mixture of the three primary colours, and are known as **trichromats**. About 8% of males and 0.5% of females differ from the majority in the proportions of the three primary colours needed to match a given colour. These fall into two classes: **dichromats** and **anomalous trichromats**. Dichromats have lost one of the three systems and therefore require only two primary colours to match any spectral colour. Anomalous trichromats have a reduction in the spectral sensitivity of one of the systems. Dichromats and anomalous trichromats are then divided into three types depending on whether the blue, green or red cone systems are defective. Loss or reduction in the red or green systems is most common and causes difficulty in distinguishing between these two colours; defects in the blue system are rare.

Colour contrast

Although colour perception depends initially on the activity of the three types of cones, colour is subsequently recoded into four colours, in two opponent pairs—red against green and blue against yellow. This colour **opponency** is illustrated by the fact that we cannot perceive reddish green or blueish yellow colours. Moreover, opponent colours enhance each other; for example, a green object stands out more against a red than a blue background. Each pair of opponent colours appears to be analysed separately, beginning in the retina and continuing in the LGN and visual cortex. This may be explained in part by the properties of double opponent cells in the visual cortex.

Colour constancy

Colour is a perception, not a measure of the wavelength of light, and the trichromat theory refers to the receptors for colour vision, not to processes in the visual cortex. The perceived 'colour' of an object is changed little when the colour or intensity of illumination is altered; for example, an apple seen in daylight or in candlelight appears red even though the wavelength of light reflected from the apple changes. Conversely, in a monochrome environment, for example an experimental room with uniform illumination at some particular wavelength, it is not possible to give an accurate description of its colour; in fact, it is likely to be described as white or light grey regardless of its illumination. Colour constancy appears to derive by comparing the relative activities of red, green and blue cones stimulated by light emitted by the object of regard with the wavelength composition of light from the surrounding visual field. Land's retinex theory (retina and cortex combined) of colour vision proposes that the brain constructs three independent images—one carried by long waves, one carried by middle waves, and one carried by short waves—and by comparing these the perception of colour is derived. Neurones in V4 display colour constancy. This property of colour vision is essential for object recognition.

Visual perception of movement

Perception of moving objects depends on specific processing within the visual system, and is the function of the magnocellular system. This system has about half the spatial resolution of the parvocellular system and is not sensitive to colour. The threshold for movement detection in humans depends on factors such as the angular velocity, the size, contrast and position of the moving stimulus, and on the duration of the movement.

The V5 cortical region is considered to be the 'movement centre' in the brain. In the monkey, most cells in this region respond to a movement in a certain direction, and preferred directions change systematically through the cortex. Other cells respond to rotating stimuli in a clockwise or anticlockwise direction. Complex movement-sensitive neurones may have very large receptive fields, responding to the same preferred direction and velocity anywhere within the visual field. Lesions in V5 lead to a specific loss of perception of

movement, without other defects in vision. For example, one patient with such a lesion said she was unable to pour a cup of tea as she could not see the moving fluid, and while she could walk between parked cars to cross the road, she could not see moving vehicles.

Development of vision

Ocular dominance columns and stereoacuity

Ocular dominance columns are not present during initial formation of projections from the LGN to V1, but appear in a dynamic fashion near the time of birth (in monkeys, and presumably human infants). Their formation and maintenance require synchronous use of both eyes, and they are fully formed in children by about 5 months of age. Similarly, depth perception is present in children by 4 months of age, and appears to be fully developed by 5 months. This may reflect the segregation of ocular dominance columns. By comparison, visual acuity improves rapidly during the first 6 months, but continues to improve for several years.

Critical periods in development

There is a period, beginning at birth, when deprivation of form vision has profound and permanent effects on visual function. In monkeys, this sensitivity reaches a peak at 2 weeks of age, and then tapers off over a period of about a year. Even a few days of deprivation at 2 weeks of age may have permanent effects. Children born with congenital cataracts that are not immediately corrected have profoundly defective vision.

In experimental animals (cats or monkeys) raised with one eye closed, lateral geniculate projections from the deprived eye form very few synaptic connections in V1. The damage is caused by form deprivation, not light deprivation, and the animal is behaviourally blind in the deprived eye. After a week or more of eye closure (at the peak critical period), opening the closed eye does not give rise to any recovery. If, at the same time, the previously open eye is closed and the monkey is still in its critical period, recovery does occur (but projections from the newly closed eye are suppressed).

Similarly, disturbances of binocular vision can occur, for example, with a squint (**amblyopia**) and have profound effects on the development of disparity-sensitive cells and hence on depth perception. Commonly in this situation, one eye becomes dominant and develops excess cortical connections while inputs from the other 'lazy' eye are suppressed.

In general the development of the visual system is tuned to visual experience. Animals raised in an environment with vertical black and white stripes, and deprived of other forms of visual experience, show an enlarged representation of the rearing orientation in V1. Animals brought up in an environment illuminated by flashes of a strobe light lack movement-sensitive neurones.

Focusing defects and eyeball size

Myopia and hypermetropia reflect anatomical defects in the size of the eye, the posterior chamber being too long or too short, respectively. At birth there is a large scatter between individuals in their ability to achieve accurate focus, with rapid growth towards emmetropia (normal eye length). This requires great accuracy in the anatomy of the eye, since depth of focus at the retina for a 5 mm pupil is only a few microns. Studies of the statistical distribution of eye focus within large groups of people show that the range is much narrower than would be expected, providing evidence for feedback control of growth of the eye.

There is much anecdotal evidence for eye growth being affected by environmental circumstances as well as the genetic background of the individual, for example, the Bedouin or American Indian with remarkable distance vision, or the extremely myopic Japanese or Talmudic scholar. There is also epidemiological evidence, such as a sudden increase in incidence of myopia in Eskimos with the coming of television, or the current 80% incidence of myopia in Taiwanese high-school pupils.

Animal experiments have demonstrated the existence of two mechanisms of developmental regulation of eye growth. One is local with a blurred image on a region of retina resulting in excessive growth in the adjacent region of the sclera. The other depends on visual feedback or a signal from brain to eye. In human eye development, both local (defocusing) and brain-dependent (over-accommodation) signals may be important.

Defects in focusing

Focusing defects arise from too short (hypermetropia) or long (myopia) an eyeball, incorrect curvature of the cornea and lens (astigmatism), and loss of lens elasticity (presbyopia).

Three common refraction errors in eyes are hypermetropia, myopia and astigmatism. In addition, all normal eyes eventually suffer from presbyopia.

1 Hypermetropia (long-sightedness). In this condition, the horizontal axis of the eye is too short and even with full accommodation, images of close objects are focused behind the retina (Fig. 7.18a). This can be corrected with a **convex lens**.

2 Myopia (short-sightedness). The axis of the eye is too long, and even with full relaxation, images of objects at infinity are focused in front of the retina (Fig. 7.18b). This can be corrected with a **concave lens**.

3 Astigmatism. Here, the curvature of the cornea (or occasionally the lens) is different in one plane from that in another, giving different degrees of refraction in different planes. This can be corrected with a **cylindrical lens** to give additional refraction in the required meridian, or by contact lenses with spherical surfaces.

4 Presbyopia. The near point of vision is the distance between the eye and the closest object that can be brought to a clear focus. It recedes with age, being approximately 10 cm from the eye at 20 years and receding to about 80 cm by about age 50–60 when all accommodative power is lost. With ageing, the inelastic crystalline core (lens nucleus) increases in size, and the surrounding lens capsule loses its elasticity.

Opacities of the lens, called **cataracts**, are a common eye disorder, especially in the elderly. A localized cataract may interfere only slightly with vision because all parts of the lens contribute to the

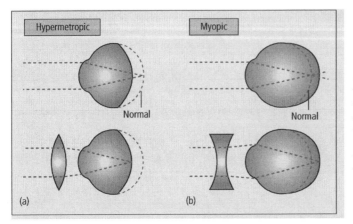

Hypermetropic	Myopic

Normal

Normal

(a)

(b)

Fig. 7.18 Defects in focusing. Light rays from a distant source are shown focusing on (a) a hypermetropic and (b) a myopic eye. The horizontal axis of the hypermetropic eye is too short for accurate focusing and the defect may be corrected with a convex lens; the myopic eye is too long and the defect may be corrected with a concave lens. The position of the normal (emmetropic) eye is shown by the broken line at the back of the eye.

formation of an image; it will, however, reduce its brightness. When vision is severely impaired, the lens may be replaced with an artificial one.

7.2 Taste

The sense of taste (gustation) is important in the selection and enjoyment of food, but full appreciation of flavour requires not only taste but also smell (olfaction), touch (texture), temperature (thermoreception), common chemical sense (chemoreception) and visual inputs as well. Taste cells occur in taste buds on the tongue and oral mucosa. They are activated by a variety of chemicals such as sugars, acids, salts, glutamate and organic compounds such as quinine. Such activation provides the basis for the sensations of sweet, sour, salty, umami and bitter. Taste cells use a variety of transduction mechanisms.

Gustatory receptors

Taste, or **gustation**, refers to the sensation experiences following the stimulation of oral chemoreceptors, and includes the stimulation of specialized receptor cells in the taste buds as well as stimulation of free nerve endings in the oral cavity (**common chemical sense**).

Taste buds are effectively **gustatory end organs**; they are embedded in the stratified epithelium of the tongue, soft palate, pharynx, larynx and epiglottis and are unevenly distributed around

these regions. The lingual taste buds are almost exclusively associated with three of the four types of **papillae** on the surface of the tongue (Fig. 7.19). They are 50–70 μm in diameter and open on to the surface of the tongue at the taste pore (Fig. 7.20). Those associated with the other structures are found on the smooth epithelial surfaces. In humans the number of taste buds varies considerably from 2000 to 5000, on average (but can be as low as 500 and as high as 20 000), with no significant age or gender differences.

Most taste buds are located on the sides of the **vallate** (circumvallate) papillae, which are found at the back of the tongue (Fig. 7.19). The smaller **fungiform** and **foliate** papillae, on the dorsum and sides of the tongue also carry taste buds. Taste buds are not found on the numerous **filiform** papillae.

Each taste buds is made up of 50–150 neuroepithelial cells arranged in a compact pear shaped structure (Fig. 7.20). Besides the sensory taste cells, there are basal cells and supporting cells. Basal cells are stem cells that give rise to taste cells. Supporting cells can be divided into type 1 (dark) cells and type 2 (light) cells. While some consider type 1 and type 2 cells to be supporting cells, others suggest that they represent different stages in the cycle of the taste cell. Taste cells are constantly shed, have a half-life of 10–14 days, and are renewed by division of the underlying basal cells. Taste cells make synaptic contact with the afferent nerve fibres (intragemmal nerve fibres) (Fig. 7.20), which they

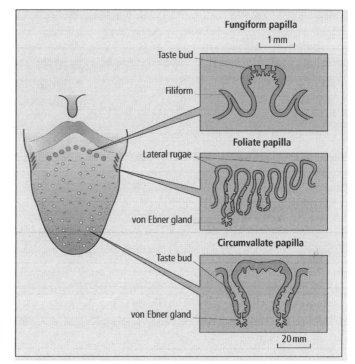

Fungiform papilla

1 mm

Taste bud

Filiform

Foliate papilla

Lateral rugae

von Ebner gland

Circumvallate papilla

Taste bud

von Ebner gland

20 mm

Fig. 7.19 Distribution of taste buds on the tongue and appearances of different papillae.

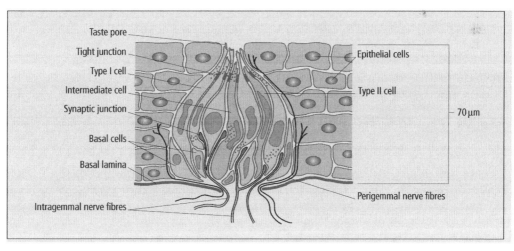

Taste pore

Tight junction

Type I cell

Intermediate cell

Synaptic junction

Basal cells

Basal lamina

Intragemmal nerve fibres

Epithelial cells

Type II cell

70 μm

Perigemmal nerve fibres

Fig. 7.20 Structure of the taste bud.

depend upon for their continual existence; denervated taste buds degenerate and new buds reappear only when the nerve regenerates.

Classically, four basic tastes have been recognized: **sweet**, **sour**, **salty** and **bitter**. A fifth basic taste, **umami**, produced by compounds like monosodium glutamate has now been added to the classical four. All complex tastes are thought to be accounted for by combinations of these basic tastes; however most of what the layperson calls 'taste' is a combination of taste and smell, touch, temperature and common chemical sense, as well as vision.

Most sugars taste sweet, for example glucose, sucrose and lactose produce the sensation of sweetness, but so too do unrelated molecules like glycine, alanine, saccharine and even certain proteins. The sensation of sourness is produced by acids and is related to the H^+ concentration, but not all acids are equally sour at equivalent pH. Salty sensations are elicited mainly by cations such as Na^+ and Li^+ but different anions (Cl^-, SO_4^{2+}, NO_3^-) alter the taste quality. Many different organic compounds are described as bitter, e.g. quinine, caffeine, nicotine, morphine and strychnine; they are often addictive or harmful.

Taste cells are chemoreceptors. Most gustatory stimuli are water-soluble and non-volatile chemicals and are either already dissolved or are dissolved in saliva during mastication.

The chemicals enter the pores of the taste buds and react with the microvilli at the apical surface of the receptor cells. The transduction process appears to involve different mechanisms for different chemicals. For example, Na^+ salts depolarize taste cells by Na^+ influx through Na^+ channels in the apical and lateral cell membrane. Similar channels may be involved for detection of H^+ ions, although the transduction mechanism for this ion shows marked species variability. Transduction of more complex molecules such as sugars and bitter substances frequently involves membrane receptors linked to G proteins (G_{gus} and G_t) and second messengers, such as cyclic adenosine monophosphate (cAMP) and inositol trisphosphate (IP_3)/diacylglycerol (DAG) (p. 26), which gate ion channels causing depolarization. Some artificial sweeteners cause depolarization by modulating ligand-gated ion channels directly. Finally, the umami response to glutamate may involve N-methyl-D-aspartic acid (NMDA) and metabotropic glutamate receptors, which appear to be similar to those in the brain (p. 81).

In most cases the depolarization leads to an action potential followed by an increase in intracellular Ca^{2+} within the taste cell, and the release of neurotransmitter (possibly serotonin or vasoactive intestinal peptide). The transmitter elicits generator potentials and hence action potentials in the afferent nerve fibres (p. 73).

Afferent nerves and central pathways in gustation

Taste buds are innervated by the chorda tympani, lingual and vagal nerves. These afferent fibres synapse in the medulla in the nucleus of the tractus solitarius before projecting to the thalamus and cortex. Most central taste cells respond to a variety of chemical stimuli.

Each taste bud receives branches from many afferent fibres. Taste buds on the anterior two-thirds of the tongue are supplied by the chorda tympani branch of the facial nerve (VII), and those on the posterior one-third by the lingual branch of the glossopharyngeal nerve (IX). The vagus nerve (X) supplies taste buds on the epiglottis. Taste profiles have been obtained from recordings from nerve fibres coming from the gustatory receptors and most single neurones respond to a number of different basic tastes. The primary afferent neurones have their first synaptic connection within the **Nucleus of the tractus solitarius** (NTS), where approximately 82% of the neurones respond to 3 or 4 basic taste stimuli. There is also convergence here between gustatory and thermal inputs, many cells responding to cooling of the tongue as well as to chemical stimuli. The second-order fibres project to the most medial part of the ventroposterior medial nucleus of the thalamus. There are also projections to the brainstem reticular formation, the parabrachial nuclei and the cranial nerve nuclei involved in reflexes associated with gustation. Thalamic neurones project to the primary gustatory cortex, which includes an area just anterior to the somatosensory area for the tongue, as well as to the nearby frontal operculum and anterior insular cortex. There is evidence for a secondary gustatory area in the orbitofrontal cortex. Responses here are modulated by hunger and are reduced when the appetite is satiated. Besides olfactory inputs, the orbitofrontal cortex also receives inputs from visual and somatosensory pathways and cells can respond to two or more modalities. The area is thought to be involved in the learning of associations between stimuli, for instance the association of the taste and smell of a food—important in our appreciation of flavour. Studies in primates suggest that the neurones that respond to specific gustatory stimuli are more numerous as one goes higher up the CNS, with 25% of neurones in the primary cortex and 74% of neurones in the secondary cortex responding to a single basic gustatory stimulus.

The **common chemical sense** has been defined as the sensation caused by stimulation of epithelial or mucosal free nerve endings by chemicals. Evidence suggests these are polymodal nociceptors and that in the mouth the major contributor to this sense is the **trigeminal (V)** nerve. The trigeminal innervates almost all regions of the mouth including the floor of the mouth, the tongue, the hard and soft palate and the mucosa of the lips and cheek. Free nerve endings are found throughout the oral cavity and can be stimulated by a number of different chemicals such as menthol, peppermint, and chemicals such as capsaicin and piperine, which are found in chilli peppers and black peppers, respectively.

Many textbooks and detailed reviews have in the past produced drawings of the dorsal view of the tongue showing areas that are sensitive to each of the four basic tastes—**the so-called tongue map**. Unfortunately, it is now thought that these tongue maps are incorrect and that their origin owes itself to a misunderstanding of the early 20th Century work (written in German) by Hänig. His work referred to the thresholds to the basic tastes and not to the exclusive nature of the loci. He showed that although there were differences, these differences in sensitivity across the loci were actually very small. Subsequent interpretations have led to the impression that the tip of the tongue detects sweet, the sides sour and salt and the back bitter. This is clearly not true.

7.3 Smell

Olfactory cells lie in a specialized region in the roof of the nasal cavity. They are modified neurones with a superficial receptor area and a fine axon passing to the olfactory bulb. Odours combine with these cells to produce depolarization and impulse activity. The sense of smell (olfaction) is important for the enjoyment and selection of food, and for warning of potentially harmful substances or places. In many species of animals, it is also used for communication. The vomeronasal organ, adjacent to the olfactory epithelium, is used to detect pheromones. Although we may not sense these consciously, pheromones may influence behaviour. Mice and bloodhounds can distinguish individuals by smell on the basis of their antigens.

Olfactory receptors

Olfactory cells lie in the olfactory epithelium (a sheet of cells 100–200 μm thick), which in humans covers an area of about 5 cm^2 in the roof of the nasal cavity. The olfactory cells are specialized bipolar neurones (Fig. 7.21). At the apical region of the cell is a modified dendrite which ends on the surface in a knob bearing 15–30 long, non-motile cilia, embedded in a layer of mucus. The ciliary plasma membrane is thought to contain the odorant receptors. The basal region gives rise to a fine (0.1–0.4 μm diameter) unmyelinated axon. The epithelium also contains supporting cells, which have apical microvilli and secrete mucus, and basal cells, which lie on the basement membrane. Recently, a fourth type of cell of unknown function, the microvillar cell, has been described. The olfactory cells are the only nerve cells in adult mammals to show continual degeneration and replacement; they are replaced by division and differentiation of the basal cells.

In contrast to the limited number of taste sensations, humans can detect about 10^4 different smells. Odoriferous compounds are mainly organic, containing 3–20 carbon atoms, but there is no simple relationship between chemical structure and odour. Threshold concentrations vary, being extremely low for certain substances; many odorants can be detected at picomolar (10^{-12} mol L^{-1}) concentrations. Odoriferous compounds reach the olfactory epithelium by diffusion and this can be aided by sniffing to increase air-flow. The molecules must dissolve in the mucus layer before they can interact with receptors on the cilia of the

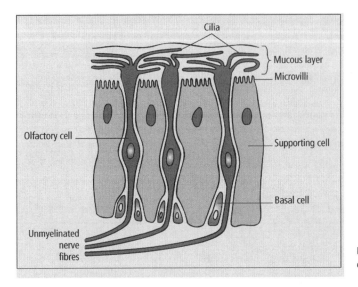

Fig. 7.21 Structure of the olfactory epithelium.

sensory neurones. An **odorant-binding protein** may bind the odorant and carry it to the receptor; it may also aid in removing the odorant.

Recent evidence indicates the existence of hundreds of different **odorant membrane receptors** located on the cilia of the olfactory cells. Olfactory neurones are thought to express only one receptor gene so that neurones have different specificities. A large family of putative odorant receptor genes (perhaps as large as 1000) have been cloned utilizing oligonucleotide probes targeted to G protein-binding motifs. Binding of the odorant to the receptor leads—probably via a GTP-binding protein (G_{olf}) and cAMP (p. 26)—to an increased conductance to Na^+, and hence to a depolarizing generator potential. In this instance cAMP directly gates a cation-selective channel. Although cAMP appears to be the major second messenger in olfactory transduction, there is increasing evidence for the involvement of phosphoinositide-derived second messengers.

Recordings from single neurones have shown that depolarization, and hence impulse activity, increases with increasing concentration of odorant. Single neurones probably contain the gene for only one odorant receptor, and are therefore selective for a particular set of odorants, which combine with that receptor. In rodents, neurones containing the same receptor are dispersed within zones in the epithelium; their distribution in humans has not yet been established. Any one odorant may activate a number of receptor types thus generating a diffuse, but unique, pattern of neuronal activity across the olfactory epithelium. The summated generator potentials of the olfactory neurones can be recorded as an **electro-olfactogram**.

The sense of smell shows marked adaptation and is subject to masking of one smell by another—the basis of air fresheners. Olfactory acuity has been shown to be best in the third to fifth decades of life and is also better in women than in men.

Afferent nerves and central pathways in olfaction

Olfactory axons terminate in synaptic regions of the olfactory bulb, termed glomeruli. From there second-order cells project to the olfactory cortex and to other regions, including the thalamus and limbic system.

The unmyelinated axons of the receptor cells form the first cranial nerve; the axons pass in bundles (olfactory fila) through the cribriform plate and enter the ipsilateral olfactory bulb where they terminate in spherical glomeruli (100–200 μm in diameter). Glomeruli are regions of synaptic contact between the afferent axons and the dendrites of mitral and tufted cells. Each olfactory neurone projects to only one glomerulus. However, each glomerulus receives inputs from several thousand olfactory neurones widely dispersed in the epithelium. There is recent evidence that each glomerulus receives inputs from neurones expressing the same receptor; thus glomeruli are functional units, responding to a particular group of odorants. Besides mitral and tufted neurones, the bulb also contains many interneurones, such as the periglomerular and granule cells. In addition it receives 'descending' projections from a variety of brain regions, which, together with the interneurones, contribute to the processing of the sensory input. For instance, there is evidence for lateral inhibition between neighbouring glomeruli, important for sharpening olfactory acuity (similar to surround inhibition; see p. 128).

Axons of the mitral and tufted cells project via the olfactory tracts to several structures, commonly referred to collectively as the primary olfactory cortex. These structures include the anterior olfactory nucleus, the olfactory tubercle and the piriform, periamygdaloid and entorhinal cortices. In addition there are projections, via the anterior commissure, to the contralateral olfactory bulb. Other areas involved in olfaction include the mediodorsal nucleus of the thalamus and the orbitofrontal cortex. There is evidence that the piriform and orbitofrontal cortices are involved in odour discrimination, but little is known about how responses are analysed to provide olfactory sensations. Olfactory pathways also provide inputs to various regions of the limbic system such as the septal area, amygdala and hypothalamus; these are thought to mediate the affective components of sensation, which are frequently associated with odours.

Disorders of smell and taste

The loss of smell and taste can be life threatening in that it impairs the ability of the person to detect smoke in a fire or identify spoiled or poisonous foods. Approximately 80% of reported taste disorders are really disorders of smell. The disorders of smell are called '-osmias' and those of taste '-geusias'. **Anosmia** is the inability to detect odours

whilst **ageusia** is the inability to detect tastes. **Hyposmia** and **hypogeusia** refer to a decreased ability to detect odours and tastes respectively and **dysosmia** and **dysgeusia** refer to a distorted detection of smell or taste. The terms **hyperosmia** and **hypergeusia** denote an increased sensitivity to some odours or gustatory stimuli. These disorders of smell and taste can be total, partial or specific to one or two selected odours or tastes.

Loss of both olfactory sensitivity and gustatory sensitivity can be attributed to three main causes: conditions that interfere with the access of the stimulus to the receptor cells (**transport loss**); conditions that injure the receptor cells and their supporting cells (**sensory loss**); or conditions that damage the nerves and their pathways to the central nervous system (**neural loss**).

In the case of the olfactory system transport loss results from swollen nasal mucous membranes in allergic rhinitis and viral and bacterial rhinitis, as well as structural alterations such as those caused by tumours, polyps and deviations of the nasal septum caused by trauma. Abnormalities of mucous secretion could also result in a loss of olfactory sensitivity.

Sensory olfactory loss is often caused by destruction of the olfactory epithelium by viral infections, inhalation of toxic substances, drugs that alter cell turnover, tumours and their treatment by radiation therapy. Neural olfactory loss can be caused by peripheral tumours of the anterior cranial fossa or more central within the central nervous system, trauma of the nasal structures including the cribriform plate area, neurosurgical procedures, administration of neurotoxic agents and a number of congenital disorders such as Kallman's syndrome in which the olfactory structures fail to develop properly.

In the case of the gustatory system the transport loss can result from bacterial colonization of the taste pore of the taste bud, inflammation of the oral cavity in general, poor oral hygiene and xerostomia (reduced saliva production). Sensory gustatory loss can be caused by a large number of different drugs, particularly those that alter cell turnover such as anti-thyroid and anti-cancer drugs. Radiation therapy, inflammatory and degenerative diseases of the mouth, including bacterial and viral infections, and endocrine and nutritional disorders can also result in sensory loss. Neural gustatory loss is caused by tumours, trauma, and surgery, in which nerves are damaged. Again damage to nerves may be either peripheral due to damage to the afferent nerve or more central due to a brainstem tumour.

7.4 Hearing

The auditory system has evolved as a survival system for warning and hunting; it also functions as the afferent part of spoken communication. To carry out these functions of recognition, location and communication, it must detect sounds of particular interest, such as human speech, and ignore irrelevant background sounds. Each ear performs a frequency analysis on the sound energy so that the auditory nerve carries information on the frequency (pitch) and intensity (loudness) of the sound components. Sound vibrations are transduced into nerve action potentials by the hair cells in the cochlea. The brain has centres specialized for analysing the relative intensity and phase of individual sounds so as to compute their direction of origin. It also has higher centres dedicated to recognizing the nature of sounds and the content of speech.

Aspects of a sound stimulus

The sensation of sound detected by the ear is caused by variation in air pressure within a specific range of frequencies and intensities. Outside this range the sensations evoked are variously described as vibration, flutter, tickle and pain.

A source of sound such as a tuning fork causes the surrounding air molecules to oscillate (Fig. 7.22). The disturbance spreads out from the source in sinusoidal waves, which consist of areas of compression of air (high pressure) alternating with areas of rarefaction (low pressure). Sound can thus be described, like all waves, in terms of both frequency and amplitude. The **loudness** of the sound is related to the amplitude of the sound wave and the **pitch** to the frequency.

Frequency

A normal young person can hear sounds ranging in frequency from 2 to 20 kHz. Higher frequencies are called ultrasound and lower frequencies infrasound. Frequency discrimination by the human ear is best at about 1 kHz, where changes of as little as 3 Hz can be detected.

Sound of only a single frequency, a **pure tone**, is uncommon in daily experience. Most sounds are composed of numerous, simultaneously occurring frequencies. Fourier first suggested that all complex waveforms could be analysed by breaking them down into simpler constituent waves of single frequencies. When subjected to Fourier analysis, musical sounds are found to be composed of a fundamental frequency plus a number of harmonically related frequencies, that is, the higher ones are integral multiples of the lowest (the fundamental). The number and intensity of each determine the tone or timbre of the sound, whilst the fundamental determines the pitch.

Amplitude

Amplitude is the objective aspect of a sound stimulus, measurable with instruments, while loudness is the subjective, conscious aspect, which is harder to quantify. The amplitude of sound waves is measured using the decibel scale (the unit of sound amplitude, the **bel**, is named after Alexander Graham Bell). This is a logarithmic scale defined as sound pressure level in decibels.

$$\text{Decibel (dB)} = 20 \log_{10} P_t / P_r$$

where P_t is the test pressure and P_r a reference pressure of $2 \times 10^{-5}\,\text{N}\,\text{m}^{-2}$, just loud enough in the range 1–3 kHz to be audible to an average listener. Alternatively, the decibel may be expressed in terms of intensity ($\text{W}\,\text{m}^{-2}$), in which case it equals 10 times the logarithm of the ratio of the intensity of the test sound to the intensity of the reference sound.

The threshold of hearing varies with the stimulus frequency and is least over the range 1–3 kHz (Fig. 7.23); that is, the human ear is most sensitive in this range. The resulting displacement of the

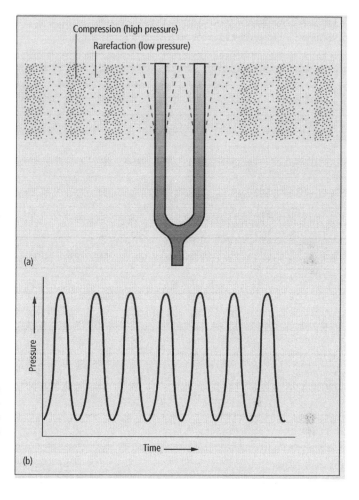

Fig. 7.22 (a) Vibration of a tuning fork causing compression and rarefaction in the surrounding air molecules. (b) The pressure changes represented as sine waves with both the frequency and amplitude of a pure tone.

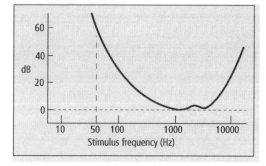

Fig. 7.23 Threshold of audibility curve.

tympanum is about the diameter of a hydrogen atom. The threshold rises to 60 dB (i.e. 10^3 times this value) at 50 Hz, and 30 dB at 10 kHz. The frequencies and intensities produced in speaking, however, lie within a narrower area of about 250 Hz to 4 kHz, and speech over the telephone must be transmitted at frequencies within this range if it is to be understood. Women's voices are about an octave higher (double the frequency) than those of men. Threshold for pain is about 120 dB, although sounds above 100 dB may damage the organ of Corti in the cochlea. Loudness discrimination is about 1 dB under the most favourable experimental conditions (but more usually 2–3 dB), so that at 1–3 kHz there are no more than about 120 steps of loudness from the threshold of hearing to the threshold of pain.

Duration

To establish a pitch requires a minimum duration of 15–20 ms, which does not appear to vary much with frequency.

Direction of sound source

At lower frequencies the direction of origin of a sound can be determined only by sensing the difference in time of arrival of the wavefront, whereas for higher frequencies (approximately 1.5 kHz) the shielding effect of the head and pinnae of the ears results in differences in amplitude of the sound between the two ears (Fig. 7.24). As a result, discrimination is best at higher frequencies where both these mechanisms can be employed. The direction of origin of a pure tone of frequency less than 1 kHZ is difficult to determine; real sounds generally contain harmonics at frequencies greater than this, allowing their position to be sensed.

Functional anatomy of the ear

The ear is divided into outer, middle and inner ear compartments (Fig. 7.25).

Outer ear

The **external auditory meatus**, about 27 mm long, conducts air pressure variations from the **auricle** (pinna or ear flap) to the **tympanum** (eardrum). The air column has a resonant frequency of about 3–4 kHz and conducts energy to the eardrum most effectively within this range.

Middle ear

The outer ear and middle ear are separated by the tympanum (Fig. 7.25). The cavity of the middle ear is air-filled and is connected to the pharynx by a narrow passage called the **Eustachian tube**, which allows the pressure of the air in the middle ear to equilibrate with the outside pressure. Vibrations of the tympanum are conveyed through the middle ear to the **oval window**, which sits between the middle ear and the fluid-filled inner ear, via a series of small bones called **ossicles**. These are the **malleus** (hammer), which is attached to the tympanum, the **incus** (anvil) and the **stapes** (stirrup), which is attached to the oval window. The ossicle chain, together with the smaller area of the oval window relative to the tympanum, operates to promote the efficient transfer of energy from air to the liquid environment of the inner ear, in other words it acts as an impedance-matching device. The reso-

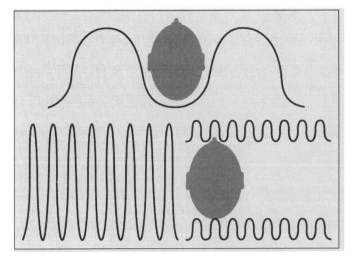

Fig. 7.24 Direction of sound source. At low frequencies (upper figure) the direction of a sound source is sensed by the difference in time of arrival of the wavefront; at higher frequencies (lower figure) the direction is also sensed by differences in amplitude due to shielding by the head and ears.

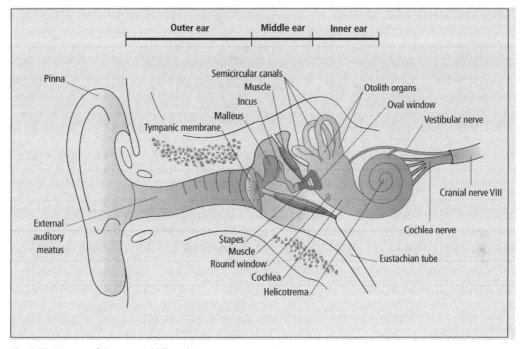

Fig. 7.25 Diagram of the outer, middle and inner ear components.

nant frequencies of the middle-ear mechanism are around 800–1200 Hz and, together with the resonance of the external auditory meatus, are mostly responsible for the low threshold of hearing in this frequency range.

The effectiveness of the ossicle chain can be modified by the activity of two small muscles in the middle ear. The **tensor tympani muscle** pulls the tympanum inwards and this results in the stapes being pushed into the oval windows. The **stapedius muscle** pulls the stapes out of the oval window and pushes the tympanum outwards. When they contract together, they stiffen the middle-ear mechanism to reduce the transfer of energy into the inner ear. They do so in response to high-intensity sounds, with a latency of about 10 ms, but soon relax again during constant stimulation. This is a protective reflex in response to loud sounds, but cannot protect against percussive sounds, such as gun shot, because of the latent period.

Inner ear

This has a bony coiled tube of two and a half turns, the **cochlea**, divided by membranes along its length into three canals or scalae, called the **scala vestibuli**, the **scala media** or **cochlear duct** and the **scala tympani** (Fig. 7.26). The scala vestibuli and scala tympani are filled with **perilymph** and join at the **helicotrema,** at the apex of the cochlea; the scala media is filled with **endolymph**. Perilymph is very close to extracellular fluid in composition while endolymph, which is continuously secreted by a plexus of blood vessels called the **stria vascularis**, is very close to intracellular fluid in composition. The scala media is separated from the upper scala vestibuli by **Reissner's membrane**, and from the lower scala tympani by the **basilar membrane**. When the stapes is pushed into the oval window, a wave is conducted along the scala vestibuli and through the flexible Reissner's membrane to the scala media. The basilar

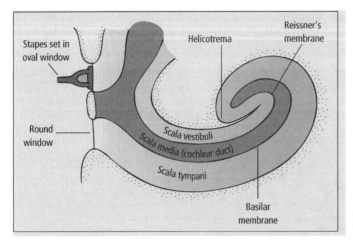

Stapes set in oval window

Helicotrema

Reissner's membrane

Round window

Scala vestibuli

Scala media (cochlear duct)

Scala tympani

Basilar membrane

Fig. 7.26 Diagram of the inner ear. (The coiling of the cochlea is reduced for simplicity.)

membrane is depressed and the round window bulges out into the middle ear where the sound energy is dissipated into the air.

The sound receptors of the ear are found in the **organ of Corti** which lies on the basilar membrane within the scala media (Fig. 7.27). The organ of Corti is composed of an epithelium of **hair cells** (Corti cells) and supporting cells. The hair cells are arranged into inner and outer groups. Each hair cell is anchored on the basilar membrane and has a bundle of hairs, called **stereocilia**, projecting from its tip and embedded in the shelf-like **tectorial membrane**. The hair cells make contact at their basal surface with afferent cochlear fibres, which pass into the bony **modiolus** where their cell bodies form the **spiral ganglion**. About 90% of the spiral ganglion cells in each ear innervate inner hair cells—about 10 axons converging on each hair cell; the remainder diverge to innervate many outer hair cells.

In addition to afferent cochlear fibres which run with the vestibular fibres in the auditory nerve (cranial nerve VIII), there is a small tract of efferent fibres ending on or close to the Corti hair cells—the olivocochlear bundle—which has an inhibitory action, reducing the afferent discharge at a given stimulus intensity. Furthermore, outer hair cells may be induced to vibrate and so actively dampen local regions of the basilar membrane.

Stimulation of Corti hair cells

The basilar membrane is a fibrous structure running from the inner core or modiolus to the outer side of the bony tube (Fig. 7.27). When the basilar membrane moves up and down, it tends to move rather rigidly, bending about an axis near the modiolus (Fig. 7.28). The tectorial membrane is pushed up and pulled down and there is a shearing motion between the tectorial membrane and the reticular lamina, bending the stereocilia to one side and the other. Bending of the stereocilia triggers the opening of mechanically gated ion channels in the hair-cell membrane (Fig. 7.29). This leads to a depolarization of the hair cell, causing the release of a chemical transmitter from the cell's basal surface, which in turn initiates action potentials in the cochlear fibres.

Hair cells are amazingly sensitive and can detect mechanical displacements as small as the diameter of a hydrogen atom. The tips of the stereocilia are connected by thin threads called tip links (Fig. 7.29), which are physically linked to ion channels. This arrangement permits very small movements to be transduced into changes in membrane potential.

The stereocilia project into the endolymph, which has a high concentration of K^+; whereas the body of the hair cell is bathed in perilymph, which

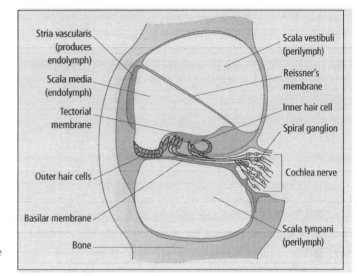

Fig. 7.27 A cross-section through the three canals of the cochlea.

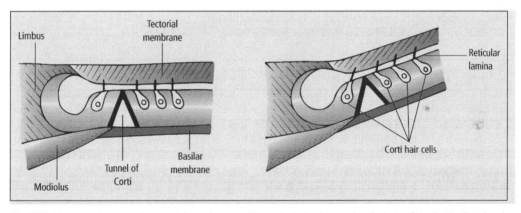

Fig. 7.28 Movement between the tectorial membrane and the reticular lamina causing the hairs of the Corti cells to bend. (From Davis, H. (1957) In: Bullock, T.H. (ed.) *Physiological Triggers and Discontinuous Rate Processes*, pp. 10–71. American Physiological Society, Washington.)

is low in K⁺ and high in Na⁺. When cilia are bent towards the tallest one, an inward K⁺ current flows through their tips, causing depolarization of the cell body, opening of voltage-gated Ca²⁺ channels and release of neurotransmitter onto the afferent nerve fibres in contact with the hair cell.

In order to get a better picture it is necessary to consider not only radial movements of the basilar membrane, but also how movements along its length from base to apex are determined by the frequency of the sound. Sound of a particular frequency causes a wave of displacement to travel along the basilar membrane. The position and properties of the basilar membrane, which at the window end is narrower and stiffer than at the apex or helicotrema, are such that the region nearest the window resonates best with high-frequency sound while more distant regions resonate best with low-frequency sound. As the membrane resonates, energy is transferred across it and is dissipated by being conducted back to the round window. So if sound containing a mixture of frequencies is passed through the oval window, its components are progressively removed with

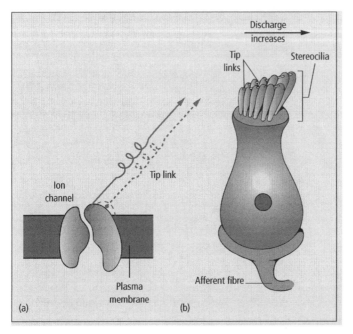

Fig. 7.29 Hair cells showing (a) tip links connected to an ion channel and (b) their position on the stereocilia. Bending of the stereocilia towards the tallest in the bundle opens ion channels and depolarizes the hair cell. Note the absence of a kinocilium in the Corti hair cell of adults.

distance along the basilar membrane, in order from high to low frequency. Figure 7.30a shows the displacement caused by a 200-Hz wave instantaneously (solid line) and the envelope of all displacements over a period of many cycles (dashed line). It can be seen that there is a region of maximum displacement over a period of many cycles and that there is a region of maximum displacement quite far from the oval window. Although all the basilar membrane from the oval window up to this point moves to a lesser degree, the amplitude falls off quickly beyond the maximum due to damping. Figure 7.30b shows the envelopes of deflection for various frequencies of sound stimuli; the peak displacement position of the basilar membrane is closer to the stapes the higher the frequency.

From the above description, it can be seen that the hair cells are mechanically stimulated at particular frequencies depending on their position in the basilar membrane—the so-called **place theory**. Furthermore, individual hair cells vary in the length and stiffness of their stereocilia; those with short stiff cilia are mechanically more sensitive to high-frequency stimuli than those with longer and

more flexible stereocilia. Finally, at least in some lower vertebrates, hair cells are electrically tuned due to spontaneous oscillations in their membrane potential, which show a characteristic frequency for each cell. In summary, each hair cell is tuned over a very narrow range by its position along the basilar membrane, by its individual mechanical properties, by active damping of local regions of basilar membrane by outer hair cells, and possibly by its electrical resonant properties.

Action potential discharges in the auditory nerve

Many single afferent fibres are spontaneously active in the absence of a stimulus. At sine-wave stimulus frequencies up to 1 kHz, the firing of single fibres can follow the sine wave in the sense of occurring only in successive cycles (Fig. 7.31). Since nerve fibres cannot carry more than about 1000 action potentials per second due to their refractory periods, when the stimulus frequency is increased beyond this, a fibre which has previously given one spike in each cycle will begin to drop out once every few cycles, and so on. At these higher

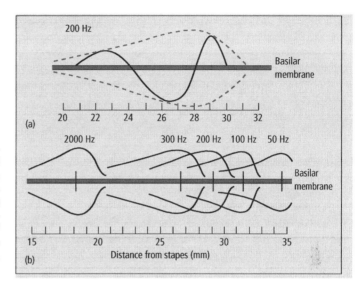

Fig. 7.30 (a) Deflections at one instant (solid line) and an envelope of all deflections over a period of time (dashed line) caused in a basilar membrane by a 200-Hz sound wave. (b) Envelopes of basilar membrane deflection for various frequencies of sound stimuli. (Adapted from von Bekesy, G. (1974) *J Acoust Soc Am*, **19**, 452–60.)

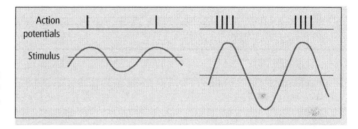

Fig. 7.31 Action potential discharges in a single afferent fibre produced by two different intensities of a fixed frequency.

stimulus frequencies, a group of fibres, in which individual fibres misfire in an independently assorted fashion, can give discharges which when recorded from the group rather than from a single fibre can keep in step up to about 3 kHz. Thus one fibre responds to cycles 1, 4, 7, and so on; a second fibre to cycles 2, 5 and 8; and a third fibre to cycles 3, 6 and 9. Above 3 kHz, no clear visible relation can be made out in the discharge of a single fibre to the stimulus waveform.

If the stimulus thresholds are determined for a single fibre at various frequencies and intensities (Fig. 7.32), it is found that they rise rapidly on both sides of one small range of frequencies (the 'best' frequency) but more steeply on the higher frequency side, so that usually some high frequencies cannot provoke discharge, however intense they are. Note that as the stimulus intensity is raised the fibre responds over a wider frequency range.

We are now in a position to describe how the auditory information is encoded in auditory nerve fibre discharges with reference to the four properties of a sound stimulus, discussed earlier.

1 Pitch discrimination is mainly determined by the area of basilar membrane occupied by firing receptors for a given stimulus frequency (the 'place theory' of hearing). High notes stimulate receptors closer to the base of the basilar membrane and low notes stimulate receptors closer to the apex (Fig. 7.30b).

2 Intensity of the sensation is derived from the total number of impulses per second in the auditory nerve fibres. At a given stimulus frequency only certain fibres will respond to a low-intensity stimulus. As the stimulus intensity is raised, the discharge frequency in these firing fibres is increased (Fig. 7.31) and previously silent fibres with higher thresholds at that stimulus frequency are recruited.

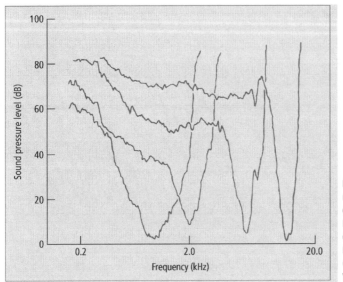

Fig. 7.32 Tuning curves of four sensory units from the cat auditory nerve. (Adapted from Kiang, N.Y.S. (1984). In: Brookhart, J.M. & Mountcastle, V.B. (eds) *Handbook of Physiology*, Section I, *The Nervous System*, Vol. III, pp. 639–74. American Physiology Society, Washington.)

3 Duration of the stimulus is signalled by the total duration of the afferent discharge caused by the stimulus.

4 Direction of the sound source is signalled by preservation in the auditory pathway of the initial time difference in receptor activation on the two sides of the head, as well as continuing intensity differences.

Central auditory pathways

Auditory inputs pass through several synaptic relays before reaching the primary auditory cortex. In the cortex responses are tonotopic and bilateral. Descending controls can modify activity at all levels of the pathway.

The auditory system as a whole is characterized by orderly segregation of nerve fibres and their cell bodies concerned with particular frequencies (tonotopic organization). A series of relay nuclei between the spiral ganglion and the auditory cortex processes this information further, allowing, for example, analysis of sound location (superior olivary nucleus) and correlations with visual location of objects (inferior colliculus).

All of the auditory fibres in cranial nerve VIII terminate in the cochlear nuclei in the medulla (Fig.

7.33). Some axons from the cochlear nuclei project to the superior olivary nucleus, the first binaural relay station. Other axons from the cochlear nuclei and those from the superior olivary nuclei ascend in either the ipsilateral or the contralateral lateral lemniscus, via the inferior colliculi, to the medial geniculate nuclei. Information is then sent to the primary auditory cortex, which lies in the superior temporal gyrus on the bank of the lateral or Sylvian fissure (Fig. 6.7). Inputs from both ears are represented in both right and left cortices. Collateral branches from the pathway travel to spinal levels, the cerebellum and reticular formation of the brainstem and to the superior colliculi. All these are for coordination with other systems.

There are also inhibitory endings derived from higher levels of the central nervous system at each afferent synaptic level so that some modification of the afferent discharge must occur in these integrating centres.

Deafness

Hearing impairment, in the sense of a raised threshold to sound stimuli, may be due to impaired sound transmission in the outer or middle ear (conduction deafness) or to damage to the re-

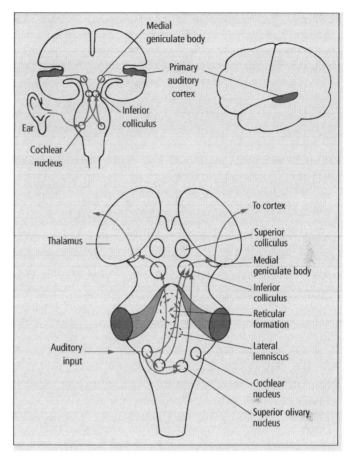

Fig. 7.33 A dorsal view of the brainstem (cerebral cortex and cerebellum removed) showing the central auditory pathways. Top left inset: simplified representation of the pathways in a roughly frontal section of the brain. Top right inset: a lateral view of the left cerebral hemisphere showing the location of the primary auditory cortex.

ceptors or to the neural pathways (sensorineural deafness).

Conduction deafness may be caused by:

1 narrowing or blockage of the external meatus, as by pus, wax, dust, etc.;

2 thickening of the tympanum following scarring or repeated middle-ear infections;

3 exudate in the middle ear (otitis media);

4 dislocation or fixation (ankylosis) of the ossicle chain; and

5 otosclerosis, which is a narrowing of the gap between the footplate of the stapes and the surrounding bone, progressing to fixation of the footplate when the gap is bridged.

Some restoration of hearing can be achieved in patients with otosclerosis by an operation in which the window is unblocked by breaking the bony bridge or by removal of the whole stapes and footplate and replacement with a prosthesis, commonly of polythene tubing.

Sensorineural deafness caused by damage to the organ of Corti results from high-intensity stimulation of long duration, predominantly of high frequencies, as in such trades as boiler-making. Ear protection is considered desirable where the ambient noise level is more than 85 dB above threshold in the range 300–2400 Hz. Other sorts of nerve deafness can be caused by certain antibiotics (streptomycin), mechanical damage to cranial nerve VIII (auditory nerve), tumour, or by diseases such as meningitis, rheumatism, malaria and syphilis.

One can differentiate diagnostically between conduction and sensorineural deafness by performing two tests with apparatus no more complex than a tuning fork. In the **Rinne test** the base of the vibrating tuning fork is placed on the mastoid bone behind the ear and then the tines are held in the air close to the ear. Subjects with conduction deafness do not hear air vibrations in the affected ear after bone conduction is over, but those with sensorineural deafness and normal hearing do. In the **Weber test** the base of the vibrating tuning fork is placed on the vertex of the skull causing energy to be conducted through the skull bones. In subjects with unilateral conduction deafness the sound is louder in the affected ear because sound energy is dissipated through the normal conduction route of the unaffected side. In subjects with unilateral sensorineural deafness the sound is louder in the normal ear because the neural pathways are damaged in the affected ear, while in those with normal hearing sound is heard equally well on both sides. An objective measure of the degree of deafness is commonly carried out with an audiometer.

Cochlear prostheses are now being used to restore hearing in patients suffering from profound sensorineural deafness due to defective sensory hair cells. These devices consist of an array of tiny electrodes connected to an external speech processor unit. The electrodes are implanted in or near the cochlea and transmit signals to stimulate the auditory nerve fibres directly. The success rate varies among devices and individual patients.

7.5 Vestibular function

The vestibular system provides information on the spatial orientation and movement of the head and plays an essential role in regulating movement of the trunk and limbs as well as the maintenance of body posture. In addition, afferent discharges from the vestibular organs influence reflex centres responsible for maintenance of a stable retinal image by controlling neck muscles and extraocular eye muscles. Rotatory movement of the head is detected by hair cells in the semicircular canals, while linear acceleration and the direction of gravity are detected by hair cells in the otolith organs.

There are two parts to the vestibular apparatus: the **semicircular canals** and the two otolith organs, the **utricle** and the **saccule** (Fig. 7.34). The ampullae of the semicircular canals contain sense organs that respond to rotatory acceleration of the head. The otolith organs are sensitive to the direction of the force of gravity and to linear accelerations of the head. All these tissues constitute the **membranous labyrinth**, a system of tubes filled with endolymph and surrounded by perilymph. This in turn is encapsulated within the **bony labyrinth**, a series of bony tubes containing both

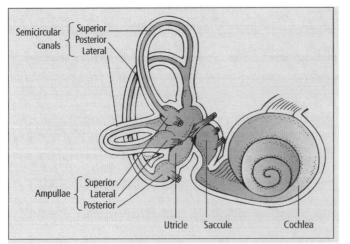

Semicircular canals
  Superior
  Posterior
  Lateral

Ampullae
  Superior
  Lateral
  Posterior

Utricle   Saccule   Cochlea

Fig. 7.34 Vestibular apparatus of the right side. (Adapted from Melloni, B.J. (1957) *The Internal Ear, An Atlas of Some Pathological Conditions of the Eye, Ear and Throat*, pp. 26–31. Abbott Laboratories, Chicago.)

the auditory and vestibular sense organs and which lies in the cavities in the temporal bone.

Stimulation of vestibular hair cells

Vestibular sensation results from stimulation of hair cells in the ampullae and otolith organs. Bundles of 40–70 **stereocilia** project from the free surface of each cell and are connected at their tips by tip links (Fig. 7.29). The stereocilia are packed hexagonally and increase progressively in length towards the side of the bundle from which the **kinocilium**—an especially long cilium with a different structure—projects (Fig. 7.35). Hair cells are polarized, so that movement of their cilia towards one side of the kinocilium causes depolarization and to the other side hyperpolarization. As they are depolarized, the hair cells release progressively more transmitter, resulting in an increased rate of firing of the afferent axons with which they are in contact. Hair cells in the resting state are typically in the mid-range of polarization so that there is a steady release of transmitter and tonic firing of sensory nerve impulses. Any slight movement of their hairs results in an increase or a decrease in the rate of firing.

The semicircular canals

The three semicircular canals lie in nearly orthogonal planes, that is, each is at right angles to the other two (Fig. 7.36). With the head erect, the lateral (horizontal) canal rises anteriorly at about 30° to the horizontal while the superior (anterior) and posterior canals are at 45–55° to both sagittal and frontal planes, respectively. The two lateral canals on the left and right side of the body are in a single plane, and the posterior canal of one side is in a plane nearly parallel to the superior canal of the other side, so that these respective pairs are stimulated similarly and at least one pair is affected by any given angular acceleration. The canals of either side alone can generate afferent impulses signalling movement in any direction.

The labyrinths are filled with endolymph, a watery fluid with ion concentrations similar to that of intracellular fluid, with K^+ ~50 mmol L^{-1} and Na^+ ~20 mmol L^{-1}. The vestibular epithelium contains **dark cells**, which are responsible for the ion transport that maintains these concentrations. Each canal is connected at both ends to the utricle (Fig. 7.34), so that the endolymph is free to circulate. At one end of each canal is an **ampulla** containing

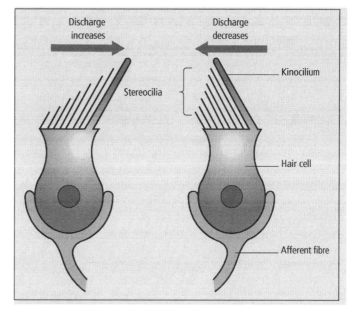

Fig. 7.35 Diagram of the vestibular hair cell. Bending the cilia towards the side of the kinocilium increases the discharge frequency; bending the cilia away from that side decreases it.

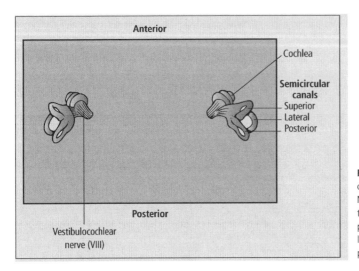

Fig. 7.36 The orientation of the semicircular canals as seen from above. Note that, while the lateral canals on the left and right side lie in the same plane, the superior canal on each side lies in almost the same plane as the posterior canal on the opposite side.

receptors, which transduce circulation of endolymph into nervous impulses. The receptor apparatus, the **crista ampullaris** (Fig. 7.37) consists of the **cupula** (or cupola), a gelatinous wedge-shaped structure running fully across the cross-section of the ampulla to form a diaphragm that effectively blocks any bulk flow of endolymph. As it has nearly the same specific gravity as the endolymph, it neither floats nor sinks and thus is almost unaffected by the direction of gravity. The cupula is mounted on a ridge carrying many hair cells that have their cilia embedded in the base of the cupula. The hair cells in each ampulla all have the same orientation; those in the ampullae of the horizontal canals have their kinocilium facing towards the utricle, while in the vertical canals they face away from the utricle. Thus, movement of fluid towards the utricle depolarizes (stimulates) the hair cells of the lateral canals, but hyperpolarizes (inhibits) those of the vertical canals.

During any angular acceleration of the head, the endolymph tends to circulate through the semicircular canals as a consequence of its inertia, and the resultant fluid pressure causes deflection of the cupula and bends the cilia projecting from the hair cells. Movement of the fluid is soon damped and during steady motion the cupula rapidly returns to its resting position and produces no further sensation.

Figure 7.38 illustrates the changes in frequency of impulses recorded from axons in the vestibular nerve when the head is rotated to the right at a constant speed. The sensation of rotation persists beyond the period of firing in vestibular axons, demonstrating that this information is integrated and stored, probably in the brainstem. There is a spontaneous resting discharge, which changes with any movement of the head. When the head accelerates to reach constant velocity, there is a sudden increase in frequency; the discharge then returns to its frequency at rest before the sensation of movement ceases in 25–30 s. When the rotation is stopped quickly, the opposite sequence takes place. The discharge frequency of the receptors changes in the opposite sense to that at the beginning of rotation and there is a feeling of rotating in the opposite direction until the cupula again returns to its resting position.

The discharge patterns from the ampullae of corresponding semicircular canals on the two sides of the body are mirror images, so that the brain receives both positive and negative sense information on any movement (Fig. 7.39).

The utricle and saccule

On the inner surface of each utricle and saccule is an otolith organ. The otolith organs are roughly

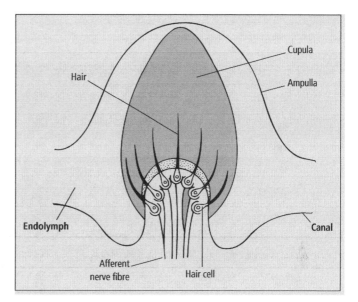

Fig. 7.37 Diagram of the crista ampullaris.

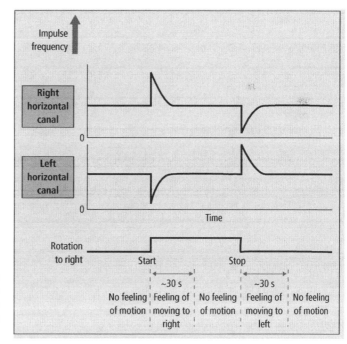

Fig. 7.38 Impulse frequency in vestibular afferent fibres when the head is rotated to the right at a constant angular velocity and then stopped.

2 mm in size and have **maculae**, thickened regions containing hair cells, and vestibular nerve terminals. The hair-cell cilia are embedded in a gelatinous mass called the **otolith membrane**, which contains a mass of calcium carbonate crystals called **otoconia** (Fig. 7.40). The specific gravity of the otoconia is about 2.9, much higher than that of the endolymph. If the head is still, the otolith membrane tends to fall to the lowest possible point, giving rise to sensation of the direction of

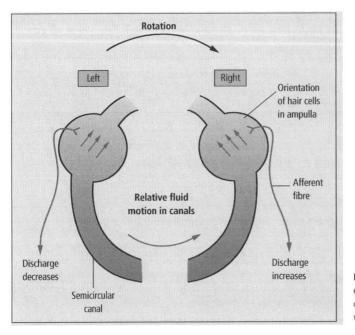

Fig. 7.39 Reciprocal changes in afferent discharge from the ampullae of corresponding semicircular canals when the head is rotated to the right.

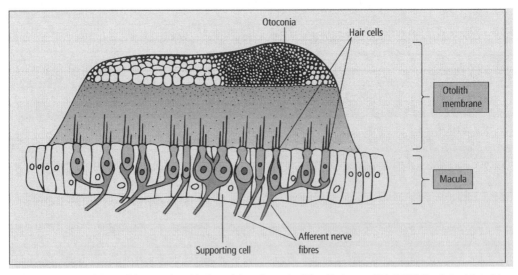

Fig. 7.40 Diagram of the otolith organ found in the utricle and saccule. (After Lindeman, H.H. (1969) *Ergeb Anat Entwicklungsgesch*, **42**, 1–113.)

the force of gravity. During movement, its equilibrium position is determined by the direction of the vector sum of all accelerations of the head—linear, centrifugal and gravitational. It should, however, be noted that conscious awareness of an accelerating force also depends on cutaneous mechanoreceptors and muscle and joint proprioceptors. Sensation of 'up' includes visual awareness of the origin of brightest light and of the horizon, as well as proprioceptive and cutaneous information.

Hair cells are arranged in each macula in a complex pattern of orientation (Fig. 7.41). There is a line of reversal in the orientation of the hair cells in the maculae of both utricle and saccule. In the macula of the saccule, the kinocilia are oriented away from each other on either side at the line of reversal rather than towards each other, as in the utricle. As a consequence of these patterns of orientation of the hair cells, each different movement of the otolith causes a different spatially organized pattern of discharge in the afferent fibres. These highly organized afferent patterns generated in different parts of the vestibular system probably account for the direction of the compensatory eye movements which occur during rotation of the body.

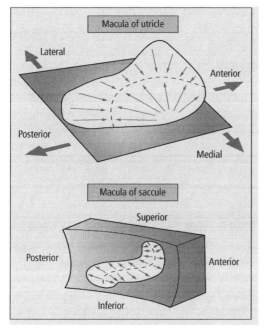

Fig. 7.41 Directions of orientation of hair cells in the maculae of the left utricle and saccule. The arrows indicate the direction of bending of the hairs for excitation. (From Spoendlin, H.H. (1966) In: Wolfson, R.J. (ed.) *The Vestibular System and its Diseases*, pp. 39–68. University of Pennsylvania Press, Philadelphia.)

Action potential discharges in the vestibular nerve

Spontaneous rates of firing in different vestibular fibres of animals vary from a few per second up to about 200 per second, averaging 90. The frequency of this discharge is altered by bending the hairs of the hair cells. To a first approximation, the ampullae of the semicircular canals are sensitive to angular acceleration and the maculae of the utricle and saccule to the direction of gravity and to linear acceleration. However, they can all respond to other modes of stimulation to some extent.

There is a small tract of efferent fibres to the vestibular apparatus whose function is probably inhibitory, as is the corresponding supply to the cochlea. These efferent fibres may play a role in **habituation** to repeated patterns of acceleration or during constant rotation.

Central vestibular pathways

Axons from the vestibular apparatus project to the vestibular nuclei in the brainstem. Vestibular inputs are involved in a variety of reflexes concerned with stabilizing the eyes (via inputs to the oculomotor nuclei), stabilizing the head (via inputs to neck motor neurones) and maintaining balance (via pathways to the cerebellum and spinal cord).

Vestibular axons on either side have their cell bodies in the vestibular ganglion (Scarpa's ganglion), which lies near the internal auditory meatus. They project to the vestibular nuclei (Fig. 7.42), which lie in the pons and the dorsorostral part of the medulla. They are components of a number of reflex arcs responsive to movement of the head and to apparent changes in the direction of the force of gravity. Such reflexes are responsible for stabilization of the eyes, holding the head erect and maintenance of body stability. They are often not consciously perceived, and awareness of head movement or the direction of gravitational force is often secondary to the automatic reflex responses to acceleratory forces on the head.

Each vestibular nucleus has a particular pattern of projections to the oculomotor system, to the

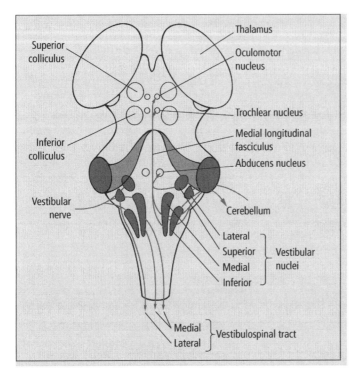

Fig. 7.42 A dorsal view of the brainstem (cerebral cortex and cerebellum removed) showing the central vestibular pathways.

spinal cord and to the cerebellum. The **lateral vestibular nucleus** (Deiter's nucleus) (Fig. 7.42) receives axons from the macula of the utricle and from the cerebellum and spinal cord. Its neurones send their axons into the lateral vestibulospinal tract that terminates ipsilaterally in the ventral horn region along the length of the spinal cord. These axons powerfully facilitate α and γ motor neurones, innervating antigravity muscles. Neurones in the lateral vestibular nucleus respond selectively to tilting of the head. Their resting discharge is increased by tilting in one direction and decreased by tilting in the other. The input from the cerebellum is inhibitory, and removal of this tonic inhibition gives rise to decerebrate rigidity. The **medial** and **superior vestibular nuclei** receive inputs from the ampullae of the semicircular canals. Outputs running in the medial vestibular tract terminate bilaterally in the ventral horn of the cervical region of the cord, making monosynaptic connections with neck muscle motor neurones. These provide for the reflex control of neck

movements to maintain the position of the head and provide a stable base for eye movements. Both nuclei also participate in vestibulo—oculomotor reflexes, having outputs which run in the medial longitudinal fasciculus to the oculomotor nuclei, and give rise to rotatory nystagmus movements. The **inferior vestibular nucleus** receives excitatory inputs from the semicircular canals and from both the utricle and the saccule, and inhibitory inputs from the cerebellum. It has vestibulospinal and vestibuloreticular outputs and also has powerful effects on the cerebellum. Although its specific functions remains controversial, this nucleus integrates input from the whole vestibular apparatus and affects higher brain centres.

Functions of the vestibular system

The vestibular apparatus evokes two interrelated categories of reflex response, **dynamic** and **static**. Oculomotor reflexes, important in stabilization of the visual image on the retina, depend primarily on the dynamic function, which is mediated principally by the semicircular canals. To maintain a stable retinal image during head movements, two quite different reflexes are involved in causing compensatory eye movements. If an object is being looked at, movements of the object or movements of the head are compensated by the **fixation reflex**, which by smooth pursuit movements of the eyes keeps the image of the object on the part of the retina giving the clearest vision, the fovea centralis. There is a limit to the amount by which an eye can be turned in the head to follow an object and to extend this it is necessary for the head to move, or for the eye to return quickly to roughly the straight-ahead position and to find another object of interest to follow as, for example, when looking out from a moving vehicle. This type of eye movement is called **optokinetic nystagmus**. The word 'nystagmus' refers to any oscillatory movements of the eyes, whether normal or pathological; in particular to the slow turn/quick return sequence of the eyes as one looks out from a moving vehicle. The direction of the nystagmus is conventionally named according to the quick phase.

The other mechanism by which the eyes are moved so as to keep an image as steady as possible on the retina is driven by the vestibular apparatus and takes place to some extent whenever the head is moved; for example, when the body is rotated in a revolving chair. This mechanism occurs even with the eyes closed or in total darkness, and is called **vestibular nystagmus** (or rotatory nystagmus). Here the slow drift is in the opposite direction to the rotation of the head and the quick phase is in the same direction. Even in the dark, this reflex may provide full compensation for head movements. In the light, this reflex collaborates with the fixation and optokinetic reflexes.

In addition to visual input the conscious sense of movement depends on the dynamic sensory components of the vestibular apparatus, and involves a part of the cerebral cortex close to the main auditory sensory area in the temporal lobe, tucked into the lateral or Sylvian fissure.

The static reflexes, mediated primarily by the utricle and saccule, are important for the maintenance of the upright position of the head and for body posture. The maintenance of balance depends on the distribution of tone in the body muscles, which is regulated via the vestibular nuclei in the medulla and their connections with the vestibulospinal tract and the cerebellum. Our awareness of the direction of gravity depends on senses in addition to the otolith organs: pressure on the soles of the feet or other parts of the body surface, proprioceptors in muscles and joints, and visual awareness of the horizon.

Disorders of vestibular function

Semicircular canal function can be tested by rotating the subject in a special chair whilst the head is held in such a posture as to stimulate one functionally-associated pair of canals selectively. One can examine the consequences of stopping rotation on either eye movements or on body muscle tone. The latter is manifested by a tendency to deviate from a straight line when walking with the eyes closed. In these procedures, both right and left canals are inevitably stimulated together.

Unilateral stimulation can be produced by running water above or below body temperature into the external meatus of the ear—the **caloric test**. The temperature difference gives rise to convection currents in the endolymph, which excite the hair cells. This produces nystagmus, which can be compared with a known normal response.

Diseases affecting the vestibule or its afferent fibres can cause abnormal discharges producing a sensation of **vertigo**, or giddiness, in which the external world may seem to move, the body may be felt to be moving, or the posture of the limbs, especially the legs, may be felt to be unsteady. Along with this there may be nystagmus, double vision, actual falling, and autonomic signs such as pallor, sweating, pulse rate and blood pressure changes, nausea and vomiting. **Ménière's disease** is characterized by attacks of vertigo and progressive impairment of hearing. The cause is unknown but on postmortem examination the endolymph-filled chambers of the inner ear are found to be enlarged.

When an often-repeated cyclical pattern of strong stimulation of the labyrinth occurs, as in sea travel or land travel in a car along a winding road, similar physiological consequences occur and are known generally as **motion sickness**. This is most marked when there is a lack of coordination between visual and vestibular information, and is often ameliorated or halted if it is possible to visualize the true horizon.

Chapter 8

Motor System

Movements are produced and postures maintained by the contraction of skeletal muscle fibres. The timing and force of contraction in turn depends on the pattern of action potentials discharged by α motor neurones innervating the muscle. Muscle tension is therefore a direct result of the recruitment and discharge frequency of α motor neurones. There are two main inputs regulating α motor neurone activity—sensory signals from the periphery and descending signals from higher centres in the neuraxis. The former are responsible for spinal reflexes and the latter for integrated postural reflexes and voluntary movement. Many of these influences, however, are directed through networks of local spinal interneurones.

8.1 Spinal cord motor system

In addition to the descending and ascending pathways, the spinal motor apparatus includes networks of interneurones converging on α and γ motor neurones, which project to the muscles. These elements together are responsible for the final patterning of muscle activities and are capable of generating some basic patterns of movement.

Motor neurones

There are two classes of motor neurones: large-diameter α cells (30–70 µm) with axons of 12–20 µm diameter that innervate skeletal **extrafusal** fibres in skeletal muscles, and small γ cells (10–30 µm) with axons of 1–8 µm diameter that innervate the **intrafusal fibres** of the muscle spindles. The cell bodies of both classes of neurones are located in the ventral horns of the spinal cord, and in analogous positions in the brainstem. The axons leave the spinal cord through ventral roots or the brain stem through cranial nerves.

α **motor neurones** (skeletomotor) are multipolar cells (many dendrites, one axon) with large somata and their dendrites spread up to 2 mm from the ventral horn to the dorsal horn and even across the midline of the cord, and also up and down a particular cord segment, thus giving many opportunities for synaptic contact. Electron microscopy has shown that the vast dendritic tree of any motor neurone is covered with tens of thousands of synaptic terminals originating from multiple sources. This extreme convergence reflects the fact that motor neurones are the final common pathway from the central nervous system (CNS) to muscle.

γ **motor neurones** (fusimotor) are scattered amongst the α motor neurones of each motor nucleus in the medial and lateral columns of the ventral horn. Their axons pass out of the ventral roots together with the larger-diameter axons of the α motor neurones, and innervate intrafusal fibres of the muscle spindles.

β **motor neurones** (skeletofusimotor) have the same size range as α motor neurones but innervate both extrafusal and intrafusal muscle fibres. Their specific role is not as clear as that of other motor neurones.

Distribution in the spinal cord and brainstem

The cell bodies of motor neurones of trunk and proximal limb muscles lie in groups with a columnar organization (**motor nuclei**) throughout the ventral horn (Fig. 8.1a), forming a long column running almost the entire length of the spinal cord (C1–L4). The rostro-caudal distribution of motor neurones corresponds to the proximo-distal distribution of muscles. In the brainstem, the column becomes discontinuous but the cell bodies of the motor neurones of the cranial nerves III, IV, VI and XII can be found in an analogous position. In the cervical and lumbar enlargements of the cord, the cell bodies of motor neurones of all distal limb muscles lie together in nuclei in the lateral part of the ventral horn (Fig. 8.1a). Generally, motor neurones innervating flexor muscles are more dorsal than those innervating extensor muscles, and motor neurones innervating more distal joints (wrist, fingers) are more lateral than those innervating proximal muscles.

The anatomical separation of medial and lateral columns of motor neurones reflects a functional distinction between the muscle groups they control. The trunk muscles, together with the proximal limb muscles, as well as those moving the feet, are involved in functions such as balance, posture and walking which require body or whole-limb movement. The muscles moving the fingers and wrists normally do not have postural functions and are more often involved in manipulatory movements, although gymnasts may use these muscles to control body position. The descending inputs reaching the ventral horn through interneurones similarly divide into those primarily influencing the medial neurones and hence posture, and those influencing the lateral neurones and hence manipulatory activity.

Preganglionic neurones subserving autonomic reflexes are located in the intermediolateral horn throughout the length of the thoracic and upper lumbar cord.

Role in regulation of muscle force

The motor neurones innervating a given muscle form a group that shares much the same afferent inputs. Therefore, the excitability of all members of the group tends to change in much the same way, at the same time. In general, however, the smallest-diameter motor neurones are more excitable because they have the highest membrane

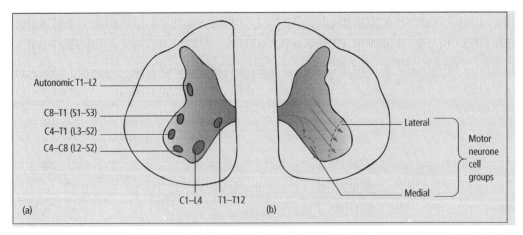

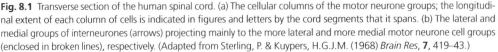

Fig. 8.1 Transverse section of the human spinal cord. (a) The cellular columns of the motor neurone groups; the longitudinal extent of each column of cells is indicated in figures and letters by the cord segments that it spans. (b) The lateral and medial groups of interneurones (arrows) projecting mainly to the more lateral and more medial motor neurone cell groups (enclosed in broken lines), respectively. (Adapted from Sterling, P. & Kuypers, H.G.J.M. (1968) *Brain Res*, **7**, 419–43.)

input resistance and so reach threshold first (see p. 79). Since the smaller-diameter motor neurones form smaller motor units, their discharge generates a small increment of tension. Initially, as each small motor neurone discharges, there is a small increment of tension, larger increments being added later in the contraction when larger-diameter cells are excited. The principle underlying this recruitment order has been termed the 'size principle'. In addition, the firing rate of each active motor neurone increases as the level of excitation increases, leading to mechanical summation of muscle activity (see p. 106). Recruitment and changes in firing rate together enable muscular tension to be varied over a wide range with a relatively small number of motor units.

Interneurones

Most inputs to the spinal motor neurones arise from interneurones dorsal to the ventral horn, which lie dorsally to them in the ventral horn. There are **excitatory** and **inhibitory** interneurones, utilizing a wide range of transmitter substances. Their topography is similar to that of motor neurones, the more medial interneurones project mainly to the medial motor nuclei and the more lateral interneurones to the lateral motor nuclei (Fig. 8.1b). The interneurones receive inputs from sensory nerves and from other motor centres. Many act locally within the same spinal segment to produce **reciprocal inhibition** (as will be seen later) or **recurrent inhibition.** In recurrent inhibition, motor neurones are inhibited by the activity of interneurones (Renshaw cells), which they themselves activate. These inhibitory Renshaw interneurones are excited by acetylcholine released from collateral branches of the motor neurone axon (Fig. 8.2). Recurrent inhibition appears to play an important role in dampening the activity of motor neurones; in particular, it appears to limit the discharge frequency of tonically active α motor neurones. However, it is often overlooked that the major source of excitation to Renshaw cells is from the brain. Moreover, an additional action of Renshaw cells is to inhibit the Ia inhibitory interneurones acting on antagonist muscles, allowing the

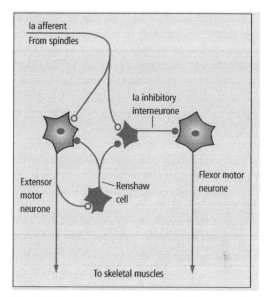

Fig. 8.2 Circuit diagram for recurrent inhibition and reciprocal inhibition. Large 1a sensory fibre from a muscle spindle of an extensor muscle makes monosynaptic contact with a motor neurone innervating the muscle from which the afferent fibres originate, and with a 1a inhibitory interneurone that inhibits the antagonist flexor motor neurone (reciprocal inhibition). The extensor motor neurone in turn excites a Renshaw cell, which inhibits the extensor motor neurone (recurrent inhibition) and also the 1a inhibitory interneurone. The control over the later permits various amounts of co-contractions between antagonist muscles.

co-contraction of antagonist muscles. Other interneurones send information across to the other side of the cord (**commissural** interneurones) or to other spinal levels (**propriospinal** interneurones) to coordinate muscle groups. Finally, other interneurones make synapses directly on presynaptic terminals from sensory afferents and can regulate the efficacy of neurotransmission in various spinal reflex pathways through a mechanism called **presynaptic inhibition**.

8.2 Regulation of motor neurone activity by sensory signals

The spinal motor system receives sensory inputs conveying information from muscle spindles about muscle length and rate of change in length, and from Golgi tendon organs about tension developed by the muscle. This information is used to regulate α motor neurone activity through various spinal reflex pathways.

The activity of α motor neurones is influenced by sensory information arising from receptors in skin (e.g. nociceptors or tactile receptors), muscles and tendons. Muscle length and tension are detected by mechanoreceptors within specialized structures known as **muscle spindles** and **Golgi tendon organs**, respectively. As in the skin, the different types of endings are supplied by nerve fibres of different diameter but they are usually referred to by the I–IV classification (p. 123). Information from these sensors is relayed to the motor neurones directly or indirectly through interneurones to produce rapid and relatively stereotyped responses to perturbations—the **spinal reflexes**. It is important to note that the same sensory information is also distributed to other regions of the CNS where it contributes to the subconscious control of posture and movement (p. 195) and to the control and conscious awareness of limb position (p. 133).

Muscle spindles

Muscle spindles (Fig. 8.3) are made up of two to 12 small-diameter striated muscle fibres termed **intrafusal** muscle fibres. Each muscle contains many muscle spindles. The whole bundle of intrafusal fibres of one spindle is enveloped in a capsule, which lies parallel to the main (extrafusal) muscle fibres and is attached to them at its ends. The middle third of the intrafusal fibres, known as the equatorial region, is non-striated and largely non-contractile. The outer thirds, known as the polar regions, are striated and contractile.

There are two types of intrafusal muscle fibres:
1 nuclear bag fibres, commonly two per spindle, which are longer and thicker and have a group of nuclei clustered around the centre of the fibre; and
2 nuclear chain fibres, commonly four to five per spindle, which are shorter and thinner and have fewer nuclei arranged in a chain along the centre of the fibre (Fig. 8.3).
Group Ia sensory axons coil around the equatorial

region of the nuclear bag and chain fibres to form **primary** receptor endings (**annulospiral endings**). There is only one Group 1a fibre per spindle. Group Ib sensory axons of similar diameter serve Golgi tendon organs as will be seen later. Group II sensory axons (smaller and slower conducting) end mainly on nuclear chain fibres to form **secondary** receptor endings (**flowerspray endings**).

The receptor endings of both group Ia and group II afferents are mechanoreceptors and are stimulated when the equatorial regions of the intrafusal fibres is stretched, as happens when the whole muscle is stretched. Conversely, activity in the spindle endings is reduced or silenced when tension is removed from the equatorial region of the spindle, as might occur when the whole muscle shortens during contraction of the extrafusal muscle fibres. This pattern of responses arises because the spindles lie adjacent and parallel to the extrafusal muscle fibres.

Responses to different degrees of stretch on the muscle spindle provide information about the current length of the muscle. They are known as the **static** or length-sensitive responses and are in some ways analogous to the indentation response of cutaneous mechanoreceptors. Both primary (Ia) and secondary (II) endings give a static response. During static firing, the frequency of impulses is proportional to the muscle length. The static response is probably associated with stretch of both bag and chain fibres.

Spindles also respond to the rate of change of length of the muscle. This is known as the **dynamic** or velocity-sensitive response. Only the primary (Ia) endings give a large dynamic response. The faster the stretch, the higher is the impulse frequency. During release from muscle stretch both primary and secondary endings commonly show a decrease in impulse frequency.

Role of γ motor neurones

In addition to the two types of sensory endings, muscle spindles also have their own motor innervation. This innervation is supplied by fusimotor or γ motor neurones. Stimulation of the γ motor neurones does not alter tension in the whole mus-

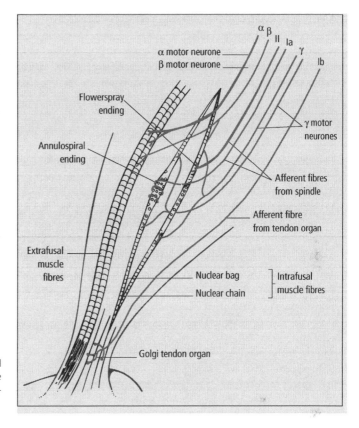

Fig. 8.3 The innervation of extrafusal muscle fibres, the muscle spindle (intrafusal fibres) and the Golgi tendon organ.

cle but it produces contraction of the polar regions of the intrafusal fibres. This, in turn, stretches the equatorial region of the intrafusal fibres, which alters the sensitivity of the spindle to stretching of the whole muscle.

The γ motor neurones have two main roles in regulating spindle sensitivity: one role is maintaining the sensitivity of the spindle during muscle contraction (shortening) and the other role is to adjust the sensitivity as required by different muscle loading conditions. First, shortening of a muscle due to active contraction of extrafusal muscle fibres would slacken the spindles, rendering them less sensitive to imposed stretches at the new muscle length. This is overcome by concurrent activation of γ motor neurones along with the α motor neurones (α–γ co-activation). This has the effect of maintaining tension on the sensory regions of the intrafusal muscle fibres during muscle shortening, and thus maintains their sensitivity. Second, the

motor control system requires that spindle sensitivity to stretch be adjusted in certain situations. For example, during the swing phase of step cycle, plantar flexor muscles of the ankle are necessarily stretched and a strong stretch reflex would interfere with the movement. On the other hand, during the stance phase, a heightened stretch reflex could assist the ongoing movement. To cope with these situations, the γ motor neurones are able to adjust spindle sensitivity at any one muscle length by variation in the level of their activity. For this, independent control of α and γ motor neurones is required.

Static and dynamic responses of spindles can be adjusted independently via two types of γ efferent fibres. These are associated with two types of ending on the intrafusal muscle fibres: **plate endings**, which are found on both nuclear bag and nuclear chain fibres at the ends or poles of the fibres, and may be associated primarily with dynamic γ efferent fibres; and **trail endings**, which are found mainly on nuclear chain fibres just next to the equatorial region of the fibres, and are associated primarily with static γ efferent fibres. Stimulation of static fibres increases the static response of both group Ia and group II afferents, while stimulation of the dynamic fibres increases both the dynamic and static responses of group Ia fibres.

Stretch reflex

Muscle spindles are the starting point for the simplest of all reflexes found in mammals—the **stretch reflex**. When a muscle is stretched, the elongation leads to a discharge in the muscle spindle afferents that is conducted into the spinal cord via the dorsal roots. Within the cord the sensory fibres branch and some terminals make **monosynaptic** excitatory contacts with α motor neurones to the extrafusal muscle fibres of the same muscle or close synergists (Fig. 8.4). Impulses generated in these motor neurones leave the cord in the ventral roots and conduct impulses back to the muscle, causing it to contract and thus oppose the change in length. Thus the stretch reflex tends to restore the initial muscle length and acts as a negative-feedback loop.

Such reflex contraction may be elicited by changes in muscle length of around 1–2 mm. Such imposed lengthening is normally caused by changes in the orientation of limbs in relation to gravity. Stretch reflexes have both phasic and tonic components, are of short latency, and are present to some extent in nearly all muscles but are best seen in the antigravity muscles (e.g. leg extensors). Feedback from stretching an agonist muscle can, under some circumstances, inhibit antagonist muscles producing what is referred to as **reciprocal inhibition**. For example, stretching the biceps (flexor) muscle spindles produces a contraction of the biceps and inhibits (via an inhibitory Ia interneurone) motor neurones to the triceps (extensor) muscle (Fig. 8.4). Reciprocally, stretching the triceps would cause a contraction of the triceps and an inhibition of the biceps.

In medical practice, simple phasic stretch reflexes are evoked by tapping muscle tendons (**tendon jerks**); this produces a brief muscle stretch which excites the dynamically sensitive spindle afferents. Changes in responsiveness can be indicative of neurological disease: for instance, the response may be reduced by a peripheral nerve lesion and exacerbated with lesions of descending pathways to α or γ motor neurones (see Fig. 8.4).

The same reflex pathway can be activated by electrical stimulation of the muscle nerve. At low

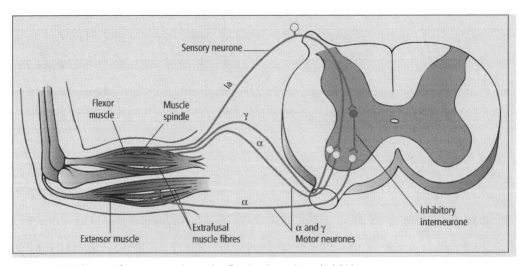

Fig. 8.4 Circuit diagram of a monosynaptic stretch reflex showing reciprocal inhibition.

stimulus strengths, the sensory Ia fibres coming from the spindles can selectively activate α motor neurones. The reflex muscle response thus induced (known as the **H-reflex** after Hoffmann, who first described it) can be recorded electromyographically as a distinct wave (H-wave), with a latency of around 35 ms. Recordings of H-reflexes in humans are useful for examining excitability changes occurring within the spinal cord, since standard repeatable stimuli can easily be applied to the nerve and changes in muscle properties or spindle sensitivity do not affect the response. Therefore, the H-reflex changes in excitability might differ from the changes in tendon jerk excitability.

Role of spindle reflexes in normal muscle tone

When a joint is passively moved a certain resistance is normally felt. This resistance or **tone** is mainly reflex, although a certain level of muscle stiffness is due to intrinsic muscle visco-elastic properties. Such a movement produces a series of reflexes in the stretched muscles, which can be seen as a series of waves in electromyographic recordings. The first, of short latency (monosynaptic), is generated by the phasic activation of primary 1a afferents resulting from the stretch of annulospiral endings. However muscle stretch also activates secondary receptor endings, which will excite α motor neurones through multisynaptic pathways involving interneurones. Finally, muscle stretch will additionally excite the motor cortex through long-loop pathways.

Golgi tendon organs

These are found on tendons, usually near the muscle–tendon junction (Fig. 8.3). Their afferents are group Ib axons which branch over several tendon fascicles. They are covered by a capsule, which, at its ends, becomes continuous with the connective tissue of the muscle or tendon.

A Golgi tendon organ responds to changes in **tension** in its muscle fascicle (and hence in the tendon); an increase in tension increases the frequency of impulses in the Ib afferents. This is due

to its position on the tendon which is in series with the muscle; the tendons do not change length but rather are exposed to the force or tension developed by the muscle. Note that in comparison with muscle spindles, Golgi tendon organs provide information about muscle performance during isometric contraction and also when a muscle actively shortens, since in both cases tension is developed in the tendon. Furthermore, this structural arrangement means that the Golgi tendon organ is much more sensitive to active muscle tension than to passive stretching of the muscle, since in the latter case much of the applied force is dissipated in lengthening the muscle. Thus, Golgi tendon organs respond not only at extreme tension but also during normal tension development.

Golgi tendon organ reflex

Information from Golgi tendon organs is utilized for reflex regulation of muscle tension, somewhat analogously to the spindle reflex control of muscle length. However, in contrast to the stretch reflex, the Golgi tendon reflex pathway operates via an inhibitory interneurone, which has synapses on α motor neurones of the muscle of origin. It is thus another example of a negative-feedback loop. The role of this loop can be most easily appreciated in maintained isometric contractions, such as holding a pen for a long period of time. The 'desired' amount of force is initially generated by a certain level of activity in α motor neurones. An inhibitory influence from the Golgi tendon organs would be exerted on the α motor neurones, but this would be matched by excitatory influences from elsewhere in the CNS. Now, if the muscle force is reduced by fatigue, then activity in the Golgi tendon organs would decline, inhibition of the motor neurones would decrease and the muscle would be excited more strongly. If, on the other hand, the force exerted is too great, the inhibitory effect will be increased and the force correspondingly reduced. It has been recently reported that during certain behaviours, such as during locomotion, the inhibitory action of the Golgi tendon organs can become excitatory and may help increase the output of extensor muscles during stance. This, of course, implies that the signal from Golgi tendon organs can also reach motor neurones through alternative pathways containing excitatory interneurones.

Role of spindle and Golgi tendon organ reflexes in ongoing motor control

It would be a mistake to think that these sensory systems act only in response to external perturbations. They are in fact of vital importance for the precise regulation of α motor neurone activity during the performance of all voluntary movements. The mechanical properties of the musculoskeletal system pose many problems for motor control systems. For example, during a movement, development of force by a muscle for any degree of α motor neurone activation will vary as the muscle changes length, due to the force–length relationship of muscles and to changes in mechanical leverage (p. 101). Similarly, the response of a muscle will differ at different times owing to fatigue. Thus a constant signal will not always produce the same increase in tension. The spinal cord circuits utilizing information from muscle spindles and Golgi tendon organs are able automatically to compensate for these variations from moment-to-moment. These control processes are best called **servomechanisms**; that is, mechanisms that modify output during performance to adapt to varying conditions. Such systems have distinct advantages as they can quickly and accurately follow command signals without the need for intervention by higher centres.

Withdrawal reflexes

Following painful, or potentially painful, stimulation (p. 227) the limb can withdraw away from the pain source. This has been described as a typical flexor reflex. The receptors are skin nociceptors, the central connections are polysynaptic, and excitation is evoked in motor nuclei of most of the limb flexor muscles while antagonistic muscles are inhibited. At the same time, contralateral motor neurones of extensor muscles are excited via interneurones, which cross to the other side of the cord (**crossed extensor reflex**), facilitating support of the body while the hurt limb is withdrawn. However, non-painful skin stimuli can also give rise to fine positioning responses of the foot and well organized specific pathways have been described to account for the multiplicity of responses triggered by the activation of different cutaneous nerves or branches following perturbations applied to various skin areas.

Although in general reflex responses are considered, by definition, as stereotypic, there are now several examples of reflex responses that can change over the various phases of complex movements such as encountered during locomotion (phase-dependent modulation of reflexes). For instance, a skin input may be excitatory for certain groups of muscles during one phase of the movement and be inefficient in the opposite phase of the movement or even be inhibitory or excitatory to the motor neurones active during this opposite phase of the movement. Such is the case for stimuli applied to the dorsum of the foot during swing (e.g. an obstacle), which generates a complex sequence of compensatory responses that bring the foot above and in front of the obstacle. When the same stimulus is applied during the stance phase, a flexion response would be inappropriate since the contralateral limb is already in flexion and unable to support the weight. In such conditions, the stimulation of the foot in stance gives rise only to a short latency inhibition, often followed by an excitatory response of the extensors.

Functions of spinal circuits in motor control

The neural circuits formed by the interneurones are responsible for the final shaping of motor neurone activity resulting from sensory or descending inputs. Most pathways to the spinal motor apparatus act by synapsing on interneurones, rather than by acting directly on motor neurones (certain notable exceptions to this include monosynaptic connections to motor neurones from muscle spindle afferents and some axons from cortical and motor brainstem structures).

Spinal networks are involved in controlling more complex aspects of motor coordination. Interneurones carry information:

1 between motor nuclei within the ventral cord to coordinate muscle activities within a limb;

2 across the cord to coordinate activity of limb pairs; and

3 up and down the cord to other spinal segments via propriospinal interneurones, enabling coordination between limb girdles.

Certain basic movement patterns such as walking, which require complex integration of activity in diverse motor neurone pools, may be organized within the cord by such intrinsic interneuronal networks, which are often referred to as central pattern generators (CPG). It is of great interest for motor control in general that, in animal preparations, such rhythmic patterns can be recorded from the spinal cord even when it is deprived of sensory afferent inputs—by section of all dorsal roots or by neurochemical paralysis which abolishes all overt movements—and deprived of all descending inputs by a complete spinal transection. Therefore, the role of descending signals from the brain and of sensory signals from peripheral structures is to initiate, stop and control the movement patterns produced by these networks so that they are adapted to the environment in which the movements take place. Thus, the walking pattern is adapted to cope with surface irregularities—reflexly by sensory inputs, and predictively (cerebral cortex) by descending inputs from the brain.

8.3 Supraspinal control of movement

Descending commands to motor neurones arise from various sites in the brainstem, and from regions of the cerebral cortex. The brainstem structures have diverse functions in motor control, many relating to less voluntary aspects such as automatic regulation of muscle tone and upright posture. Cerebral cortical involvement relates more to the control of discrete voluntary movements. In turn, cerebral cortical motor functions are modulated by important contributions from the basal ganglia and the cerebellum.

Pathways to spinal motor circuits

Inputs to spinal motor circuits arising from higher centres in the neuraxis are necessary for the instigation of coordinated movements and their postural concomitants. Most of these inputs act via synapses on spinal cord interneurones, but some synapse directly upon the motor neurones. There are six main pathways (Fig. 8.5). The corticospinal tract (comprising a large lateral part and small ventral part) originates in the cerebral cortex; the rubro-, lateral vestibulo- and reticulospinal tracts

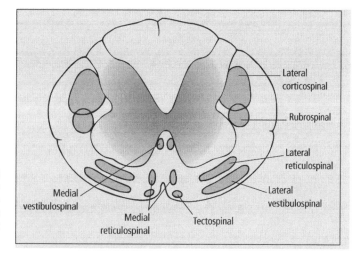

Fig. 8.5 Diagram of the descending pathways of the spinal cord in transverse section. (The small ventral corticospinal tract lying medial to the medial reticulospinal tract is not shown.)

Lateral corticospinal

Rubrospinal

Lateral reticulospinal

Lateral vestibulospinal

Tectospinal

Medial reticulospinal

Medial vestibulospinal

originate in the brainstem and extend the length of the spinal cord; the tecto- and medial vestibulospinal tracts also originate in the brainstem, but extend only through the cervical region and are primarily concerned in regulating the motor nuclei of neck muscles.

Brainstem motor systems

Role of individual nuclei in the brainstem

Regions of the brainstem that are important in controlling movements are the red nucleus, the lateral vestibular nucleus, the medial vestibular nucleus, the pontine and medullary reticular formation, the deep layers of the superior colliculus, the locus coeruleus and the raphe nuclei (Fig. 8.6).

The **red nucleus** (nucleus ruber) receives inputs from the cerebral cortex and from the dentate and intermediate nuclei of the cerebellum. In their relationship to movement, neurones of this nucleus are similar to those found in motor cortical regions (p. 197); however, they may be involved in the regulation of more automatic, well-learnt movements. Cells of the posterior or magnocellular part of the nucleus receive afferents from the intermediate nuclei and send axons to the spinal cord via the **rubrospinal tract** (Fig. 8.5). These efferent fibres cross immediately and run down the contralateral side of the brainstem and spinal cord. Their terminals are distributed similarly to those of the crossed corticospinal tract in the dorsolateral part of the intermediate zone, although some synapse directly with α motor neurones. Cells of the anterior or parvocellular part of the nucleus receive afferents from the dentate and send axons ipsilaterally to terminate in the inferior olive (often also called the inferior olivary nucleus).

The **lateral vestibular or Deiters nucleus** receives input from the otolith organs of the vestibular apparatus, i.e. dynamic information about linear accelerations and static information about head tilt. It also gets a major input from the cerebellum and the pontine reticular formation. Neurones of this nucleus project ipsilaterally into the **lateral vestibulospinal tract** (Fig. 8.5), which ter-

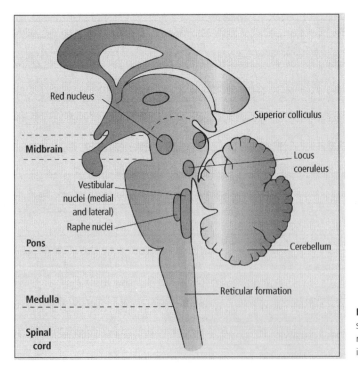

Red nucleus

Superior colliculus

Midbrain

Locus coeruleus

Vestibular nuclei (medial and lateral)

Raphe nuclei

Pons

Cerebellum

Medulla

Reticular formation

Spinal cord

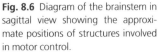

Fig. 8.6 Diagram of the brainstem in sagittal view showing the approximate positions of structures involved in motor control.

minates in the medial or anterior white matter of the spinal cord. A few fibres terminate directly on medial motor neurones. This system seems to be involved in maintaining the upright stance against perturbations associated with head movements.

The **medial vestibular nucleus** receives information about dynamic angular accelerations of the head from the semicircular canals; it projects via the uncrossed **medial vestibulospinal tract** (Fig. 8.5)—the caudal equivalent of the medial longitudinal fasciculus—and influences the oculomotor nuclei (III, IV and VI) in the brainstem and spinal cord which control eye and neck muscles. This system is involved in the **vestibulo-ocular reflex** (p. 182) that stabilizes eye position on visual targets during head rotation; it also activates neck muscles in response to vestibular stimulation to keep the head stable during body movements.

The **reticular formation** is a diffuse aggregation of cells in the core of the brainstem, permeated by a tangle of fibres running in all directions. These fibres give it a reticular (net-like) appearance histologically. Some components of this system are concerned with somatic motor control, regulating eye, neck, trunk and limb movements. They receive somatic and proprioceptive sensory signals, as well as descending inputs from the cerebral cortex and limbic system. They are also interconnected with the fastigial and intermediate nuclei of the cerebellum. The reticular system can be divided into pontine and medullary parts: the pontine part projects ipsilaterally down the spinal cord, while the medullary part sends axons down both sides of the cord. The **reticulospinal fibres** (Fig. 8.5) terminate on the ventromedial group of interneurones and to a small extent on medial motor neurones. The pontine part is important for automatic maintenance of the upright stance, through facilitation of antigravity reflexes; the medullary part seems to suppress spinal reflexes during sleep and also to allow descending controls to override them during voluntary movement.

The **superior colliculus** (tectum) is the dorsal region of the mesencephalon that receives inputs conveying visual information; it seems to be important in generating head movements that help direct one's gaze (i.e. coordinated eye and head

movements) to a particular point. It may also be important in mediating very fast orientation movements in response to visual stimuli. Tectospinal fibres from this region join the **medial vestibulospinal tract in the medial longitudinal fasciculus** (Fig. 8.5) to form a bilateral pathway terminating on interneurones in the cervical cord.

The **locus coeruleus** is located near the floor of the rostral part of the fourth ventricle. It projects widely in the CNS, including the cerebral cortex and the spinal cord. Neurones in the locus coeruleus contain the neurotransmitter noradrenaline. Neurones from the **raphe nuclei** also project to both the cerebral cortex and the spinal cord. They are a narrow continuous collection of cells in the middle of the brainstem, which contain the neurotransmitter 5-hydroxytryptamine (serotonin). The locus coeruleus and raphe nuclei are activated in a non-specific way by external stimuli and internal states, such as sleep and wakefulness, and the monoamines released appear to modulate the responsiveness of neurones to set their background excitability level in relation to demands likely to be made of them.

Role of brainstem motor systems in postural control and movement

By **posture** we mean the maintenance for a period of time of position of the head, limbs, and trunk in space, as a prelude or background to movement. Fundamentally, posture implies maintenance of a particular distribution of muscle tone, to achieve a particular disposition of the body usually against the omnipresent force of gravity. Postural control includes a wide variety of motor acts and is a function of all levels of the motor system. For instance, postural activities occur with or even in advance of voluntary movements to maintain balance. These **postural adjustments** are triggered by the cerebral motor cortex, often in **anticipation** of changes in the body's centre of mass accompanying voluntary movements. At the other extreme, the spinal cord networks and the various spinal reflexes are responsible for more simple, immediate reflex responses to peripheral perturbations of individual limbs. In between, there are more complex responses, some of which are controlled by motor structures of the brainstem. An important source of descending inputs which trigger the spinal circuits into action is the **pedunculopontine nucleus** (see Fig. 8.9), often called the mesencephalic locomotor region (MLR). Stimulation of this nucleus in decerebrate animals will induce locomotion on a treadmill. The pedunculopontine nucleus is connected to neurones of the reticular formation, which send signals to the CPG to induce locomotion. The pedunculopontine nucleus is regulated in turn by the subthalamic nucleus of the basal ganglia (Fig. 8.9), which receives input from the motor cortex.

The vestibular nuclei contribute to postural reflexes in response to changes in head position. For instance, when the head is dorsiflexed, the otolith organs (p. 180) are stimulated and pathways from the vestibular nuclei activate appropriate motor neurones to promote extension of all four limbs (assisting postural support), and the eyes 'counter-roll' downwards. The eye movement responses are most clearly seen in severely brain-damaged, comatose patients with an intact brainstem where the eyes counter-rotate in the opposite direction to passive rotations of the head (**doll's eye phenomenon**). However, a major additional component of limb and eye responses to changes in head position arises from activation of neck proprioceptors (e.g. muscle spindles of neck muscles), which produces tonic neck reflexes. Normally, the vestibular and neck muscle reflexes interact with each other and with ongoing motor activities; they are most clearly demonstrated in isolation in preparations which are not producing spontaneous movements, and in which only the neck or vestibular systems are intact.

Linear acceleration also stimulates the otolith organs, and the reflexes that follow are organized by the lateral vestibular nuclei which give rise to the vestibulospinal tracts. An example of this type of reflex is the **vestibular placing reaction**. This can be evoked by suddenly tipping a blindfolded cat head-down, whereupon its forelegs extend. If the blindfold is removed, a cat will still extend its legs even if its utricles are destroyed—a **visual placing reaction**. In general, visual stimuli can substitute

for labyrinthine stimuli in postural reflexes. Thus, animals and humans with bilateral labyrinthine damage have normal posture if they can use their eyes.

Angular acceleration stimulates the semicircular canals (p. 177) and the ensuing reflexes involve the medial (and other) vestibular nuclei, which contributes to the medial longitudinal fasciculi and the medial vestibulospinal tracts. Eye movements evoked by prolonged angular rotation are called **vestibular nystagmus** (p. 183), comprising a slow phase in the direction of rotation followed by a rapid saccade in the opposite direction. Limb muscle responses are subtle, but involve a biasing of limb muscle tone that would tend to counter any imposed rotation.

The role of the brainstem in postural control is most clearly demonstrated in quadrupeds, where the brainstem alone is capable of organizing entire sequences of postural responses into coherent adaptive behaviour. This was revealed in experiments in which the brain and spinal cord of quadrupeds were transected at various levels. When the spinal cord is isolated from higher centres (a spinal preparation), the animal cannot remain upright for any length of time, although it will exhibit stepping motions. If the cut is made at the level of the upper medulla, such an animal can stand for long periods but cannot right itself if laid on its side, while a cut through the midbrain will permit such righting responses. Thus the complex integrated response of standing up can be organized in the brainstem in such species. In primates, however, descending inputs from higher centres are required for full expression of these behaviours.

Voluntary movements

More than one hundred and fifty years ago the pioneering English neurologist, Hughlings Jackson, categorized movements along a continuum from automatic to voluntary. At the lowest level, were automatic movements; simple stereotyped reactions largely under immediate sensory control. At the highest level, were voluntary movements known to be varied, purposeful and requiring the integrity of the cerebral cortex. In somewhat altered form, this continuum is recognized even today and the term voluntary movement still implies purposeful movements that are the results of a long, and not necessarily linear, process of transformations from stimulus to response. The simple act of reaching for an object involves transforming the visual stimulus which is initially represented in the retina and visual system in terms of a retinotopic coordinate system into a muscle and limb-based coordinate framework based on the timing and appropriate force commands associated with reaching and grasping. For this reason it is not surprising that many cortical motor areas have now been identified as involved in different stages of this complex sequence and the degree to which they function in sequence or in parallel is currently the subject of much research. In fact, the entire nervous system may be viewed as a multipurpose movement controller.

Motor cortex

The motor cortex consists of several regions in the cerebral cortex, which are directly involved in the regulation of brainstem and spinal cord motor systems. In general terms, the motor cortex is important in the control of voluntary movements, particularly those accurately performed. The cortical regions (Fig. 8.7) involved include:

1 the **primary motor cortex**, which lies in the precentral gyrus immediately rostral to the primary sensory areas;

2 the **premotor** and **supplementary motor** areas, which lie laterally and medially, respectively, in front of the primary motor cortex;

3 the **frontal eye field**, which lies further rostrally again; and

4 additional areas in the **cingulate gyrus** close to the supplementary motor area.

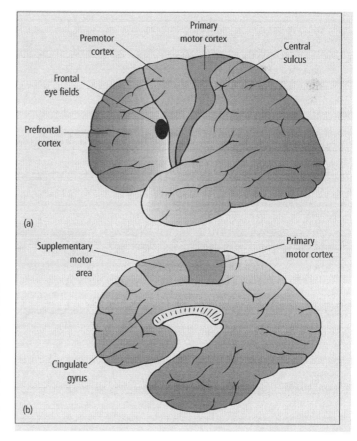

Fig. 8.7 Motor areas of the brain. (a) Lateral surface of the left cerebral hemisphere showing the primary motor cortex (precentral gyrus), the premotor cortex and the frontal eye field. (b) Medial view of the surface of the right cerebral hemisphere (with the left hemisphere removed), showing the medial extension of the primary motor cortex and also the SMA in front of the primary cortex.

These areas are identified as being important in motor control on several grounds. For example, neuronal activity in these areas is found to accompany voluntary movements, and electrical stimulation of these regions can evoke discrete movements involving a single muscle or a small number of muscles. Damage to the cortical motor regions may disturb movement control in various ways. Each of these regions contain neurones which send efferent fibres into the cerebral peduncle that ultimately terminate either in the spinal cord **(the corticospinal tract)** (Fig. 8.5) or in the motor nuclei of the cranial nerves in the brain stem (the **corticobulbar tract**).

The origin of the names for some of the regions requires explanation. The **primary** motor cortex was the first recognized, and is most clearly implicated in the immediate control of discrete movements. Lesions here produce a localized paralysis of the contralateral body called hemiplegia. Electrical stimulation is able to elicit discrete movements at very low intensities and its organization reveals a more detailed somatotopic map (see below) than any of the other areas. Neuronal activity recorded in this region during voluntary movements is closely coupled to the speed and force with which these movements are executed. Stimulation of the **supplementary** motor area (SMA) reveals a smaller, less ordered somatotopic map. The cells are somewhat less tightly coupled to movement, and lesions produce only transient deficits. The **premotor** area was at first not considered to have any direct influence on the spinal motor apparatus, but direct projections have now been found. Electrical stimulation produces some movements, at a rather high intensity of stimulation.

Corticospinal (pyramidal) tract

Axons projecting from the cortex to the brainstem or spinal cord arise in layers III and V of both motor and sensory regions of cortex, in almost equal proportions. Neurones within the sensory areas project to the dorsal cord and presumably modulate sensory systems predominantly, although they will not be considered further here. The axons of the motor cortex descend through the posterior

limb of the internal capsule and the cerebral peduncles to pass through the ventral pons and medulla. In the midbrain and medulla, some axons (corticobulbar fibres) leave the tract and pass to the motor nuclei of cranial nerves. These are crossed pathways but no definite tracts can be seen as the axons pass across the brainstem in small separate bundles. Axons also terminate in the red nucleus and the reticular nuclei, both of which give rise to spinal projections themselves.

The majority of corticospinal fibres cross or decussate to the opposite side in the caudal medulla, forming a pyramidal-shaped structure which gives the tract its alternative name. The crossed fibres thereupon enter the spinal cord, forming the lateral corticospinal tract (Fig. 8.5). A few fibres (15%) do not cross at this level and pass down ipsilaterally in the anterior fasciculus of the spinal cord.

The fibres of the lateral corticospinal tract terminate on the lateral group of interneurones in the dorsolateral part of the intermediate zone. In primates, and in particular humans, about 10% of the fibres also terminate directly on motor neurones—mostly in motor nuclei in the lower cervical cord, which serve more distal muscles such as of the forearm and hand.

Somatotopic maps in the motor cortex

Electrical stimulation of discrete parts of the cerebral hemispheres of humans and experimental animals evokes movements on the opposite side of the body. Experiments in which the cortex is systematically stimulated millimetre-by-millimetre reveal at least two representations or maps of the body in terms of movements evoked: one within the precentral gyrus (primary motor cortex), and another on the medial surface of the brain (SMA).

In the primary motor cortex, also known as the MI, the movements evoked are always only brief twitches rather than complex series of movements. Leg movements are elicited from regions extending on to the medial surface of each hemisphere, while movements of the trunk, arm, hand and head muscles are elicited in a fairly ordered (**somatotopic**) sequence across the mediolateral extent of the hemisphere. The somatotopic representation of the body is similar to that in the postcentral gyrus (see p. 129), except that the size of the representation in the precentral gyrus is proportional not to the density of receptors but to the precision of voluntary control over muscles in a particular body region.

The basic plan of the somatotopic representation within the primary motor cortex arises because each region is connected via the corticospinal tracts with the appropriate interneurones and motor neurones to produce muscle contraction of that part of the body. However, the details, especially boundaries between body parts, are highly variable between individuals and even flexible over time within a single individual. The boundaries seem to be controlled by local cortical inhibitory connections, and by patterns of thalamic inputs relaying sensory information from the periphery. In addition, neurones within the motor cortex receive afferents from the somatosensory cortex (the postcentral gyrus) conveying stimuli from skin, muscle and tendon receptors. These afferents are segregated into a caudal zone extending from the fundus deep within the central sulcus to the cortical surface, which is largely cutaneous and a rostral zone extending from the convexity of the sulcus forward to the premotor area where the afferents originate mainly from muscles and tendons.

The map within the supplementary motor cortex extends rostrally from, and is continuous with, the primary motor cortex leg representation. Although also broadly somatotopic, in that arm and head movements tend to be evoked from more rostral regions, the map is much smaller, extending for only about 2–3 cm, and the areas are less well defined. When it was identified first in humans using very high electrical currents, stimulation produced complex synergistic movements of the contralateral limbs and body, often with vocalization. However, since responses similar to those seen in MI have been found, there is still no definitive agreement about the deficits associated with lesions restricted to the SMA (see below).

Functions of motor cortical subregions

Primary motor cortex

As noted above, stimulation of this area of brain reveals a fairly detailed map or representation of the movement of the body. However, each joint, and in fact each muscle, is represented several times at different sites within the map, perhaps reflecting organization at the cortical level in terms of combinations of muscles required for different movements, rather than of muscles *per se*.

Neurones within each region are found to be active in relation to movement of the same joint or muscle; a proportion of these neurones project to the spinal cord (**corticospinal cells**). Pyramidal tract neurones show a variety of discharge patterns in relation to voluntary movements. Some cells, called phasic cells are silent at rest and only discharge at the initiation of movement. Others are spontaneously active and modulate their discharge frequency up or down depending on the speed and force of the muscle contraction. Many cells change their activity just before muscle activation, and this is believed to be one of the efferent signals, along with others arising from the cerebellum and postcentral gyrus that initiate voluntarily controlled muscle action. The activity of some cells also specifies the force produced by the muscles during the ensuing contraction. Although the majority of corticospinal cells act by way of connections with spinal interneurones, some of them, particularly those related to the digit muscles, synapse directly on α motor neurones and often control several muscles, which work together (**synergists**). These special neurones are called **corticomotoneuronal cells** and are thought to be especially important for achieving fractionated movements of individual digits (e.g. of the fingers during precision grip). This function is the most severely affected by damage to the primary motor cortex or the pyramidal tract.

In addition to a role in control of individual muscle action, large numbers of MI neurones act together to specify movement direction, by selectively stimulating muscle groups acting at a particular joint—as for example at the shoulder. In fact, during a shoulder movement, most cells in the shoulder region of the cortex change their activity in some way partly because the shoulder is one of the few joints that is held in place by tonic muscle activity. This coding of movement direction by a large number of cells (**population coding**) means that an infinite variety of movement directions can be specified by changing the mix of activity in a large but finite number of cells. It also means that no individual cell has to specify the movement accurately because the precision arises out of the summed activity of many cells. In addition, no one cell is indispensable and individual cells can die, but the population will still be able to specify the movement. However, if a sufficient number of cells die within the shoulder region such as after a trauma or stroke, the shoulder is paralysed and a painful condition called subluxation often results.

Primary motor cortex neurones in turn are regulated by inputs which arise from other regions of the motor cortex, from the sensory cortex of the postcentral gyrus, and from the parietal cortex. In addition, inputs are relayed through the thalamus from the cerebellum and basal ganglia. Traditionally, the primary motor cortex has been seen as the final common path through which most of the higher motor control is routed; now, however, it is realized that many regions of the wider motor cortex have direct access to the spinal cord, and thus act to some extent in parallel to the primary motor cortex.

Frontal eye field

This region is in front of the premotor cortex on the lateral surface of the brain (Fig. 8.7). Stimulation in the frontal eye field evokes movements of the eyes and sometimes turning of the head in the direction of movement. The commonest movement elicited is a conjugate deviation of the eyes to the contralateral side. The frontal eye fields are probably the primary motor cortex for the eyes, since no eye movements are evoked by stimulation within the precentral gyrus. Neuronal activity in the frontal eye fields is enhanced during voluntary eye movements and destruction of this area causes failure to inhibit saccadic eye movements to any new visual stimuli.

Supplementary motor area (also known as MII)

As noted above, the SMA is found on the medial surface of each hemisphere above the cingulate gyrus and in front of the leg area of the primary motor cortex (Fig. 8.7). There is debate over the function of the SMA. On the one hand, it may have higher-order functions, such as in planning or programming of movements generated internally, rather than in response to external cues. Patients with lesions here are reported to show a lack of spontaneous movement and speech, and recent studies of regional blood flow in humans have shown that when only thinking about a motor task there is an increased blood flow in the SMA of both sides, while an increase in the contralateral MI only occurs if the movement takes place. Electrical signs of cortical activity before movement recorded from human subjects (Fig. 8.8) are also suggestive of a preparatory role for the SMA. In these experiments, subjects perform the same movement many times, and the tiny electroencephalogram signals recorded from the subject's scalp are averaged before and during the movement. Prior to movement a very early negative potential (the **readiness potential**)—presumably indicative of excitation of cortical neurones—is recorded, which can begin more than 0.5 s before the movement. It then merges with a potential associated with the movement itself (the **motor potential**). The readiness potential can be recorded widely over the skull but is maximal over the SMA and is assumed to originate there. It is found to be largest in internally driven rather than in externally cued movements. It is also larger when a complex, rather than simple, series of repetitive movements is performed.

Neurones in the SMA are more likely to be active very early prior to movement than are MI neurones. Recently, neurones have been found in the SMA that seem to be active only when an animal is performing a remembered sequence of movements, rather than the same movements in response to visual signals.

On the other hand, a role for the SMA in more direct motor control is also presumed, because of the projections from the SMA to the spinal cord, the

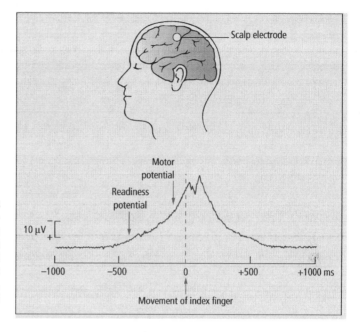

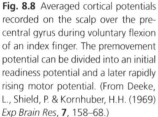

Fig. 8.8 Averaged cortical potentials recorded on the scalp over the precentral gyrus during voluntary flexion of an index finger. The premovement potential can be divided into an initial readiness potential and a later rapidly rising motor potential. (From Deeke, L., Shield, P. & Kornhuber, H.H. (1969) *Exp Brain Res*, **7**, 158–68.)

presence in the SMA of MI-like responses to cortical stimulation and of MI-like neurones active in relation to simple, triggered movements. The actual direct motor control function of the SMA is unknown. It may be important in suppressing unwanted movements, since lesions of the area in humans do affect the ability to inhibit movements, such as 'forced-grasping' a neurological sign in which patients involuntarily grasp any object placed in the hand. However, the lesions associated with forced grasping may have extended deeper to include the cingulate motor area as well as the SMA. Alternatively, the SMA may have a special role in facilitating coordinated movements between both sides of the body. Evidence for this includes the fact that ablation of the SMA in monkeys brings about a disturbance of bimanual coordination. Also, neurones, found in the SMA, discharge in relation to whether the hands are used together or singly, rather than in relation to activity of a particular muscle.

Premotor cortex

This lies between the precentral gyrus and the prefrontal cortex on the lateral surface of the brain and is frequently divided into a dorsal premotor area medial to the arcuate sulcus and a ventral premotor area that lies more laterally (Fig. 8.7). It shows a limited response to brain stimulation at rather high stimulus levels. It is possible that several subregions exist. Overall, it is postulated to be important in planning for movements, particularly those performed in response to external cues.

Other areas involved in movement control

Other areas, including parts of the cingulate gyrus and parietal cortex, have recently been included within the motor cortex on the basis of connections with the primary motor cortex and spinal cord, and the relation of their neuronal activity to movement. Functions of the cingulate areas are at present obscure, but seem similar to those ascribed to the SMA and premotor cortex. The parietal cortex has long been known to be important in movement performance; a person who suffers a left-sided parietal lobe lesion may be unable to carry out actions requiring a series of sequential movements on command, though quite capable of the individual movements. This condition is termed **apraxia**. However, it eventually becomes partly a subjective decision where motor cortex begins and ends; for instance, lesions of visual processing areas in the parieto-occipital cortex can produce specific movement deficits called **visuomotor apraxias**, the most common of which is dressing apraxia. Lesions of this region also cause uncoordinated reaching movements known as **optic ataxia**. These movement abnormalities are not seen in acutely blind patients, suggesting that some aspect of movement control must already be processed in these regions. In the end, it can be argued that all of the brain is involved to some extent in movement control!

Role of the ventrolateral thalamic nuclei

The ventral division of each thalamus consists of anterior, lateral and posterior nuclei. It is the lateral group that is concerned with motor function. It is well established that the neurones of the ventrolateral nucleus project to and receive projections from the ipsilateral motor cortex. The thalamic neurones are in turn excited by axons from the contralateral deep cerebellar nuclei (see Fig. 8.12) and also receive input from the basal ganglia (Fig. 8.9) (p. 204). This input is topographically distributed. There is thus the potential for complex integration of signals from the basal ganglia and cerebellum with signals from the motor cortex representing recent motor commands.

Effects of damage to the descending motor pathways

Effects on control of posture, tone and some rhythmic processes

The projections of the brainstem and cortex systems to the spinal motor apparatus are very important in regulating the excitability of the α motor neurones, which in turn is an important determinant of the reflex response to muscle to stretching (muscle tone). Immediately following a spinal transection, for example in the cervical region below the level of the phrenic motor neurones, there ensues a state of profound torpor: the muscles lie inert, the strongest stimulation of a sensory nerve evokes no response, reflexes are unobtainable, the blood vessels dilate, the blood pressure falls, thermal sweating is absent, the bladder distends leading to urinary overflow and the viscera in general are quiescent. This condition is known as **spinal shock**. It is not due to the trauma or low blood pressure, but to interruption in the normal flow of impulses down the long descending tracts of the cord that impinge on interneurones and motor neurones, so that their excitability is lowered. The lateral vestibular and pontine reticulospinal tracts are most important in this respect and spinal shock follows any section caudal to the lateral vestibular nucleus. The course of recovery varies with the species from a few minutes in frogs to some weeks in humans. There is a gradual increase in excitability; first, flexor withdrawal reflexes return with extensor inhibition, then the bladder and rectum empty reflexly, the blood pressure rises, and after some months (in humans) extensor activity returns and tendon jerks can be elicited. In several animal species, there is a gradual reappearance of spinal locomotor patterns when hindquarters are put on a treadmill belt. Although these locomotor movements are involuntary they have several characteristics of the normal locomotor hindlimb movements. Soon after the spinal section, such locomotor movements can be triggered by monoamines.

The recovery of excitability of the motor neurones, which underlies the reflex recovery, may be due to sprouting of the terminals of their remaining inputs. This may enable the input fibres to excite the motor neurones more readily. There may also be an increase in sensitivity of the motor neurones to the transmitter released by the remaining inputs, so that the same quantity of transmitter is now more effective. This would be akin to the post-denervation supersensitivity of skeletal muscle.

Complete brainstem section just rostral to the vestibular nuclei causes the tone to be exaggerated instead of lost. The exaggeration of tone is so extreme in antigravity muscles that a particular posture is maintained—**decerebrate rigidity**. Humans in this condition have arms and legs extended, the back arched and the head dorsiflexed. The feet are ventroflexed and the arms pointed. The wrists are flexed but the fingers little affected. The rigidity is due, essentially, to the removal of inhibitory influences with the maintenance of facilitatory influences, and can be made more extreme by making a more rostral transection, in the midbrain, leaving the pontine reticular nuclei intact. Neurones in this nucleus, like the neurones of the lateral vestibular nucleus, excite the motor neurones of antigravity muscles.

Decorticate rigidity occurs when the motor systems above the brainstem are severely damaged, e.g. removal of most of the cerebral cortex. It differs from decerebrate rigidity in that it can be modified by reflexes, and shows great variation in severity in different species. Cats, for instance, can walk about in a decorticate condition, but a human being in this condition is unconscious, with legs extended and arms in a position determined by the head position (through neck reflexes). Thus, if the head is turned to the right, the right arm is extended and the left arm flexed and if the rotation is to the left the opposite is seen.

Effects on voluntary movement

A complete transection of the spinal cord will cause permanent loss of all voluntary movement controlled by motor neurones caudal to the plane of section. People with a spinal-cord transection above the lumbar but below the cervical enlargement are paralysed in both legs and are said to be **paraplegic**. A section above or in the cervical enlargement below C4 will give rise to paralysis of all four limbs. Such people are called **quadriplegics**. A transection above C4 can lead immediately to death unless respiratory assistance is provided.

Paralysis or weakness of one side of the body (**hemiplegia**) commonly results from a sudden interruption of the blood supply to an area of the nervous system, causing disruption of the cortical motor pathways to the spinal cord. This is commonly referred to as a **stroke**. Because of the crossed nature of this motor innervation, a hemiplegia signals a lesion of pathways on the opposite side of the brain.

Although reflexes in humans are regained 2–4 weeks after interruption at any level of the pathways from the motor cortex, recovery of voluntary movements takes much longer and is rarely complete. In particular, finger and hand movements are seldom completely regained.

The signs commonly displayed by a patient with hemiplegia, on examination, include the following.

1 Muscle **weakness** without wasting, particularly of distal muscle groups, e.g. finger muscles are more affected than shoulder. Also the arm muscles are commonly more affected than the leg muscles. Because of their bilateral innervation, the muscles that move the eyes, the muscles of the upper third of the face and the trunk muscles, are spared in unilateral lesions.

2 Changes in muscle tone. For weeks or months there is commonly reduced resistance to movement—**hypotonia**. In many patients, this is then replaced by **spastic tone** in which the resistance to movement typically increases as the muscles are stretched. Spasticity is a velocity-dependent increase in muscle tone with exaggerated tendon jerks, resulting from hyperexcitability of the stretch reflex. After stretching the muscle, there is a brisk return to the original position, contrary to rigidity seen in Parkinsonian patients (see later).

3 Changes in reflexes. For weeks or months reflexes are lost or diminished in amplitude, but eventually in many patients the amplitude of reflexes such as the jaw, biceps, knee and ankle jerks is increased. **Clonus**, i.e. repeated responses to a single stimulus, may be present.

4 Absence of superficial reflexes. The abdominal reflexes—a brisk contraction of the abdominal muscles following stroking of the overlying skin—are lost.

5 Extensor plantar response (**Babinski's sign**). Normally, the big toe and all the other toes turn down when the lateral border of the foot is stroked. With interruption of the corticospinal pathway the big toe dorsiflexes instead. This is reminiscent of the alternative cutaneous reflex responses mentioned above. The Babinski's sign is said to be the most important sign in clinical neurology. In babies of a few months old, Babinski's sign is present, but as myelination of nervous pathways proceeds and the corticospinal input takes control, the reflex disappears. Its return in hemiplegia is thus no surprise.

This constellation of signs is known to neurologists as the **upper motor neurone syndrome**. In addition, the hemiplegic will display other signs that will indicate the level of the lesion. For example, difficulties with speech with a right hemiplegia suggest a left-side cortical lesion, while the presence of visual field defects and disorders of sensation may indicate a lesion in the internal capsule, and the presence of a third-nerve palsy may indicate a midbrain lesion.

The neurological basis of the signs of hemiplegia is to some extent obvious. For instance, the loss of movement and its distribution, and the initial loss of tone and reflexes reflect the interruption of the cortical output to motor neurones. The spastic tone and brisk tendon jerks indicate an increase in excitation of α motor neurones. This may arise as the result of changes in the spinal cord. These changes include a slowly increasing effectiveness in the excitation of motor neurones by the primary endings of muscle spindles and a slowly decreasing effectiveness of the reciprocal inhibition of antagonist motor neurones.

8.4 Basal ganglia

The basal ganglia are a group of interconnected nuclei deep to the cerebral cortex in each hemisphere (Fig. 3.19). They comprise the **neostriatum**, made up of the caudate nucleus and putamen, the **globus pallidus, claustrum, subthalamic nucleus** and the **substantia nigra**, a darkly pigmented nucleus lying in the midbrain.

The basal ganglia is important in regulating the function of the cerebral cortex. All regions of cortex project to the basal ganglia, which, via the thalamus, eventually project back upon the cortex (Fig. 8.9) through direct and indirect loops. The net effects of these loops are excitatory or inhibitory in the cortex. Indeed, activity through these loops is modulated by circuitry within the basal ganglia, so that only specific pathways are active while others

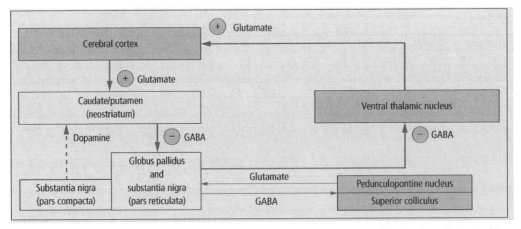

Fig. 8.9 Some basal ganglia pathways involved in the control of movement. Components of the basal ganglia are in white boxes. The known neurotransmitters involved are indicated. The loop, which begins and ends at the cerebral cortex, is important in the control of voluntary movement of the body and limbs. The dominant synaptic effect of each link in the loop is given by the signs in the circles; the presence of two inhibitory links in series means that the net effect of cortical input to the neostriatum will be enhanced excitability in the cortex. The output to the pedunculopontine nucleus may be involved specifically in locomotion, while the superior colliculus has a role in directing neck and eye movement. The projection from the pars compacta of the substantia nigra to the neostriatum (dashed line) is formed by cells that use the neurotransmitter dopamine, and it is this projection which degenerates in Parkinson's disease. Note that structures which in some species are anatomically distinct (caudate and putamen; globus pallidus and substantia nigra, pars reticulata) form single functional entities. Another component of the basal ganglia, the subthalamic nucleus (not shown), also receives input from the cortex and globus pallidus, and may act to modify output of the neostriatum, globus pallidus, and substantia nigra.

may be inhibited. Thus, rather than simply amplifying cortical activity as a whole, the basal ganglia may be important in selecting certain patterns of cortical activity to be promoted, at the expense of others. In circuits involving motor control regions of cortex, this may play a role in the selection and reinforcement of **motor programmes**—patterns of cortical activity responsible for generating movements.

Circuits within the basal ganglia

Afferent pathways

The neostriatum is the input structure of the basal ganglia. The latter receive projections from all regions of the cortex (which are known to be excitatory); there are also inputs from the thalamus and the substantia nigra. Afferents to the neostriatum make direct synaptic contact with the cells that project out of this structure. However, the responses of these cells are modulated by circuits within the basal ganglia. First, the output cells influence each other via recurrent axon collaterals. These are inhibitory to neighbouring output cells, since they use **γ-aminobutyric acid** (GABA) as the transmitter. Second, local interneurones are present in low numbers; an important group of these use **acetylcholine** as their transmitter. Third, the **nigrostriatal pathway** from the substantia nigra to the neostriatum (Fig. 8.9) releases **dopamine** into the striatum; this modulates the activity of output cells and interneurones, either directly, or by modulating the effectiveness of cortical inputs. This dopamine system is disordered in **Parkinson's disease**.

Efferent pathways

Output neurones of the neostriatum pass to and inhibit neurones in the globus pallidus and the substantia nigra (Fig. 8.9). Neurones in these target organs are tonically active; they project to and inhibit cells in the ventral group of thalamic nuclei, which in turn project upon and excite neurones in the cortex. Note that around the loop there is first excitation of neostriatal cells; these inhibit globus pallidus and substantia nigra cells, which normally inhibit thalamic cells. Thus activation of the neostriatum will inhibit cells that are inhibiting the thalamic cells, i.e. the thalamic cells will be released from inhibition, resulting in activation of their cortical targets.

In addition to the cortex–basal ganglia–cortex loop, which may be of particular importance for control of limb movements, there are some projections from the basal ganglia to brainstem motor structures, for instance to the pedunculopontine nucleus (Fig. 8.9) in the midbrain which is involved in the control of locomotion, and from the substantia nigra to neurones in the superior colliculus which control neck and eye movements. Output to the pedunculopontine nucleus is both inhibitory (from the globus pallidus and substantia nigra) and excitatory (from the subthalamic nucleus). The subthalamic nucleus seems to be particularly important in locomotor control; it receives direct excitatory cortical inputs, as well as inhibitory inputs from the globus pallidus.

Functions of the basal ganglia

Neurones in basal ganglia of experimental animals discharge in relation to movement of the contralateral limb, as is the case for the majority of motor cortical neurones. In fact, basal ganglia neurones have similar properties to those in the motor cortex, apart from their activities being poorly correlated to force production. There are thus cells that are activated by sensory instruction signals, during delay periods, in advance of voluntary movements and in association with movement. Recently it has been suggested that each of the cortical–basal ganglia–cortical loops from different cortical regions acts in parallel, structuring activity in each cortical region rather than funnelling information from non-motor cortex to motor cortex, as was once thought. This structuring is thought to be mediated both by the recurrent inhibitory collaterals in the striatum, and by the dopamine input from the substantia nigra. This latter function reflects the postulated role of the dopamine system in **reward**. Dopamine cells are selectively activated by stimuli and actions which are potentially rewarding to the animal, and their activity may be necessary to allow rapid selection of appropriate motor programmes likely to result in achieving the reward.

Diseases affecting the basal ganglia

The association of the basal ganglia with the control of movement was first proposed as the result of studies on patients with diseases of, or injuries to, this region. Lesions of the neostriatum or subthalamic nucleus produce disorders characterized by excessive, abnormal involuntary movements such as **athetosis** (slow writhing movements), **chorea** (involuntary jerky movements of the extremities and facial muscles) and **ballismus** (violent flailing movements usually of one limb involving the proximal muscles). Ballismus is a characteristic sign of damage to the subthalamic nuclei, while **Huntington's chorea** is a genetic disease associated with degeneration of the neostriatum.

On the other hand, degeneration of the dopamine cells of the substantia nigra which project to the neostriatum produces **Parkinson's disease**, a syndrome which includes: **bradykinesia** (a slowness in initiating and changing movement); **resting tremor**, which is characteristically involuntary, occurs at rest and disappears during movement; Paradoxically, Parkinsonian patients also show **rigidity**, due to abnormally high tone in both agonists and antagonists acting about joints. Flexing or extending a rigid limb gives the impression of manipulating a lead pipe. Rigidity is not velocity-dependent as is the case with spasticity. When tremor is superposed upon rigidity, the rigidity also fluctuates rhythmically, giving rise to a characteristic **cogwheel rigidity**.

The symptoms of Parkinson's disease can be alleviated by treatment with a dopamine precursor, l-dopa, which crosses the blood–brain barrier and is able to increase levels of dopamine in the striatum to substitute for the reduction of dopamine release by the degenerating substantia nigra. This treatment can be effective over several years. In non-responsive patients, deep brain stimulation of the globus pallidus or the subthalamic nucleus, using a chronically implanted electrode with a pacemaker, is also a current successful therapy. Neurosurgical approaches can be envisaged in certain cases to de-stroy hyperactive areas (i.e. pallidotomy or ventrolateral thalamotomy). Cellular implants of dopamine-releasing cells or stem cells have been used, but much work is needed in this area.

8.5 Cerebellum

The gross anatomy of the cerebellum is discussed in Chapter 3 (p. 56 and Fig. 3.17). All the lobes of the cerebellum have a three-layered cortex covering white matter in which are embedded the deep nuclei.

Cerebellar cortex

Histologically, the cerebellar cortex displays a remarkable degree of uniformity (Fig. 8.10). The three layers comprise:

1 a molecular layer containing a large number of granule cell axons (parallel fibres) which run along each folium parallel to its long axis, and which intersect Purkinje dendritic trees at right angles;

2 a thin Purkinje cell layer containing the cell bodies of the large Purkinje cells; and

3 a granular layer containing 20 billion granule cells, afferent mossy and climbing fibres, and the elaborate synaptic complexes between incoming mossy fibre axons and granule cell dendrites.

In addition to Purkinje and granule cells, there are Golgi cells, basket cells and stellate cells.

Purkinje cells are about 15 million in number. Their dendritic trees pass up into the molecular layer to intersect with granule cell parallel fibres (Fig. 8.11). The parallel fibres form excitatory synapses with spines on the Purkinje cell dendrites. A second type of excitatory synapse is made by cells originating in the inferior olive and which terminate as climbing fibres that wind round the Purkinje cell dendrites to form powerful synaptic contacts. The axons of the Purkinje cells project mainly out of the cortex to the deep cerebellar nuclei. All Purkinje cells have an inhibitory action and use the neurotransmitter GABA.

Granule cells are **excitatory** neurones that receive excitation from incoming mossy fibres and send their axons up to the molecular layer to form the parallel fibres (Fig. 8.11).

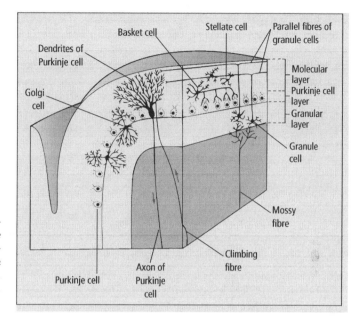

Fig. 8.10 Organization of the cerebellar cortex. The arrows indicate the direction of action potential conduction. (Modified from Johnson, T.B. & Willis, J. (eds) (1949) *Gray's Anatomy*, 30th edn, p. 956. Longmans, London.)

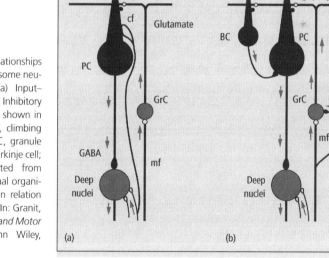

Fig. 8.11 Synaptic relationships within the cerebellum and some neurotransmitters involved. (a) Input–output circuits (arrows). (b) Inhibitory circuits (inhibitory cells are shown in black). BC, basket cell; cf, climbing fibre; GoC, Golgi cell; GrC, granule cell; mf, mossy fibre; PC, Purkinje cell; pf, parallel fibre. (Adapted from Eccles, J.C. (1966) Functional organization of the cerebellum in relation to its role in motor control. In: Granit, R. (ed.) *Muscular Afferents and Motor Control*, pp. 19–36. John Wiley, New York.)

Golgi cells, basket cells and stellate cells are all **inhibitory** interneurones (Fig. 8.11b). **Golgi cells** have their cell bodies near the Purkinje cell layer. They inhibit granule cells and their dendrites receive excitation in both the molecular and granular layers. Their role would appear to be to reduce

the level of excitation on Purkinje cells. **Basket cells** have their cell bodies in the molecular layer close to the Purkinje cells. Their dendritic trees intersect the parallel fibres that excite them, and their axons form a dense meshwork around the initial segment of each Purkinje cell. The Basket cells exert the most direct and powerful inhibitory control over Purkinje cells, and each Basket cell is capable of inhibiting approximately 10 Purkinje cells. **Stellate cells** (Fig. 8. 10) resemble basket cells but they lie more superficially in the molecular layer and their axons terminate on the distal dendrites of Purkinje cells and as a result their impact on Purkinje cell excitability is considerably less than that of basket cells.

Deep intracerebellar nuclei

These are four masses of grey matter embedded in the white matter of each half of the cerebellum (Fig. 8.12). They lie in a line from lateral to medial. The largest, the **dentate nucleus**, lies most laterally and the **fastigial nucleus** lies most medially under the vermis, forming part of the roof of the fourth ventricle. Between the fastigial and dentate nuclei on each side are smaller masses of grey matter—the **globose** and **emboliform nuclei** in humans, but which in other species form the two nuclei known as the anterior and posterior **interpositus nuclei**. The vestibular nuclei also receive direct inhibition from Purkinje cells and, although they are situated beyond the cerebellum below the fourth ventricle, their physiology bears considerable similarity to that of the deep cerebellar nuclei.

The computations performed in the cerebellar cortex influence movement and posture via these nuclei. Their neurones receive excitatory impulses

continuously from branches of all types of incoming afferent fibres on their way to the cerebellar cortex (Fig. 8.11). Superimposed on this activity are periods of inhibition of varying length produced by the inhibitory output of the Purkinje cells related to the particular nucleus. The functioning unit in the cerebellum comprises a group of neurones in a deep intracerebellar nucleus and a group of neurones in a related region of the cerebellar cortex. Figure 8.13 summarizes these relationships and indicates the final destinations of the intracerebellar nuclear axons. Although the histology of the cerebellar cortex is uniform, it can be divided into longitudinal zones on the basis of function and the target nuclei of Purkinje cell projections (Fig. 8.14). In the most medial zone (equivalent to the vermis) the Purkinje cells all project to the fastigial nuclei; in the intermediate zone (medial part of the cerebellar hemisphere), they project to the globose, emboliform and vestibular nuclei; and in the lateral zone (the bulk of the cerebellar hemisphere) they project to the dentate nucleus. The functional roles of these regions are to some extent defined by their input and output connections (Fig. 8.13). Thus, the lateral zone is also known as the **cerebrocerebellum**, by virtue of its relationship with the cerebral cortex; it is considered important for accurate planning and execution of voluntary movements, and may have a role in learning and memory functions. The intermediate and medial zones, which have strong

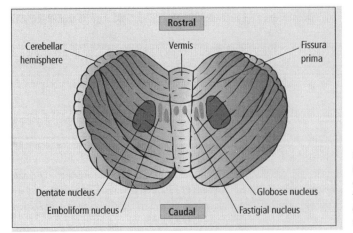

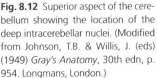

Fig. 8.12 Superior aspect of the cerebellum showing the location of the deep intracerebellar nuclei. (Modified from Johnson, T.B. & Willis, J. (eds) (1949) *Gray's Anatomy*, 30th edn, p. 954. Longmans, London.)

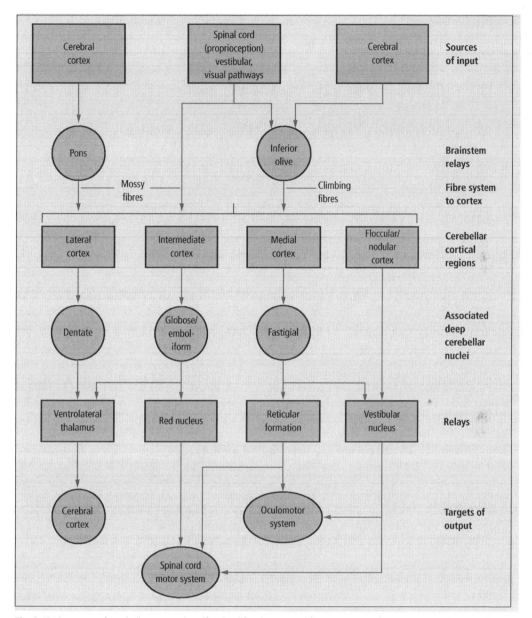

Fig. 8.13 Summary of cerebellar connections (for simplification, several features are not shown). In particular, note that: (i) different inputs to the cerebellum are differentially distributed, to some extent, within the cortical regions; (ii) the mossy and climbing fibre systems have side branches that synapse within the deep nuclei; and (iii) some of the cerebellar outputs reach structures which are sources of input, forming information-processing loops through the cerebellum.

links to the brainstem and spinal cord motor systems are together sometimes called the **spinocerebellum**, and are thought to be important for the regulation of ongoing movement. The flocculus and nodulus together form a separate region, the flocculo-nodular lobe, which receives input from the vestibular apparatus, and regulates postural and eye movements through outputs to the

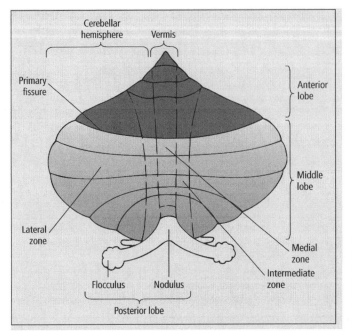

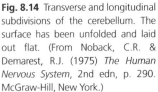

Fig. 8.14 Transverse and longitudinal subdivisions of the cerebellum. The surface has been unfolded and laid out flat. (From Noback, C.R. & Demarest, R.J. (1975) *The Human Nervous System*, 2nd edn, p. 290. McGraw-Hill, New York.)

vestibular nuclei. It has recently been shown that within these broad anatomical zones, multiple, narrow longitudinal bands, or 'microzones', can be identified on the basis of their enzyme cytochemistry and the somatotopic relations of climbing fibre inputs.

Cerebellar afferents

Mossy fibres send information from the spinal cord to the cerebellum by direct and indirect pathways. Of at least 10 tracts, four are sufficiently large and well known to be described here. The **dorsal spinocerebellar tracts** in the dorsal quadrants of the spinal cord and the **ventral spinocerebellar tracts** in the lateral quadrants arise in the thoracolumbar segments of the cord and terminate as mossy fibres in a lower limb representation area of the cerebellar cortex. The **cuneocerebellar** and **rostrospinocerebellar tracts** are the rostral or upper limb equivalents of these tracts and also terminate in the cerebellar cortex as mossy fibres. The information carried by the dorsal spinocerebellar and cuneocerebellar tracts is proprioceptive, i.e.

about muscle length and tension, joint position and skin deformation. Each half of the cerebellum thus receives information during limb movement about the phase and strength of contraction of individual muscles, the joint angles and the time at which the limb extremity touches the ground. In contrast, the ventral spinocerebellar and rostrospinocerebellar tracts are thought to convey information mainly about the activity of the anterior horn cells in the execution of motor commands, such as the rhythm generation, which underlies walking. Other spinocerebellar tracts give rise to mossy fibres indirectly by terminating on the lateral reticular nucleus in the medulla. The axons of this nucleus in turn form mossy fibre afferents relayed to the cerebellar cortex through the inferior cerebellar peduncle.

Information is sent to the cerebellum from many areas of the cerebral cortex, including the visual and auditory areas and the motor cortex. The pathways project along with the corticospinal and corticobulbar fibres and terminate on the ipsilateral pontine nuclei. The axons of the **pontine nuclei** form mossy fibres and are the largest source of such fibres. Collaterals from corticospinal and cortico-bulbar fibres also terminate here. These inputs are excitatory. Vestibular input to the cerebellum is both direct from the vestibular ganglion and indirect, arising from cells in the vestibular nuclei, which give rise to mossy fibres.

Climbing fibres are axons of neurones of the **inferior olivary nucleus**, a prominent nucleus in the medulla at the level of the pyramids. This nucleus has many subdivisions, each with a particular pattern of input, and each subdivision projects to Purkinje cells in a particular part of the cerebellar cortex. The largest inputs to the inferior olivary nucleus come from the premotor cortex, the vestibular nuclei and the spinal cord, but there are other inputs, such as from the superior colliculus that conveys information about the direction of visual movement.

Functions of the cerebellum

Although the cellular architecture of the cerebellum is fairly well known, an equivalent level of understanding of its function has not been achieved. There is general agreement, however, that the complex cellular and network architecture, consisting of a basic circuit (Fig. 8.11) repeated a large number of times to form a regular array, seems suited to some type of specific computational function. The cerebellum may use this computational power in the service of whatever information brain systems send to it. Thus the cerebellum has a major role in processing proprioceptive and other sensory information necessary for generating and regulating movements. However, in some situations, notably the electrosensory system of certain fish, the cerebellum appears to process information about movements of objects sensed in the external environment. Although it has been suggested that the cerebellum is involved in some higher cognitive functions it is not clear whether the cerebellum plays a role in cognition or thinking as such or whether it is merely involved in strategically planned voluntary movements. Thus, while it is clear that the cerebellum is important in the coordination of movements, it is not clear exactly how it is involved or

whether this is all that the cerebellum does. One theory suggests that the cerebellum controls muscle synergies especially those that involve either the co-contraction or reciprocal inhibition of antagonist muscles to adaptively regulate joint, limb and trunk stiffness during voluntary movement. Another theory suggests that the cerebellum controls the flow of relevant sensory information into other regions of the brain that are involved in controlling, perceiving or imagining things that move, and that it adjusts activity in these regions to ensure that the information they contain about movements is accurate. According to this theory the cerebellum is not a movement controller *per se*, but is necessary for generating accurate movements and for correcting faulty movements. Both theories are consistent with the fact that cerebellar dysfunction usually presents as an ataxia or a deficit in coordinating rapid muscle activities both spatially (multi-joint movements) and temporally (rapidly alternating reciprocal movements).

Role of the cerebellum in motor learning

There is increasing evidence that quite apart from its importance in movement execution, the cerebellum also plays an important role in the learning of new motor skills that are acquired through repetition and practice. For example, wearing magnifying or reducing lenses before the eyes can significantly change the gain of the vestibular-ocular reflex. Lesions of the cerebellum or of the olivo-cerebellar connections result in a loss of this plasticity, although the basic vestibular-ocular reflex remains intact. Other experiments have demonstrated cerebellar involvement in conditioned eye blink responses, and increased neuronal discharge related to the preparation for predictable perturbations. Further studies have shown that cerebellar lesions impair the ability to adapt visually-guided reaching movements while wearing lateral displacing prisms. On a more molecular level, the climbing fibres of the inferior olive are thought to be able to selectively depress certain parallel fibre inputs to cerebellar Purkinje cells, by a process referred to as long-term depression or LTD. Depression of the Purkinje cell inhibition of the cerebellar nuclei is thought to result in increased excitability of the nuclear cells related to movement performance of complex motor skills. Destruction of the climbing fibre system impairs the ability to acquire new motor skills.

Disorders of the cerebellum

Cerebellar dysfunction can produce a wide variety of movement disorders ranging from clearly impaired voluntary movements to subtle differences in muscle tone. The deficits usually appear on the same body side as the lesion, because although the cerebellum activates the contralateral thalamus and motor cortex, the corticospinal tract is itself crossed, and therefore influences muscles ipsilateral to the corresponding cerebellar region. One of the most common signs of cerebellar impairment is **ataxia**—which literally means 'lack of order', and refers to the disordered timing of contractions in agonist and antagonist muscles. Reaction times are increased by only a few tenths of a second after cerebellar damage, which is not clinically observable. However, during fast movements this slight delay in recruiting the braking action of an antagonist muscle can produce **hypermetria**, or a movement that dramatically overshoots its in-

tended target. When the particular regions of the cerebellum concerned with posture and locomotion are affected then both gait and balance are severely impaired, as for example the wide based stance and unsteady gait associated with severe alcohol intoxication. When the tongue and glottal muscles are involved speech becomes slurred and inarticulate. Ataxic movements frequently are associated with an action or **intention tremor**, which only appears during movements and disappears when the limb is at rest. Another abnormality associated with cerebellar lesions is **dysrhythmia**, or the inability to execute rapidly alternating movements such a finger tapping or pronation–supination of the hand. These movements accentuate the difficulty cerebellar patients have in the rapid excitation and inhibition of antagonist muscles to attain a steady frequency and amplitude. A number of eye movement abnormalities are also associated with cerebellar lesions, including ocular dysmetria (eye movements that overshoot or undershoot their intended target) and nystagmus. In general after cerebellar damage there is a reduction in resting muscle tone and, although this is difficult to demonstrate clinically, tendon reflexes tend to have a pendular quality.

Chapter 9

Higher Nervous Functions

Our behaviour is guided by the higher nervous functions of the brain through perception and learning. Perception is not simply the passive receiving of sensory information, but rather the active gathering and processing of information from different sensory systems, which must be merged to generate a single percept of the world around us. This percept is strongly influenced both by our past experience and by the current sensory input. Learning is therefore a key element in perception and also in the governing of goal-directed behaviour. Our most complex behaviours involve language and social communication.

9.1 Sensory perception

At any given time we have a unique percept of our environment that derives through an interaction between the actual ongoing peripheral sensory input and our internal high-level representation of the environment. Sensory perception is an active process combining past experience, current sensory information and expectation. Our perception can therefore be altered both by changes in our external environment and in our internal brain state.

Sensory input changes from two different sources; either it is actively induced by self-generated motor commands, or is passively evoked by external forces. For example, for the visual system we are constantly moving our eyes, even when looking at an unchanging scene. For auditory in-

formation, our own speech or chewing generates noises actively, in contrast to passively listening to sounds in our environment. Self-generated sensory input is processed differently from external input, since motor areas of the brain communicate with the area of the brain primarily involved in processing sensory information. In general, for all sensory systems a feed-forward efferent copy of the motor commands are believed to be signalled from motor to sensory areas. So if we actively move our hand to touch an object, the somatosensory areas of our cortex are informed of the expectation of contact with the object, and many of its likely features are known from past experience of touching similar visually identified objects. From these examples it should be clear that the processing of peripheral sensory information to obtain a percept is a highly dynamic process, integrating the senses together with expectations derived from past experiences.

Visual perception

Studies of the visual system have been particularly informative. Vision is much more than taking a picture. When we open our eyes we see objects and this task of identifying objects is so complex that as yet no machine can perform a comparable task. To identify an object we need to separate the visual scene by extracting and grouping the boundaries of separate objects. Different observers looking at the same scene may have different percepts, because they focus on different aspects of the scene or because they have different experiences; they might for example never have encountered similar objects. Equally, the same scene can evoke different percepts in an individual by grouping different elements together. Interestingly although a given picture can give rise to different percepts, at any given time there is a single unique percept. One well-known example of a picture evoking bi-stable perception is shown in Figure 9.1. Viewed over a long time, our percept of the picture changes back and forth between seeing two faces looking at each other and seeing a vase. If you look at the picture for long enough, you may be able to influence which you perceive. Such observations highlight that perception is a complex process depending on the ongoing activity in your brain as well as the sensory input arriving from the periphery.

Sensory areas of the neocortex are active even in the absence of sensory input

In support of profound influences of the higher brain on the processing of sensory information it is

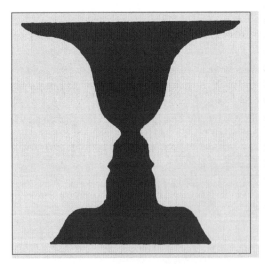

Fig. 9.1 Bi-stable perception. The image can be perceived either as a vase or two faces looking at each other. The switch in perception occurs without change in the peripheral visual input. Visual perception is an active constructive mental process.

interesting to note that electrical activity of primary sensory cortical areas does not disappear in the absence of stimuli. So in the absence of light the visual cortex does not become silent, but rather it is spontaneously active. This can be demonstrated most easily by recording the eletroencephalogram (EEG) over the occipital pole (overlying the visual cortical areas). When the eyes are open the EEG shows small rapid fluctuations, but when the eyes are closed a large amplitude, 8–10 Hz α rhythm is obvious (Fig. 9.2).

Activity in the primary sensory cortices is therefore not exclusively driven by sensory input from the thalamus. Anatomical studies provide support for massive cortico–cortical synaptic connectivity, far outweighing the synaptic input from the sensory thalamus. Such synaptic input connecting different cortical areas is likely to provide the top-down influences involved in sensory processing. The interactions between different visual cortical areas in the primate are thus beginning to be mapped out (Fig. 9.3).

Parallel processing of sensory information

Different aspects of the visual scene are processed in different pathways. Motion processing is thought to occur predominantly in area MT (middle temporal area; located posterior bank of the superior temporal sulcus), whereas colour and form processing occur in area IT (inferior temporal cortex). It can be summarized that information about 'what' is in a visual scene is encoded in area IT, and information regarding 'where' is processed in area MT. Lesions in patients confirm such parallel processing streams of visual information. Patients with localized damage to the temporal cortex can lose colour vision, whilst nonetheless having good vision for form.

The fact that different aspects of the visual scene—which form a single percept—are processed in different brain areas highlights a major unsolved problem in neuroscience: how can the brain activity encoding information relating to an object be grouped and kept separate from information relating to a different object. For example, if we are

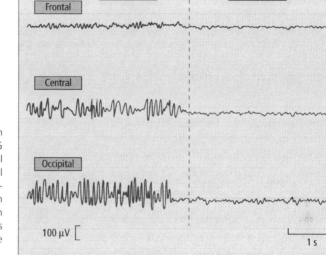

Fig. 9.2 EEG recorded from a human scalp. The traces show typical EEG waveforms recorded over the frontal and occipital poles and in the central region between them. Note the appearance of the 8–10 Hz α rhythm in the central and occipital traces when the subject has his eyes shut and its disappearance (α blocking) when the eyes are opened.

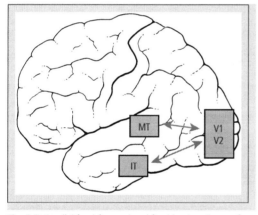

Fig. 9.3 Parallel feed-forward and feed-back pathways for processing visual information. Visual input from the thalamus is initially processed in primary visual cortex (V1). 'Where' information is processed in pathways leading to the middle temporal (MT) area, and 'what' information is processed in a stream leading to inferior temporal (IT) area. Higher order visual areas have strong feedback or top-down influences on the earlier stages of visual processing. V2, secondary visual cortex.

looking at a red square and a blue circle, how does our brain keep red and square perceptually grouped and separate from blue and circle. Or as a more extreme example, how do the colour, shape, smell and texture of a lemon—which are processed separately in visual, olfactory and somatosensory areas—become united into a single percept. Such issues and many other, related questions have given rise to the 'binding problem' of how sensory information is bound together to form a single percept. One hypothesis is that information relating to the same percept is grouped by synchronized neural activity at the millisecond time-scale. The relative strength of such synchronization might also regulate the level of attention given to the percept.

Perception is affected by many factors, including attention, fear and emotion. Perceptions can undergo dramatic deviations from reality during hallucinations induced by drugs, or by brain diseases such as schizophrenia. Indeed we all experience a daily dramatic transformation of perception as we fall asleep or wake up.

9.2 Sleep and wakefulness

Sleep is a state of being, distinct from the waking state. It is actively controlled by the reticular formation of the brainstem and does not resemble the unconsciousness that results from brain damage. There are two types: slow-wave (SW) and rapid eye movement (REM) sleep. Every night we spend our sleep cycling between these states, which can be defined by EEG. The physiological function of sleep is currently unknown.

Slow-wave sleep

As one goes to sleep, the α rhythm—characteristic of the drowsy state—appears and is later replaced by low-amplitude θ waves of a slower frequency (4–6 Hz), which characterize stage 1 sleep (Fig. 9.4). When sleep becomes deeper (as judged by the difficulty of awakening the sleeper), occasional bursts of fast waves (12–15 Hz) are seen—sleep spindles—signalling stage 2 sleep. Stage 3 is characterized by the presence of high-amplitude δ waves with a frequency of 1–2 Hz, and by the presence of K complexes (bursts of more rapid waves on top of δ waves). Stage 4 is characterized by a trace consisting almost entirely of large δ waves. Similar phenomena are seen in recordings from all mammals, and are referred to as slow-wave (**SW**) sleep. When people are awake their eyes are constantly moving (Fig. 9.5a), but during SW sleep eye movements are much reduced in amplitude and so too is muscle tone (Fig. 9.5b). Also, during SW sleep the pupils of the eye are constricted (miosis).

Rapid eye movement sleep

At times during sleep the EEG shows a desynchronized pattern resembling that recorded in the waking state (Fig. 9.4). When the EEG from the cortex shows this desynchronized pattern, large-amplitude rapid (60–70 Hz) saccades in eye movement are recorded, which have given it the name rapid eye movement (**REM**) sleep (Fig. 9.5c). A total postural relaxation is also found due to an almost complete loss of muscle tone (Fig. 9.5c), although sudden jerks of limbs are very common. Sleepers are more difficult to arouse from REM sleep than

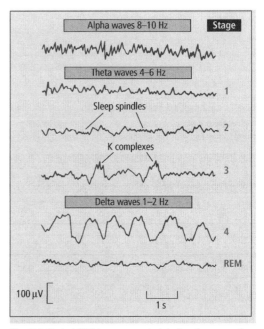

Fig. 9.4 Typical EEG traces recorded during the successive stages (1–4) of SW sleep, and during REM sleep.

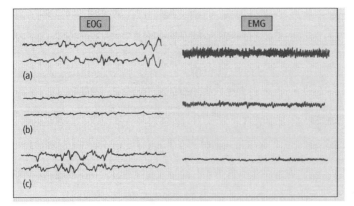

Fig. 9.5 Records of electrical activity from extraocular muscles (electro-oculogram, EOG) and from limb muscles (electromyogram, EMG): (a) in the awake state, (b) during stage 2 of SW sleep and (c) during deep REM sleep. Note in REM sleep the characteristic activity in the EOG and the flat trace in the EMG.

from SW sleep, and sudden dilation of the pupils (mydriasis) may accompany REM.

Closer examination has shown that the REM state is accompanied by a number of signs of excitement and stress. For instance, there is a marked variation in the pulse and blood pressure and irregularity in respiration, accompanied by secretion of corticosteroids. Furthermore, in males, a cycle of penile erections occurs, beginning and ending with each REM period; testosterone secretion is also increased at night in association with REM sleep.

Duration of SW and REM sleep

The majority of people sleep 7–8 h a night but there are also short (5–6 h) and long (8–9 h) sleepers. When compared with long sleepers, short sleepers go to sleep more quickly, spend less time in stages 1 and 2 and in REM sleep, but spend the same amount of time in the deepest stages (3 and 4) of SW sleep. The first REM period normally lasts about 20 min; later periods become progressively longer (Fig. 9.6). SW sleep develops with maturation of the nervous system. Those newborn animals whose central nervous system (CNS) is not completely developed at birth show only alternations between waking and the REM state. Human babies at birth spend some 18 h asleep, of which 45–65% is in the REM state. A 2-year-old is still spending 40% sleep-time in REM sleep, but a 5-year-old approaches the young adult figure of 20%. For those over 50 the period spent in REM sleep forms about 15% of total sleep.

Dreaming and mental activity during sleep

Subjects awakened from REM sleep almost invariably report that they have been dreaming. Apparently, we all dream, although we do not always recall our dreams.

It is attractive to suppose that the eye movements, limb twitches and penile erections, together with the alternations of pulse, arterial blood pressure and respiration which occur during the REM state of sleep, are associated with the acting-out of dreams. There is some evidence for this view, which is largely drawn from correlation of the content of dreams and the observed signs. Dreams, of course, may be distressing, and it is of interest that angina pectoris may also occur at this time, while sufferers from duodenal ulcers, migraine and partial seizures, especially those of frontal or temporal lobe origin, tend to have exacerbations of their symptoms during periods of REM sleep. Sufferers of obstructive lung disease are also adversely affected by REM sleep, presumably, because of the lack of muscle tone (atonia).

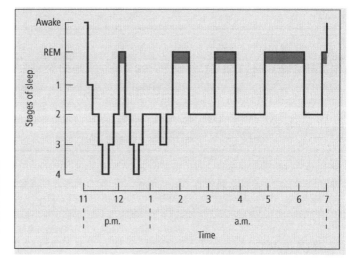

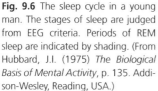

Fig. 9.6 The sleep cycle in a young man. The stages of sleep are judged from EEG criteria. Periods of REM sleep are indicated by shading. (From Hubbard, J.I. (1975) *The Biological Basis of Mental Activity*, p. 135. Addison-Wesley, Reading, USA.)

Mental activity continues during SW sleep; approximately 20% of subjects awakened from this state say they have been thinking—or even deny being asleep. Evidently, the mental activity is akin to everyday mental activity, and lacks the hallucinatory aspect of dreaming.

Recordings of neuronal activity from experimental animals indicates that patterns of activity related to experience in the period before sleep are replayed during sleep. Such replayed patterns of neuronal activity might underlie dreams and/or processes of memory consolidation.

The need for sleep

The working hypothesis of many investigators is that SW sleep is needed for bodily repair. There is evidence, for instance, that marathon runners have more SW sleep after their race than before, and it is well established that growth hormone is only secreted during SW sleep. The idea has also been investigated that REM sleep, on the other hand, is concerned with recovery from mental tiredness.

Neural basis of sleep

The circadian rhythms underlying the sleep-wake cycle are regulated by genetic pacemakers of neurones in the suprachiasmatic nucleus within the hypothalamus. Transcription of several genes is internally regulated through positive and negative feedback loops to maintain the 24-hour cycle, which can also be entrained by the light-dark cycle through information from the retina. The suprachiasmatic nucleus signals to other hypothalamic neurones, basal forebrain and brainstem, all of which are closely involved in regulating brain states. These areas interact in complex positive and negative feedback networks through release of neurotransmitters including acetylcholine, serotonin, orexin/hypocretin and noradrenaline. Lesions in the forebrain preoptic region can make animals permanently sleepless. Equally, stimulation of several areas—including the preoptic region—can induce sleep, and neuronal activity correlates with the sleep/wake cycle. During sleep

neurones in the preoptic region are active. The preoptic region has substantial efferent projections to the midbrain, particularly to its reticular formation. These are known to be predominantly inhibitory, suggesting that the preoptic region, as well as inducing behavioural and EEG signs of sleep, also puts the machinery for wakefulness and attention out of action.

Sleep disorders

The most common sleep disorder is **insomnia**. This may affect 20% of the population at one time or another, but in most cases no physiological problem with the sleep-generating mechanism can be identified. Insomnia is usually a symptom of an underlying psychological disturbance (e.g. depression, anxiety or excitement), or due to a physical cause such as the discomfort associated with disease or injury.

The opposite of insomnia is **narcolepsy**, in which there is an irresistible urge to sleep during daytime activities. Most patients suffering from narcolepsy have reduced levels of the neuropeptide orexin/hypocretin in the cerebrospinal fluid. Dogs with a mutation in the orexin/hypocretin receptor gene suffer from narcolepsy. There is therefore growing evidence that narcolepsy results from deficiency in the orexin/hypocretin-signalling pathway. Orexin/hypocretin signalling originating in the lateral hypothalamus may be involved in maintaining wakefulness through a dense projection to the locus coeruleus.

Some people have severely disturbed sleep due to **sleep apnoea**, periods where respiration stops completely. The sufferer awakes, takes a few breaths and then falls asleep again, only to awaken soon after with another apnoea attack. Sleep apnoea can arise from intermittent airway obstruction, as in snorers, or from lesions of the CNS. Another disorder leading to disturbed sleep is **nocturnal myoclonus**, in which there are sudden repeated contractions of muscles, commonly in the legs, during sleep. This disease is thought to be akin to epilepsy.

Sleep-walking (**somnambulism**) and bedwetting (**nocturnal enuresis**) have been shown to occur during periods of SW sleep. Somnambulists walk with their eyes open and avoid obstacles, but when awakened they cannot recall the episode. These problems are more common in children than in adults.

Whereas our dreams evoke strong percepts and can seem very real momentarily, they do not usually remain long in our memories. Learning is therefore largely confined to the awake state.

9.3 Learning and memory

Perhaps the most important feature of the nervous system is our ability to learn from our past experience in order to guide our future actions. Thus our behaviour is not pre-programmed genetically, but can adapt according to our needs and environment. Short-term memory is likely encoded in ongoing electrical activity of neurones, but longer-term memories involve structural changes at synapses.

All but the most simple and stereotyped behaviours are based upon learned experiences. Learning allows actions to be adapted for each particular situation and specific goal. Learning and memory are therefore fundamental aspects of neurophysiology. Over the last decades significant progress has been made in the understanding of how we learn and how memories may be stored in the brain.

Studies of the normal type of memory for verbal material indicate that there are short-term (primary) memories for snippets of information looked up immediately before use (e.g. telephone numbers), longer-term (secondary) memories of much-rehearsed material, and memories which last a lifetime (tertiary memory), such as for one's name and important life events.

Short-term memory

The characteristics of short-term, working, or primary memory are that it has a small capacity, short duration and employs storage as words.

1 Relatively few items can be recalled immediately after a short exposure (visual or aural). For instance, when photographs, printed letters or drawings are flashed on a screen for very short, precisely controlled intervals of time (tachistoscopic experiments) subjects can recall only five to nine items.

2 In this type of experiment, primary memory decays in a few seconds.

3 A study of errors in primary memory suggests that the material is coded in words. Volunteers in tachistoscopic experiments were found to be rehearsing the material they had learned, by mumbling either overtly or covertly. In remembering, mistakes were made between letters that sounded alike. The sounds were confused, although the subjects were shown only the letters. Indeed, the same mistakes were made if the subjects were shown the material or if it was spoken. Thus, mistaking 'cat' for 'hat' was possible, but not 'cat' for 'kitten'.

Primary memory is thought to be represented in the nervous system by circulating nerve impulses, because an insult that disrupts the functioning of neurones prevents any memory of events which take place a short time before. Thus, after head injury causing loss of consciousness, or after electroconvulsive shock therapy (ECT), there is a short but persistent loss of memory (**amnesia**) for the period immediately preceding it. A permanent reduction in the capacity of short-term memory may occur after lesions in the cerebral cortex. For instance, a reduction in verbal and short-term memory has been described in a patient with a parietal lobe lesion. The neural activity of working memory is likely to be distributed across different brain areas with the prefrontal cortex playing a prominent role.

Declarative and non-declarative memory

We are all intuitively aware that there are different types of memories. Non-declarative memories involve repetition over many trials with gradual improvement in performance. Improving perceptual and motor skills are examples of non-declarative learning. A different sort of learning involves conscious processing to encode and retrieve information. Such declarative memory is involved for example when we recount the events of yesterday. These different types of memories also seem to have different neural bases.

Role of the medial temporal lobe

Within this area, the hippocampus and nearby perirhinal cortex, appear to be the most important structures for normal memory function. There are patients suffering from epileptic seizures apparently originating in the temporal lobes who have had the medial part of one temporal lobe cut away, together with the underlying hippocampus, to try to cure the epilepsy. Unfortunately, in one patient the operation was performed bilaterally and he developed global amnesia. He could not form any new memories and had only patchy memories of the decade preceding the operation. When asked about his house, his family or the city he lived in, the patient did not even seem to understand these questions, as if their objective was entirely unknown to him. He appeared to feel completely isolated, with neither a past nor a future. Long after the operation, a grave memory defect persisted, although there was some improvement in the ability to pay attention.

Analysis of many case histories confirms that patients with damage to the hippocampal system show no loss of motor skills acquired preoperatively, and that intelligence, as measured by formal tests, is unimpaired. But, with the possible exception of the acquiring of new motor skills, they seem largely incapable of adding new information to their long-term store. The immediate registration of new input (short-term memory) appears to take place normally and material that can be rehearsed verbally is held for many minutes. Interruption of the rehearsal, however, produces immediate forgetting of what has gone before. Material already in long-term storage is unaffected by the lesion.

Further evidence for the importance of the hippocampus comes from the effects of stimulation of the brains of conscious patients during operations. For instance, in 1954 the Canadian neurosurgeon Penfield described that, when he stimulated particular points in the temporal lobes overlying the hippocampus, his patients reported that fragments of past experiences seen, heard or felt long ago were being re-experienced and, moreover, at the same rate as originally. Things not in the focus of the patient's attention at the time of the original experience were not present in the hallucinations. Many of these patients suffered from epilepsy. Their attacks were preceded by flashbacks consisting of the recall of experiences from their past similar to those evoked by brain stimulation. It is important to note that patients reported that the material either elicited by stimulation or coming into consciousness before an epileptic attack was much more distinct than anything they could normally recall. Penfield was convinced that his patients had records of their experiences in their brain, which were normally not completely available to them.

These striking observations might suggest that each hippocampus is a site at which memories are stored. However, this cannot be completely true, because patients with bilateral hippocampal damage can acquire motor skills and also verbal long-term memories by special techniques in which they are given part of the information but have to supply the rest. In both types of learning, they are as effective as normal subjects. Memory formation is now thought to require concurrent activity in the hippocampus and other brain sites.

Classification of amnesias

Damage to the hippocampus and related structures results in memory impairment in which there is an inability to add new memories following the lesion, although older memories remain relatively intact. This is called **anterograde amnesia**. It is also seen in some chronic alcoholics (**Korsakoff's psychosis**). In contrast, temporary disruption of brain function, for example after severe head injury, may result in **retrograde amnesia**, in which there is loss of memory of events that occurred over a considerable period prior to the injury. The events before the accident are often very dramatic and must have been registered by the nervous system, yet quite often the subject has no memory of them. During recovery the length of the period of retrograde amnesia shrinks markedly.

Clinical experience also suggests that **suppression** of memory occurs, for example, following ECT for depression. After treatment many patients forget their anxieties and are able to function normally again, although when interviewed later under the influence of a barbiturate they can recall their troubles, showing that these were not permanently forgotten but simply not recalled in the normal waking state.

Reward system

Animals are able to learn from experience to select those behaviours which produce favourable outcomes (**reward**), and to avoid those that are unfavourable. This learning is promoted by activation of a brain pathway, the 'reward system', which signals to the animal that the outcome of behaviour was favourable. The reward system has been mapped in animal studies in which electrical stimulation through implanted electrodes was used to reward appropriate behaviour. In 1954 Olds and Milner found that rats thus prepared could be trained to press a lever that turned on stimulating current. Regions of the brain could be classified according to the percentage of time the animals spent pressing the lever. Areas with high scores were found in the septal nuclei, and to a smaller extent in the cingulate cortex and the hypothalamus. Self-stimulation of the hippocampus occurred less often but was still at rates above control levels. The most remarkable area was the **median forebrain bundle** in the lateral hypothalamic area, which, among its other functions, connects the hypothalamic nuclei with the septal nuclei rostrally and with the midbrain caudally. If a rat had a stimulating electrode implanted there, it continually pressed the bar, suggesting that the ensuing brain stimulation was experienced as a reward. Indeed, given a choice between feeding and pressing, the rat would rather stimulate its median forebrain bundle than eat. Recent evidence points specifically to a central role of dopaminergic neurones of the ventral tegmental area in the reward/error system. By pairing sensory input with electrical stimulation of the ventral tegmental area or the associated median forebrain bundle it is possible to induce large-scale changes in the response properties of cortical areas. Since learning is thought to rely upon changing neural activity, such experiments support a prominent role for the reward/error system in learning.

Emotion

Memories of events involving strong emotion are remembered particularly well. The emotional consequences of an action or situation signal some aspect of the value and seriousness of that event, which is used to govern subsequent behaviour. Furthermore the outward expression of emotion is very important in the organization of social interactions between individuals of the same species. It allows the value and seriousness of one individual's situation to be understood by others, and so guides their behaviour.

The **limbic system** (p. 59) is thought to be the site of generation of emotional tone, but emotional expression resulting from limbic system activity is mediated by the hypothalamus through the autonomic and somatic systems. In people, stimulation of the limbic structures may enhance and lesions reduce emotional tone. For instance, aggressive behaviour has been reported in a patient during stimulation of one of the amygdaloid nuclei through implanted electrodes, while bilateral amygdalectomy has resulted in an apathetic individual. Undercutting of the cingulate gyrus (cingulotractotomy) has been used to treat severe chronic depression that does not respond to any other form of treatment. Enthusiasm for such operations should be tempered by the possibility that the improvement may not be permanent. In some studies, half of the patients initially improved by cingulotractotomy relapsed within 3 years of the operation and were left with permanent brain damage.

Cellular and molecular mechanisms of information storage

There are several stages involved in storing information in the brain. Initially, recurrent neural activity involving the prefrontal cortex can hold information for short periods. However, for the information to be stored for longer periods, the brain changes its internal structure. These structural changes can affect which neurones signal information to other neurones, and under which conditions. This can therefore serve to store information. Several mechanisms by which the communication between neurones in many different brain regions can be altered have been discovered.

The most prominent candidates for memory storage involve long-term synaptic plasticity to regulate the efficacy of a synapse to evoke activity in the postsynaptic neurone. Long-term potentiation (LTP) was discovered by Bliss and Lomo in 1973, and is a mechanism for increasing synaptic strength. Long-term depression (LTD) is a mechanism to decrease synaptic strength. Both of these mechanisms can be evoked in animals *in vivo* using particular stimulation paradigms. The cellular and molecular mechanisms underlying LTP have been studied in detail. LTP requires activation of postsynaptic glutamate receptors of the *N*-methyl-D-aspartic acid (NMDA) subtype (see p. 81). Pharmacological or genetic blockade of NMDA receptors has been shown to block certain forms of spatial learning in rodents, thus supporting a role for LTP as a component of learning. NMDA receptor activation evokes a localized calcium influx in the postsynaptic specialization. The calcium signal activates kinases that promote insertion of glutamate receptors into the postsynaptic density and

initiate further signalling pathways. Information is also relayed to the presynaptic component of the synapse and to the nucleus to regulate gene transcription and translation. Altogether enhanced synaptic transmission between neurones following LTP (Fig. 9.7) is likely to occur through coordinated increases in receptor density postsynaptically, increased neurotransmitter release presynaptically and structural modifications. Our memories depend upon the synthesis of new proteins, as can be demonstrated in experimental animals. It is also likely that new synapses are formed and others eliminated during learning, in addition to the modification of existing synapses.

9.4 Speech and language

Speech, together with its associated activities (reading and writing), is a most complex phenomenon. Basically, it is the conveying of meaning by the spoken word. It has a motor output, which has specialized control regions in the brain, usually in the dominant hemisphere (the left side in most people).

It is necessary to distinguish the production of voice (**phonation**), the shaping of voice into words (**articulation**), and speech as language, which implies meaning and understanding. In one sense,

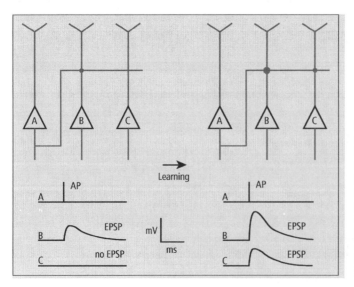

Fig. 9.7 Some types of synaptic changes that might accompany learning. Before learning, cell A might be synaptically connected to cell B, meaning that an action potential (AP) in cell A might evoke an excitatory postsynaptic potential (EPSP) in cell B. After learning, the synaptic connection of cell A onto cell B is strengthened and a new synapse onto cell C has formed. Memories may be stored through such synaptic changes.

speech is a motor activity involving control of the labial, lingual, pharyngeal, palatal and respiratory muscles. Motor activities in general result from plans made in the frontal lobe, which are further elaborated by the basal ganglia and cerebellum and relayed to the ventrolateral thalamus. A final relay to the motor cortex brings appropriate motor neurones—and thus muscles—into action. The motor aspects of speech do not differ from other motor activities except in the planning stage, which is complex.

The sounds made by animals as the result of strong emotion are akin to the expressions made by humans in similar excited states. The production of such sounds is controlled from the limbic system in animals.

Dominant hemisphere

It has long been known that speech is unique among motor activities, in that its higher control depends on the integrity of only one of the two cerebral hemispheres—the **dominant hemisphere**, which, in most people, is the left. This hemisphere also controls the right hand, but cerebral dominance is not necessarily paralleled by appropriate handedness. Tests have shown that 95% of right-handed and 50% of left-handed people have their speech centre on the left.

Dysarthria and dysphasia

The production of speech involves subcortical and motor cortical components and also a component from association areas. Disturbance of any component will cause a difficulty in speaking. Such difficulties are termed **dysarthrias** if they involve the motor apparatus in the strict sense, and **dysphasias** if they involve the unique one-sided cerebral control. A characteristic dysarthria occurs in many diseases, such as the scanning speech of cerebellar disease and the slow, slurred speech of Parkinson's disease. While there may be some temporary disturbance of articulation, a permanent dysarthria does not commonly occur with the hemiplegia following a cerebral vascular accident, because the motor nuclei of the vagus and

glossopharyngeal nerves supplying the palate, pharynx and vocal cords are bilaterally innervated. Bilateral loss of cerebral control of the medullary cranial nerves, on the other hand, causes a severe dysarthria as well as numerous other signs and symptoms (**pseudobulbar palsy**).

Dysphasia

Following brain lesions in the cortical areas shown in Fig. 9.8, patients have a difficulty in speaking, which differs from dysarthria. There is no impairment of the muscular apparatus or its control; rather, the difficulty is in the higher processes connected with the selection and ordering of words. This type of disturbance is commonly called an aphasia, which literally means 'without speech'. However, strictly speaking, such patients should be said to have a **dysphasia**, since they can speak, although with difficulty.

Non-fluent aphasia

A French physician, Broca, noticed in 1861 that patients with a right-sided hemiplegia had poorly-articulated speech which was produced slowly and with great effort, and was abnormal in rhythm and intonation. For these reasons, this is termed a **non-fluent** aphasia and is the commonest form of aphasia. The speech content has been compared to a

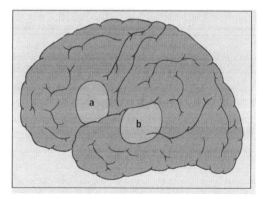

Fig. 9.8 A lateral view of a human brain showing areas important for the generation of speech. (a) Broca's area; damage here may cause motor aphasia. (b) Wernicke's area; damage here may cause sensory aphasia.

telegram in that patients can name objects and produce single words, but have difficulty with sentences and they are unable to utilize connecting words. These patients have trouble in reading and find writing difficult or impossible. Their comprehension appears unimpaired, but formal testing reveals deficits. At postmortem, such patients may have lesions involving the frontal lobe (Fig. 9.8a). An older name for this sort of aphasia is **motor** aphasia.

Fluent aphasia

In 1874 a German neurologist, Wernicke, described patients with normal articulation, rhythm and expression, and correct grammar, who had great difficulty in finding the correct words. The patients were unable to understand spoken or written language; that is, unlike the patients with nonfluent aphasia, their comprehension was obviously severely impaired. In severe cases, they might produce a grammatically correct but meaningless flow of language. This form is termed **fluent** or **sensory** aphasia. At postmortem such patients may have lesions involving the posterior part of the temporal lobe (Fig. 9.8b).

Other forms of aphasia are known in which patients are thought to have lesions in the white matter underlying and connecting the areas described by Broca and Wernicke (Fig. 9.8). Patients with such **conduction** aphasia can, for instance, comprehend the speech of others but cannot repeat it. Their own speech is fluent, but full of circumlocutions and of errors in word use.

More restrictive language defects arise when the speech area is disconnected from the cortical representation of one particular modality. In these cases, a patient may be able to name an object presented in one sensory modality but not when presented in another (**anomic** aphasia). Speech itself is fluent and comprehension intact.

9.5 Brain diseases

Genetic studies have begun to point to the underlying pathology and molecular biology of some brain disorders like Alzheimer's, Huntington's and Parkinson's diseases. Progress has also been made with understanding other brain diseases such as schizophrenia and epilepsy.

Alzheimer's disease

Impairment in making new memories is the first obvious symptom of Alzheimer's disease; but over time there is a general cognitive decline. The definitive diagnosis shows extracellular plaques containing amyloid mainly in the neocortex and hippocampus. Accompanying the amyloid plaques, there are also neurofibrillary tangles and there is massive cell loss in the hippocampus, neocortex and the cholinergic nucleus basalis. It is currently unclear what mediates this neurodegeneration.

There is a clear genetic component to Alzheimer's disease, as the risk is elevated for near relatives. This is particularly clear for early onset Alzheimer's, which affects people in their 40s or 50s. Genetic linkage analysis has shown that the amyloid precursor protein is mutated in early onset Alzheimer's disease. The mutations are thought to enhance production of one form of amyloid, known as Aβ42 peptide, which is known to participate in plaque formation. There is therefore increasing evidence supporting a causative role of amyloid plaques in Alzheimer's disease, but there remains much that is unknown and there are currently no treatments for the disease.

Huntington's disease

Patients suffering from Huntington's disease may suffer initially from clumsiness and depression, but as the disease progresses the uncontrolled movements gradually increase until the patient is confined to bed or a wheelchair. During the course of the disease there is a massive loss of GABAergic and cholinergic striatal neurones, resulting from aggregates containing the protein huntingtin. The huntingtin gene contains a series of glutamines near its N-terminal. The number of glutamines encoded in this repeated region of the gene varies between individuals due to polyglutamine expansion. If there are more than 36 repeated glutamines then the risk of disease increases; the longer the repeat then the earlier the onset of disease. Current research is aimed at understanding the link between huntingtin protein aggregates and neurodegeneration, so that treatments for the cause of this disease may be developed in the future.

Parkinson's disease

Tremor and difficulty in the initiation of movement are characteristic features of Parkinson's disease. Patients have dramatic reductions in dopamine levels, which are paralleled by neurodegeneration in the substantia nigra, one of the most important areas in the brain containing dopaminergic cells. Remarkably, treatment with a dopamine precursor L-DOPA improves symptoms, and ongoing research aims to target the drugs enhancing the dopamine pathway. Another strategy that appears useful in alleviating disease symptoms is the implantation of stimulating electrodes into the thalamus. Some people suffering from Parkinson's disease carry mutations in the gene encoding the protein α-synuclein. Abnormal folding of this protein forms toxic aggregates termed Lewy bodies.

Schizophrenia

The delusions, hallucinations, memory deficits and general cognitive decline associated with schizophrenia commonly occur during teenage years or in early adulthood. The psychotic aspects of the disease can be effectively treated using classes of drugs acting on dopaminergic signalling pathways. Such treatment means that patients suffering from schizophrenia need not be hospitalized. However, the treatments to date do not help with the associated cognitive impairment, for which new medication must be developed.

Susceptibility for schizophrenia is inherited. However, it is likely that several or many genes are involved hindering straightforward analysis. If one identical twin suffers from schizophrenia then the chance of the other suffering from schizophrenia is high, but it is still less than 50%. This indicates that genetic predisposition only accounts for part of the disease and that other environmental factors, perhaps involving stress during childhood, are important.

Epilepsy

Epilepsy may be defined as a recurrent, paroxysmal, transitory disturbance of the CNS that is characterized by uncontrolled neural discharge. Epileptic seizures generally involve total or partial loss of consciousness and may be accompanied by uncontrolled motor activity. A significant proportion of people have at least one mild brief epileptic event during their lives. Epilepsy appears to result from an imbalance of excitatory and inhibitory neuronal activity, and some drugs that prevent excessive excitation are clinically useful in preventing and treating epileptic seizures. A fraction of epileptic seizures are resistant to current pharmacological therapy.

In the most common cases of adult epilepsy, the seizure spreads out from a well-defined focus, often a part of the temporal lobe. If the focus of the seizure remains stable then surgical removal of the epileptic focus can help.

Generalized epilepsy

Two varieties of generalized epilepsy are relatively common—grand mal and petit mal. **Grand mal** seizures are characterized by an abrupt loss of consciousness and violent involuntary contractions of skeletal muscles. Together these phenomena are termed a **convulsion**. Many patients have mild symptoms that precede the attack—the **aura**. Many forms of aura have been described: tingling or numbness in the limbs, visual or auditory hallucinations or sudden emotional changes, such as fear. The aura is followed by the convulsion, and it is usually the last thing the patient remembers.

The convulsion has several prominent phases. First, the patient stiffens and is apparently thrown to the floor; respiration stops and the pupils dilate. This is the **tonic phase**. It lasts 10–30 s, during which the patient often lies with the legs fully extended and the arms flexed and abducted, as if

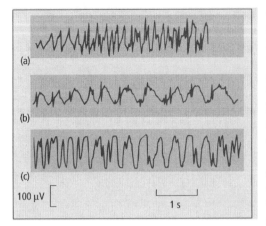

(a)

(b)

(c)

100 μV

1 s

Fig. 9.9 EEG during epileptic seizures. (a) Tonic and (b) clonic phases of grand mal seizure; (c) petit mal seizure.

decorticate. It is followed by a **clonic phase** with severe jerking movements and, commonly, emptying of the bladder. After the convulsions the patient appears relaxed and drowsy, and may complain of headache. This stage lasts 30–60 min and is often followed by sleep. During a seizure, the EEG usually shows high-voltage spiking during the tonic phase; during the clonic phase this becomes mixed with a high-voltage slow component (Fig. 9.9). ECT produces convulsions of a grand mal type but the motor components are in practice prevented by anaesthetizing the patient and administering a muscle relaxant.

Petit mal usually affects children rather than adults; in this type of epilepsy there is no warning (aura) prior to periods of unconsciousness, or altered consciousness during which the patient may stare blankly—the eyes may roll upwards until the pupils are hidden under the lid. Episodes last 5–30 s and a patient may stop what he or she is doing and restart after the seizure without apparently being aware of what has happened. The EEG of petit mal shows a characteristic waveform (Fig. 9.9c). There is an alternation between high-voltage waves of short and of long duration (spike-and-dome complex).

Chapter 10

Pain

10.1 What is pain?

Pain has been described as an unpleasant sensory and emotional experience associated with actual or potential tissue damage. However, it is difficult to accurately define pain because it has qualitative aspects that require subjective assessment and if quantitative changes are measured, autonomic activity may interfere with measurements *in vivo*. There is increasing evidence, based on clinical observations, that long-term pain is a disease rather than a symptom. The type of pain sensations that are difficult to explain include:

1 spontaneous pain, i.e. without tissue damage;

2 pain that is reported as pleasant;

3 when, for the same stimulus, some people may experience pain but others may not;

4 phantom pain, where a limb or organ is removed yet spatial pain sensations are reported; and

5 loss of sensation from a wound in an accident/war, until some time later.

Pain, as a sensation, is considered to be protective in the short-term. The function of the nervous system to respond to a potentially harmful stimulus is called **nociception**. Nociception is part of the somatosensory nervous system and it serves an exteroceptive function; e.g. to avoid tissue damage by reflex withdrawal of a limb when heat is applied to it. There is no requirement for consciousness in this process; however, many of our concepts of pain mechanisms are developed from nociceptive experiments in animals, where the conscious perception of pain is inferred through behavioural or physiological effects in the central nervous system (CNS). The interpretation of such knowledge has to be via application to clinical situations and through pharmacological manipulations.

The basis of nociception is a series of steps that transform a stimulus into a nerve signal that moves into the CNS and activates the centres in the brain that respond to that stimulus (Fig. 10.1). Transduction changes the stimulus into electrical energy; transmission moves the nerve activity along to the spinal cord via the afferent neurone and its cell body in the dorsal root ganglion (DRG). Further transduction occurs at synapses in the dorsal horn (DH) of the spinal cord, and the nerve impulses are then passed rostrally to the brain centres—first to the thalamus and then to the cortex. Modulation of this activity occurs at all levels and depends on other on-going activity, previous experiences or other modulators such as hormones, drugs, etc. For example, a minor injury in football may not be felt until the end of the game, or endometriosis may alter the response to a kidney stone.

The **types of stimuli** that initiate nociceptive responses can cause tissue damage at different levels: mechanical (e.g. cutting), electrical, thermal (heat, cold) and chemical stimuli can cause damage superficially, at the skin surface; ischaemia, distension (stretch) and inflammation can damage deeper tissues; and trauma, ischaemia and chemical

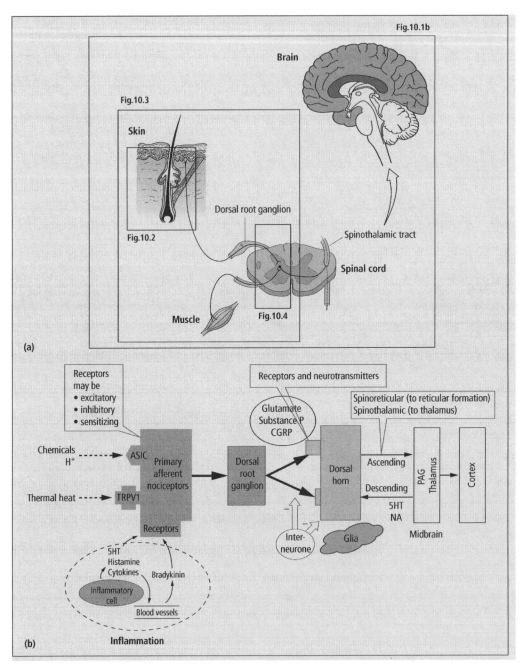

Fig. 10.1 (a) A diagram of the anatomical locations of the figures in this chapter. (b) Schematic diagram of nociceptive activity from receptors on the peripheral primary afferent nociceptor (solid black arrows) to the spinal cord and central nervous system. The inhibitory interneurones can release GABA and enkephalin. PAG, periaqueductal grey; 5-HT, 5-hydroxytryptamine; NA = noradrenaline; CGRP, calcitonin gene-related peptide; ASIC, acid-sensing ion channel; TRPV1, transient receptor potential vanilloid.

stimuli can cause damage to nerves. Therefore, different stimuli may generate nociceptive responses from different tissues. Superficial stimuli have been most commonly studied and their mechanisms thus predominate in the literature, but may not be relevant to many patients.

The psychological responses that are associated with pain include emotion (i.e. how people feel—both negative and positive, e.g. anger, anxiety), mood (a longer-term factor), cognitive elements (e.g. how people think), and behaviour (i.e. how people act). In measuring pain sensations, a common approach is to include emotive responses as part of a multidimensional assessment; e.g. the McGill Pain Questionnaire (MPQ). The MPQ asks patients to describe the following: what the pain feels like (a sensory assessment, e.g. shooting, sharp); how it changes mood (an affective assessment, e.g. fearful); and its character (a quantitative measure, e.g. unbearable).

Primary afferent neurone

The main molecular events that control initial transduction, that is the excitability of a primary afferent neurone, are shown in Fig. 10.2. The normal control of cell excitation is by the opening and closing of voltage-gated sodium or potassium channels. The combined effects result in membrane depolarization and impulse propagation. The potassium ion is responsible for the stage of hyperpolarization, which tends to prevent firing until the membrane potential is back to normal. The calcium-activated potassium ion channel is both voltage- and ligand-gated; when cytoplasmic calcium binds to the inside of the channel, the channel opens and increases potassium efflux. Where there are opioid receptors on the nerve cell surface, these G protein-coupled receptors also enhance potassium efflux and result in hyperpolarization, and hence closure of the voltage-sensitive calcium channels.

Primary afferent sensory neurones are characterized as Aδ or C fibres. C fibres respond in a polymodal fashion to mechanical, thermal and chemical stimuli. The C fibres are non-myelinated, small diameter and slow conducting ($<2\,\text{ms}^{-1}$), and

they have a mainly nociceptive function, demonstrate a high threshold of response, and have a large receptive field. In contrast, the Aδ fibres are myelinated, larger diameter, faster conducting ($>2\,\text{ms}^{-1}$), and they respond to a variety of stimuli. In consequence, in response to a noxious stimulus, the Aδ fibres produce sharp, fast-onset 'first' pain, and the C fibres produce dull, slow-onset, so-called 'second' pain.

The C fibres are classified according to their neurochemistry as:

1 **peptidergic** due to the chemicals they synthesize (in the DRG) and release, which include calcitonin gene-related peptide (CGRP), substance P (SP), somatostatin (SOM), vasoactive intestinal peptide (VIP) and galanin (GL); and

2 **non-peptidergic** expressing the lectin IB4 and purinoceptors, e.g. P_2X_3.

The chemical mediators that can alter sensitivity or directly excite receptors act on nociceptive neurone surface receptors (Table 10.1). These receptors are either **ionotropic**—one whose activation results in the flow of ions, e.g. transient receptor potential vanilloid (TRPV1) and P_2X_3, or **metabotropic**—coupled to a metabolic reaction, e.g. G protein-coupled receptors and tyrosine kinase-coupled receptors.

Differences between receptor activities include:

1 speed of activation when ionic fluxes can occur much faster than G protein-coupled receptor responses (milliseconds versus seconds);

2 long-term changes in receptor density, controlled by gene expression and protein synthesis; and

3 desensitization, that is loss of effect of a ligand (i.e. a molecule binding to a receptor), as may occur through internalization and other mechanisms.

The binding of an endogenous ligand to the receptor may induce rapid internalization of the receptor so that it is no longer part of the membrane. The process allows the ligand to be removed from the receptor and the receptor to be recycled.

During development of the nervous system in fetal life, primary neurones develop under the influence of **neurotrophic factors**—e.g. nerve growth factor (NGF). Postnatally, sensitivity to these factors remains in peptidergic C fibres

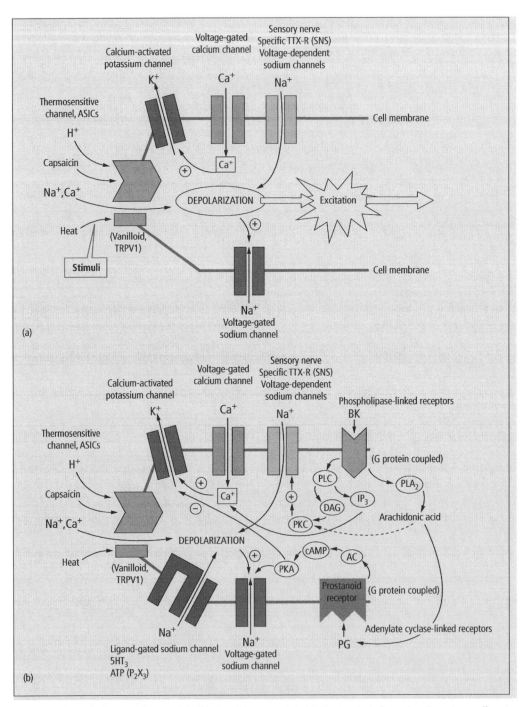

Fig. 10.2 Schematic diagram of some of the initial excitatory events inside the terminal of a nociceptive primary afferent neurone after stimulation: (a) the basic events and (b) additional responses to ligands and associated intracellular messenger systems. AC, adenylate cyclase; ATP, adenosine triphosphate; DAG, diacyl glycerol (from membrane precursor); BK, bradykinin (releases calcium from intracellular stores through IP$_3$); PG, prostaglandin; PL, phospholipase; PK, protein kinase; ASIC, acid sensing ion channel; TTX-R, tetrodotoxin receptor.

Table 10.1 Receptors involved in nociception.

Types of receptors	Ligand
Ligand-gated ion channels (ionotropic)	
γ aminobutyric acid (GABA$_A$) [Cl$^-$ channel]	GABA
Transient receptor protein (vanilloid; TRPV1)	Capsaicin, H$^+$, >43°C
α-Amino-3-hydroxy-5-methylisoxazole-4-propionic acid (AMPA)	Glutamate
N-methyl-D-aspartate (NMDA)	Glutamate, nitric oxide
Acid sensing ion channel (ASIC)	H$^+$
Purinergic (P$_2$X$_3$)	ATP
Tyrosine kinase (Trk)-coupled receptors (metabotropic)	
TrkA	Nerve growth factor (NGF)
G protein-coupled receptors (metabotropic)	
Opioid (MOR, KOR, DOR)	Endorphin, leu-/met-enkephalin, dynorphin
Nociceptin (NOR)	Nociceptin (N/OFQ)
5-Hydroxytryptamine (serotonin; 5-HT) [except 5-HT3 = ligand gated]	5-HT
Tachykinin (NK1, 2, 3)	Substance P (SP), neurokinin (NKA, NKB)
Kinin (BK1, BK2)	Bradykinin
Calcitonin gene related peptide (CGRP)	CGRP
GABA$_B$	GABA
Glutamate (mGlu)	Glutamate
Adrenoceptors (e.g. α_2)	Noradrenaline (norepinephrine), adrenaline (epinephrine), dopamine
Cannabinoid (CB$_1$, CB$_2$)	Arachydonylethanolamide (anandamide; AEA)

through the NGF receptor—tyrosine kinase A (TrKA), in non-peptidergic C fibres through the glial cell-line-derived neurotrophic factor receptor, and in A fibres through TrKC receptor. Nociceptive neurones thus retain a mechanism for sensitivity after injury or inflammation. NGF also degranulates mast cells and releases more chemicals that amplify the inflammatory signal.

Nociception from primary afferent fibres in deeper tissues is less well understood. Pain from muscles, joints, bone and viscera is more diffuse and difficult to localize. There are no fast or slow components that characterise superficially-induced cutaneous pain. However, sensation is often accompanied by autonomic nervous system activity (e.g. through C fibres) such as sweating, increased blood pressure, raised heart rate, and increased respiratory frequency. Under inflammatory conditions a group of afferent neurones in deeper structures that normally do not respond to noxious or non-noxious stimuli become respon-

sive. These neurones are called **silent nociceptors**. Their activation will increase the barrage of nociceptive activity reaching the DH of the spinal cord when tissues are inflamed.

When a tissue-damaging heat stimulus activates superficial nociceptors in the skin, the area of injury becomes tender and has a lower threshold for stimulus-induced pain. This is termed **primary hyperalgesia**. Sensitization occurs due to the release of chemicals from damaged cells as part of the inflammatory reaction to heal injured tissue (Figs 10.1 and 10.2). Some of the chemicals act on blood vessels, triggering the release of mediators from mast cells and basophils. These mediators include adenosine triphosphate (ATP), bradykinin, 5-hydroxytryptamine (5-HT, serotonin), noradrenaline (norepinephrine), prostaglandin E$_2$ and NGF. The receptors present on the primary sensory neurones that respond to a noxious heat stimulus include TRPV1—a receptor that responds not only to heat but also capsaicin, purine P$_2$X$_3$ receptors for

ATP, acid-sensing ion channels (ASIC), sodium channels, e.g. Na1.8 (PN3, SNS), bradykinin receptors, 5-HT$_{2A}$ and TrKA receptors (Fig. 10.2). Prostaglandins increase cyclic adenosine monophosphate (cAMP) levels within the nociceptor, possibly by phosphorylating a sodium channel; hence by reversing this mechanism, non-steroidal anti-inflammatory agents can reduce firing and provide analgesia.

Methods to reduce activation of sensitization mechanisms include:

1 reducing inflammatory activity (e.g. cyclo-oxygenase inhibitors);

2 altering receptor function (e.g. antagonists at excitatory receptors such as NMDA); and

3 modifying signalling pathways (e.g. those that elevate intracellular calcium and cyclic AMP, such as phospholipase C).

Afferent transmission from deep tissues and viscera

Musculoskeletal pain is common in the general population. Aδ and C fibres innervate muscles and joints and, in normal joints, extreme pressure can elicit nociceptive responses through receptors in the joint capsule, ligaments, bone and perivascular sites. In experimental joint inflammation, sensitization occurs through a similar mechanism to that employed by cutaneous nociceptors, so that small movements activate afferents. One clinically relevant change is the up-regulation of opioid receptors. After tissue damage, opioid receptors are transported from the DRG to the periphery by retrograde (antidromic) transmission and become activated. In addition, immunocompetent cells liberate endogenous opioids.

Skeletal muscle makes up a large proportion (up to 30%) of body mass and is richly innervated. Muscle nociceptors are stimulated by pressure, heat, and by chemicals such as hypertonic saline. Ischaemia can also initiate pain sensations. Local muscle tenderness may result from sensitization, following endogenous chemical release induced by muscle trauma or unaccustomed exercise. Clinically, a local vicious cycle can cause this problem to spread. In experimental muscle pain, excitation is

generated centrally by neurokinin receptors (the ligand for which is SP), N-methyl-D-aspartic acid (NMDA) receptors (whose ligands are glycine and glutamate), and by a reduction in nitric oxide synthesis. Muscle pain is often associated with hyperalgesia and referred pain. The pattern of referred pain from muscle is relatively constant and predictable. For example, the referred pain sites from a gluteus medius muscle hypersensitive site (called a trigger point) is in the distribution of the sciatic nerve.

Visceral afferents are either Aδ or C fibres, and these respond to low or high threshold stimuli. The fibres activated at a low threshold are involved in normal functions such as peristalsis; high threshold fibres have a lower rate of spontaneous activity and act as mechanosensitive nociceptors. Furthermore, there are nociceptors that respond to chemicals that may be activated in inflammation. Thus, compared with cutaneous nociceptors, visceral nociceptors are fewer in number and respond to different stimuli—distension, inflammation, ischaemia and chemicals. In female animals, the high threshold mechanosensitive fibres have been demonstrated to change their threshold during the different phases of the reproductive cycle.

The afferent nociceptors from viscera occur close to blood vessels; these vessels can contribute to pain by releasing chemical mediators, or by their own nociceptors being activated (e.g. puncture of an artery is painful). Organs considered to be visceral include the internal structures of the thorax and abdomen (e.g. heart, blood vessels, lungs, gastrointestinal tract, spleen, renal and reproductive organs), and the cranium (e.g. brain and meninges). In headache nociceptive stimuli often originate in the blood vessels within the dura and meninges. The trigeminal nerve can become sensitized and extracranial phenomena may be the result of trigeminal nerve activation. One aspect of visceral nociception is that it is possible for pathology in an organ not to be recognized because pain sensations are not felt. Examples include silent myocardial infarction and silent kidney stones. The mechanism postulated for these effects is an inhibition generated by long-term changes in the CNS.

The patterns of pain sensations associated with

deep structures are of two types: referred pain (Fig. 10.3), which has vague boundaries (e.g. pain from an inflamed appendix is felt diffusely in the abdomen); and muscle and skin sensitivity, which has defined boundaries and is in the segmental region of the deep structure. A common example of the former, which may be interpreted as 'flu-like' symptoms by a patient, is referred pain after abdominal laparoscopy when central diaphragmatic irritation is referred from the cervical segments C3 & 4 through phrenic nerve innervation to the neck and shoulder.

Modulation

One of the most important concepts in the perception of pain is that of modulation. At all levels of the nervous system modulation can change perception: in tissues during inflammation; at the distal nociceptor via the transduction process; through transmission in the primary afferent nerve; at transduction within the synapses of the spinal cord; through transmission in the nerves of the spinal cord; and more widely, in CNS processes. This dynamic milieu may be altered by previous experiences of pain, by time (e.g. circadian variations, age), hormonal state (e.g. reproduction, stress), disease, drugs and psychosocial factors.

Dorsal horn

A classical modulatory system is present in the dorsal horn of the spinal cord. As shown in Fig. 10.4, input from peripheral large nerve fibres (Aβ) can

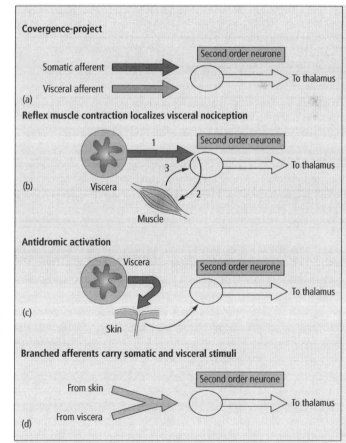

Fig. 10.3 Mechanisms for referred pain. (a) Convergence-projection. (b) Reflex muscle contraction localizes visceral nociception (1, visceral afferent impulse; 2, reflex efferent generating muscle contraction; 3, nerve fibre activity generated from muscle contraction). (c) Antidromic activation. (d) Branched afferents carry somatic and visceral stimuli.

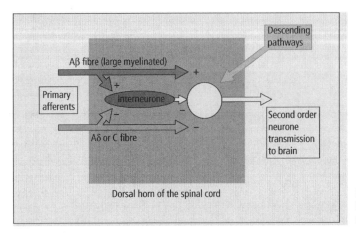

Dorsal horn of the spinal cord

Fig. 10.4 Basic gate modulation of input through the dorsal horn of the spinal cord to the brain.

inhibit input into the spinal cord. Such a modulatory system can explain how transcutaneous electrical nerve stimulation (TENS) functions: as large fibres are electrically stimulated by high frequency current using a battery-operated machine they inhibit the activity of the small nociceptive fibres at the spinal cord in the same segment. Hence the therapy is used in the same segment as the site of the pain, and primary afferent nerve fibre activity is required; where sensory nerves are not present, e.g. in de-afferentation where nerves are destroyed, TENS is unable to modulate pain sensations.

Transmission through the dorsal horn can be suppressed either through descending inhibition from the CNS, or at the level of the spinal segment involved (Fig. 10.1). Descending inhibition can act pre- or postsynaptically on the second-order neurone projecting to the CNS. Presynaptic inhibition decreases excitatory neurotransmitter release (e.g. glutamate) from the primary afferent nerve, and subsequently reduces the electrical activity of the second-order neurone. Thus there is less amplification of the stimulus from the periphery. Numerous other cells in the dorsal horn (e.g. interneurones and glia) act locally and modulate on-going nerve activity through inhibitory mechanisms. The inhibitory neurotransmitters that can be released include γ-aminobutyric acid (GABA), endogenous cannabinoids and opioids. The superficial laminae in the spinal cord have a dense system of opioid-containing interneurones containing naturally-occurring opioids such as enkephalin and dynorphin. Their receptors are expressed presynaptically on the terminals of the primary afferent neurone and postsynaptically on the projection second-order neurones.

Supraspinal modulation

Descending inhibitory pathways from the brain modulate nociceptive activity in the spinal cord. The two key structures from which these pathways originate are: the periaqueductal grey (PAG) that surrounds the cerebral aqueduct in the midbrain, and the rostroventral medulla (RVM) in the brainstem. The neurochemicals controlling activity in these structures are opioids, cannabinoids, 5-HT and noradrenaline. These systems partly mediate the analgesia associated with stress, e.g. during trauma; naloxone, an opioid antagonist, can block such stress-related analgesia. Such pharmacological intervention confirms that this inhibitory system includes endogenous opioid activity.

Using brain imaging, multiple centres of activity have been observed during a noxious stimulus. The primary centres include the thalamus and the somatosensory cortex. The cortical centres determine sensory discrimination, e.g. site of pain. Other key areas are the limbic system that is activated during emotional responses such as anger, the anterior cingulate that processes affective responses, and motor regions that generate appropriate movement. Pain modulation in the CNS is linked to other functions such as attention, emotional state, cognition and past experience. Research can identify these through experiments, such as distraction tests to investigate attention.

Specific functional areas

Dorsal root ganglion (DRG)

The DRG (Fig. 10.1) lies within the vertebral column and contains virtually no synapses. It contains the cell bodies of the primary afferent fibres. It has been thought to have a mainly nutritive function but this is now questioned because the DRG can generate spontaneous firing, express a large variety of neurochemicals (e.g. substance P, somatostatin, CGRP) and through transcription mechanisms it can manufacture receptors. In addition, it differs from the peripheral nerves that are its extensions in that it lacks a blood-nerve barrier, i.e. in function the cells are similar to those in the CNS chemosensory areas.

Spinal transmission from the dorsal horn to the thalamus

The nociceptive axons (second order neurones) projecting to the thalamus ascend in two fairly distinct locations, one laterally and the other anteriorly (ventral). As they approach the thalamus they divide into medial and lateral divisions. They terminate in distinct regions of the thalamus (e.g. ventroposterior nuclei) and then synapse and project to the somatosensory cortex.

If the anterolateral quadrant of the spinal cord is destroyed there is a loss of pain and temperature sensation on the side opposite the lesion and about four segments below the level of the deficit. Sensation from superficial (skin) and deep (muscle and viscera) tissues is lost. However, from other clinical evidence, crude information from the ipsilateral side can be processed and some deep sensation may be retained. The neurones in the anterolateral quadrant terminate finally at the thalamus (the spinothalamic tract) but other connections may occur below the thalamus (e.g. in the spinoreticular tract, which is part of the spinobulbar projec-tions to the four main areas of the brainstem including the PAG).

Destruction of part of this system in the spinal cord or brain can cause an imbalance of modulatory activity that has variable effects. For example, it may generate central pain after a stroke that is characterized by a burning quality and referred to an area of the body where there is a paradoxical loss of cutaneous pain sensitivity (i.e. analgesia). The inhibitory interneurones in the thalamus are GABAergic and many second order neurone terminals release excitatory amino acids (e.g. glutamate, glycine) onto brain stem or thalamic neurones, with NMDA receptors involved in mediating excitatory responses. Other neuromodulators from the brainstem acting on the thalamus are serotonin (5-HT), norepinephrine (NE) and cholinergic neurones. In addition endogenous opioid activity in the thalamus has also been observed.

Endogenous ligands

Opioids

The three receptor subtypes for opioid analgesia are μ (MOR), δ (DOR), and κ (KOR). Their endogenous ligands are endorphins, enkephalins (leu- and met-enkephalin; both small 5-amino acid compounds) and dynorphin, respectively. Their activation—through a G protein-coupled receptor—leads to inhibition of adenylate cyclase activity, which subsequently reduces cyclic AMP, stimulates potassium efflux, and inhibits voltage gated calcium channels. The net effect is to hyperpolarize the cell membrane so that it is less likely to reach the threshold value of potential difference needed for excitation. Opioid modulation acts via presynaptic inhibition at the DH, to prevent the release of excitatory peptides from the primary afferent neurones, and via direct postsynaptic inhibition of the second-order (projection) neurones.

Endogenous opioids are rapidly formed from precursors—propiomelanocortin for β endorphin that acts on MOR, KOR and DOR receptors, proenkephalin for leu- and met-enkephalin, and prodynorphin for dynorphin A and B. Enkephalins are present in many parts of the CNS and are of importance in the descending inhibitory pathways. They are broken down rapidly by neural endopeptidase to remove them from the site of action. Endorphins act mainly in the brainstem at the PAG, the nucleus raphe magnus and in the DH, and their breakdown is mediated in part by angiotensin converting enzyme. A further opioid—nociceptin, acts supraspinally to induce hyperalgesia. In the spinal cord the nociceptin receptor, NOR, is expressed by interneurones in laminae I, II and V, and produces presynaptic inhibition and analgesia.

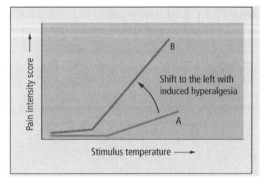

Fig. 10.5 The relation of stimulus intensity to pain intensity in (A) normal subjects and (B) after induced hyperalgesia.

Cannabinoids

There are two main types of cannabinoid receptors; CB1 is located mainly in the CNS and CB2 mainly in immune cells, but also in glial cells. Endogenous cannabinoids are not potent agonists at cannabinoid receptors and may have other functions such as activating the vanilloid receptor TRPV1. The endogenous cannabinoids are arachydonoyl ethanolamide (anandamide; AEA), 2-arachydonoylglycerol (2-AG) and palmitoylethanolamide (PEA). They are short-acting and are rapidly broken down by fatty acid amide hydrolases (FAAH). CB1 receptors are located in the skin on Aδ fibres where they modulate SP, nitric oxide and CGRP release, and are antinociceptive. Both CB1 and CB2 are G protein-coupled receptors and are found at all levels in the CNS where nociception is modulated.

Hyperalgesia

When the curve relating stimulus intensity to pain intensity is drawn (Fig. 10.5), its position can be moved to the left by the phenomenon of hypersensitivity. The curve illustrates a lower threshold to pain and, for the same suprathreshold stimulus, a higher pain intensity response. Sensitization is the neural process that occurs in relation to hyperalgesia and differs with tissue and injury type.

Primary and secondary hyperalgesia

Hyperalgesia is a common event and features in pain from superficial and deep structures. For example, during a urinary tract infection micturition is painful, in arthritis slight movement is painful, and after a burn the skin is painful if nociceptors have not been lost. Hyperalgesia at the site of injury is called **primary hyperalgesia**, and in the uninjured skin around the injury it is termed **secondary hyperalgesia**. In general, the mechanism for secondary hyperalgesia is considered to be in the CNS (i.e. the brain and spinal cord).

In the spinal cord after injury a state of hyperexcitability exists where DH neurones will respond to weaker electrical signals from afferent fibres, which therefore expands the receptive field of neurones and increases the number of DH cells responding to the stimulus. These changes result in a non-noxious stimulus releasing SP, and the phenomenon of 'wind-up'. Wind-up refers to the situation when the stimulus strength does not change, but if it is repeated there will be a measured increase in the response from DH neurones—e.g. in output of excitatory neurochemicals. The whole system is dynamic, but the key factor is the NMDA receptor. For this receptor to function, certain events have to occur. First the normal glutamate release from nociceptors occurs. This amino acid binds to α-amino-3-hydroxy-5-methyl-isoxazolepropionic acid (AMPA; a sodium selective ion channel) and produces a short-acting postsynaptic depolarization. If the noxious stimulus persists, peptides are released—e.g. tachykinins (such as substance P and neurokinins A and B) and

CGRP. This delay is inbuilt (because the peptides are stored at some distance from the nerve terminal) and opportune (because the calcium released by the NMDA receptor opening has major intracellular activities). The tachykinins induce membrane depolarization that differs from AMPA activity by being slower to rise and longer lasting. Finally the membrane becomes sufficiently depolarized to remove the magnesium block of the NMDA receptor. At this point the available glutamate can activate the NMDA ligand-gated calcium channel, and a large influx of calcium occurs.

The intracellular events that follow effectively maintain open the NMDA channel. The main effect is mediated through protein kinase C (PKCγ, in contrast with PKCε in the peripheral nerve), via tyrosine kinases, PKA and brain derived neurotrophic factor (BDNF), all of which can enhance NMDA receptor function. The elevated calcium activates phospholipase A_2 (PLA_2) so that cyclo-oxygenase products are formed and prostaglandin E_2 released.

Visceral hyperalgesia

Tenderness in skin and muscle may be the result of visceral hyperalgesia. It can exist long after the initial stimulus has gone. The hyperalgesia is a result of central sensitization, but there are some unresolved issues. For example, some visceral disorders cause an excessive amount of pain and other visceral pain disorders occur repeatedly with other pain conditions, e.g. interstitial cystitis and irritable bowel syndrome. One proposed mechanism is the convergence of somatic and visceral afferents at the DH; another is that there is convergence of visceral afferents from different organs. However, visceral organs have a broader segmental spread than just one segment, so the effects observed through DH interactions may be more diverse than these theories suggest.

Allodynia

When Aβ primary afferents switch phenotype from touch sensory fibres to nociceptors and express SP and BDNF, then low-intensity stimula-tion induces tactile allodynia (when touch becomes painful). Such a situation follows a superficial burn. On recovery from acute tissue damage, the allodynia disappears—in hours or days.

In neuropathic pain, i.e. pain from nerve damage, the allodynia becomes persistent. In this state there is a maintained alteration in transcription factors, and these long-term changes make the primary afferent cells more excitable. Thus although normally only C fibre activity can induce central sensitization, Aβ fibre activity becomes involved in nociceptive processing, either in the short- or long-term.

Peripheral nerve damage

During normal function nociceptors only become activated when stimulated by noxious conditions. When nerves are cut or inflamed or their blood flow is reduced and abnormal responses occur. These include spontaneous activity and increased sensitivity to stimuli, i.e. they activate at a lower threshold. The CNS thus receives an abnormal afferent input from ectopic foci along the nerve, as well as spontaneous activity within the DRG and increased firing from sensitization. At the molecular level the changes in electrical activity are accompanied with an increased expression of ion channels (e.g. sodium) and receptors. It is at the site of the ectopic activity that these receptors and ion channels are located and these changes make spontaneous and ectopic electrical potentials more probable.

Where C fibre input into the DH is lost as a result of degeneration or de-afferentation, there is a reduction in synaptic contacts, and Aβ afferents that normally synapse in deeper laminae (III and IV) grow and sprout into more superficial lamina (II) and directly contact the de-afferented cells. This synaptic re-organization occurs in a small group of patients and may induce altered painful sensations.

In the normal state nociceptors do not respond to sympathetic stimulation or catecholamines, but after injury interaction occurs in the distal nerve (e.g. where there may be a neuroma), in intact nociceptors and in the DRG. The latter site is interesting because the ganglia contain blood vessels whose sympathetic nerves sprout. Thus the application of catecholamines can induce or exacerbate pain, and their antagonists can relieve this pain.

Phantom pain

There are clinical conditions such as phantom rectum (after abdomino–perineal resection) or phantom limb (after amputation), where an organ or limb has been removed yet pain is sensed in the body part that no longer exists. A related phenomenon occurs when part of the sensory cortex is stimulated during neurosurgery, and a sensation is created that mimics a stimulation in the body part with the corresponding cortical representation. Similar sensations can be induced by local anaesthesia of a limb when nerves are blocked adequately for surgery yet a mental image of the arm's position remains (and can be incorrect if the eyes are closed).

Chapter 11

Endocrine System

The endocrine system, acting through blood-borne chemical messengers (**hormones**), is involved in coordinating the body's responses to environmental stimuli. This coordination involves the control of the storage and utilization of energy substrates, and results in the maintenance of the internal environment (homeostasis). In addition, the endocrine system plays an essential role in the regulation of growth, development and reproduction. The actions of the endocrine system are slower in onset, more prolonged and generally more diffuse than those of the nervous system. The two systems are linked through the **hypothalamus**, which controls secretion from many of the endocrine glands.

Hormones are secreted not only by organs classically termed as endocrine glands, but also by specialized cells in several other organs. In fact, the first hormone to be discovered—by Starling in 1902—was secretin, which is produced by the duodenum. Hormones, released (secreted) into the blood by endocrine cells, exert their biological effect on remote tissues at extremely low concentrations (between 10^{-6} and 10^{-12}M).

The principal endocrine glands in mammals are the **hypothalamus, pituitary, thyroid, parathyroids, adrenals, pancreatic islets, gonads** and **placenta**. Hormones and hormone-like substances are also produced in the cardiovascular system (p. 405), kidney (p. 573), and certain cells of the gastrointestinal tract (p. 499). The hormones produced in these organs often exert only a local (paracrine) effect. Many substances which were first identified as hormones produced in endocrine glands are now also known to be synthesized in the nervous system, where they act as neurotransmitters or neuromodulators (p. 80).

11.1 Hormones

Hormones are carried in the circulation at low concentrations and bind to specific receptors in their target tissues to elicit specific cellular responses. Peptide hormones and adrenaline bind to receptors in the plasma membrane and their actions are usually mediated by intracellular messengers (e.g. cyclic adenosine monophosphate (cAMP), cyclic guanosine monophosphate (cGMP), inositol 1,4,5-trisphosphate (IP_3) and diacylglycerol). These messengers either directly or indirectly stimulate protein kinases or protein phosphatases, which regulate specific cellular responses. Steroid and thyroid hormones most often bind to intracellular receptors to induce (or repress) gene activation and the synthesis of specific proteins which, in many cases, are enzymes.

Basic concepts

A hormone can be defined as a chemical substance that is synthesized and secreted by a specific cell type, is transported in the circulation and, at very low concentrations, elicits a specific response in distant target tissues. Not all hormone-like substances meet these criteria. For example, some cells release substances that diffuse into surrounding regions and act locally on neighbouring cells (paracrine). Sometimes cells secrete enzymes that act on plasma proteins to produce hormones, e.g. the renin–angiotensin system.

Hormones may be classified according to their chemical structure into:

1 **peptide hormones**, e.g. growth hormone, insulin and vasopressin (AVP);

2 **steroid hormones**, e.g. aldosterone, ooestrogen and testosterone; and

3 **tyrosine derivatives**, e.g. thyroxine and adrenaline.

Because of the low concentration of hormones in the blood, their presence was difficult to detect by chemical analysis, and so **bioassays** and later, **radioimmunoassays**, were devised for measuring hormone levels.

Hormone synthesis and secretion

As discussed in Chapter 23, peptide hormones, similar to other peptides destined for secretion, are synthesized on the rough endoplasmic reticulum as part of larger precursor proteins called preprohormones, which are subsequently modified by splitting off peptide sequences and, in the case of glycoproteins, by the addition of carbohydrate moieties (p. 23). The peptide hormones are stored in vesicles and released by exocytosis in response to elevated cytoplasmic Ca^{2+} concentrations (Ca^{2+} signal), evoked by the appropriate stimuli.

Steroid hormones are lipophilic; they are not encapsulated in vesicles for secretion and their rate of release is determined by their rate of synthesis. They are synthesized from cholesterol in a series of steps that take place in the mitochondria, smooth endoplasmic reticulum and cytoplasm (p. 23). As they are synthesized, they diffuse across the plasma membrane of the cell into the interstitial fluid and then into the blood stream.

Synthesis of hormones that are derivatives of tyrosine occurs by specific pathways in thyroid and adrenal medullary cells.

Hormone transport and inactivation

Once released into the blood stream, lipid-soluble hormones, e.g. thyroid and steroid hormones, are carried bound to various plasma proteins. The **free** form is usually only a small fraction of the total hormone in the blood and exists in dynamic equilibrium with the **bound** form. Generally speaking, only the free hormone can enter the target cell. The concentration of the active hormone in the blood is therefore determined by the dynamic relationship between its rate of secretion, its rate of inactivation and the degree to which it is bound to plasma proteins.

Hormones have a half-life in the body of minutes to days. Inactivation may occur in the blood, in the liver or kidney, or in some cases in the target tissues. Hormones may be inactivated by degradation, oxidation, reduction, methylation or by conjugation to glucuronic or sulphuric acid, and are then excreted in the urine or bile. Peptide hormones generally have short half-lives (minutes) because they are rapidly degraded by peptide cleavage.

Hormone actions

Hormones affect the growth, development, metabolic activity and function of tissues. The responses are often the result of the actions of several hormones. Actions may be **stimulatory** or **inhibitory**. A hormone, which has no effect *per se* but is necessary for the full expression of the effects of other hormones, is said to have a **permissive** action. Most commonly the key step in hormone action is a change in enzymatic activity, either due to activation (or inactivation) of pre-existing enzymes or to an altered rate of enzyme synthesis. Whereas activation (or inactivation) of enzymes — usually that of a rate-limiting enzyme in a critical reaction pathway — may be preceded by modification of the membrane permeability to specific ions (leading, for example, to depolarization) and is finally achieved by a change in the phosphorylation state of the enzyme protein, the synthesis of enzyme (or non-enzyme) proteins may be controlled at the transcriptional or more rarely, translational, level.

The first step in the action of a hormone is its binding to a specific cell **receptor**. Peptide hormones, which do not penetrate cells readily, act by binding to specific receptors in the plasma membrane. The receptor of a few hormones (growth hormone (GH), prolactin, erythropoietin, leptin) is a relatively simple membrane protein containing a single transmembrane domain. Binding of the appropriate ligand to such a receptor, termed cytokine receptor, induces a conformational change in the protein that results in the binding and activation of cytosolic protein tyrosine kinase(s). Other protein or peptide hormones bind to a so-called G-protein-coupled receptor (GPCR) that has seven transmembrane domains. Upon activation of the receptor, a cytosolic loop between two transmembrane segments binds a specific G-protein which, in turn, may activate enzymes (e.g. cAMP—producing adenylyl cyclase or IP_3—producing phospholipase C), or may change the activity of transmembrane ion channels and thereby the membrane potential, etc.

In contrast, steroid hormones readily cross the plasma membrane and bind either to **cytoplasmic** receptors, which are then translocated to the nucleus, or to **nuclear** receptors in their target tissues. The hormone–receptor complex induces (or suppresses) gene activation altering the transcription of mRNA species and, consequently, the synthesis of specific proteins. Nevertheless, quite a few steroid actions have recently been found to occur at **plasmalemmal** receptors; these are non-genomic actions. Thyroid hormones, which cross the plasma membrane readily, regulate gene transcription by binding to **nuclear** receptors that are already bound to DNA in their target tissues.

Hormone-induced changes in receptor function modify the efficiency of a maintained or repeated hormonal stimulus. This mechanism may prevent the excessive, often harmful, increase of hormone secretion, and may also serve as an adaptation to the general hormone status of the organism. The regulation of G-protein-coupled receptors involves homologous and heterologous desensitization, receptor internalization, and down-regulation. Desensitization and internalization are rapid phenomena that can occur within minutes, or in

some cases seconds, following the stimulation of GPCR; whereas down-regulation is a much slower process, mediated by a decrease in the total cellular receptor pool. Homologous desensitization of a GPCR involves agonist-induced phosphorylation of the receptor, followed by uncoupling of the receptor from its cognate G-protein. This mechanism limits the duration of the signal generation after receptor activation and therefore it is an essential element of the termination of stimulation. If continuous supply of plasma membrane receptors (e.g. via new receptor synthesis or receptor recycling) is not available, prolonged agonist stimulation may lead to depletion of the non-desensitized plasma membrane receptor population, and homologous desensitization of the tissue may occur. Heterologous desensitization is caused by phosphorylation of GPCR during stimulation of the cell via agonist(s) that target different receptors. This process is mediated by second messenger-induced stimulation of protein kinases, and is important in regulating the agonist sensitivity of hormone target tissues. Whereas the term 'internalization' is applied to the translocation of cell surface receptors into intracellular compartments with no major change in total receptor number, down-regulation signifies a decrease in the total cellular receptor pool. This decrease may result from both increased receptor degradation and reduced receptor synthesis, and usually develops over hours or days.

Control of hormone secretion

The immediate stimulus for the secretion of a hormone may be neural, hormonal, or change in the level of some metabolite or electrolyte in the blood. Secretion rates are usually influenced by **negative feedback** mechanisms, whereby increased levels of hormone in the blood lead to the inhibition of further hormone secretion. A unique case of positive feedback control is found with hormonal regulation of ovulation during the female reproductive cycle. However, it should be emphasized that the control mechanism consists of both the hormonal feedback and the neural mechanisms.

Analysis of hormones

There are several methods for assaying hormone concentrations in serum or urine—bioassay, radioimmunoassay, and enzyme-linked immunosorbent assay (ELISA)—although the level of some hormones, e.g. catecholamines and steroid hormones, may also be estimated by chemical analysis. Traditionally, the activity of newly-discovered hormones was estimated by **bioassay**. This involves quantifying the responses of tissues to various concentrations of a hormone (standard or unknown), either *in vitro* or *in vivo*. For example, chorionic gonadotrophin was formerly assayed by its ability to induce ovulation in rabbits. A standard curve was plotted and the concentration of the unknown was extrapolated from it. Such assays are often cumbersome to perform and variable in their response. However, they do measure the biological activity of the hormone.

Radioimmunoassay depends on the availability of radioactively-labelled hormone and of antibodies that react with it. A competition assay is set up in which the unlabelled standard or unknown hormone competes with the labelled hormone for a site on the antibody; as the concentration of unlabelled hormone increases, then the proportion of labelled hormone bound to the antibody decreases. The hormone-bound complex is then separated from the free hormone by various physicochemical means (e.g. filtration, precipitation, charcoal exclusion), and the radioactivity of the complex determined. A standard curve is prepared and the concentration of the unknown is extrapolated from this. Radioimmunoassay is an extremely sensitive (in the femtomole range) and specific technique. However, it does not necessarily specifically measure the biological activity of the hormone, since it can also detect precursors and degradation products, thus leading to an overestimation of the hormone concentration.

Enzyme-linked immunosorbent assay (ELISA) was developed to eliminate the need for radioactive-labelling and to automate procedures for hormone assay. Instead of the hormone (antigen) being labelled with a radioisotope, in an ELISA it is linked to an enzyme marker, e.g. horseradish

peroxidase or alkaline phosphatase, which generates a coloured product when the appropriate substrate is added. Alternatively, an antibody against the hormone may be linked to an enzyme marker. A further refinement of this type of assay is that it is usually carried out with the reactants bound to a 'solid phase' (e.g. polyvinylchloride plastic) to facilitate the washing steps involved. Small quantities of proteins, such as hormones and antibodies, are readily adsorbed onto the surfaces of plastic tubes or wells when solutions are incubated in them. Excess adsorption sites can then be blocked, and after each reaction step the tubes are washed with detergent solutions. There are a number of variations of such assays (Fig. 11.1). In an antibody-capture assay the hormone is immobilized on a solid support and an enzyme-linked antibody is allowed to bind; in an antigen-capture assay an antibody is attached to a solid support and the labelled hormone (antigen) is allowed to bind. A third type of assay is the two-antibody assay in which an antibody is immobilized on a solid support and the hormone allowed to bind; a second antibody labelled with an enzyme marker is then allowed to bind to the hormone, and the level of bound enzyme can then be quantified.

11.2 The hypothalamo–adenohypophyseal system

The **pituitary** (hypophysis) is a small gland, weighing approximately 0.5 g in humans, and is situated at the base of the skull, connected to the brain by the pituitary stalk. It consists of an anterior part (adenohypophysis) and a posterior part (neurohypophysis). During embryonic development the neurohypophysis, which includes the pars posterior (pars nervosa), is derived from a downward evagination of the brain.

The adenohypophysis secretes six hormones. Secretion of anterior pituitary hormones is controlled by hypothalamic neurohormones, which reach the anterior pituitary via the hypothalamo–hypophyseal portal system. Release of the trophic hormones is also controlled by negative feedback via hormones released from their target gland.

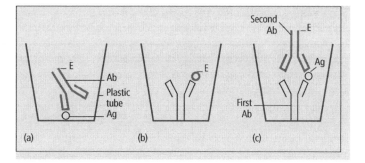

Fig. 11.1 Various types of ELISA: (a) antibody-capture assay; (b) antigen-capture assay; (c) two-antibody assay. The enzyme tag is indicated by E. Ab, antibody; Ag, antigen.

The **adenohypophysis**, which includes the pars anterior (pars distalis) and the pars intermedia, comes from an outgrowth of the roof of the mouth known as Rathke's pouch. In the adult human, the pars intermedia is only a remnant. The anterior pituitary synthesizes and secretes at least six hormones (some of which are referred to by different names). Some of these are trophic hormones, which regulate the secretion of hormones from other endocrine glands. (The suffix 'trophin' is usually used in English texts while 'tropin' is used in American texts.) Thyroid-stimulating hormone (TSH) stimulates the secretion of thyroxin from the thyroid gland, adrenocorticotrophic hormone (ACTH) stimulates cortisol secretion from the adrenal cortex, while follicle-stimulating hormone (FSH) and luteinizing hormone (LH) control gonadal function. FSH and LH are known collectively as the gonadotrophins. Two other hormones, GH and prolactin (PRL) act directly on target tissues: GH acts on several peripheral tissues, whereas prolactin stimulates milk production and influences gonadal function and sexual behaviour. Each of these hormones is produced by a specific cell type, although gonadotrophs secrete both FSH and LH. These different cell types are interspersed throughout the pars anterior and their hormones are secreted in response to stimulation by the corresponding hypothalamic neurohormones (releasing hormones).

Structurally the pituitary hormones may be grouped in three classes. Belonging to the same class may result in cross-talk, which means that a hormone, present at high concentration, activates the receptor of another hormone of the same class (showing related structure). Having a common **ancestral** gene, GH (containing 191 amino acid residues) and PRL (198 amino acid residues) are simple proteins, showing about 80% identity at the amino acid level. Oversecretion of GH may result in a PRL-like effect on gonadal function. The glycoprotein hormones TSH, FSH and LH consist of an identical α chain (96 amino acid residues) and a similar β chain, containing 112 (TSH), 114 (FSH) or 116 (LH) amino acid residues. The gene of the placental hormone **human chorion gonadotrophin** (hCG) derived from the common **ancestral** gene of the glycoprotein hormones; it contains an identical α chain and 146 amino acid residues in its β chain. Due to its structural similarity to LH, it exerts its actions on LH receptors. ACTH derives from the prohormone **proopiomelanocortin** (POMC), which contains the sequences of a number of bioactive compounds; in addition to that of ACTH, it contains the sequences of melanocyte-stimulating hormones (MSH) and of endorphins (p. 235). POMC is expressed in several organs, including the brain, spinal medulla and the testes. The POMC-derived compound(s) secreted by a particular cell type will therefore depend on that cell's repertoire of proteolytic enzymes. The pars intermedia of the pituitary gland secretes β-**endorphin, met-enkephalin and MSH.** The first two of these peptides are endogenous opiates. In amphibia and fish both types of MSH, the identical α-MSH and β-MSH (polypeptides of M_r ~2000), cause the skin to darken by dispersing melanin granules within the melanophores; this therefore enables these animals to blend their skin colour with the environment. The structural sequence of α-MSH corresponds to residues 1–13 of ACTH. Due to structural similarities ACTH and the various types of MSH bind to related receptors, termed melanocortin receptors. This is the reason why excess production of ACTH in humans can cause an increase in melanin synthesis and hyperpigmentation. In the human, the pars intermedia is a rudimentary tissue, it occupies only 1% of the pituitary and it is probably functionally redundant.

GH acts on many tissues to stimulate growth and metabolism, while prolactin stimulates lactation in the mammary glands, and influences gonadal function and sexual behaviour. The trophic hormones stimulate the growth and secretion of other endocrine glands in the body: TSH acts on the thyroid gland, ACTH acts on the adrenal cortex, and the gonadotrophins, FSH and LH, act on the testes and ovaries. Not only do the trophic hormones influence the secretion of their target glands, they also influence their size and development and maintain normal function. Removal of the pituitary (hypophysectomy) therefore results in an inhibition of growth (in children), in atrophy and functional insufficiency of the thyroid gland and adrenal cortex, and in infertility and sexual dysfunction. However, removal of the pituitary is not incompatible with life, although hypophysectomized animals have a low tolerance to cold, hypoglycaemia, infections and other forms of stress.

Control of anterior pituitary hormone secretion

The function of the hypothalamo–adenohypophyseal system is controlled both by neural and humoral factors. The hypothalamus is served by ascending afferents from the vital centres in the brainstem, and by descending afferents from the forebrain. Some hypothalamic neurones are especially sensitive to blood glucose level, blood temperature or circulating toxins. This way the hypothalamus obtains information about parameters of the internal environment (e.g. blood pressure, pO_2, glucose level) as well as dangerous changes in the environment (perceived by the sensory organs). Inputs from the limbic system result in the activation of the hypothalamic neurones during emotional reactions. The hypothalamic integration of these neural effects (together with the accidental humoral effects) is the basis of the control of the adenohypophysis as well as important vegetative centres (those of body temperature, thirst and appetite) located in the hypothalamus.

The hypothalamus exerts its controlling function on the anterior pituitary through **neurohormones** which are elaborated in small (parvocellular) neurones in specific nuclei of the hypothalamus. These neurohormones are released at the level of the median eminence. They diffuse into a primary plexus of capillaries and are transported down large portal veins in the pituitary stalk to a secondary set of capillaries or sinusoids in the anterior pituitary — the **hypothalamo–hypophyseal portal system** (Fig. 11.2). The neurohormones comprise both releasing and release-inhibiting hormones.

GH-releasing hormone (GHRH) and **thyrotrophin-releasing hormone** (TRH) stimulate

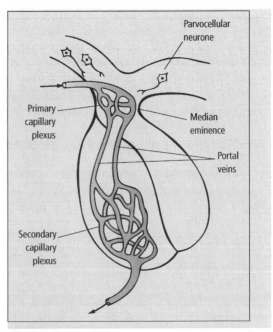

Fig. 11.2 The hypothalamo–hypophyseal portal system of blood vessels.

the release of growth hormone and TSH, respectively. **Corticotrophin-releasing hormone** (CRH) and **arginine vasopressin (AVP)**, secreted by the parvocellular neurones of the supraoptic nucleus, both stimulate the secretion of ACTH. **Gonadotrophin-releasing hormone** (GnRH) stimulates the release of LH and FSH. Finally, **vasoactive intestinal peptide** (VIP), present in the central nervous system as a neurotransmitter, enhances the secretion of prolactin. The release-inhibiting hormones secreted by the hypothalamus are **GH release-inhibiting hormone (somatostatin)** and **prolactin release-inhibiting hormone**, which has been identified as **dopamine**. Thus, secretion of GH and that of prolactin are subject to dual control by the hypothalamus. As a result of the predominant effect of releasing hormones, following the removal of the pituitary gland (hypophysectomy) the secretion of pituitary hormones falls significantly lower than control level. An exception to this is that prolactin secretion increases, since, under resting conditions, its inhibition by dopamine was stronger than its stimulation by VIP. TRH is a tripeptide (pyroglutamylhistidyl–proline amide). The other hypothalamic neurohormones are also peptides; except dopamine, which is a precursor of noradrenaline.

Humoral control of the hypothalamo–adenohypophyseal system also involves negative feedback effects of the hormones, which are secreted by the peripheral endocrine glands under pituitary control. These hormones inhibit the secretion of their respective releasing hormone and/or pituitary trophic hormone. Thus, cortisol inhibits the secretion of CRH and ACTH, whereas thyroxin inhibits the secretion of TRH and TSH. The negative feedback may have a buffering role under stressful conditions, preventing excessive hormonal responses. Removal of an adrenal gland or partial removal of the thyroid gland is followed by enlargement (compensatory hypertrophy) of the contralateral adrenal cortex and remaining thyroid tissue, respectively; this phenomenon is due to a decrease in the tonic negative feedback. Chronic administration of a steroid hormone suppresses secretion of the respective trophic hormone (e.g. long-term administration of a synthetic glucocorticoid depresses ACTH secretion), leading to atrophy of the endocrine gland (adrenal cortex). Testosterone and estradiol inhibit the secretion of GnRH and LH but, under well-defined temporal conditions, estradiol may exert positive feedback effects on FSH and LH release. The ovarian cycle is based on a complex feedback control, involving both negative and positive feedback effects.

There are factors, other than the peripheral (target) hormone acting on the hypothalamus, which also influence feedback mechanisms. Pituitary hormones, which reach the hypothalamus via special vessels from the pituitary, may exert so-called short-loop feedback effects. The somatomedin insulin-like growth factor-1 (IGF-1), released from the liver in response to GH, has a negative feedback effect on GH secretion (by stimulating somatostatin release from the hypothalamus).

The action and control of secretion of ACTH, TSH, the gonadotrophins and PRL will be discussed in detail in the sections dealing with the adrenal cortex, thyroid gland and reproduction, respectively. However, we will concentrate on GH in the next section.

Growth hormone

The processes that control growth are complex. In addition to an adequate food supply and to genetic endowment, a number of hormones are involved, including **GH**, **sex hormones**, **thyroid hormones** and **insulin**. There are two periods of accelerated growth: the first occurs in the first two years of life and the second at the time of puberty. The period of accelerated growth at puberty is associated with increased levels of sex hormones. Although both androgens and oestrogens can stimulate GH secretion, their role in the enhancement of GH secretion during puberty has not yet been established. The cessation of growth around 18–20 years of age is due to oestrogens, which cause fusion of the growing ends of bones (**epiphyseal closure**). Thus, the effect of excessive or deficient GH secretion depends on whether it occurs before or after closure of the epiphyses. Excess GH secretion in young people causes **gigantism**, but in adults it leads to **acromegaly**, in which there is a general coarsening of the features due to thickening of bone and soft tissue. On the other hand, a deficiency of GH in children leads to **dwarfism**. Humans respond only to GH of human (or other primate) origin.

GH, also known as somatotrophin, is a species-specific protein (M_r ~22 kDa) secreted in the anterior pituitary by specific cells called somatotrophs. It has close structural similarities with a placental hormone, chorionic somatomammotrophin, and, to a lesser extent, with prolactin, which suggests their evolution from a common progenitor molecule. In addition to the effects of GH in promoting the growth of muscle and bone, it also has metabolic effects on most of the tissues of the body. Its actions are counter-regulatory to insulin as it increases blood glucose and mobilizes free fatty acids. Its growth-promoting actions (and some of its other actions) are mediated by specific growth factors (termed somatomedins). The secretion of GH occurs in bursts in response to dual control by GHRH and somatostatin; it is stimulated by low blood glucose, high blood amino acids, and ghrelin.

Actions of GH

The most prominent effect of GH in the infantile and juvenile organism is the promotion of growth of both the bones and soft tissues. In bones, GH enhances the proliferation of cartilage cells (chondrocytes), the synthesis of mucopolysaccharides and collagen, and the deposition of calcium. GH also stimulates the proliferation and differentiation of subperiosteal osteoblasts. In the soft tissues GH promotes mitosis and the incorporation of amino acids into proteins, resulting in the growth of several, although not all, organs. Excessive secretion of GH leads to gigantism, whereas insufficient secretion is one of the causes of dwarfism (nanosomia). After epiphyseal closure at the end of puberty linear growth is no longer possible; however, the proliferative effect of GH on subperiosteal osteoblasts and soft tissues is maintained, and therefore hypersecretion of GH in adult humans results in acromegaly, characterized by coarsening of the features. Typically one may observe enlargement of

the jaw, superciliar arc, nose, ear, and of the hand and foot.

In contrast to the long-term effects of GH, as described above, the acute metabolic effects of the hormone subserve protection against hypoglycaemia. It antagonizes the effects of insulin (that reduces blood glucose level) probably by several mechanisms. Following a lag-time of 1–2 hours GH induces glycogenolysis and gluconeogenesis in the liver, and inhibits glucose uptake by muscle and fat cells. Therefore, more glucose is provided to the brain and the heart. Simultaneously, GH stimulates lipolysis in the fat cells, providing free fatty acid to the heart and the active skeletal muscle. When exogenous GH is repeatedly applied to an otherwise healthy human (e.g. a body-builder), the ensuing hyperglycaemia evokes a compensatory hypersecretion of insulin. This leads to the exhaustion of beta cells in the pancreatic islets and diabetes mellitus develops.

Mode of action of GH

The action of GH begins with its binding to specific GH receptors, belonging to the superfamily of cytokine receptors. Upon binding their ligands on their extracellular domain a conformational change occurs in the whole receptor molecule. Due to this change, the cytosolic domain can then bind a cytosolic tyrosine, leading to a cascade of protein phosphorylation. There are probably several molecular pathways leading to the acute metabolic effects of GH; for example, intracellular translocation of a G-protein and a block in the action of activated insulin receptor. The long-term effects are due to the formation of somatomedins, a family of growth factors, tissue-specifically produced in GH target organs. These growth factors induce mitosis and, consequently cell proliferation, in the respective organ. The somatomedin produced by liver in response to GH is IGF-I, and its release from the liver raises IGF-I concentration in the plasma. This led to the general view that GH influences bone metabolism via hepatic IGF-I secretion. However, somatomedins are paracrine factors rather than hormones, and hence exert their effect where they are produced, probably at high concentration. Moreover, more than a single species of so-matomedins may be produced in response to GH in a given organ, and other hormones may also induce the production of somatomedins. In carti-lage GH induces the synthesis of basic fibroblast growth factor (bFGF), and in bone tissue it induces the synthesis of epidermal growth factor (EGF). IGF-I is also formed in the bone, in response to parathyroid hormone (PTH) and estradiol; howev-er, it is unclear as to whether GH can also induce this effect. The precise molecular mechanism for the hormonal control of bone growth remains to be clarified.

IGF-I is structurally related to insulin and, accordingly, it is capable of increasing glucose utilization and reducing lipid utilization. These effects are opposite to those of the acute, anti-in-sulin, actions of GH. However, both starvation (i.e. low blood glucose) and high cortisol (occurring during stress) inhibit GH-induced formation of IGF-I, which means that insulin-like effects develop in non-stressed, well-fed organisms only; hence, continuous starvation leads to the retarda-tion of body growth.

Control of GH secretion

The level of GH in the blood exhibits a pulsatile pattern. The integrated daily concentration of GH is high in childhood; sex steroids are claimed to re-sult in an increase in GH to maximal levels during puberty, whereas only about a quarter of this level is demonstrated in adults (Fig. 11.3). The secretion of GH is under hypothalamic control via **GHRH** and **somatostatin**, which stimulate and inhibit se-cretion, respectively. The secretion of GHRH and consequently, of GH, is increased during fasting, in stress, exercise and during stages 3 and 4 of sleep. Hypoglycaemia (Fig. 11.3) and high plasma amino acid concentrations, especially lysine and arginine, are efficient stimuli of GH secretion. The stimula-tory effect of fasting on GH secretion is also medi-ated by the gastrointestinal peptide hormone, ghrelin. The stimulatory effect of noradrenaline, acting at α_2 adrenergic receptors in the hypothala-mus, has been utilized in the treatment of some forms of dwarfism. In contrast, IGF-I, released from

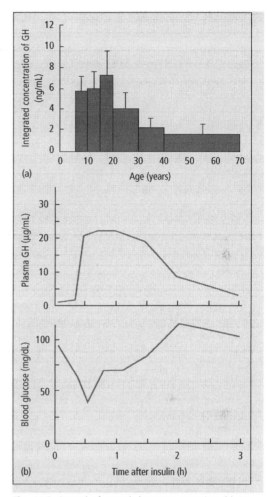

Fig. 11.3 Control of growth hormone secretion. (a) 24-hour integrated plasma concentration of GH as a function of age. (From Zadik, Z., Chalew, S.A., McCarter, R.J. Jr. *et al.* (1985) *J Clin Endocrinol Metab*, **60**, 513–16.) (b) Changes in plasma GH concentration in response to insulin-induced hy-poglycaemia. (From Roth, J., Glick, S.M., Yalow, R.S. & Berson S. (1963) *Science*, **140**, 987–8.)

the liver, stimulates the secretion of somatostatin from the hypothalamus, leading to reduced secre-tion of GH.

When insufficient secretion of GH leads to retarded growth or dwarfism, substitutional therapy may be applied before the epiphyseal clo-sure. In the case of hypothalamic insufficiency, treatment with either GHRH or GH may be effective in accelerating growth. Treatment with an α_2 adrenergic agonist may also be effective. In pituitary insufficiency GH should be administered. (GH can be produced using gene technological methods.) A defect in either GH or IGF-I receptors (e.g. as occurs in African pygmies) cannot currently be treated.

11.3 The hypothalamo–neurohypophyseal system

The posterior lobe of the pituitary, also termed the neurohypophysis, secretes two nonapeptide hormones, **AVP (identical with antidiuretic hormone, ADH)** and **oxytocin**, each with a molecular mass of approximately 1000. These hormones are synthesized in the hypothalamus in the cell bodies of large (magnocellular) neurones of the supraoptic and paraventricular nuclei. Each hormone is synthesized as part of a prohormone containing the corresponding **neurophysin** (oxytocin, neurophysin I; ADH, neurophysin II), and then packaged into granules. Neurophysin is cleaved from the hormone as the granules are transported down the axons to their terminals in the posterior pituitary, where they are stored prior to their release into the circulation. Release of each hormone, together with its corresponding neurophysin, is triggered by nerve impulses originating in the respective hypothalamic nuclei, in response to appropriate stimuli. No function for the released neurophysins has yet been reported. AVP is required for the formation of concentrated urine and is also a potent vasoconstrictor. Oxytocin contracts smooth muscle and plays an essential role in inducing the contraction of myometrium and milk ejection.

Vasopressin (AVP)

AVP controls the reabsorption of water by the kidneys and also constricts arterioles. In mammals, there are two types of AVP, which differ by a single amino acid—arginine (in humans; hence the abbreviation AVP) or lysine. AVP has a half-life of approximately 5 min in the plasma and is metabolized by the liver and kidneys.

Two types of receptor for AVP have been identified: V_1 receptors found in vascular smooth muscle and V_2 receptors found in the distal tubules and collecting ducts of the kidney. Binding of AVP to V_1 receptors induces a Ca^{2+} signal that triggers muscle contraction. Activation of V_2 receptors brings about increased cAMP formation.

AVP increases the **reabsorption of water** by the kidneys and so reduces the excretion of water from the body. It acts on the distal nephron, induces the translocation of water channels (**aquaporin**-2) into the luminal plasma membrane of the collecting tubules, thus increasing their permeability to water (p. 562). Water moves passively out of the nephrons along an osmotic gradient and so urine volume is decreased. AVP also promotes the reabsorption of urea from the lumen of the inner medullary collecting tubules. This is an important process in the formation of high interstitial osmotic concentration, required for water rebsorption. AVP is a potent **vasoconstrictor**. It acts on V_1 receptors in vascular smooth muscle to increase cytoplasmic Ca^{2+} via IP_3, and triggers muscle contraction. The vasoconstrictor effect of AVP is important in the maintenance of arterial pressure in hypotensive conditions, such as haemorrhage.

Consistent with the dual role for AVP, changes in osmotic concentration and blood pressure both influence its release. The strongest stimulus of AVP secretion is dehydration, characterized both by hyperosmosis and hypotension. Although the magnocellular neurones of the supraoptic nucleus of the hypothalamus also sense osmotic concentration, the osmoreceptors are found in the circumventricular organ (around the third ventricle). An increase of extracellular osmotic concentration by as little as 3 mOsm evokes depolarization of these neurones, which in turn connect synaptically to, and induce depolarization in, the AVP-producing hypothalamic neurones. In this way they trigger the release of the hormone from the neurohypophysis, where the axon terminals of the magnocellular neurones are located.

AVP is released in response to decreased stimulation of atrial stretch receptors, decreased stimulation of arterial baroreceptors, and increased release of angiotensin II. The hypotension- and/or hypo-volaemia-induced AVP secretion is especially important after blood loss when AVP contributes to the immediate maintenance of blood pressure via vasoconstrictor effects and, in the longer term, promotes the restoration of water balance by increasing renal water reabsorption. (The circumventricular osmoreceptors also induce thirst and drinking; this is essential in dehydration and after haemorrhage. The restoration of blood volume also requires increased aldosterone secretion, for retaining sodium, and erythropoietin, for increased formation of red blood cells.)

Pain, exercise and various stressors also stimulate AVP secretion. Alcohol is a powerful inhibitor of secretion, causing the well-known diuretic effect, even without increased additional fluid intake.

Diabetes insipidus

Damage to AVP-producing neurones in the hypothalamus may result in the condition known as **diabetes insipidus**, which is characterized by the voiding of large volumes of dilute urine (polyuria) and excessive thirst (polydipsia). This condition can be treated with synthetic AVP administered through skin patches. Diabetes insipidus may also arise from failure of the kidneys to respond to AVP. This latter form of the disease, termed nephrogenic diabetes insipidus, may be the consequence of a genetic defect in either the V_2 receptors or in aquaporin-2. Inappropriately high levels of AVP can also occur as a result of ectopic production of the peptide by a tumour.

Oxytocin

The synthesis and metabolism of the nonapeptide oxytocin are similar to those of AVP.

Oxytocin stimulates the myoepithelial cells of the mammary gland, causing **milk let-down**. Milk let-down is a reflex action in response to suckling at the breast. A neuroendocrine reflex pathway is involved, in which impulses initiated by suckling are relayed to the hypothalamo–pituitary axis, causing the release of oxytocin. In lactating women, a conditional reflex may also lead to oxy-tocin release and milk ejection when she sees another woman feeding her baby.

Oestrogen-stimulated myometrium contracts in response to oxytocin. Sexual intercourse occurring during the follicular phase of ovarian cycle evokes such **uterine contraction**, which may assist in the rapid passage of sperm into the uterine cavity. There is also a marked elevation of plasma oxytocin levels during parturition in response to stretching of the uterus and cervix, leading to uterine contraction. Oxytocin is used clinically for the induction of labour. There are no known disorders due to abnormal secretion of oxytocin.

11.4 The thyroid gland

The thyroid gland lies in front of the trachea just below the larynx and has a very rich blood supply. It is composed of many spherical follicles of about 50–500 μm diameter. Each follicle is composed of a single layer of epithelial cells surrounding a cavity in which the thyroid hormones are stored as integral components of the storage protein, **thyroglobulin**.

The main hormones secreted by the thyroid gland are iodinated derivatives of tyrosine, T_4 and T_3, collectively known as the thyroid hormones (Fig. 11.4). The thyroid gland also secretes the peptide hormone, **calcitonin**, which lowers plasma calcium concentrations and is discussed later (p. 258). Sufficient T_3 and T_4 is stored in the gland to last 2–3 months. There is approximately 50 times more T_4 than T_3 in the plasma. In the tissues, T_4 may be converted to T_3 or to reverse T_3 (3,3′,5′-tri-iodothyronine) by deiodination (Fig. 11.4). T_3 is the major hormone active in target cells; reverse T_3 is inactive.

The hormones T_4 and T_3 play an essential role in the control of gene expression. Through this action they influence growth and development, particularly of the nervous system, and control metabolic activity in the body. They are synthesized in the lumen of the thyroid follicle by iodination and coupling of tyrosine molecules attached to thyroglobulin, which is then taken up by the surrounding follicle cells and thyroid hormones are subsequently released into the circulation. The

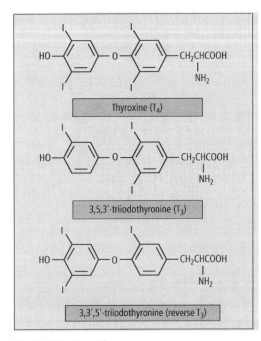

Fig. 11.4 The thyroid hormones.

synthesis and release of thyroid hormones are controlled by TSH, which in turn is controlled by TRH and by feedback inhibition of the thyroid hormones.

Thyroid hormone deficiency in the fetus and early childhood produces the condition of **cretinism**, which is characterized by a failure to grow and severe mental retardation. This condition is caused by failure of the thyroid gland to develop properly. A closely related condition associated with enlargement of the thyroid gland (**goitre**) may occur in regions where the content of iodine in the soil and water is low. This was not uncommon for example in the Alps; however here endemic cretinism and goitre have been prevented by the introduction of iodized salt. This type of thyroid deficiency rarely occurs in coastal regions because of the high iodine content of fish and other sea foods.

Synthesis and secretion of thyroid hormones

Iodide is taken up and accumulated by epithelial

cells lining the cavity, with secondary active transport, performed by both Na^+–I^- co-transporters and Na^+,K^+–ATPase (which removes Na^+ from the cell) (Fig. 11.5). Due to the activity of a specific nicotinamide adenine dinucleotide phosphate (NADPH) oxidase (called duox) and superoxide dismutase, hydrogen peroxide (H_2O_2) is formed which, utilizing thyroperoxidase, oxidizes iodide to atomic iodine; the iodine then immediately iodinates tyrosine residues contained in thyroglobulin (Fig. 11.5). Thyroglobulin is a large protein (M_r 670 000) which is synthesized in the follicle cells and secreted into the follicular cavity. The iodinated tyrosine residues in thyroglobulin undergo coupling to form T_4 and T_3. Iodination and coupling take place at the cell surface bordering the follicular cavity, and the thyroid hormones are stored in the cavity as integral amino acids in the thyroglobulin molecule.

The synthesis of the thyroid hormones can be blocked at several sites, as follows.

1 Iodide uptake is blocked by thiocyanate and perchlorate.

2 Oxidation of $I^- \rightarrow I + e$ is blocked by propylthiouracil and carbimazole.

3 Iodination of tyrosine molecules in thyroglobulin by atomic iodine is blocked by propylthiouracil and carbimazole.

4 Coupling of the two iodinated tyrosine residues to form T_4 or T_3 is inhibited by propylthiouracyl and carbimazole.

The **antithyroid** compounds, by reducing the negative feed back effect of T_4 on the hypothalamo–adenohypophyseal system, induce increased secretion of TSH which, in turn, stimulates cell proliferation of the thyroid tissue, leading to goitre. Of these **goitrogen** compounds, thiocyanate may be ingested with food, e.g. in cabbage and turnip; excessive consumption of these vegetables may hence cause goitre. Paradoxically, excess iodide also inhibits biosynthesis of the thyroid hormones. Pertechnetate competes with iodide for the Na^+–I^- co-transporter; the isotopic form of pertechnetate is applied in scintigraphy of the thyroid.

The first step in secretion is the uptake of small globules of colloid into the follicle cells by endocy-

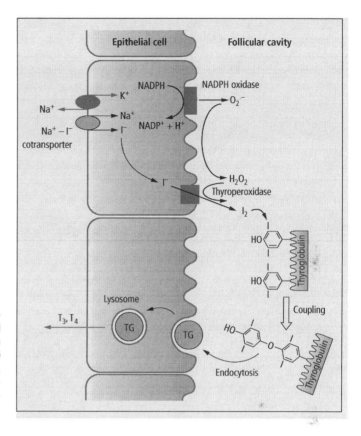

Fig. 11.5 Iodide transport and thyroxin synthesis. Synthesis of thyroid hormones (T$_3$, T$_4$), their storage in association with thyroglobulin (TG) and their secretion are shown. H$_2$O$_2$, hydrogen peroxide; NADP, nicotinamide adenine dinucleotide phosphate; NADPH, NADP reduced.

tosis. The globules then fuse with lysosomes and their contents are digested, thus liberating the thyroid hormones which diffuse out of the follicle cells into the blood.

Proteolytic degradation of thyroglobulin within the follicular cells causes the liberation of monoiodotyrosine (MIT) and di-iodotyrosine (DIT), as well as T$_3$ and T$_4$. A specific iodotyrosine deiodinase enzyme in the follicular cells allows the iodine to be removed from MIT and DIT (but not from T$_3$ and T$_4$) so that the iodine and the tyrosine can be recycled. This reaction is important for conserving supplies of iodine in the thyroid, and a genetic abnormality of the deiodinase can cause iodine deficiency because of loss of iodotyrosine in the urine.

Transport and inactivation of thyroid hormones

Most of the circulating T$_4$ is bound to plasma proteins, mainly to **thyroxin-binding globulin** (TBG) and, to a lesser extent, to prealbumin and albumin. T$_3$ is less firmly bound to plasma proteins than is T$_4$, which is reflected in the finding that, although the concentration of total T$_4$ in the plasma (about 100 nmol L^{-1}) is much higher than that of total T$_3$ (about 1.5 nmol L^{-1}), the concentrations of the free hormones are similar (about 0.04 nmol L^{-1} for T$_4$ and 0.02 nmol L^{-1} for T$_3$). Similar to other plasma proteins, the synthesis of TBG is under hormonal control. It is important for everyday medical practice (pregnancy and application of oral contraceptives) that oestrogens raise TSH concentration in the plasma, thus reducing the concentration of free thyroid hormones. This is compensated for by an increase in the secretion of TRH and TSH, and the ensuing enlargement of thyroid then ensures a normal level of free T_4; i.e. normal T_4 supply of the target cells.

The thyroid hormones are broken down in several tissues, particularly the liver and skeletal muscle. T_4 has a half-life of 7 days, T_3 about 1 day. Much of the iodide that is released is reclaimed, but about 500 µg of iodide is lost in the urine and faeces daily and must be replaced in the diet.

Actions of thyroid hormones

T_4 is a lipophylic molecule, it therefore diffuses easily into the target cells, where it is converted to T_3 and hence binds to nuclear receptors. Such binding modulates transcription of mRNA from a variety of genes coding for enzymes and structural proteins. The resulting change in protein synthesis has a lag time of several hours but the effect is long-lasting in that it may only attain its peak after several days and may not decay until after a week or later.

One of the principal effects of thyroid hormones is to stimulate oxidative metabolism and thereby increase the production of heat in warm-blooded animals, which occurs in all tissues of the body except the brain, lungs, spleen and sex organs. The **thermogenic effect** of T_4 is very strong in brown adipose tissue, which is present in newborn but absent in adult humans. A protein uncoupling mitochondrial oxidation and phosphorylation (uncoupling protein-1, UCP-1) seems to be responsible for this latter effect. The increase in basal metabolic rate produced by a single injection of T_4 begins after a latency of several hours and lasts several days. The basal metabolic rate may increase by as much as 100%, while after thyroidectomy it may fall by 50%. T_3 and T_4 may cause a slight increase in body temperature, but increased secretion of hormone does not occur in adult humans as part of an acute response to cold. However, the hormones may act in a permissive manner to allow other mechanisms, such as increased sympathetic activity, to accelerate production of heat. It appears that the action of thyroid hormones on oxidative metabolism is due, at least in part, to an increase in the synthesis of Na^+,K^+–ATPase, and hence in the activity of the Na^+–K^+ pump.

Thyroid hormones are essential for normal **growth** in childhood. In amphibia, the thyroid hormones act as a trigger for metamorphosis, and premature metamorphosis can be induced in tadpoles by feeding them pieces of thyroid gland. T_3 and T_4 appear to stimulate growth by a direct effect on tissues, but they also have a permissive effect on GH action.

The thyroid hormones are essential for normal myelination, dendritic arborization and formation of synapses in the **nervous system** in childhood. In the absence of early treatment with replacement thyroid hormones, then congenital thyroid insufficiency results in a severe retardation of neural and mental development, and may even lead to cretinism. In the adult, a deficiency of thyroid hormones may lead to a prolonged reflex time, listlessness, and blunting of intellect; conversely, excessive production can cause restlessness and hyperexcitability.

Excess production of thyroid hormones causes an increased cardiac stroke volume and tachycardia. These effects are partly a direct response to the thyroid hormones, which increase sensitivity to catecholamines, and are partly secondary to increased demands for oxygen associated with their thermogenic action. The thyroid hormones have less well-defined effects on carbohydrate and lipid metabolism, including the lowering of plasma cholesterol concentration. Hyperthyroidism may lead to wasting of skeletal muscle proteins and a negative nitrogen balance. The thyroid hormones also influence calcium metabolism, and demineralization of the skeleton is common in severe hyperthyroidism. Adequate secretion of hormones is also necessary for gonadal function and lactation.

Control of thyroid hormone secretion

For normal thyroid hormone secretion, there must be adequate intake of iodine in the diet. The immediate stimulus for the release of thyroid hormones is **TSH** secreted by the anterior pituitary. TSH acts through cAMP to stimulate every step in the production and secretion of T_3 and T_4. In addition, it controls the size of the gland; if the pituitary is removed, then thyroid atrophy occurs.

Secretion of TSH is stimulated by **TRH**, which is secreted by neurones in the hypothalamus and transported to the anterior pituitary in the hypophyseal portal vessels. The actions of TRH appear to be mediated by a rise in cytosolic Ca^{2+}, triggered by IP_3, although some of them are mimicked by cAMP. TSH secretion is also regulated by feedback inhibition of T_3 and T_4 on the anterior pituitary, where they may reduce the number of cell receptors for TRH. The thyroid hormones may also act at the level of the hypothalamus to affect the output of TRH.

Although the feedback control of TRH–TSH secretion is very effective and maintains a stable plasma concentration of the thyroid hormones, certain environmental stimuli enhance the activity of the TRH–TSH axis. Cold is an effective stimulus in newborns and in experimental animals, but not in adult humans, except for people living permanently under arctic conditions. Stress and starvation diminish the function of the thyroid gland.

Disorders of thyroid function

Hypothyroidism may result from disease of the pituitary or of the thyroid gland (**autoimmune thyroiditis** or **Hashimoto's disease**), or from severe deficiency of iodine in the diet. Severe hypothyroidism in the fetal period and early childhood results in impaired longitudinal growth; thus ossification is impaired and the development of teeth is abnormal. The characteristic altered body proportions (wide and flat nose, protruding tongue, potbelly), together with mental retardation, is termed **cretin dwarfism**. Substitution therapy begun at birth can prevent the development of these symptoms; a few months later the somatic but not the mental damage can be prevented.

Severe hypothyroidism in the adult is called **myxoedema** because of the puffiness of the hands and face due to an abnormal accumulation of mucoproteins in the subcutaneous layers. Other signs are low metabolic rate, bradycardia, cold intolerance, mental and physical lethargy and slow, hoarse speech.

Hyperthyroidism results from the overproduction of thyroid hormones and is characterized by a high metabolic rate, tachycardia, heat intolerance, hyperexcitability, restlessness and weight loss. A common form of hyperthyroidism is **Graves' disease** which is also characterized by protruding eyeballs (exophthalmos) and goitre. Graves' disease is caused by abnormal thyroid stimulators in the blood. Long-acting thyroid stimulator was the first of these to be discovered, and it is now clear that this is one of a group of autoantibodies, called **thyroid-stimulating antibodies**, responsible for this condition.

Goitre is often associated with hyperthyroidism. However, it may also be a manifestation of hypothyroidism in which there is a compensatory increase in TSH secretion, as occurs within iodine deficiency (endemic goitre) or in diseases of the thyroid gland which result in defective T_3/T_4 synthesis or secretion. In the diagnosis of disorders of thyroid function the physician is guided by estimates of plasma levels of free T_3 and T_4 and of TSH, by measuring the response to test doses of TRH, or by the pattern of thyroid uptake of radioactive iodine measured externally. Radioactive technetium, given as the pertechnetate, is now commonly used instead of radioactive iodine for imaging of the thyroid gland.

11.5 The parathyroid glands and calcium metabolism

PTH and the vitamin D-derived calcitriol and calcitonin are termed **calciotropic** hormones. Parathyroid glands on the dorsal surface of the lobes of the thyroid gland secrete PTH, which raises plasma calcium and lowers plasma phosphate concentration. Calcitriol, produced by the kidney, stimulates calcium and phosphate absorption in the gut and promotes bone mineralization. The parafollicular or C-cells of the thyroid gland secrete calcitonin, which lowers the plasma calcium concentration.

The calciotropic hormones have also actions independent from calcium and bone metabolism. GH, cortisol and sexual steroids also influence bone metabolism; their effect and role is discussed in relation to the respective endocrine gland.

Calcium metabolism

Calcium has a number of essential physiological functions in the body. In addition to its vital role as a second messenger in all cells, it has several extracellular actions, including the control of excitability of nerve and muscle, and formation of bone. Approximately 99% of body calcium and 80% of body phosphorus is found in bone. The concentration of calcium in plasma is about 2.4 mmol L^{-1} (range 2.1–2.6 mmol L^{-1}), of which about 1.2 mmol L^{-1} is ionized, about 1.1 mmol L^{-1} is bound to protein and a small amount is present as complexes with anions, such as citrate, bicarbonate or phosphate. Phosphorus occurs in plasma within a number of organic constituents, including lipids and nucleotides, and is also present as

inorganic phosphate at a concentration of about 1 mmol L^{-1}. The solubility product of calcium and phosphate is such that the product of the concentrations of the free ions is low and remains relatively constant.

On a typical diet, about 25 mmol (1 g) of calcium is ingested daily, but individuals vary greatly in their intake. Most of this calcium is in the form of calcium phosphate derived especially from milk and other dairy products. There is abundant phosphorus in the diet to meet daily needs. For calcium balance to be maintained, an intake of 12.5–20 mmol day^{-1} is recommended for infants and adults. A higher daily intake (25–37.5 mmol day^{-1}) is recommended for rapidly growing adolescents and for women during pregnancy and lactation, and after the menopause. Net intestinal absorption of dietary calcium depends heavily upon nutritional needs and vitamin D (calcitriol) effects, and is influenced by faecal losses of calcium in intestinal secretions (Fig. 11.6). Intestinal absorption occurs mainly in the duodenum by active transport; this transport cannot be enhanced by increased

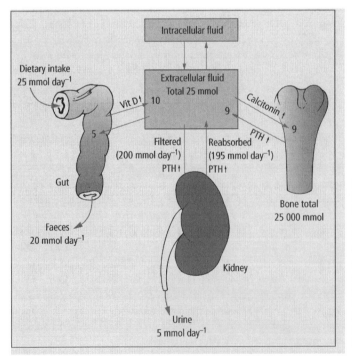

Fig. 11.6 Calcium balance in the body and its regulation by parathyroid hormone (PTH), calcitonin and vitamin D. The plasma Ca^{2+} concentration in young men was increased or decreased by infusion of calcium gluconate and the calcium chelator ethylenediamine tetra-acetic acid (EDTA), respectively. Means ± S.E.M. are shown. (Modified from Portale, A.A., Lonergan, E.T., Tanney, D.M. & Halloran, B.P. (1997) *Amer J Physiol*, **272**, E139–E146.)

calcium intake, but it is stimulated by calcitriol. Some concentration-dependent passive absorption of calcium occurs throughout the small intestine; this absorption is not hormonally controlled. Urinary excretion is also important in regulating calcium homeostasis and PTH increases calcium reabsorption in the distal nephron. Due to these hormonal effects, under normal conditions calcium intake equals urinary and faecal calcium loss. There is also steady-state exchange of Ca^{2+} between the interstitial fluid and the bone, as detailed below. When calcium intake is less than calcium loss, as may occur in lactating women, calcium is withdrawn from the bones and the bone mass decreases.

Bone

Bone is composed of an organic matrix of collagen in a ground substance consisting largely of mucopolysaccharides and non-collagen proteins (including thrombospondin, osteocalcin, osteonectin and proteoglycans), within which crystals of a complex salt of calcium and phosphate very similar to hydroxyapatite $(Ca_{10}(PO_4)_6(OH)_2)$ are deposited. A more amorphous form of calcium phosphate is also present, as well as small amounts of Na, Mg, Cl and F. The main protein of bone matrix is collagen (type I); this is responsible for providing the bone with mechanical strength, and presents a binding surface for inorganic salt crystals. Newly formed bone matrix, termed osteoid tissue, is unmineralized. At the local pH in osteoid tissue, calcium and phosphate ions are present in a supersaturated solution due to the solubilizing effect of pyrophosphate, which is also present. An increase in calcium or phosphate ion concentration or decrease in pyrophosphate concentration triggers the precipitation of hydroxyapatite crystals on the surface of collagen; this process is completed several days after the formation of osteoid tissue. Mineralization requires calcitriol, and the lack of its parent compound — vitamin D — results in insufficient mechanical strength, as is seen in **rickets** in childhood and **osteomalacia** in adults.

Three types of cells appear to function in the formation and resorption of bone, namely osteoblasts, osteoclasts and osteocytes. The **osteoblasts** synthesize and secrete collagen fibres and promote the deposition of calcium phosphate crystals. **Osteoclasts**, which are specialized macrophages, cause resorption of bone. Bone resorption depends on the destruction of collagen by lysosomal enzymes and phagocytosis, and on the dissolution of bone mineral by an increase in lactate and citrate production. **Osteocytes** are the most numerous cells in mature bone and are formed from osteoblasts, once surrounded by calcified matrix. Osteocytes have long cytoplasmic processes that make contact with their neighbouring osteoblasts by tight junctions. Osteocytes sense mechanical forces imposed on the bone, specifically mechanical distortion, which initiates bone remodelling. Osteocytes play an essential role in the exchange of calcium between extracellular fluid and bone. This role depends upon the activity of PTH, calcitriol and calcitonin. Only about 1% of the calcium and phosphate of bone is in equilibrium with the extracellular fluid through the activity of osteocytes — the so-called exchangeable pool of bone mineral which acts to buffer short-term changes in blood calcium ion concentration. The remaining 99% comprises the non-exchangeable pool, from which the mineral can be released only by osteoclastic resorption, as occurs in normal remodelling or in certain disease states.

Osteoblasts also send signals to the osteolytic osteoclast cells via direct cell-cell contacts, or via paracrine mediators; these signals are required for the full differentiation and activity of osteoclasts. Two membrane-bound and one soluble protein(s), which are essential for this intercellular signalling, have recently been identified. In this process, the membrane receptor **RANK** (abbreviation for receptor activator of nuclear factor κB) on osteoclasts binds to **RANK ligand** (RANKL) (also termed **osteoclast differentiation factor**) on the surface of osteoblasts. This contact or binding of released RANKL promotes osteoclast activation. However, if a soluble product of osteoblasts and other cell types (e.g. bone stromal cells, monocytes, endothelial cells), termed **osteoprotegerin** (OPG), is also present, it competes with RANK (on osteoclasts) for binding to RANK ligand on osteoblasts.

In this way, soluble OPG inhibits osteoclast activity and the resulting osteolysis (Fig. 11.7).

Bone formation and resorption form a continuous cycle and, under steady-state conditions, the two processes are in equilibrium. The overall process, termed **remodelling** of bone, is influenced by many hormones. If bone resorption exceeds bone formation, **osteoporosis**, a widespread, disabling disease of the elderly occurs; whereas excess bone formation over bone resorption results in **osteopetrosis**. PTH and calcitriol, as well as several paracrine factors (among them several interleukins), up-regulate osteoclast differentiation factor (RANKL) on the osteoblast cell membrane, thereby promoting osteolysis. Glucocorticoid excess, occurring in Cushing syndrome or during long-term therapeutic administration of synthetic glucocorticoids, also favours bone resorption. Osteoporosis developing under such conditions is due to suppressed formation of soluble OPG and increased expression of RANKL. On the other hand, oestrogens inhibit the secretion of osteoclast-activating cytokine production by osteoblasts, and also OPG synthesis, therefore conserving bone mass (Fig. 11.7). The lack of oestrogens in postmenopausal women (and also in elderly men) is responsible for the high frequency of osteoporosis in these groups. Any dysregulation of RANK, RANKL or OPG expression leads to pathological alterations in bone metabolism. In this respect, the discovery of the OPG/RANK/RANKL triad presents novel therapeutic opportunities for diseases characterized by excessive bone resorption.

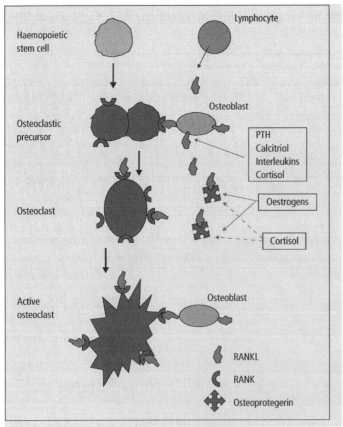

Fig. 11.7 Hormonal control of the differentiation and activation of osteoclasts. Stimulatory hormonal effects are shown by a solid blue arrow, inhibitory effects are shown by a dashed blue arrow. PTH, parathyroid hormone; RANK, receptor activator of nuclear factor κB; RANKL, RANK ligand.

Vitamin D

Vitamin D is essential for proper bone development, and a deficiency of this vitamin in children causes **rickets**, a disorder characterized by stunted growth and bowing of the limbs due to failure of mineralization of bone. In adults, vitamin D deficiency can cause a failure in bone mineralization (**osteomalacia**). Vitamin D is a lipid-soluble, steroid-like compound, existing in two forms. One is vitamin D_2 (ergocalciferol), a derivative of the plant sterol ergosterol, found in a limited number of plant foods. The other form, vitamin D_3 (cholecalciferol) can be found in milk and dairy products, but it is mainly produced in the skin. It derives from 7-dehydrocholesterol in response to UV light. As the two forms of vitamin D are equally active, the generic term vitamin D will be used when referring to either. Vitamin D deficiency occurs when the food is deficient in vitamin D and the body is not exposed to sun (or arteficial UV) light. Cod liver oil is the richest food source of provitamin D.

Conversion to calcitriol

Vitamin D is converted to the hormone **calcitriol** which controls calcium and phosphorus metabolism. It is first converted to a 25-hydroxyvitamin D in the liver, and the rate of this conversion depends on vitamin D supply only. Then, in the kidney, this intermediary compound is converted to 1,25-dihydroxyvitamin D (calcitriol), if extracellular concentrations of calcium or phosphate are low (Fig. 11.8). The renal enzyme 1α-hydroxylase, which catalyses this conversion, is stimulated by PTH and low plasma phosphate; a direct negative feedback is the repression of the renal 1α-hydroxylase gene by calcitriol. A protective mechanism against vitamin D overdose is provided by the renal enzyme 24-hydroxylase: if the concentrations of calcium and phosphate are normal, most of the vitamin is transformed in the kidney to the 24,25-hydroxy and 1,24,25-trihydroxy derivatives which are inactive.

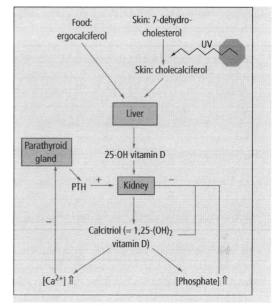

Fig. 11.8 Control of the metabolism of vitamin D.

Actions of calcitriol

Calcitriol acts on the **small intestine** to promote the **absorption of calcium and phosphate,** which are necessary for bone formation, and it facilitates bone mineralization by increasing the extracellular fluid concentration of calcium and phosphate. It has also been shown, together with PTH, to have the reverse effect on bone mineralization *in vitro*, causing release of these ions from bone. This action may be important in bone remodelling. Calcitriol has receptors in the nucleus. The action of calcitriol–receptor complex on gene expression in bone leads to the synthesis of the matrix proteins osteocalcin and osteopontin in the osteoblasts; calcitriol also induces the expression of RANKL in osteoblasts. In the intestine it increases the synthesis of a calcium-binding protein, which may promote calcium absorption. It can also reduce PTH synthesis by directly inhibiting expression of the PTH gene.

Parathyroid hormone

Four **parathyroid glands** are usually found

embedded in the thyroid gland. PTH, an 84-amino acid polypeptide (M_r 9500) is secreted by the 'chief' cells of the parathyroid glands. This circulating hormone is then rapidly metabolized in the liver and the kidney. Removal of the parathyroid glands causes plasma calcium levels to fall and leads to **hypocalcaemic tetany**. This is characterized by extensive spasms of skeletal muscle and can lead to asphyxiation due to laryngeal spasm.

Actions of parathyroid hormone

PTH **increases ionized plasma calcium** and **lowers plasma phosphate** concentration. It acts on bone, the kidney and, indirectly, on the gastrointestinal tract; its actions on bone and kidney are mediated by cAMP. PTH increases the rate of bone resorption by stimulating the activity of osteocytes and osteoclasts. Within a lag-time of 2–3 hours PTH increases the permeability of osteocytes, enabling their Ca^{2+} uptake from the bone interstitial fluid and the subsequent release of Ca^{2+} towards the capillaries. A slower-developing but more striking effect of PTH is the induction of RANKL with the ensuing increase in the number of active osteoclasts. The osteoclasts acidify their microenvironment, bringing about the dissolution of hydroxyapatite crystals of the matrix. The released Ca^{2+} and phosphate will traverse the osteocytes and enter the capillaries. The actions of PTH on the kidney are more important in compensating for short-term changes. In the kidney, PTH **decreases** the reabsorption of phosphate in the proximal tubule. Phosphate ions bind Ca^{2+}, and therefore the ensuing fall in plasma phosphate concentration will increase the ionized fraction of plasma Ca^{2+}. PTH also **increases** the reabsorption of calcium in the distal tubule. An indirect but significant effect of PTH on calcium metabolism is the induction of 1α-hydroxylase activity in the kidney (see above). Thus, the absorption of calcium in the gastrointestinal tract is increased as a consequence of an increase in calcitriol. In the long-term, increased secretion of PTH may result in a net loss of calcium from the body through the kidney. Under these conditions, the increase in ionized plasma calcium increases the filtered load by an amount that exceeds the additional calcium reabsorbed in the tubules.

Control of parathyroid hormone secretion

PTH secretion is regulated by plasma calcium acting on the parathyroid glands. The chief cells of the parathyroid gland express a Ca^{2+}-binding receptor, termed 'Ca^{2+}-sensing receptor', on their plasma membrane. These receptors belong to the superfamily of 7-transmembrane domain, G-protein-coupled receptors. They have an exceptionally long extracellular N-terminus, which serves as a Ca^{2+} binding site. Ca^{2+} binding activates G_q, and the resulting Ca^{2+} signal reduces PTH secretion. So PTH secretion varies inversely with the level of ionized calcium in the plasma, in the range of 1.1 to 1.3 mmol L^{-1} (Fig. 11.9). Calcitriol, the formation of which is also enhanced by PTH, also inhibits PTH secretion (Fig. 11.10). This is an additional negative feedback mechanism that has a lag-time of several hours, in contrast to the immediate inhibitory effect of Ca^{2+}.

Calcitonin

Calcitonin is a polypeptide (M_r 3500) secreted by the parafollicular or C-cells of the **thyroid gland**. The C-cells have calcium-sensing receptors, similar to the chief cells of the parathyroid gland. However, whereas binding of Ca^{2+} to such receptors inhibits PTH secretion in the parathyroid gland, it stimulates calcitonin secretion by C-cells. Calcitonin decreases plasma calcium and phosphate

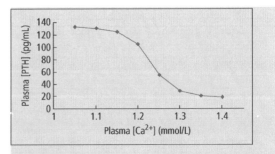

Fig. 11.9 Function of parathyroid hormone (PTH) in maintaining plasma ionized calcium concentration.

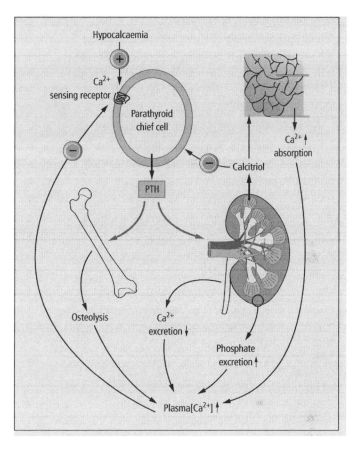

Fig. 11.10 Control of parathyroid hormone (PTH) secretion and actions.

levels by inhibiting bone resorption. Calcitonin is probably the only hormone directly acting on osteoclasts—it inhibits their function. It also increases the urinary loss of calcium and phosphate by decreasing their reabsorption in the kidney. The release of calcitonin is stimulated by an increase in plasma calcium (Fig. 11.10). Removal of the thyroid gland does not cause hypercalcaemia in humans, whereas hypocalcaemia regularly follows removal of the parathyroid glands. Therefore, the physiological significance of calcitonin has not yet been generally accepted. Cancer of the parafollicular cells (medullary thyroid carcinoma) may be associated with extremely high calcitonin levels, yet, plasma [Ca^{2+}] is normal. Although this finding may be accounted for by down-regulation of calcitonin receptors, it also challenges the significance of calcitonin in human endocrinology. Calcitonin is used clinically in the treatment of

Paget's disease to reduce the accelerated rate of bone turnover.

Disorders of calcium metabolism

Hypocalcaemia causes excessive neuromuscular irritability. A rapid decrease of ionized plasma calcium to below 1 mmol L^{-1} results in spontaneous firing of peripheral nerves. On the afferent side, this causes unusual sensations such as tingling (paraesthesia); on the efferent side, muscular twitching, spasm and cramps can develop, causing **manifest tetany**. If ionized calcium decreases more slowly or to a lesser extent, then stimuli such as localized ischaemia, hyperventilation or pressure over a nerve may be required to elicit the motor events. This is termed **latent tetany**. A low ionized plasma calcium may be consequent upon decreased levels of PTH or calcitriol in the body. It may also result from increased plasma pH, e.g. in respiratory alkalosis, due to the release of hydrogen ions from plasma proteins making additional negatively charged binding sites available for calcium. Tetany may also occur when ionized magnesium concentration in plasma is reduced, and in metabolic alkalosis associated with potassium depletion.

Osteomalacia, due to a deficiency of calcitriol, is characterized by a normal bone mass but the newly synthesized matrix fails to calcify. In **osteoporosis**, the bone is normally calcified but bone mass is decreased to a greater degree than in **osteopenia** which accompanies ageing. Oestrogen deficiency leads to osteoporosis, which most commonly occurs in women after the menopause. Genetic susceptibility to osteoporosis has been shown to be linked to variation in the structure of the calcitriol-receptor protein. Osteoporosis also occurs with prolonged immobilization and with excess glucocorticoid secretion or administration.

Hypercalcaemia is seen most frequently in hyperparathyroidism. A common cause of hypercalcaemia is the secretion of **PTH-related peptide**, which is produced by a wide variety of tumours. Increased calcium mobilization from bone leads to painful softening and hence fractures of bones, and the increased calcium and phosphate excretion in urine may result in nephrocalcinosis and renal stones. Increased plasma calcium may also cause headaches and decreased tone (hypotonia) in skeletal and intestinal muscle.

11.6 The adrenal medulla

There are two adrenal glands, situated one on top of each kidney. Each adrenal gland comprises two endocrine organs—the adrenal medulla and the adrenal cortex. The two parts of the adrenal gland have different embryonic origins and are anatomically quite distinct. The adrenal medulla secretes **catecholamines** while the adrenal cortex secretes a number of **steroid hormones**.

The chromaffin cells of the adrenal medulla secrete the catecholamines, adrenaline and noradrenaline. These hormones are released by splanchnic nerve stimulation in response to emergencies. They circulate in the blood stream and complement the noradrenaline released locally in tissues. Their actions are numerous and include the stimulation of heart rate and contractility, inhibition of gut motility, bronchodilation, and the stimulation of glycogenolysis.

The medulla is a modified nervous tissue derived from the neural crest, and can be regarded as a collection of postganglionic sympathetic neurones in which the axons have not developed. Catecholamines are produced in chromaffin cells of which there are two types, one secreting **adrenaline** (epinephrine) and the other **noradrenaline** (norepinephrine). In humans, adrenaline constitutes about 80% of the catecholamines produced by the medulla under resting conditions. Small collections of chromaffin cells are also located outside the adrenal medulla, usually adjacent to the chain of sympathetic ganglia. The organization of the blood supply of the adrenal gland is such that the medulla receives blood from the cortex rich in corticosteroids, which enhances the synthesis of the enzyme that converts noradrenaline to adrenaline. In addition to catecholamines, the chromaffin cells also secrete enkephalins, dynorphins, neurotensin, somatostatin and substance P. The role of these adrenal peptides has not yet been elucidated.

Catecholamines are synthetized from tyrosine (p. 240). They are stored in membrane-bound granules and their secretion is initiated by acetylcholine released from **sympathetic fibres** that travel in the splanchnic nerves. The catecholamines have only a short half-life in the blood stream (minutes). They are rapidly taken up into extraneuronal tissues to be degraded by catechol-*O*-methyltransferase, or into nerve terminals to be recycled or degraded by monoamine oxidase. The degradation products eventually appear in the urine.

Actions of catecholamines

The actions of adrenaline and noradrenaline are complex and depend on their binding to various adrenoceptors. Both bind to α and β adrenoceptors, but their affinities differ according to the type of adrenoreceptor and its subclass (p. 390). Noradrenaline causes widespread vasoconstriction and a marked increase in peripheral resistance, while adrenaline causes vasoconstriction in skin and viscera but vasodilation in skeletal muscles, so that total peripheral resistance may decrease. Both catecholamines increase heart rate and contractility directly, but overall the increase in peripheral resistance and mean arterial pressure caused by noradrenaline administration leads to reflex bradycardia. Catecholamines have pronounced effects on metabolic processes and increase basal metabolic rate, stimulate glycogenolysis and mobilize free fatty acids. They also cause bronchodilation (particularly adrenaline) and relaxation of the gastrointestinal tract.

Control of catecholamine secretion

The secretion of catecholamines is initiated by sympathetic activity controlled by the hypothalamus and occurs in response to such stimuli as pain, excitement, anxiety, hypoglycaemia, cold and haemorrhage. Increased secretion is part of the 'fight or flight' reaction described by Cannon in 1921. In an emergency, catecholamines released by the adrenal medulla are disseminated in the blood stream while noradrenaline is also released from sympathetic nerve terminals locally. In frightened or stressed animals, there is a general increase in sympathetic activity in which the sympathetic nerves appear to play the dominant role, as removal of the adrenal medulla does not seriously impair an animal's ability to cope with stress.

Tumours of chromaffin cells called **phaeochromocytomas** can secrete catecholamines in excess. This may cause hypertension (noradrenaline) or hyperglycaemia (adrenaline).

11. 7 Adrenal cortex

The adrenal cortex secretes glucocorticoids (cortisol and corticosterone), which affect the metabolism of carbohydrates, fats and proteins and are important in mediating the response of the body to fasting and stress, mineralocorticoids (mainly aldosterone), which are essential for the maintenance of sodium balance and consequently extracellular fluid volume, and androgens, which play a role in sexual maturation and participate in the control of protein metabolism. The secretion of glucocorticoids and androgens is controlled by ACTH, while that of aldosterone is controlled mainly by the renin–angiotensin system.

The cortex is organized into three zones—the outer **zona glomerulosa** which secretes **aldosterone**, the middle **zona fasciculata** which secretes **glucocorticoids** and the inner **zona reticularis** which secretes **glucocorticoids** and **androgens**. During fetal life, the cortex has a large inner fetal zone which produces precursor steroids for the synthesis of oestrogens by the placenta.

The adrenocortical steroids have the same basic structure as other steroids—the glucocorticoids and aldosterone contain 21 carbon atoms, and the androgens 19 (Fig. 11.11). They are derived from cholesterol, which may be synthesized directly by the adrenocortical cells or taken up from low-density lipoproteins in the circulation and stored as cholesterol esters in lipid droplets in the cytoplasm. Cholesterol is released from the lipid droplets by the action of cholesterol esterase which is stimulated by ACTH or angiotensin II. It is then converted to pregnenolone in the mitochondria. This step, which is also regulated by ACTH or angiotensin II, is the rate-limiting step in steroid biosynthesis. The actions of ACTH appear to be mediated by cAMP, and those of angiotensin II by Ca^{2+}. Pregnenolone is then transferred to the smooth endoplasmic reticulum. It undergoes further modifications here and in the mitochondria to form the three main classes of steroids (Fig. 11.11).

The steroid hormone produced depends on which hydroxylases and other enzymes are expressed in the tissue concerned. For example, formation of cortisol requires 17-hydroxylation of pregnenolone to 17-hydroxypregnenolone, or of progesterone to 17-hydroxyprogesterone. 17-hydroxylation takes place in the zonae fasciculata and reticularis, but the respective enzyme is not expressed in the zona glomerulosa. Conversely, aldosterone synthase, converting

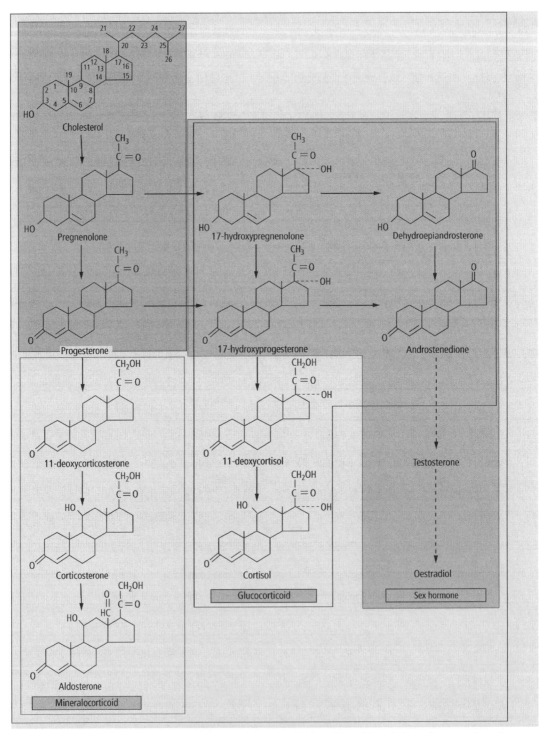

Fig. 11.11 Synthetic pathways for steroid hormones. The steps occurring in each steroid-producing cell type are shown in the grey-tinted area; those occurring in the zona glomerulosa only are shown in the blue frame; the steps confined to the deep adrenocortical zones (fasciculata and reticularis cells) are shown in the black frame; and the steps specific to gonads are shown in the blue-tinted area.

11-deoxycorticosterone (DOC) to aldosterone (via corticosterone), occurs in glomerulosa cells only. These steps require NADPH and O_2. There is no appreciable storage of these hormones in the adrenal cortex and the rate of release corresponds to the rate of synthesis. In humans, approximately 20 mg of cortisol and 0.2 mg of aldosterone are secreted per day. (No cortisol is produced in the rodent adrenal; the rodents' glucocorticoid hormone is corticosterone, produced mainly by fasciculata cells.) The adrenal cortex also secretes significant amounts of androgens, particularly dehydroepiandrosterone and androstenedione. Although these are only weakly androgenic but, due to their high concentration, their activity has biological significance at the onset of puberty (so-called **adrenarche**, preceding the maturation of the gonads) and in women.

The corticosteroids are transported in the circulation mostly bound to the plasma protein **corticosteroid-binding globulin (transcortin)**. Aldosterone has no specific binding protein and is found loosely bound to albumin. About 90% of cortisol and 60% of aldosterone exists in the bound form, which acts as a reserve and protects the steroids from degradation. The half-life of cortisol is about 1 h, whereas that of aldosterone is about 20 min. Inactivation of the steroid hormones by reduction to tetrahydro derivatives, or conjugation with glucuronic acid or sulphate, occurs in the liver and the kidney and these metabolites are excreted in the urine and bile.

Glucocorticoids

Cortisol is the main glucocorticoid in humans; corticosterone has a slight additional effect. Glucocorticoids play an important role in the control of the intermediary metabolism of carbohydrate, fat and protein throughout the body. Their mode of action is the regulation of the synthesis of specific enzymes. In many instances these enzymes are key regulators of metabolic functions or are required to mediate the actions of other hormones, such as adrenaline, glucagon and GH. Hence they are said to have a 'permissive' action on the effects of other hormones.

In the normal state glucocorticoids promote **glycogen storage** in the liver by stimulating the synthesis of the glycogenetic enzymes (pyruvate carboxylase, phosphoenolpyruvate carboxykinase and diphosphofructophosphatase). These are the enzymes activated (via cAMP-dependent phosphorylation) by the glucose-mobilizing hormones glucagon and adrenalin; therefore cortisol plays a permissive role in the action of these hormones. During fasting they stimulate **gluconeogenesis** in the liver to provide glucose for brain metabolism. The main substrates for gluconeogenesis are amino acids derived from **protein catabolism** in skeletal muscle. Glucocorticoids also stimulate this process, and excess production (or administration) of these hormones causes severe muscle wasting. Protein synthesis (except for specific, mostly intracellular proteins) is also inhibited. The inhibition of collagen synthesis retards wound healing, an effect often neglected during administration of glucocorticoid-containing ointments. The glucocorticoids also have a counter-regulatory effect on insulin, in that they **raise blood glucose** effectively by inhibiting glucose uptake in muscle and adipose tissue. They also enhance **fatty acid mobilization** from adipose tissue by potentiating the lipolytic effects of catecholamines, glucagon and GH.

Glucocorticoids are essential for the maintenance of normal **myocardial contractility** and **vascular resistance**. Their action is a permissive one in that they potentiate the expression of β_1 adrenergic receptors in the heart and α_1 adrenergic receptors in vascular smooth muscle.

Glucocorticoid is required for surfactant production in the lung. A defect in surfactant production, due to insufficient cortisol secretion in the **premature newborn**, leads to condition known as **respiratory distress syndrome**. Glucocorticoids present at pathological (Cushing's syndrome) or therapeutic concentrations lead to **osteoporosis**; the reduction in bone mass results from an induction of osteoblast apoptosis, depressed collagen synthesis in bone and reduced calcium absorption from the gut.

Glucocorticoids exert a very small mineralocorticoid effect, increasing sodium reabsorption and potassium excretion in the kidney. Considering, however, that the concentration of cortisol in the human plasma is three orders of magnitude higher than that of aldosterone, the mineralocorticoid effect of cortisol is not negligible and becomes significant in cases of excessive secretion of cortisol, typically observed in Cushing's syndrome. Cortisol is required for normal glomerular filtration, and a lack of cortisol results in renal insufficiency.

Stress

Stress is the non-specific response of the organism to any effect (termed stressor) that **endangers** the integrity of the organism. Painful stimuli, blood loss, hypoxia, bacterial infection, hypoglycaemia, extreme cold, trauma, seeing or hearing a predator enemy, as well as negative social factors, all act as stressors. As originally observed by Selye shortly before World War II, such states are associated with increased activity of the adrenal cortex, and atrophy of the thymus and lymphatic tissues; adrenalectomy may be fatal under such circumstances. Common to all these situations is the increase in cortisol secretion seen. The adrenocortical response in stress occurs simultaneously with Canon's **alarm reaction**—the catecholamine secretory response of the adrenal medulla to factors endangering the organism. Both the adrenocortical and adrenomedullary response are initiated in the hypothalamus.

Cortisol is required for the expression of adrenergic and angiotensin II receptors in the cardiovascular system, thus it exerts a permissive role in the cardiovascular response to hypotension and/or hypovolaemia. Similarly, cortisol-induced enzyme synthesis in the liver and adipose tissue is required for the development of the hyperglycaemic and lipolytic effect, respectively, of adrenalin, glucagon and GH. Increased plasma level of cortisol will be responsible for the inhibition of glucose uptake by the non-vital peripheral tissues (e.g. muscle and fat).

In large doses, the glucocorticoids **suppress the immune response**. They decrease the number of circulating lymphocytes and eosinophils, cause in-volution of the thymus and lymph nodes, and may depress the antibody response. They inhibit the synthesis or antagonize the action of several inflammatory cytokines (e.g. prostaglandins, leukotrienes, histamine, nitric oxide) and prevent the release of proteolytic enzymes from the lysosomes. In addition to suppressing extreme immunological (e.g. anaphylactic) reactions, corticol also suppresses the hypersecretion of other hormones (e.g. AVP), thus preventing the often fatal side-effects of several defence responses. Synthetic corticosteroids are widely used therapeutically to suppress rejection of transplanted organs and to treat allergies. They also have **anti-inflammatory** properties and are used in the treatment of rheumatoid arthritis and related diseases.

Control of glucocorticoid secretion

The secretion of cortisol and corticosterone (and androgens) is controlled by **ACTH** produced by the anterior pituitary. The secretion of ACTH is regulated by hypothalamic secretion of **CRH** and **AVP** into the hypophyseal–portal system. In this instance, the AVP is secreted by the same cells (**parvocellular** neurones of the paraventricular nucleus) as those that release CRH, which are distinct from the AVP-secreting, **magnocellular** cells that project to the posterior pituitary. CRH and AVP are released in response to neural or humoral inputs to the hypothalamus, informing this neural centre of any effect endangering the integrity of the organism. Cortisol and synthetic glucocorticoids exert a negative-feedback effect on the hypothalamus and on the pituitary. The concentration of plasma cortisol follows a diurnal pattern, peak levels occurring in the morning just before waking.

Mineralocorticoids

Aldosterone is the main mineralocorticoid produced by the adrenal cortex. It acts on epithelial cells, chiefly on the distal tubules of the **kidney** to promote the **reabsorption of Na$^+$ in exchange for K$^+$ and H$^+$**, which are excreted. Excess production of aldosterone in conjunction with Na$^+$ retention leads to expansion of the extracellular fluid volume and hence hypertension, hypokalaemia and alkalosis. Adrenalectomy leads to a fall in extracellular Na^+, hypotension and eventually death. Recent observations indicate that aldosterone, produced within the heart under pathological conditions, is responsible for the development of cardiac fibrosis.

Control of mineralocorticoid secretion

ACTH is not the major regulator of aldosterone secretion, in contrast to the other corticosteroids, but it does play a supportive role. The primary regulators of aldosterone secretion are angiotensin II produced by the renin–angiotensin system and extracellular K^+.

Disorders of adrenocortical function

In **Addison's disease** there is deficient secretion of all adrenocortical hormones, commonly due to autoimmune destruction of the gland. This disease usually develops slowly and is characterized by lethargy, weakness, weight loss and hypotension. Dehydration, circulatory failure and metabolic disturbances may all lead to death (Fig. 11.12). Sudden stress can precipitate a crisis requiring emergency medical treatment. A common feature of this disease is hyperpigmentation of the skin due to excessive secretion of ACTH, leading to stimulation of melanocyte activity in the skin. The elevation of ACTH concentration is brought about by removal of the negative feedback provided by cortisol. Patients with Addison's disease require replacement therapy with both a glucocorticoid and a mineralocorticoid. Haemorrhage of the adrenal gland may acutely lead to adrenocortical insufficiency, a condition which is lethal in the absence of rapid treatment.

Cushing's syndrome is a general term for conditions associated with prolonged elevation of plasma glucocorticoids, resulting from excess ACTH secretion (a specific condition known as **Cushing's disease**), tumours of the adrenal cortex, or overadministration of glucocorticoids in the course of therapy. Cushing's syndrome is characterized by

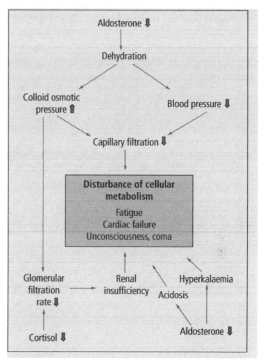

Fig. 11.12 The pathogenesis of adrenocortical insufficiency.

redistribution of body fat, a 'moon face', severe muscle wasting, osteoporosis and a predisposition to diabetes and hypertension. Chronic oversecretion or excess administration of glucocorticoids leads to functional atrophy of the CRH–ACTH axis and recovery may take a considerable time after removal of the suppressive influence.

Primary aldosteronism (Conn's syndrome) is due to excess mineralocorticoid secretion caused by a tumour of the adrenal cortex. This leads to K^+ depletion and Na^+ and water retention, resulting in hypertension, muscle weakness, tetany and hypokalaemic alkalosis.

Adrenogenital syndrome is associated with excessive androgen secretion which may cause masculinization in the female and precocious puberty in the male. This may be due to an androgensecreting tumour or it may be congenital. The latter is known as congenital adrenal hyperplasia in which one of the enzymes involved in cortisol synthesis is deficient. This leads to increased ACTH

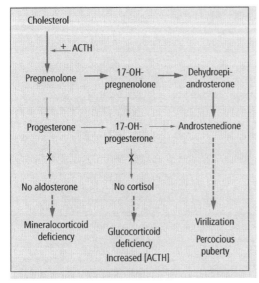

Fig. 11.13 Increased formation of androgen steroids in the 21-hydroxylase deficiency form of adrenogenital syndrome. ACTH, adrenocorticotrophic hormone.

secretion by the pituitary and hence excess production of adrenal androgens. The most common form is due to a defect of 21-hydroxylase, which occurs in one out of 10 000 newborns. The altered steroid synthetic pathway in this defect is shown in Fig. 11.13. Treatment with glucocorticoids corrects the deficiency and also suppresses excess ACTH secretion.

11.7 The pancreatic islets

The pancreatic islets produce insulin and glucagon. Insulin is secreted in response to high blood glucose; it lowers blood glucose levels and stimulates the synthesis of glycogen, fat and protein. In contrast, glucagon, which is secreted in response to low blood glucose, increases blood glucose by stimulating glycogenolysis and gluconeogenesis. During feeding insulin promotes glucose utilization and storage as glycogen and fat, while during fasting the actions of glucagon (and some other hormones) help to maintain adequate supplies of glucose, which are essential for the function of the brain.

The pancreas is both an endocrine and an exocrine gland. The endocrine cells of the pancreas are localized in the **islets of Langerhans** which constitute only 2% of the mass of the pancreas. **Insulin** is produced in the B (β) cells and **glucagon** in the A (α) cells of the islets. **Somatostatin**, also secreted as a neurotransmitter by the hypothalamus, is produced in the islets from D (δ) cells. Insulin was successfully extracted by Banting and Best in 1921 from the dog pancreas after they had first depleted it of proteolytic enzymes by ligating its exocrine ducts. The disease known as **diabetes mellitus** is due to a deficiency of insulin or to insulin resistance.

Insulin

Insulin is a small protein (M_r 5800) consisting of two peptide chains, called A and B, which are linked by two disulphide bonds. The A chain contains 21 amino acid residues and the B chain 30 residues. Beef and pig insulin differ from human insulin in only a few residues and were once used in the treatment of diabetes mellitus but have now been replaced by human insulin produced by recombinant DNA technology. Insulin is stored as an inactive prohormone, **proinsulin** (Fig. 11.14) in secretory vesicles. Proinsulin is converted to insulin by cleavage of a connecting peptide (C-peptide) to form the two peptide chains, attached by two disulphide bridges. Insulin is released from the cell by exocytosis in response to cytoplasmic Ca^{2+}. Its half-life in the blood is only a few minutes.

Actions of insulin

Insulin **lowers blood glucose** by facilitating glucose uptake and utilization while shifting the metabolism of fats and proteins from breakdown (catabolism) to building (anabolism) and storage. Insulin receptor is a plasmalemmal tyrosine kinase receptor, composed of two α subunits, which bind the hormone, and two β subunits, which contain the kinase activity. Binding of insulin results in autophosphorylation of the receptor. The now fully active receptor docks and phosphorylates cytosolic protein kinases and phosphatases, which, in turn,

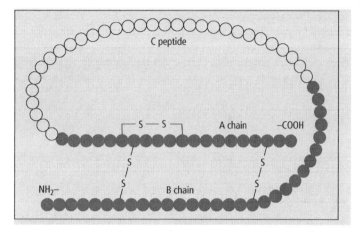

Fig. 11.14 Structure of proinsulin (insulin shown in blue).

regulate diverse metabolic cascades. One of the more rapid responses, requiring a few minutes of lag-time only, is increased uptake of glucose by muscle and adipose cells; insulin stimulates the translocation of the transporter protein (GLUT-4) from cytoplasmic vesicles to the plasma membrane. (Physical exercise also enhances the translocation of GLUT-4 to the plasma membrane—an effect to be considered at the prevention and treatment of diabetes.) Another rapid effect is the post-translational covalent modification of pre-existing enzymes. The most important action within this group is the activation of cAMP-phospodiesterase. The resulting decrease in cAMP levels in the target tissues is efficient in antagonizing the effects of the hyperglycaemic hormone glucagon and adrenaline. Insulin has long-term effects on gene expression. In addition to its mitogenic action, it controls the expression of several enzymes involved in intermediary metabolism. One of its genomic actions is the repression of the synthesis of glucagon.

Insulin down-regulates its own receptor by stimulating its endocytic uptake and subsequent degradation in cells, and this may play a role in the decreased insulin sensitivity associated with obesity.

The most important target tissues of insulin are the liver, muscle and fat. In the liver it stimulates glycogen and fat synthesis and inhibits glycogen breakdown and ketone body formation. In muscle,

it stimulates glucose and amino acid uptake, and glycogen and protein synthesis. In adipose tissue it inhibits lipolysis and stimulates glucose uptake and triglyceride synthesis (Fig. 11.15). Altogether, these effects bring about the enhanced oxidation of glucose as well as its incorporation into storage molecules (glycogen, triglycerides) after carbohydrate feeding. Lipolysis is suppressed simultaneously. By reducing blood glucose level the loss of glucose with the urine can also be avoided. Insulin increases K^+ uptake into cells and consequently can lower plasma K^+, an effect to be considered during infusion of insulin.

Ketone bodies (acetoacetic acid and β-hydroxybutyric acid), formed from fatty acids in the liver, are taken up by the skeletal muscle and oxidized there in the tricarboxylic acid cycle, provided the capacity of the cycle is maintained at a sufficient level by insulin. A lack of insulin (action) results in elevated plasma concentrations of ketone bodies (**ketonaemia**).

Control of insulin secretion

An increase in plasma **glucose** concentration provides the major stimulus for insulin secretion. Glucose enters the β-cells through the facilitative glucose carrier GLUT-2 and is phosphorylated by glucokinase. Both the carrier and the enzyme has low affinity for glucose, therefore the amount of glucose entering the metabolic pathway will be

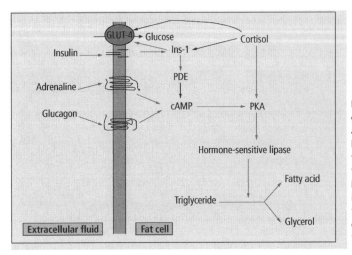

Fig. 11.15 The actions of the hyperglycaemic hormones glucagon and adrenaline and the hypoglycaemic hormone insulin on the metabolism of fat cells. Grey arrows indicate stimulation, blue arrows indicate inhibition. Ins-1, insulin-substrate-1 (one of the identified molecules within the signal transducing pathway of insulin); PDE, cAMP phosphodiesterase; PKA, protein kinase A.

related to the extracellular glucose concentration. Consequently, adenosine triphosphate (ATP) production will also depend on glucose concentration. The increase in the ATP/ADP ratio will result in the closing of ATP-sensitive K^+ channels, and the subsequent depolarization and Ca^{2+} signal will trigger insulin exocytosis. (The **sulphonylurea drugs** such as tolbutamide, used in the treatment of type II diabetes, which usually occurs in the elderly, enhance insulin secretion by closing ATP-sensitive K^+ channels.)

Carbohydrate-loading induces an initial rapid phase of secretion (Fig. 11.16), due to release of preformed hormone, followed by a second slower phase of sustained secretion due in particular to the release of newly synthesized hormone. Arginine, lysine and leucine significantly potentiate the effect of glucose on insulin release. Free fatty acids also contribute to the stimulation of insulin secretion. After feeding, the level of insulin may rise even before that of blood glucose because **gastric inhibitory peptide (GIP) and glucagon-like peptide-1 (GLP-1)** can also stimulate insulin release. Parasympathetic activity also enhances insulin release, resulting in insulin secretion prior to the beginning of food intake.

There are also efficient inhibitory mechanisms participating in the control of insulin secretion. **Somatostatin**, produced in the D-cells of the islets, inhibits insulin release. Hyperglycaemia following

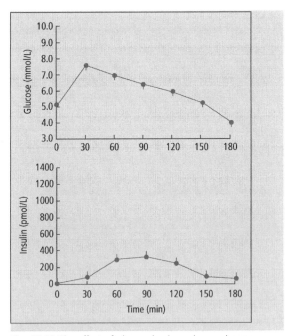

Fig. 11.16 The effect of glucose load on plasma glucose and insulin concentration as a function of time. 75 g glucose was taken orally in adult humans. (Modified from Ehrmann, D.A., Breda, E., Cavaghan, M.K., Bajramovic, S., Imperial, J., Toffolo, G., Cobelli, C. & Polonsky, K.S. (2002) *Diabetologia*, **45**, 509–17.)

carbohydrate intake induces insulin secretion, which, in turn, suppresses blood glucose level below the fasting value (**postalimentary hypoglycaemia**). The fact that this hypoglycaemic effect is small and of short duration is probably due to the paracrine action of somatostatin. Catecholamines, acting at α_2 adrenergic receptors, inhibit insulin secretion. Accordingly, sympathetic activity inhibits the function of β-cells, and this effect prevents the energy-storing action of insulin when energy mobilization is required, for example during physical exercise. **Leptin**, the product of the *ob* gene (a mutation which may cause obesity), inhibits basal and glucose-stimulated insulin release.

Glucagon

Glucagon is a polypeptide (M_r 3500) which is secreted by the α-cells of the pancreatic islets in response to low blood glucose. Elevation of glucose level suppresses glucagon secretion. Glucose uptake by the α-cells is insulin-dependent, therefore reduced insulin concentrations (imitating a condition of low blood glucose for the cell) will enhance glucagon secretion. This mechanism is especially important in diabetes mellitus, where hyperglycaemia is brought about not only by the lack of insulin action but also by the associating high glucagon level.

In contrast to insulin, glucagon **increases blood glucose** levels. Glucagon acts on the liver (via cAMP) to stimulate **glycogenolysis** (breakdown of glycogen) and **gluconeogenesis** (synthesis of glucose from lactate, amino acids or glycerol). Glucagon secretion is also stimulated by amino acids, as is insulin release. This ensures that, when there is a high intake of amino acids, a precipitous fall in blood glucose due to elevated insulin is prevented by the action of glucagon.

Control of energy utilization and storage

The brain uses glucose almost exclusively as an energy source and it is necessary to maintain an adequate blood glucose concentration at all times or convulsions and coma will ensue. Blood glucose is normally maintained at fairly constant levels of 4–6 mmol L^{-1} by the interactions of several hormones, namely **insulin, glucagon, GH, adrenaline** and **cortisol**. Of these, insulin acts to lower blood glucose, whereas the other four act to raise blood glucose. During the **absorptive state** following a meal, there are adequate glucose supplies and this causes the secretion of insulin which enhances the utilization of glucose and the storage of energy as glycogen and fat. During the **postabsorptive** or **fasting state**, blood glucose falls and insulin secretion decreases in relation to that of the hyperglycaemic hormones. The ratio of insulin to glucagon is probably the most important factor in controlling the shift from the absorptive to the postabsorptive state. This ensures that during fasting adequate glucose levels are maintained for the brain, initially by glycogenolysis, and then by gluconeogenesis in the liver and by glucose-sparing reactions in other tissues. A further account of energy storage and utilization is given in Chapter 22.

Effects of insulin deficiency

Diabetes mellitus is a major health problem; according to WHO statistics approximately 150 million people have diabetes mellitus worldwide, and this number may well double by the year 2025. Much of this increase will occur in developing countries and will be due to population growth, ageing, unhealthy diets, obesity and sedentary lifestyles. A predisposition to diabetes is inherited, but the genetic factors are complex. Two types of diabetes are recognized clinically — type 1 (formerly known as **insulin-dependent** or juvenile-onset diabetes mellitus; IDDM) and type 2 (formerly **non-insulin-dependent** or maturity-onset diabetes mellitus; NIDDM). Type 1 patients have low plasma insulin and require injections of insulin, although type 2 patients may also become temporarily insulin-dependent. Type 1 diabetes is an autoimmune disease, possibly triggered in childhood by a viral infection. Type 2 patients may have normal or elevated levels of insulin but show decreased sensitivity to insulin, often correlating with a reduction in insulin receptor concentration. These patients are often obese and generally show improvement with weight reduction. For experimental purposes, diabetes can be simulated in animals by treatment with alloxan or streptozotocin, which destroy the β cells of the islets of Langerhans.

Insulin deficiency is often accompanied by excess glucagon secretion; this imbalance causes hyperglycaemia due to reduced glucose uptake into cells and enhanced glycogenolysis and gluconeogenesis. In uncontrolled diabetes the capacity of the renal tubules to reabsorb glucose is exceeded and excess glucose is excreted in the urine. The inhibition of complete glucose reabsorption is associated with NaCl and water loss (**osmotic diuresis**), resulting in polyuria and polydipsia (thirst). Whereas glucosuria means a loss of energy-containing nutrient, the loss of salt leads to dehydration and hypotension. Due to increased utilization of fatty acids and limited capacity of the tricarboxylic acid cycle (see above), the ensuing ketonaemia evokes **metabolic acidosis** and osmotic diuresis. If left untreated, the patient may become unconscious (**diabetic coma**) (Fig. 11.17). The administration of too much insulin can also lead to coma because of the sudden lowering of blood glucose, which the brain depends upon as an energy source. There are also long-term effects of the disease: in particular, atherosclerosis in the coronary and leg arteries, and capillary abnormalities in the eyes, kidneys and nerves. The latter effects may be caused by the high glucose levels leading to abnormal protein glycosylation and to the production of sorbitol which causes osmotic damage. Diabetics

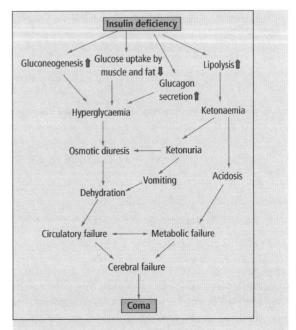

Fig. 11.17 The pathogenesis of diabetic coma.

are also prone to infection, and injuries take longer to heal than normal.

In the diagnosis of diabetes, the physician is guided by the fasting blood glucose concentration and the presence of glucose and ketones in the urine. In response to a glucose load (**glucose tolerance test**), the blood glucose concentration rises higher in diabetics than in normal subjects and returns to baseline more slowly.

Chapter 12

Reproduction

From a physiological point of view a fundamental difference between the female and the male is that the former undergoes obvious cyclic variations in reproductive activity. **Female** mammals have an **ovarian cycle** with a characteristic mean frequency for each species, e.g. 4 days in rats and 28 days in women. In women and in some other primates, the cycle is marked by a period of menstrual bleeding, which is due to the shedding of the endometrial lining of the uterus. Other female mammals do not menstruate, although they show a phase called **oestrus**, or 'heat' as it is commonly known, when the female becomes receptive to the male just before ovulation. In some species, e.g. the cat and rabbit, ovulation is triggered by copulation. In most mammals, however, ovulation is regulated by an intrinsic rhythm controlled by interactions between the hypothalamus, pituitary and gonads.

12.1 Sexual development

At an early stage of development the fetus has primordial genital ducts for both the male and the female forms. In the genetic male testosterone promotes the development of the male ducts, while Müllerian-inhibiting hormone causes the regression of the potential female ducts. In the genetic female the absence of these hormones allows the opposite to occur. At puberty sexual maturity occurs, and is accompanied by increased secretion of the gonadal hormones.

The sexual differences between male and female depend ultimately on differences in their chromosomes. In most mammalian species, the female has two X sex chromosomes while the male has one X and one Y sex chromosome, in addition to the autosomal chromosomes (22 pairs in humans). The sex-chromosomal pattern is best evaluated by the study of chromosomal spreads from leucocytes isolated from blood and the resulting preparation is called a karyotype. Most sex-chromosome abnormalities, such as XXY (Klinefelter's syndrome) and XO (Turner's syndrome), result in infertility due to the failure of germ cells in both sexes to survive. Such conditions are also associated with hormonal disturbances which result in defective development and function of the reproductive system. The XXX (superfemale) and XYY (supermale) patterns, however, do not result in abnormal sexual development.

In humans, the 'indifferent' gonads of both sexes are identical until differentiation begins at about the sixth week of fetal life. At this stage, the primordial germ cells have migrated from the yolk sac to invade the gonadal ridge formed from the intermediate mesoderm. In the genetic male, the presence of the testis-determining gene—termed *SRY*—located on the Y chromosome, causes differentiation of the gonads into testes, resulting in the incorporation of the primordial germ cells and supporting cells to form seminiferous cords. In genetic females, in the absence of *SRY*, the primordial germ cells are surrounded by cells to form primordial ovarian follicles which then proceed to undergo the early stages of meiosis. In mice, a critical step in the development of the female pattern is the expression of follistatin in the female gonad but not in the male. If this does not occur, there is a significant loss of germ cells leading to premature ovarian failure. (A few women have the Y chromosome but lack the testis-determining gene; a few men lack the Y chromosome but have the testis-determining gene on another chromosome.) At this stage, the fetus has primordial genital ducts for both the male (**Wolffian ducts**) and the female (**Müllerian ducts**). In the male fetus, testosterone secreted by the developing testes causes the Wolffian ducts to develop into the internal genitalia (epididymis, vas deferens, seminal vesicles and prostate) and a protein hormone called **Müllerian-inhibiting hormone**, also secreted by the testes, inhibits the development of the Müllerian ducts. In the female fetus, the absence of testosterone and Müllerian-inhibiting hormone allows the opposite to occur. The external genitalia of both sexes also have the potential to develop into the organs of either sex at this stage. In males, the androgenic hormone testosterone is produced by the testes and is converted to dihydrotestosterone, which acts on the external genitalia causing them to develop into the male form; whereas external genitalia develop into the female form in the absence of these androgens.

The secretion of testosterone and Müllerian-inhibiting hormone is necessary but not sufficient for the development of the male phenotype. The tissues must also have the essential androgen receptors to enable them to respond; otherwise a defect known as **testicular feminization** (androgen-insensitivity syndrome) will result, in which genetic males appear as phenotypic females with abdominal testes. Moreover, some fetal tissues require testosterone for differentiation while others, e.g. the prostate and the penis, require dihydrotestosterone. The conversion of testosterone to dihydrotestosterone is catalysed by the enzyme, 5α-reductase. In **5α-reductase deficiency**, the affected males at birth have testes but lack a prostate gland, and their external genital organs resemble those of the female. Another defect caused by an inborn error of metabolism is **congenital adrenal hyperplasia**, which is associated with masculinization of the female fetus (p. 265).

Animal studies indicate that the potential for developing cyclic reproductive activity is present in both sexes at the fetal stage. In some species (e.g. rat) the secretion of testosterone in the male appears to abolish this intrinsic rhythm, because if testosterone is injected into the genetic female at a critical period within a few days after birth, then the sexual rhythm is not generated. However, similar experiments in primates have failed to demonstrate the abolition of cyclic reproductive activity by testosterone injection around the time of birth.

Immediately after birth in human males, for a period of 6–12 months, the testis secretes testosterone and the supporting cells in the seminiferous cords, called Sertoli cells, produce a protein hormone called inhibin. After this time in males, and from birth in females, reproductive development is dormant until **puberty** when the reproductive organs in both sexes are reactivated by increased secretion of gonadotrophins due to maturation of the hypothalamo–pituitary axis. Puberty coincides with accelerated growth of the body and the development of the **secondary sexual characteristics**. The onset of puberty usually occurs at about 11 in girls and 12 in boys, although this may vary considerably depending on genetic and environmental influences. Sexual maturity is signified by the **menarche** or first menstrual bleeding in the female, and by the first ejaculation in the male. At about 50 years of age in women the **menopause** occurs: the ovary ceases to respond to gonadotrophins due to the absence of ovarian follicles, menstruation ceases, and symptoms relating to oestrogen deficiency frequently occur. In contrast, the production of sperm and testosterone in males continues throughout life, but testosterone levels decline at about 1.5% per year from about 30 years of age.

11.2 The male reproductive system

Once puberty has been reached, testosterone production and spermatogenesis in the testes occur continuously. These two functions are controlled by the hypothalamo–pituitary axis through the release of the glycoprotein gonadotrophins, follicle-stimulating hormone (FSH) and luteinizing hormone (LH). Testosterone, a steroid hormone, has a negative feedback effect on the secretion of the gonadotrophins; it also promotes the development of the male reproductive system, the production of sperm and the characteristics of maleness.

The primary reproductive organs or gonads of the males are the **testes**, which produce **spermatozoa** and also secrete the male sex hormone, **testosterone**. In addition, there are the reproductive ducts, the epididymis and vas deferens (Fig. 12.1), and accessory secretory glands (**seminal vesicles**, **prostate gland** and **bulbourethral glands**), which are involved in the secretion of seminal fluid. A few weeks before birth the testes pass out of the abdominal cavity into the scrotal sac. Failure of the testes to descend into the scrotum (**cryptorchidism**) will result in infertility, because **spermatogenesis** is disrupted since this process depends on a temperature about 4°C below body temperature. The lower temperature is maintained

by a counter-current heat exchange between the testicular artery and the surrounding plexuses of veins that are filled with blood at a lower temperature draining from the scrotally-placed testes. The scrotum can contract or relax to move the testes closer to or further away from the body so that this temperature is maintained.

Spermatogenesis

Spermatozoa are produced in the **seminiferous tubules** of the testes (Fig. 12.2a). These tubules are lined with germ cells and **Sertoli cells**. The latter closely surround the developing germ cells (Fig. 12.2b) and provide them with nutrients and stimulating factors, hence they are sometimes referred to as nurse cells. They also secrete a number of substances, including androgen-binding protein and the hormone inhibin.

At puberty, in response to gonadotrophic hormones released by the anterior pituitary, spermatogenesis is initiated and occurs continuously thereafter. Primordial germ cells that enter the fetal testes divide and become **spermatogonia**, the

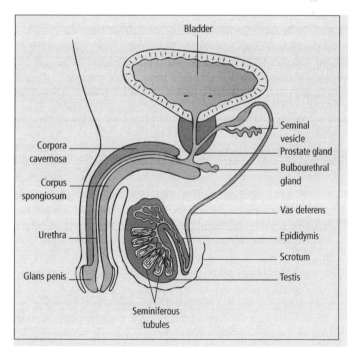

Fig. 12.1 The male reproductive system.

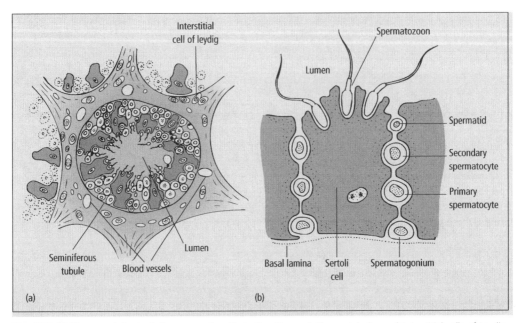

Fig. 12.2 (a) Diagram of the testis in cross-section illustrating the seminiferous tubules and interstitial cells of Leydig. (b) Structure of the wall of a seminiferous tubule showing the intimate relationship between the Sertoli cells and the developing germ cells.

stem cells of the testes that divide by mitosis. Subsequently groups of these cells become **primary spermatocytes**, which undergo the first meiotic division. This is a complex process during which homologous chromosomes derived from maternal and paternal sources pair and exchange genetic material before completing this division to form **secondary spermatocytes**. The secondary spermatocytes, which contain a haploid number of duplicated chromosomes, then undergo a second meiotic division to form haploid **spermatids**. During meiosis, there is a reduction in the number of chromosomes from 46 to 23. Finally, spermatids differentiate to give rise to **spermatozoa**. The process of spermatogenesis, from spermatogonia through to the release of spermatozoa into the lumen of the seminiferous tubule, takes about 70 days.

When spermatozoa are released into the seminiferous tubules, they are non-motile and incapable of fertilizing an ovum. From the seminiferous tubules, spermatozoa pass into the **epididymis** where they mature and are stored until ejaculation

takes place. The production of spermatozoa is a continuous process, and spermatozoa not ejaculated sometimes pass out into the urine (spermaturia) or eventually deteriorate and are reabsorbed within the epididymis.

The **mature sperm** consists of a head, middle piece and long tail (Fig. 12.3). The head is composed mainly of the nucleus and is covered by a cap known as the **acrosome**. The acrosome is a large vesicular structure containing lytic enzymes that help the sperm to penetrate the outer coat of the ovum. The middle piece consists of a helical sheath of mitochondria surrounding a core of contractile microtubules, called the axoneme, which extend to the tip of the tail. The mitochondria provide energy for motility of the spermatozoon, which is generated by sliding of the microtubules to produce wave-like movement of the tail. The structure of the sperm tail shows many of the characteristics of cilia and genetically based syndromes, such as the immotile cilia syndrome, involve infertility due to immotile sperm and bronchiectasis, a respiratory disorder due to recurrent infection in the bronchial tree due to the failure of the cilia in the respiratory epithelium to function.

Testosterone

Testosterone is the principal androgenic hormone produced by the testis (Fig. 12.4). It is a C19 steroid synthesized from cholesterol, as illustrated in Fig. 11.11. This steroid hormone is secreted by the **interstitial cells of Leydig**, which lie scattered between the seminiferous tubules (Fig. 12.2a). Most of the androgens in the male are synthesized here,

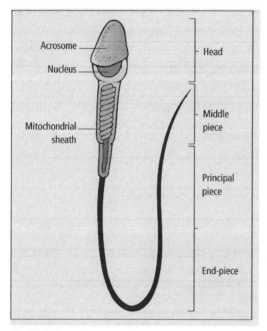

Fig. 12.3 The mature spermatozoon.

although a small amount is produced in the adrenal cortex (p. 263). Once released into the blood, testosterone is bound to a binding protein called sex hormone-binding globulin. In most of its target tissues (except muscle), testosterone is converted to a more potent androgen called **dihydrotestosterone** (Fig. 12.4). Both androgens act via nuclear receptors to promote gene activation and the synthesis of specific proteins (p. 33). The hormone is metabolized in the liver by reduction and conjugation with glucuronic acid, and the metabolites are then excreted by the kidneys.

Testosterone promotes the development of the reproductive system and of the **secondary sexual characteristics** of the male and has important anabolic effects in skeletal muscle and bone. The most obvious effects of testosterone are seen at puberty, namely, enlargement of the penis and testes, increased rate of growth of muscle and bone, appearance of facial, axillary and pubic hair, and change in the pitch of the voice. Castration or removal of the testes in childhood prevents most of these changes from occurring.

Castrated males do not become bald and the presence of testosterone is necessary for baldness to occur in males genetically predisposed to this condition. Testosterone also promotes libido (sexual drive) and aggression.

Control of male reproductive activity

The gonadotrophic hormones **FSH** and **LH** control spermatogenesis and synthesis of testosterone, respectively (Fig. 12.5). FSH and LH are glycoproteins, each composed of two subunits called α and

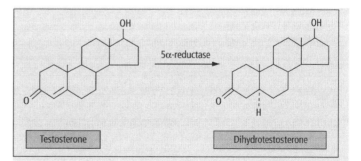

Fig. 12.4 Testosterone and its conversion to dihydrotestosterone.

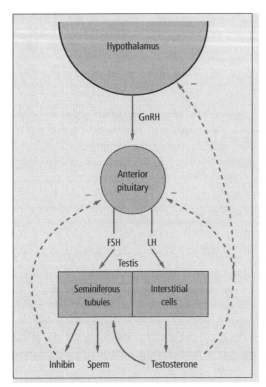

Fig. 12.5 Control of spermatogenesis and testosterone secretion. FSH, follicle-stimulating hormone; GnRH, gonadotrophin-releasing hormone; LH, luteinizing hormone.

β. The α subunits of FSH and LH are identical in structure, and specificity is determined by the β subunit. Their actions are mediated by cyclic adenosine monophosphate (cAMP). The pulsatile release of the gonadotrophic hormones is controlled by a single hypothalamic neurohormone—**gonadotrophin-releasing hormone** (GnRH), also known as **luteinizing hormone-releasing hormone**. Both testosterone and FSH are necessary for normal spermatogenesis. Testosterone inhibits secretion of LH in a typical negative feedback manner, acting mainly on the hypothalamus, but has less effect on FSH secretion. **Inhibins** are glycoprotein hormones secreted by the Sertoli cells in the testes, have a negative feedback effect on the secretion of FSH, acting at the pituitary. Inhibins are disulphide-linked dimers of two peptide chains, α and β. There are five forms of the β chain—β_A to β_E—but only β_A and β_B, in combination with the α

chain, are active (equally) in inhibiting FSH secretion. These form inhibin A ($\alpha\beta_A$) and inhibin B ($\alpha\beta_B$); inhibin B is the major circulating form in adult males. Dimers of the β chains, $\beta_A\beta_A$, $\beta_A\beta_B$ and $\beta_B\beta_B$, termed **activins** A, AB and B, respectively, are all potent stimulators of FSH secretion. Activins are paracrine growth factors, controlling cell proliferation, differentiation and apoptosis in a wide variety of tissues. They regulate testicular steroidogenesis and spermatogenesis, ovarian folliculogenesis and atresia, erythroid differentiation, neuronal development, etc. The activin-binding protein follistatin is a glycoprotein expressed in a wide range of tissues. **Follistatin** can neutralize all of the actions of activin and hence has significant FSH-suppressing activity within the pituitary gland, where it inhibits the action of locally produced activin B resulting in a decrease in FSH secretion. The physiological roles of the β_C–β_E chains have yet to be established.

Semen

The ejaculated fluid or semen contains spermatozoa and secretions of the seminal vesicles, prostate gland and bulbourethral glands. The average volume of ejaculate in man is about 3 mL and contains approximately 100 million spermatozoa per millilitre. The secretions of the accessory glands comprise about 95% of semen volume and assist in the transport and nourishment of the sperm. The seminal fluid contains high concentrations of **fructose**, which serves as an energy substrate for the spermatozoa, and also high concentrations of **prostaglandins**, which may increase motility of the uterus, thus promoting transport of spermatozoa. Fertility depends on the quality of the semen, the most important factors being the number, motility and morphology of the spermatozoa. Decreased sperm production (**oligozoospermia**) reflected as a sperm count of less than 20 million/mL is a common cause of infertility in the male and is often accompanied by low motility (<50%) and a high percentage of abnormal sperm. However, it is important to realize that many pregnancies occur in the presence of low counts, but usually after a prolonged duration of infertility.

Erection

Penile erection, which is necessary for coitus and delivery of semen to the female, is caused by engorgement of the penis with blood. Erection may be initiated by psychic stimuli and by tactile genital stimulation. Failure of erection, i.e. **impotence**, may be due to psychological as well as organic disturbances. In erection, a spinal reflex arc is involved in which impulses pass along afferent nerves to integrating centres in the **sacral spinal cord**, to initiate impulses which travel back along **parasympathetic fibres**. Excitation of the parasympathetic fibres releases nitric oxide through a cyclic guanosine monophosphate (cGMP) mechanism, which causes **arteriolar dilation** in the penis so that the sinusoids of the corpora cavernosa and corpus spongiosum (Fig. 12.1) become engorged with blood. This, together with compression of draining veins against the fibrous tunica and by the ischiocavernosus muscle, produces penile erection. The cGMP is produced locally at the nerve endings and is rapidly inactivated by the enzyme type V phosphodiesterase, a mechanism inhibited by drugs such as Viagra, Cialis and Levitra, thereby facilitating erections.

Ejaculation

This is a reflex action involving movement (**emission**) of spermatozoa and glandular secretions into the **urethra** followed by the sudden ejection of the semen from the urethra. Emission of the glandular secretions occurs in a definite sequence. During erection, the secretion of the bulbourethral glands is discharged to lubricate the urethra. Prostate secretions are followed by testicular secretions containing sperm, and subsequently by secretions from the seminal vesicles, which contribute the alkaline component of the ejaculate. Consequently, in men with congenital absence of the vas deferens, which is accompanied by absence of the seminal vesicles, the volume of the ejaculate is reduced and has a pH of 6.9–7.1, in contrast to the alkaline pH (>7.8) of semen from normal men.

Ejaculation is triggered by stimulation of tactile receptors in the glans penis causing impulses to pass along afferent nerves to centres in the **lumbar spinal cord** and initiate impulses which then return along sympathetic fibres. This **sympathetic activity** leads to contraction of the smooth muscle of the epididymis, vas deferens and secretory glands propelling spermatozoa and glandular secretions into the urethra. At the same time, the internal sphincter of the urethra constricts, preventing semen from entering the bladder; failure of this contraction results in retrograde ejaculation. Contraction of the bulbospongiosus and ischiocavernosus muscles due to reflex activity in **somatic motor nerves** then leads to pulsatile emission of the seminal fluid from the urethra.

Vasectomy

This procedure, in which the vasa deferentia are cut, is a permanent and effective means of contraception in the male. Spermatogenesis continues after vasectomy and the spermatozoa bank-up, often distending the epididymal duct, the site at which the sperm degenerate, and are reabsorbed by the combined action of macrophages and the epididymis. Since spermatozoa represent less than 5% of semen volume, the volume of the ejaculate is not altered by vasectomy. While spermatogenesis continues after a vasectomy, studies reveal that there is a decrease in spermatogenesis such that reversals performed more than 10 years after a vasectomy have lower sperm outputs and lower pregnancy rates. Further, about 70% of men develop antibodies to sperm after a vasectomy and these proteins may impair sperm motility and fertility. Given the more frequent break up of marriages in modern society, men contemplating a vasectomy should be made aware that sperm can be stored frozen for in excess of 10 years.

11.3 The female reproductive system

Activity in the female reproductive system is regulated by periodic changes in the secretion of FSH and LH by the anterior pituitary, and subsequently oestrogen and progesterone by the ovaries. A central event in the female cycle is ovulation, which is

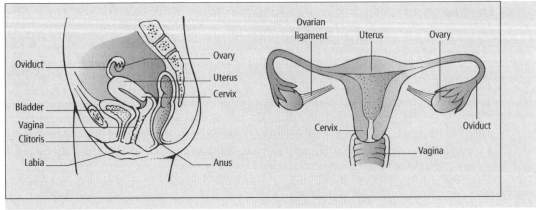

Fig. 12.6 The female reproductive system.

triggered by a surge in LH secretion. An external manifestation of the cycle is menstruation, when a fall in oestrogen and progesterone causes the shedding of the endometrial lining of the uterus. Since the ovarian hormones suppress the release of FSH and LH, their removal coincides with a rise in FSH, which allows a new cycle to begin again.

The primary reproductive organs of the female (Fig. 12.6) are the two **ovaries**, which produce ova and secrete the sex hormones, **oestrogen** and **progesterone**. The accessory reproductive structures comprise the two **uterine tubes** (fallopian tubes), and the **uterus**, **cervix** and **vagina**. At the opening of the vagina lie the external genitalia (the vulva).

Oogenesis and follicular development

The primordial germ cells migrate from the region of the yolk sac to the gonadal ridge and, in the female, multiply and become surrounded by primitive follicular cells. The germ cells, now called **oogonia**, commence the first meiotic division, which is arrested at diakinesis without completing division to form diploid **primary oocytes**. These oogonia and their surrounding single layer of follicular cells are called **primordial follicles** and, at birth, number approximately 1 million. Some of these degenerate and at puberty less than about 400 000 remain. In groups of these follicles, the oogonia enlarge and their follicular cells secrete a

complex mixture of mucopolysaccharides and glycoproteins to form the **zona pellucida**, with the follicles being termed **primary ovarian follicles** (Fig. 12.7). Although the first stage of meiosis begins before birth, completion of the first meiotic division does not occur until just prior to ovulation when the **secondary oocyte**, containing a haploid number of duplicated chromosomes, is formed. In this process, most of the cytoplasm is retained by the oocyte and a smaller rudimentary cell, called the first polar body, is split off. The entry of a sperm triggers the onset of the second meiotic division and occurs in the uterine tube; a second polar body is eliminated and the mature **ovum** is formed.

In the ovary at puberty, groups of primary ovarian follicles enlarge by division of follicular or **granulosa** cells in response to a rise in the gonadotrophic hormone FSH at the beginning of each cycle. Normally, only one of these reaches the stage of ovulation; the rest degenerate by a process of programmed cell death called atresia. Only about 400 of the primary follicles develop into ova during the reproductive life of a woman.

As a follicle matures, it becomes surrounded by a capsule of ovarian tissue containing capillaries, made up of an inner cellular layer, the **theca interna**, and a more fibrous outer layer, the **theca externa**. With further maturation fluid accumulates amongst the granulosa cells to form a central cavity filled with fluid called the **antrum**. These

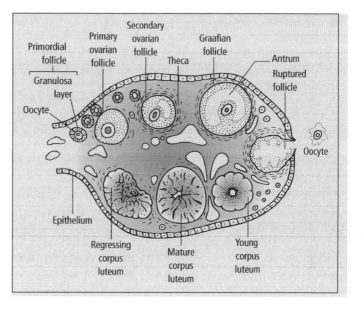

Fig. 12.7 Diagram of the ovary in cross-section illustrating the different stages in the development of a follicle and corpus luteum during one ovarian cycle. (The sequential arrangement is not an actual representation.)

antral follicles are also called **Graafian or secondary ovarian follicles**, in which the oocyte is embedded in a mass of granulosa cells and protrudes into the antrum (Fig. 12.7). The theca interna cells synthesize androstenedione (see Fig. 11.11), which is converted by the granulosa cells into the oestrogenic hormones, **oestradiol** and **oestrone**. About the middle of the ovarian cycle, ovulation occurs: the follicle ruptures and the secondary oocyte, together with its surrounding granulosa cells, is extruded into the peritoneal cavity. It is then swept by the movement of cilia into the open end of the oviduct, which is closely applied to the ovary.

After ovulation, the granulosa cells remaining in the ruptured follicle, together with cells of the theca interna, proliferate and become invaded by blood vessels to form a new endocrine structure— the **corpus luteum**. This continues to secrete oestrogens but also produces the hormone **progesterone**. The corpus luteum is functional for about 12 days after ovulation, after which it regresses, unless fertilization of the ovum and implantation have occurred. The regression of the corpus luteum causes a decline in the secretion of oestrogen and progesterone and this withdrawal results in sloughing of the endometrium as the menstrual blood flow.

Gonadotrophic hormones

Maturation of follicles in the ovary requires the presence of the **gonadotrophic hormones**, FSH and LH, which are secreted by the anterior pituitary. The secretion of both gonadotrophic hormones is stimulated by **GnRH**, which is produced in the medial basal area of the hypothalamus and secreted pulses with a periodicity of 1–2 h. Secretion of the gonadotrophins is regulated by feedback actions of oestrogen, inhibins and progesterone (see below and Fig. 12.10). Inhibin A and B and oestradiol are secreted by the granulosa cells under the stimulus of FSH and act on the pituitary to inhibit the release of FSH, a negative feedback effect. Whereas FSH stimulates the conversion of androstenedione to oestradiol, the production of androstenedione by the theca interna is regulated by LH. The rapidly rising oestradiol levels exert a positive feedback action on both the pituitary and hypothalamus to promote a sudden peak of LH secretion at mid-cycle that **triggers ovulation**. Ovulation can be induced in infertile women by treatment with recombinant FSH to induce follicular maturation and, when the follicle has reached a level of maturity judged by its size and level of oestradiol secretion, ovulation is induced by recombinant LH or human chorionic gonadotrophin (hCG). LH is also required for normal corpus luteum function.

Menstrual cycle

The monthly loss of blood for 3–5 days during the reproductive life of women is termed the menstrual cycle, which has an average length of 28 days but may vary considerably among different women. The first signs of bleeding signal the start of a new menstrual cycle. During this time and until ovulation, the **ovarian follicles** develop and secrete increasing quantities of **oestrogen**. Oestrogen acts on the uterus to stimulate regeneration and growth of the **endometrium** from the remnants left after the previous menstrual cycle, causing a two- to threefold increase in the thickness of the endometrium. The first 2 weeks of the menstrual cycle are therefore referred to as the **follicular phase** with respect to the ovary, and as the **proliferative phase** with respect to the uterus (Fig. 12.8). Ovulation occurs at about the mid-point of the cycle, i.e. around day 14. The variation that occurs

in the duration of the menstrual cycle is usually due to variation in this first half of the reproductive cycle.

During the second half of the reproductive cycle, the **corpus luteum** develops and secretes both **oestrogens** and **progesterone**. Oestrogens continue to promote proliferative activity in the endometrium while, under the action of progesterone, the endometrial glands become distended with secretory products, including **glycogen**, which is an important nutrient for the developing embryo should implantation take place. Endometrial blood flow increases and the spiral arteries become more tightly coiled and twisted. The second half of the cycle is therefore referred to as the **luteal phase** with respect to the ovaries and as the **secretory phase** with respect to the uterus. If implantation does not occur, the corpus luteum regresses, there is a rapid fall in secretion of oestrogen and progesterone and the endometrium undergoes shrinkage due to loss of extracellular water and constriction of the spiral arteries. This causes a reduction in blood flow to the endometrium with cell death and weakening of the walls of blood ves-

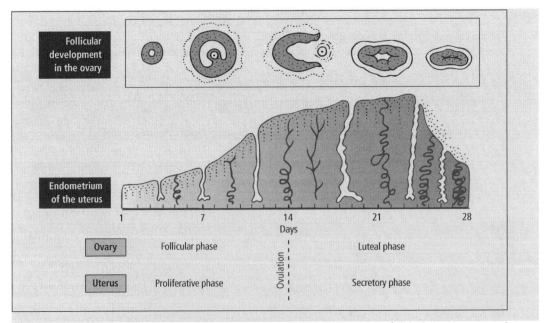

Fig. 12.8 Diagram showing the changes occurring in the endometrium and in an ovarian follicle during the menstrual cycle.

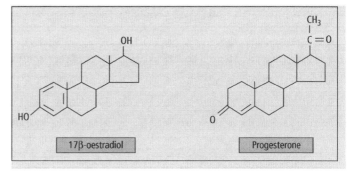

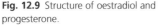

Fig. 12.9 Structure of oestradiol and progesterone.

sels. As the phase of vasoconstriction wears off, blood leaks from the damaged vessels to initiate **menstrual bleeding** and eventually all but the basal layer of endometrium are detached from the uterus. A second phase of vasoconstriction of the spiral arteries minimizes loss of blood.

Ovarian hormones

The ovary secretes two steroid hormones, **oestrogens** and **progesterone** (Fig. 12.9), and the protein hormone **inhibin**. 17β-oestradiol is the main oestrogen produced but oestrone, which has less biological activity than oestradiol, is also secreted in significant amounts. Androgens, produced in low but significant concentrations in the adrenal cortex and ovaries of women, have a role in the promotion of libido.

Oestrogens and progesterone are C18 and C21 steroids, respectively, and are synthesized from cholesterol as outlined in Fig. 11.11. These steroid hormones are transported in the blood bound to plasma proteins. Like other steroid hormones, oestrogen and progesterone produce their effects in responsive tissues by combining with nuclear receptors to promote gene activation with a subsequent increase in synthesis of the effector proteins (p. 33). They are metabolized by reduction and hydroxylation in the liver, and their metabolites (particularly oestriol and pregnanediol conjugated with glucuronic acid) are then excreted by the kidney.

Oestrogen is produced by the granulosa cells of the follicle from the precursor androstenedione, a weak androgen produced by the cells of the theca interna under the action of LH and, after ovulation, it is produced by the corpus luteum. The peak of LH that occurs at ovulation is preceded by a steep rise in oestrogen secretion, which stimulates LH secretion. Thus a rise in oestrogen levels at this point in the cycle has a **positive feedback** effect on LH (and FSH) secretion (Fig. 12.10) and is thought to act on GnRH secretion by the hypothalamus. During the secretory phase of the menstrual cycle, oestrogen and progesterone act synergistically to exert a **negative feedback** effect on the secretion of the gonadotrophic hormones. The primary site of the negative feedback action of oestrogen is the pituitary (Fig. 12.10). The negative feedback effect diminishes as the concentrations of oestrogen and progesterone fall with regression of the corpus luteum.

The present model of positive oestrogen feedback is that, in the follicular phase, oestrogen in the absence of progesterone acts by increasing the frequency and amplitude of GnRH secretory pulses, thus stimulating LH release and both FSH and LH synthesis. This effect is inhibited by progesterone; thus, there is no positive feedback in the luteal phase, despite comparable or greater levels of oestrogen in the follicular phase.

In addition to its positive and negative effects on gonadotrophin secretion, oestrogen:
1 sensitizes the ovaries to the effects of gonadotrophins by stimulating the synthesis of FSH and LH receptors;
2 stimulates growth of the endometrium and contractility of the myometrium;

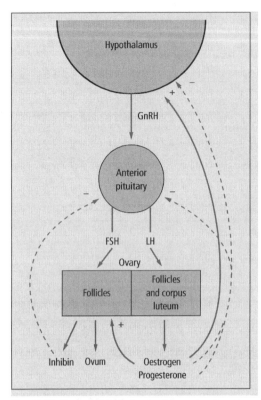

Fig. 12.10 Control of follicular development and oestrogen secretion. FSH, follicle-stimulating hormone; GnRH, gonadotrophin-releasing hormone; LH, luteinizing hormone.

3 stimulates the output of mucus from the cervical glands and causes changes in the properties of the mucus which assist entry of spermatozoa;

4 causes the vaginal epithelium to proliferate and show increased cornification;

5 stimulates the growth and development of the breasts, particularly of the lactiferous ducts;

6 promotes the growth of bones and skeletal muscle and helps to bring about the characteristic female patterns of distribution of body hair and adipose tissue;

7 promotes closure of the epiphyses at the end of the period of linear skeletal growth; and

8 helps to conserve bone (p. 256); osteoporosis is a common condition in postmenopausal women.

Progesterone, which is present in significant amounts only during the luteal phase of each men-

strual cycle, acts on tissues that have already been stimulated by oestrogen. In addition to having inhibitory effects on gonadotrophin secretion and follicular development during the luteal phase, progesterone:

1 transforms the endometrium to its secretory phase and decreases the spontaneous electrical activity of the myometrium;

2 modifies the composition of cervical mucus, making it more viscous and resistant to penetration by spermatozoa;

3 causes further changes in the vaginal epithelium with regression of cornification;

4 promotes development of the breasts, particularly of the secretory units; and

5 causes an increase in basal body temperature after ovulation, which may be useful clinically to indicate that ovulation is occurring.

The principal role of **inhibin** is to suppress FSH secretion by pituitary gonadotrophs (Fig. 12.10).

Control of the female reproductive cycle

The blood levels of the gonadotrophic and ovarian hormones throughout the ovarian cycle are shown in Fig. 12.11. A marked peak in the level of gonadotrophins, particularly LH, occurs at the midpoint of the menstrual cycle and coincides with the time of ovulation. (Because it is difficult to pinpoint the time of ovulation, the peak in blood LH has been arbitrarily designated as day 0 in Fig. 12.11, but in clinical practice the beginning of menstruation is taken as day 1 of the menstrual cycle.) Just before the beginning of each cycle there is a small rise in FSH. This rise in FSH stimulates follicular development and, together with LH, leads to an increase in oestrogen and inhibin A and B secretion. Oestrogen plays an important role in the maturation process because it sensitizes the granulosa cells to the effects of gonadotrophins and thus increases their capacity to produce oestrogen. The surge in oestrogen secretion that occurs just prior to ovulation has a positive feedback effect on both the anterior pituitary and the hypothalamus, causing a marked rise in LH and FSH secretion. The peak in LH secretion triggers ovulation. After ovu-

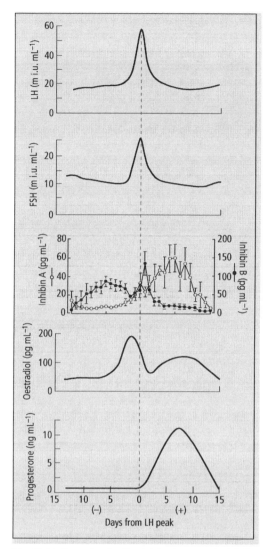

Fig. 12.11 Plasma levels of luteinizing hormone (LH), follicle-stimulating hormone (FSH), oestradiol, progesterone, inhibin A and inhibin B during the ovulatory cycle centred on the mid-cycle LH peak (day 0). (After Groome, N.P. *et al.* (1996) *J Clin Endocrinol Metab*, **81**, 1401–5.)

menstruation. The corpus luteum also secretes inhibin A and the fall in this glycoprotein, as well as oestrogen and progesterone secretion also removes the negative feedback influence on the secretion of the gonadotrophic hormones. The resultant rise in output of FSH triggers the development of a new batch of follicles and the beginning of a new cycle of uterine and ovarian function.

Sexual response

Sexual arousal in the female is similar to that of the male, with reflex arteriolar dilation and congestion leading to erection of the clitoris and the tissue around the vaginal opening. Orgasm produces reflex contractions of the vagina and uterus, but does not appear to be connected to, or essential for, sperm transport or conception. The posterior pituitary hormone oxytocin appears to be the hormone most closely associated with sexual activity in the female. In both sexes, orgasmic intensity is strongly correlated with plasma oxytocin concentrations. Central nervous system administration of oxytocin induces maternal and sexual behaviours in rats, and it has been suggested that oxytocin influences affiliation and social bonding in humans.

Menopause

The termination of reproductive function in the female occurs at the menopause, which is the time of the last menstrual period. The period of time leading up to this is termed the **climacteric**, which is often characterized by irregular menstrual cycles, hot flushes, sweating, vaginal dryness and urethral irritation. The menopause results from the absence of any remaining ovarian follicles that are capable of responding to FSH and LH, leading to a fall in oestrogen and progesterone levels. The reduction in the negative feedback effects of oestrogen and progesterone causes plasma FSH and LH to rise to high levels. In postmenopausal women, bone loss is accelerated and may develop into osteoporosis, a disorder characterized by a reduction in bone density and an increased incidence of bone fractures.

lation, the increase in oestrogen and progesterone that coincides with the development of the corpus luteum prepares the endometrial lining of the uterus for implantation. If implantation does not occur, the levels of oestrogen and progesterone fall in parallel with the demise of the corpus luteum and their decreasing concentrations results in

Hormone replacement therapy with oestrogen helps to conserve bone mass, the benefits being greatest soon after menopause. It also reduces or eliminates menopausal symptoms. A progesterone-like steroid (progestogen) should also be administered because of the increased risk of endometrial cancer associated with unopposed oestrogen therapy.

Hormonal contraception

The oral contraceptive pill is a very effective means of preventing pregnancy and is based on the negative feedback effects of oestrogenic and progestagenic compounds on the secretion of FSH and LH by the pituitary gland. 17β-oestradiol and progesterone have largely been replaced by synthetic oestrogens and progestagens that are more slowly degraded in the gut and liver. The most commonly used contraceptive pill is a combination of a synthetic oestrogen and a synthetic progestagen taken daily to suppress FSH and LH thereby prevent ovulation and, when withdrawn at the end of the month, to result in menstruation. Preparations containing only a progestogen also produce changes in the cervical secretions, making it more difficult for sperm to penetrate the uterus and to undergo capacitation (p. 282). These appear to be the main actions of the progestogen-only contraceptive, although many women who take it do not ovulate. It is administered continuously, either orally or by the slow release of hormone from a vaginal suppository, intramuscular injection, or by a subcutaneous implant. Some synthetic steroids may also induce changes in the endometrium, preventing successful embryonic implantation. The new abortion pill RU 486 is an antagonist of progesterone that binds competitively to progesterone receptors. Its actions prevent implantation in the uterus and enhance myometrial contractions, thereby expelling the embryo.

Prolactin

Prolactin is required in mammals for breast development and lactation (p. 243). In some rodents it prolongs the life of the corpus luteum and so has been called luteotrophic hormone. Although the production of prolactin is controlled principally by the inhibitory influence of dopamine, a stimulatory influence is exerted by prolactin-releasing factors, such as thyrotrophin-releasing hormone, and by oestrogen during pregnancy. Prolactin, in turn, enhances the secretion of dopamine at the median eminence and so acts in a negative feedback manner to inhibit its own secretion. Because prolactin secretion is stimulated by oestrogen, it increases in girls at puberty, but not in boys. In pregnancy the rise in oestrogens stimulates further secretion of prolactin, which prepares the breast for lactation and, after birth, suckling induces prolactin secretion thereby maintaining lactation.

Hyperprolactinaemia occurs when prolactin secretion is excessive, as for example in certain pituitary tumours. Elevated blood prolactin concentrations cause anovulation and amenorrhoea in women, and low testosterone and impotence in men. In these conditions, prolactin appears to inhibit the actions of LH and FSH on the ovary and testis, respectively. Dopamine agonists are capable of effectively suppressing the growth of these adenomas, thus decreasing prolactin secretion, which greatly reduces the need for surgery.

Pineal gland

This gland, situated in the centre of the brain, secretes the hormone **melatonin**. The secretion of melatonin fluctuates in relation to light (and hence day length) and it is thought that the pineal gland plays a role in determining the seasonal breeding patterns of animals.

In humans and other species the secretion of melatonin is elevated at night and suppressed during the day. Melatonin is synthesized from serotonin in a reaction which is entrained to the light–dark cycle via a circuitous pathway from the eye, relaying in the suprachiasmatic and paraventricular nuclei of the hypothalamus, then descending to the thoracic spinal cord and superior cervical ganglion to innervate the pineal gland. At night, melatonin synthesis is stimulated by noradrenaline released by postganglionic sympathetic nerve fibres from the superior cervical ganglia. Noradrenaline (via cAMP) stimulates the synthesis and activity of *N*-acetyltransferase, one of the enzymes involved in the synthesis of melatonin. During the day, light suppresses noradrenaline release by the postganglionic sympathetic nerve fibres innervating the pineal gland and melatonin synthesis decreases. The function of the pineal gland in humans is uncertain. Melatonin probably influences circadian rhythms and can reduce the symptoms of jet-lag.

Infertility

Between 10 and 15% of couples are infertile, due to a number of causes that affect either the male or female in about equal numbers. In most cases the cause in females can be diagnosed. The failure of ovulation can be successfully treated with ovarian stimulants such as the anti-oestrogen clomiphene citrate or, less frequently, FSH and LH/hCG. In other cases surgery can correct tubal obstructions. In males, while a semen analysis can provide some quantification of the degree of infertility, in about 40% of men with defective spermatogenesis the cause of this abnormality is unknown. The view that many such cases may be caused by a genetic defect has been supported by the finding that, in about 3–6% of such men, large deletions of genetic information from the long arm of the Y chromosome have been found. In many men with spermatogenic defects there is no method of raising sperm counts. For such men, where sperm are present, albeit in very low numbers, pregnancies can be achieved by the injection of a single sperm into an ovum, a process known as **intracytoplasmic sperm injection (ICSI)** and embryo transfer, techniques broadly classified as assisted reproductive technologies. These technologies include *in vitro* **fertilization** (IVF), a process originally developed to treat women with tubal obstruction in which oocytes are retrieved from the ovaries after superovulation by transvaginal ultrasound-directed aspiration, and then fertilized *in vitro* with sperm or sperm introduced by ICSI. The resulting embryos are implanted transcervically into the uterus. Most IVF programs now transfer a maximum of two embryos and achieve pregnancy rates of about 30% with a twin pregnancy rate of about 20%.

11.4 Pregnancy

After fertilization in the uterine tube, the fertilized ovum is transported down the oviduct and implanted in the uterine wall. Implantation occurs about 7 days after fertilization, during which time the fertilized ovum develops to form the blastocyst. Part of the blastocyst forms the chorion, which subsequently becomes incorporated into the placenta. The placenta forms not only a transporting organ between mother and fetus, but also is an endocrine organ, which secretes a number of hormones essential for the maintenance of pregnancy.

The duration of pregnancy (or gestation) in women is approximately 38 weeks, or 40 weeks when taken from the last menstruation. Sperm survive for a few days in the female reproductive tract and the ovum remains fertile for less than a day. Therefore, fertilization can occur if sperm are deposited in the female reproductive tract a few days before ovulation. Sperm need to spend some period of time in the female reproductive tract before they are capable of fertilizing the ovum. This process, which involves changes in surface glycoproteins, is known as **capacitation** of the sperm. Sperm are transported to the uterine tubes by contractions of the uterus and the beating of ciliated epithelium. After ovulation the ovum is swept into the tube, also by the actions of ciliated epithelium and only one of many millions of sperm deposited in the vagina can fertilize the ovum.

Fertilization occurs in the oviduct and the **zygote** begins to divide as it makes its way to the uterus. By the time it reaches the uterus (about 3 days), it is a small mass of cells called a **morula**. Identical twins may arise if the morula separates into two parts during this stage. (Non-identical or fraternal twins may occur when two ova are released at ovulation.) The morula develops into the blastocyst, which is composed of an outer layer of trophoblastic cells separated from an inner mass of embryonic cells (Fig. 12.12). Implantation of the

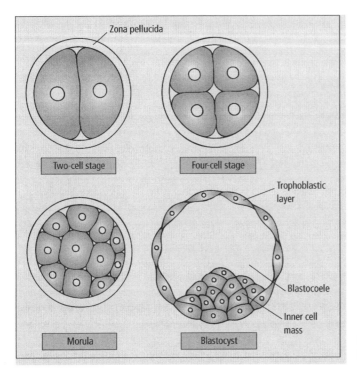

Fig. 12.12 Stages in the early development of the embryo.

blastocyst in the uterine wall occurs about 7 days after fertilization but occasionally it may implant in the wall of the uterine tube, or rarely in the abdominal cavity, and such **ectopic pregnancies** will require surgical intervention.

The trophoblastic layer forms the **chorion** which gives rise to the fetal part of the placenta. At about 9 days after fertilization, the trophoblastic layer begins to secrete the hormone **chorionic gonadotrophin** (CG) that prolongs the life of the corpus luteum leading to the continued secretion of oestrogens and progesterone, thus enabling the continuation of pregnancy during the first trimester. Thereafter, the role of the corpus luteum is supplanted by the placenta that acts as an endocrine gland, secreting both oestrogen and progesterone as well as other protein hormones required for the successful completion of pregnancy. The **placenta** also serves as a means for exchanging respiratory gases, nutrients and waste products between fetal and maternal circulations.

Placental hormones

The placenta secretes at least four hormones. Two of these hormones are proteins, namely CG and chorionic somatomammotrophin (CS), as well as oestrogen and progesterone. The maternal plasma levels of these hormones during pregnancy are shown in Fig. 12.13.

Chorionic gonadotrophin

CG is a glycoprotein (M_r 38 000) secreted by the trophoblastic cells of the placenta and which is chemically and biologically similar to LH. It is secreted in large quantities during the first trimester (Fig. 12.13) and its main role is to maintain the corpus luteum during the early part of pregnancy. Since CG is secreted as early as 9 days after fertilization, its detection by radioimmunoassay provides a simple test for pregnancy. In addition, it stimulates the formation of the fetal generation of

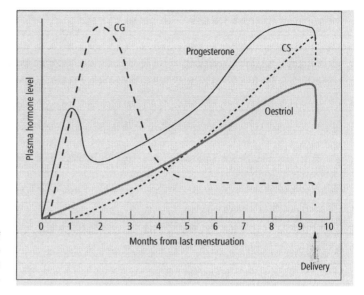

Fig. 12.13 Maternal plasma levels of placental hormones during pregnancy. CG, chorionic gonadotrophin; CS, chorionic somatomammotrophin.

Leydig cells in the testis and the production of testosterone.

Chorionic somatomammotrophin

Originally named placental lactogen, this protein (M_r 18 500) secreted by the trophoblastic cells is structurally similar to the human growth hormone family. CS levels in the maternal circulation increase steadily throughout pregnancy (Fig. 12.13), but its functions are not well defined. Like growth hormone, it has a counter-regulatory action to insulin, promoting free fatty acid mobilization and inhibiting glucose uptake in the mother. As its name implies, it also promotes mammary development in preparation for lactation.

Progesterone

During pregnancy the maternal plasma levels of progesterone reach a peak 3 weeks after fertilization and then decline before increasing up until the time of parturition (Fig. 12.13). The initial peak reflects the development of the corpus luteum and the later rise is due to secretion by the placenta. Progesterone maintains the endometrium and suppresses spontaneous contractions of the my-ometrium of the uterus. Progesterone has relaxant effects at other sites in the body and also stimulates the development of the mammary glands.

Oestrogen

Oestriol is the main oestrogen secreted by the placenta; the maternal plasma levels of this hormone are shown in Fig. 12.13. The placenta cannot form the precursor steroid, 17-hydroxyprogesterone, and depends on the availability of dehydroepiandrosterone sulphate by the fetal adrenal gland. This steroid is desulphated by the placental sulphatase and converted to oestradiol, the levels of the latter and its metabolite oestradiol, provide an indication of the function of the **fetoplacental unit**. It is possible to monitor the well-being of the fetus by measuring the maternal urinary levels of oestriol but better information is obtained now by ultrasound scans. Although the total circulating levels of oestrogens increase some 50-fold during pregnancy, the levels of free oestrogens are not greatly increased because of a corresponding rise in the sex hormone-binding globulin. Oestrogens are required during pregnancy for the uterus to develop to accommodate the growing fetus and also for the development of the mammary glands.

Maternal changes during pregnancy

The mother's physiology adapts to provide for the growing fetus within her. By the end of the first **trimester** (3 months), her cardiac output has increased by 25–50%, through an increase in basal heart rate and a fall in the total peripheral resistance. There is also an increase in the total plasma volume early in pregnancy. Increased concentrations of circulating progesterone in pregnant women lead to increased ventilation and breathlessness in 60–70% of cases. The partial pressure of CO_2 in the maternal serum drops and plasma bicarbonate and sodium are reduced through renal excretion, leading to a drop in the osmolarity of the plasma. This decreases the secretion of antidiuretic hormone from the posterior pituitary, which causes both increased diuresis (frequency of urination) after fluid intake and increased thirst, especially in the first trimester. Over 60% of pregnant women suffer from morning sickness, a term used to describe symptoms that range from nausea upon rising, through to constant vomiting and dehydration due to an inability to retain food and fluid. Morning sickness is most prevalent in the first trimester of pregnancy. A significant number of women are hospitalized by this sickness, the causes of which remain obscure. Many pregnant women develop varicose veins as the pregnancy progresses. The growing weight of the fetus compresses the inferior vena cava, increasing the venous pressure in the legs. This results in the blood pooling in the legs and pelvic veins, forming varicosities. The compression may also lead to hypotension and fainting, as well as to oedema of the ankles.

Parturition

The exact trigger for parturition in women has not been established and the process is complex involving multiple mechanisms. While **progesterone** concentrations in the circulation do not fall immediately prior to delivery, there is evidence that locally within the myometrium there is an effective progesterone withdrawal. This decrease increases myometrial contractility. **Oxytocin** levels are increased in labour and this modest rise is augmented by a marked increase in oxytocin receptors in the myometrium and decidua and the combination leads to a stimulation of uterine contractions. Oxytocin is indeed used clinically to induce labour. Nevertheless, parturition can still be initiated in women with hypothalamic damage who lack oxytocin. **Prostaglandins** will also induce labour but again there is insufficient evidence that they provide the trigger for parturition in women. Their effective concentrations are a balance between the effects of progesterone and glucocorticoids. In sheep, however, it has been established that the fetus determines the time of delivery by increasing its release of **adrenocorticotrophic hormone** (ACTH) and hence cortisol. The increase in fetal cortisol secretion causes a change in placental steroid synthesis (increased ratio of oestrogens to progesterone) and stimulates prostaglandin synthesis leading to a facilitation of uterine contractility. The stimulation of ACTH probably results from the progressive increase in corticotrophin-releasing hormone (CRH) from placental sources and a decrease in its binding protein, resulting in an increase in ACTH secretion. Such a mechanism has been implicated as the way in which stress can initiate premature labour. These studies are reaching the point where the mechanisms, described above, can be modulated in effort to prevent the onset of premature labour.

Towards the end of pregnancy **relaxin**, a polypeptide hormone, can be extracted from the ovary, uterus and placenta. Relaxin and other similar polypeptides appear to play a role in parturition by promoting relaxation of the birth canal and the pubic symphysis and other pelvic joints.

Lactation

Mammary glands provide both milk for nourishment and antibodies for protection of the young. Milk is produced by epithelial cells lining the alveoli, which then drain into slender ducts. Development of the alveoli and ducts requires the presence of several hormones—oestrogen, progesterone, cortisol, CS and growth hormone. During the latter part of pregnancy, prolactin is required for full maturation of the mammary glands and eventually milk production. It also stimulates the production of calcitriol (p. 257) and so may help in maintaining calcium balance during pregnancy and lactation.

The initiation of copious lactation occurs shortly after parturition. It requires a fall in the concentrations of oestrogens and progesterone and a rise in prolactin. The steroids inhibit the effect of prolactin on milk production. Consequently, when the source of these steroids, the placenta, is removed, milk production is initiated.

While prolactin stimulates milk production, milk let-down depends on the release of oxytocin which is induced by suckling (p. 249). Suckling is also necessary for the continued release of prolactin because it stimulates nerve endings in the nipples, which in turn send impulses to the hypothalamus to inhibit the release of dopamine, the prolactin release-inhibiting hormone, and to stimulate the release of putative prolactin-releasing factors. In the absence of suckling, prolactin secretion is reduced and lactation ceases. The suckling stimulus and high prolactin levels also inhibit secretion of gonadotrophins, which presumably accounts for the suppression or delay in ovulation that occurs in nursing women.

Chapter 13

Blood

Blood is the fluid contained within the cardiovascular system; it is composed of cellular elements and plasma. The cellular elements comprise red blood cells (red cells, **erythrocytes**), white blood cells (white cells, **leukocytes**) and platelets (**thrombocytes**). The plasma is a complex aqueous solution containing electrolytes, protein, lipids, carbohydrates and many other organic constituents.

Blood circulates through the body distributing blood cells, nutrients, waste products, water, chemical messengers and heat thus helping to maintain homoeostasis and coordinate the activities of the different organs. The red cells are essential for the transport of the respiratory gases: O_2 from alveolar air to tissues, and CO_2 from tissues to alveolar air. White cells have important phagocytic and immunological functions. By transporting white cells and antibodies (**immunoglobulins**) to the tissues, the blood promotes defence against pathogenic organisms and foreign substances. The platelets and coagulation proteins in the plasma participate in blood clotting and stop bleeding (**haemostasis**) after injury.

If a sample of blood is collected in a tube containing anticoagulant and the tube is centrifuged, the blood will separate into cells and plasma (Fig. 13.1a). It is possible to estimate, from the lengths of the columns of red cells and plasma, the fraction of a volume of blood occupied by the red cells ($x/(x + y)$ in Fig. 13.1a). This is the **haemat-ocrit** or **packed cell volume** (PCV) (see Table 13.3).

The total volume of blood varies with body weight and is normally in the range of 60 to 80 mL per kg, so that a 70 kg subject would be expected to have about 5 L of blood. About 90% by weight of plasma is water, 8% is plasma proteins (Fig. 13.1b)—albumin, globulins (α, β, γ) and fibrinogen—and the remaining 2% consists of other organic compounds and electrolytes (see Table 1.1). Gamma globulins are synthesized by plasma cells in lymphoid tissue (p. 308) and form the antibodies that function in immunity. All other plasma proteins are synthesized in the liver. Albumin is the major contributor to the colloid osmotic (oncotic) pressure of the plasma responsible for maintaining the fluid volume within the intravascular space. Several hormones, bilirubin, fatty acids and Ca^{2+} are transported in the blood bound to albumin and globulins. Plasma coagulates when the soluble plasma protein fibrinogen is converted into insoluble fibrin (p. 320) forming a gel-like mesh. The liquid outside the clot is called **serum**, similar in composition to plasma except for fibrinogen and other coagulation factors.

13.1 Blood cell production

Blood cells are formed in the red bone marrow (as opposed to yellow bone marrow which is mainly fat) through lines of developing precursors, which

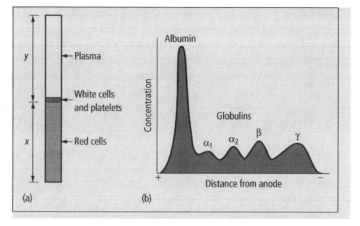

Fig. 13.1 (a) Fluid and cellular constituents of a sample of blood as seen after centrifugation. The fraction occupied by the red cells ($x/(x + y)$) is the haematocrit. (b) Separation of serum proteins by electrophoresis.

can be identified in samples of bone marrow. These immature cells arise in turn from populations of self-renewing, progenitor stem cells. Production of blood cells (**haematopoiesis**) is controlled by haematopoietic factors, which are cytokines released by supporting cells in the bone marrow, and by the hormone erythropoietin, secreted by the kidneys.

Sites of production

Haematopoiesis begins during the first few weeks of gestation with the appearance of primitive haematopoietic cells in the mesodermal tissues of the yolk sac. From about 6 weeks to 7 months blood cells are formed mainly in the liver but also in the spleen. During the fifth month, haematopoiesis begins in the red marrow of the bones. At birth, and throughout adulthood the bone marrow is the main site of haematopoiesis, with lymphocyte production continuing also in the spleen and other lymphoid tissues.

At first, red marrow occupies the cavities of all bones but from the age of 5–7 years, fat begins replacing the marrow of the limb bones. In adults, red marrow is normally confined to the bones of the trunk, the skull and the upper ends of the humerus and femur. Even at these sites about 50% of the marrow consists of fat but if there is increased demand for blood cells, the red marrow can expand into fatty spaces. The adult bone marrow consists of fat and developing blood cells in

clusters held together by fine reticulin fibres, separated by a network of sinusoidal capillaries, which drain into a central venous sinus. New cells are released into the blood through gaps in the endothelium of the marrow sinusoids.

Although red cells outnumber all other cell types in the blood by over 600 times, in the red marrow red cell precursors represent only about 25% of all precursor cells. This is because the turnover of red cells is far slower than that of all other blood cells. The life-span of red cells is about 120 days, whereas that of white cells in the circulation, and that of platelets, is generally less than ten days.

Samples of red marrow can be obtained for cytological examination by **aspiration** with a syringe and marrow-puncture needle, or by means of a **trephine**, with which a small core of marrow is cut from the bone for histological examination.

Stem cells and haematopoiesis

All types of blood cells produced in the bone marrow derive from uncommitted, pluripotent **haematopoietic stem cells** that are capable of **self-renewal**. Some of the daughter cells differentiate into committed **progenitor stem cells** that in turn differentiate into **precursor cells** for each of the different types of blood cell lineage. Precursor cells undergo terminal differentiation into mature blood cells (Fig. 13.2) and show recognizable morphologic features characteristic of each cell lineage. Current knowledge of progenitor populations

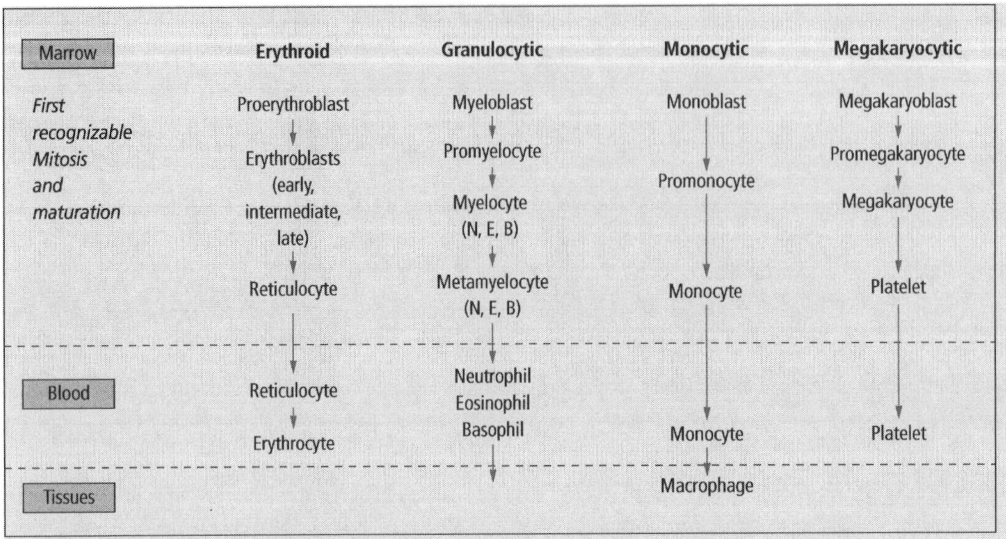

Marrow	Erythroid	Granulocytic	Monocytic	Megakaryocytic
First recognizable Mitosis and maturation	Proerythroblast ↓ Erythroblasts (early, intermediate, late) ↓ Reticulocyte	Myeloblast ↓ Promyelocyte ↓ Myelocyte (N, E, B) ↓ Metamyelocyte (N, E, B)	Monoblast ↓ Promonocyte ↓ Monocyte	Megakaryoblast ↓ Promegakaryocyte ↓ Megakaryocyte ↓ Platelet
Blood	Reticulocyte ↓ Erythrocyte	Neutrophil Eosinophil Basophil ↓	Monocyte ↓	Platelet
Tissues			Macrophage	

Fig. 13.2 Bone marrow production lines. B, basophil; E, eosinophil; N, neutrophil.

suggests that there is a common progenitor cell for megakaryocytes and erythrocytes, and for granulocytes and monocytes. Lymphocytes arise from a separate progenitor cell. Some lymphoid progenitor cells migrate from the bone marrow to the thymus and other lymphoid structures where they complete their development.

Haematopoietic cellular proliferation, differentiation, and lineage commitment are controlled by a variety of **haematopoietic factors** (often referred to as **growth factors**) that bind to specific receptors on the cell membrane. Most of these factors are **cytokines** (p. 307)—small proteins with paracrine activity—produced in the bone marrow by stromal cells, endothelial cells, leukocytes and macrophages. The main haematopoietic factors described comprise **colony-stimulating factors (CSF)**, interleukins, erythropoietin (p. 294), and thrombopoietin.

Stem cells cannot be recognized by microscopy in films of bone marrow but it is possible to grow them in culture where they give rise to colonies of descendant cells. Colony-stimulating factors are able to stimulate committed progenitor stem cells to proliferate *in vitro*, forming cell colonies of specific cell lineage(s). Macrophage-

CSF, granulocyte-CSF and granulocyte–macrophage-CSF promote, respectively, the development of either macrophages, granulocytes, or both. The colony-forming progenitor cells, often called **colony-forming units (CFU)**, are specified by the name of the cell(s) each colony comprises. For example, CFU-GEMM is a CFU with a potential for developing granulocytic, erythroid, monocytic and magakaryocytic lines; CFU-E gives rise to erythrocytes. The proliferation and commitment of haematopoietic stem cells is regulated by **stem cell factor** and by certain interleukins and CSF.

13.2 The red blood cell

Production of red cells (**erythropoiesis**) in the bone marrow involves overlapping stages of mitosis and maturation, with release of reticulocytes into the blood. Renal secretion of erythropoietin stimulates the rate of red blood cell production to keep pace with the rate of destruction. Erythropoiesis requires essential dietary constituents, particularly iron, vitamin B_{12} and folic acid. Depletion of the body stores of these substances can reduce red blood cell production.

Erythropoiesis

The process of red cell production (Fig. 13.3) begins with the differentiation of progenitor stem cells along the erythroid lineage. The first recognizable erythrocyte precursor is the **proerythroblast**, a large cell with loose chromatin, visible nucleoli and basophilic cytoplasm, indicating an abundance of polyribosomes. The proerythroblast follows a sequence of differentiation and maturation stages that include basophilic erythroblast (early basophilic), polychromatophilic erythroblast (intermediate polychromatic), orthochromic erythroblast (late pyknotic orthochromatic), reticulocyte, and erythrocyte. During this process the cell size progressively decreases and the organelles gradually disappear; there is a gradual decrease in the number of polyribosomes and a gradual increase in the haemoglobin content of the cytoplasm, reflected by a steady increase in cytoplasmic acidophilia; the capacity for mitosis ceases with the basophilic erythroblast, after which there is increasing nuclear condensation, and finally, nuclear extrusion preceding the reticulocyte stage. Reticulocytes contain remnants of RNA and polyribosomes, and continue synthesizing haemoglobin. After remaining in the bone marrow for 1–2 days, reticulocytes are released into the peripheral blood where within 1–2 days they lose their residual polyribosomes and mature into erythrocytes.

Reticulocytes can be identified in blood films with supravital stains, such as methylene blue or cresyl blue, which react with the polyribosomes to form precipitates visible as dark blue granules or filaments. The **reticulocyte count** (see Table 13.3) is a useful index of the erythropoietic activity of the bone marrow.

The process of erythropoieses from proerythroblast to the release of reticulocytes into the circulation, takes about 7 days. It involves overlapping

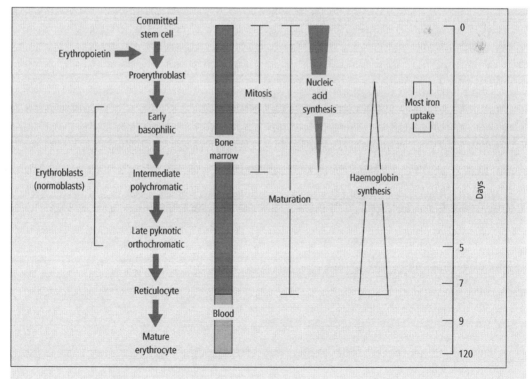

Fig. 13.3 Normal erythropoiesis.

biochemical events, with early uptake of iron by erythroblasts, decreasing synthesis of nucleic acids, and increasing synthesis of haemoglobin (Fig. 13.3).

Control of erythropoiesis

In health, the rate of red blood cell production by the bone marrow balances the rate at which old cells are destroyed. This steady state is controlled by the glycoprotein hormone **erythropoietin** (M_r 33 000), which is secreted mainly by the kidneys in response to local hypoxia. About 10–15% of the erythropoietin in adult blood is made by the liver. Erythropoietin is normally present in the plasma at low concentration (about $10 \, pmol \, L^{-1}$). It has a half-life in the circulation of about 5 h, and is inactivated in the liver. The hormone acts on the red bone marrow to stimulate the differentiation of committed progenitor stem cells into the erythrocyte lineage; it also increases the rate of mitosis of red cell precursors and shortens their maturation time. The result is an increased output of erythrocytes until the rise of blood haemoglobin concentration restores normal delivery of O_2 to the tissues.

Recombinant erythropoietin is available for therapeutic use. Its major therapeutic value is in the treatment of the otherwise intractable anaemia which occurs in chronic renal failure.

Growth factors secreted by cells in the bone marrow, and various other hormones besides erythropoietin, also stimulate erythropoiesis. Among them, corticosteroids, androgens, growth hormone and thyroxine. Some of these hormones may act by stimulating release of growth factors in the bone marrow.

Synthesis of haemoglobin and erythropoietic factors

Normal human **haemoglobin** consists of four iron-containing porphyrin rings—the **haem** moiety—each attached to a polypeptide chain. Together, the four polypeptide chains are referred to as the **globin** moiety. Proerythroblasts in the bone marrow initiate the synthesis of haemoglobin,

which continues until the reticulocyte stage. The **haem** and **globin** moieties are synthesized separately and then combined to form the haemoglobin molecule (Fig. 13.4). Certain dietary constituents such as iron, vitamin B_{12}, folic acid, vitamin B_6 (pyridoxine) and amino acids are required for the normal production of DNA and haemoglobin (Fig. 13.4). Deficiencies of any of these can decrease haemoglobin production and erythropoiesis. Haemoglobin synthesis may also be defective because of a fault (often genetic) in the production of haem or of globin.

Synthesis of haem begins in the mitochondria (Fig. 13.4) with the binding of succinyl coenzyme A to glycine, forming δ-aminolaevulinic acid (δ-ALA). This step requires vitamin B_6 as co-factor and is inhibited by haem. After several further reactions, protoporphyrin IX is formed, which then combines with ferrous iron to form the haem moiety. Iron is brought to the erythroblasts bound to the plasma protein **transferrin**. The iron–transferrin complex is endocytosed into the cell where the iron is released and the transferrin is returned to the extracellular fluid (Fig. 13.4). Some of the cellular iron is stored as **ferritin**, an iron–protein complex formed by the combination of iron with the protein apoferritin.

Iron

In adults, the total amount of **iron** in the body is between 2 and 5 g. About 60–70% of this iron is in haemoglobin (Table 13.1), and 4–5% in myoglobin of muscle. Small amounts of iron are present in some enzymes and in the cytochrome proteins of mitochondria. Most of the remaining body iron is

Table 13.1 Representative values of iron in adults.

	Men	Women
Haemoglobin iron (mmol L^{-1} blood)	8–11	7–10
Stored iron (mmol)	5–27	0–18
Serum iron (µmol L^{-1})	14–32	11–30
Serum iron-binding capacity (µmol L^{-1})	50–70	50–70
Serum ferritin (µg L^{-1})	40–340	15–140

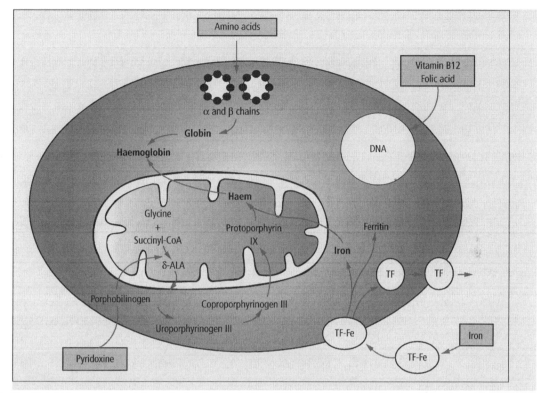

Fig. 13.4 Dietary requirements for synthesis of haemoglobin and DNA in erythroblasts. δ-ALA, δ-aminolevulinic acid; CoA, coenzyme A; TF, transferrin.

stored in hepatocytes and in macrophages of the liver, spleen and bone marrow, as **ferritin**. Smaller quantities of iron are stored as **haemosiderin** — an insoluble complex of iron and protein. Ferritin is also present in the blood (Table 13.1) at concentrations that reflect the level of iron stores. Normally, women have less iron than men because of the periodic iron loss during menstrual bleeding.

In the plasma, iron is transported bound to **transferrin**, a protein synthesized in the liver at a rate that varies directly with the level of stored iron. Transferrin is normally only one-third saturated with iron so that **serum iron** concentrations are lower than the total **iron-binding capacity** (Table 13.1). The total iron-binding capacity increases when the serum iron concentration is low and decreases with iron overload. It is useful in monitoring certain clinical conditions with altered iron levels, such as iron deficiency anaemia.

The concentration of serum ferritin is usually a more accurate index of the state of the body iron stores than the serum iron and total iron binding capacity. Iron intake and absorption, and the factors affecting these, are discussed in Chapter 19 (p. 532).

Iron exchanges and requirements for balance
The iron in plasma, about 70 μmol in a 70-kg man, turns over between five and ten times a day. Of this turnover, about 80–85% arises from movement of iron from the extracellular fluid to the bone marrow for haemoglobin synthesis, and from phagocytic cells in the liver, spleen and bone marrow to the extracellular fluid, as iron is released from degraded haemoglobin (Fig. 13.5). The remaining movements of iron through the plasma are accounted for by exchanges of iron with non-erythroid tissues, including absorption from the

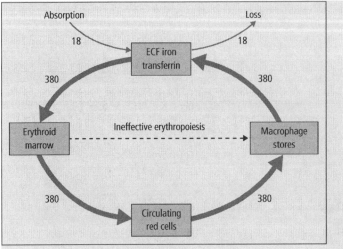

Fig. 13.5 Daily iron exchanges. Values (μmol) for a 70-kg man with a haemoglobin concentration of $150\,g\,L^{-1}$ and red cell life-span of 120 days. Iron exchanges from ineffective erythropoiesis are omitted. ECF, extracellular fluid.

small intestine and loss in exfoliated intestinal cells.

The daily loss of iron in adults, mainly from the gut, is between 9 and 18 μmol. Small amounts are also lost in sweat and urine. Women lose, in effect, an extra 9–18 μmol^{-1} day^{-1} due to menstruation and require an additional 18–36 μmol day^{-1} during pregnancy. Adolescents and infants require extra iron for growth. **Negative iron balance** occurs if these daily needs are not met by absorption of iron from the diet.

Iron from the breakdown of red cells is reused for erythropoiesis. Stored iron is available to meet extra demands.

Iron deficiency

A continuous net loss of iron will lead to exhaustion of the iron stores and a fall in serum iron, despite a compensatory rise in iron-binding capacity. When the saturation of transferrin falls to less than 15%, delivery of iron to the bone marrow is impaired and **iron-deficiency anaemia** develops.

Physiological and pathological conditions may cause a negative iron balance and iron deficiency. **Increased physiological demands** for iron occur during periods of rapid growth, pregnancy and lactation. Menstrual blood loss may increase the requirements for iron. A low dietary iron intake would contribute to iron deficiency. By far the most common cause of iron deficiency in adults is pathological **blood loss**, especially when the bleeding is chronic. The gastrointestinal tract and the uterus are the main sources of blood loss. Blood with a haemoglobin concentration of $150\,gL^{-1}$ contains about 9 μmol of iron per millilitre. An average daily loss of more than 10 mL of blood is likely to cause a negative iron balance because this volume will contain more iron than can be maximally absorbed (about 90 μmol), from a normal daily diet containing about 270 μmol of iron.

Vitamin B$_{12}$

Vitamin B$_{12}$ (cobalamin) is a cobalt-containing molecule synthesized by bacteria. The chief dietary sources of cobalamin are protein-rich foods of animal origin—liver, kidney, muscle, eggs, cheese, milk. The ingested vitamin combines with **intrinsic factor**, a protein secreted by parietal cells in the stomach, and the complex is absorbed in the terminal ileum (p. 533).

Aspects of vitamin B$_{12}$ balance are summarized in Table 13.2. An adult loses about 1.5 nmol of vitamin B$_{12}$ each day, mainly in the urine and the faeces, and needs to absorb a similar amount daily to stay in balance. Body stores, mainly in the liver, are enough to meet requirements for 3–4 years, if dietary intake were to cease completely.

Table 13.2 Vitamin B_{12} and folic acid.

	Vitamin B_{12}	Folic acid
Daily diet supplies	4–22 nmol	900–2300 nmol
Absorption limit	2.5 nmol day^{-1}	50–100% of intake
Absorption site	Ileum	Duodenum, jejunum
Daily needs	1.5 nmol	220 nmol
Adult store	1500–2200 nmol	14–45 µmol
Time for depletion	3–4 years	2–7 months
Serum concentration	150–700 pmol L^{-1}*	4–20 nmol L^{-1}*
Red cell concentration	—	300–1500 nmol L^{-1}*

* Radioimmunoassay; values for normal range depend on method.

Deficiency of vitamin B_{12} is almost always the result of impaired absorption; only rarely does it arise from inadequate dietary intake (e.g. in strict vegetarians). Impaired cobalamin absorption may be caused by a lack of intrinsic factor—in gastrectomy, with loss of parietal cells; or in pernicious anaemia. Cobalamin absorption may also be affected by a reduced absorptive capacity of the ileum (in ileal disease), ileal resection, or competition for the vitamin by intestinal parasites or bacteria.

Folic acid

Folic acid (pteroylglutamic acid) is a vitamin normally available in the diet, mainly as a polyglutamate. The highest concentrations of folate are found in liver, yeast, green vegetables, nuts and fruit. Dietary folate may provide as much as 2.3 µmol daily. The amount available varies widely depending on the type of food eaten and the method of preparation, since folic acid is easily destroyed by cooking. Absorption of folate occurs in the duodenum and jejunum (p. 533).

Handling of folate in the body is summarized in Table 13.2. An adult requires about 220 nmol of folic acid daily and up to 660 nmol or more per day during pregnancy. Folate and its breakdown products are lost in the urine and sweat. In contrast to the ample storage of vitamin B_{12}, the stores of folic acid, mainly in the liver, are small relative to the daily requirement. In the absence of folate intake, body stores can become exhausted in several months (Table 13.2), so that severe deficiency of folate can develop rapidly.

Inadequate dietary intake of folate will contribute to folate deficiency caused by: defective absorption (in small intestinal mucosal disease); drugs (anticonvulsants, alcohol); or increased demands for the vitamin when cellular turnover is rapid, as in physiological states (pregnancy) or in certain pathological conditions (malignant tumours).

Megaloblastic erythropoiesis

Deficiency of vitamin B_{12} or folic acid leads to decreased DNA synthesis in proliferating tissues and produces characteristic morphological abnormalities in the bone marrow. The erythroid precursors are larger than normal (megaloblasts) and impaired synthesis of DNA leads to a delay in maturation of the nucleus relative to the cytoplasm; similarly, circulating red blood cells are enlarged (macrocytes). The production of white cells and platelets is also affected, and a macrocytic anaemia is often accompanied by low granulocyte and platelet counts in the blood.

Characteristics of red cells

The mature red cell lacks nucleus and organelles. It is a biconcave disc, 7–8 µm in diameter, 2.5 µm thick near the rim and 1 µm thick at the centre. The flat shape, with a large area : volume ratio, is optimized for rapid diffusion of the respiratory gases into and out of the cell. Gas transport is mediated by two specialized molecular machines: a Cl^-:HCO_3^- exchange carrier (the anion exchanger) in the red cell membrane, and haemoglobin. The anion exchanger is expressed with 1.1 million copies per cell, and is critical for the transport of CO_2 (see p. 20). The haemoglobin concentration in cell water is about 7 mM, one of the highest soluble protein concentrations of any cell. Keeping the volume of a water-permeable cell with a high haemoglobin concentration constant, in a plasma environment that has a much lower protein concentration, is not a trivial challenge: the formidable oncotic pressure created by the high haemoglobin concentration would lead to rapid swelling and lysis of the red cell unless somehow balanced. The general strategy that red cells have evolved to live for a relatively long period of time, and to prevent bursting, is to maintain an extremely low membrane permeability to cations, particularly Na^+, the most abundant extracellular solute. Minor residual cation leaks can be balanced by small numbers of sodium and calcium extruding pumps in the membrane, with only minute metabolic demands. Thus, cation-tight red cells efficiently transport O_2 and CO_2 during long life-spans at minimal metabolic cost, sustained exclusively by a low-level glycolytic metabolism.

Electronic cell counters are now generally used to measure standard red cell and reticulocyte parameters. Table 13.3 lists ranges of normal values.

These ranges represent variations in mean values observed in blood samples from different normal subjects. In each sample, the values of individual red cells fluctuate around the mean within remarkably narrow limits, particularly so for haemoglobin concentration. Thus, red cell volume and haemoglobin content variations have a standard deviation of about 13% around the mean, whereas haemoglobin concentration, which represents the ratio of haemoglobin content to volume in each cell has a standard deviation of only 6% around the mean. This uniformity is particularly extraordinary if one takes into consideration that about 2×10^{11} red cells are produced and destroyed per day in a normal adult.

The red cell membrane

The membrane of the red cell is composed of a lipid bilayer with its embedded proteins, and an underlying, mesh-like, filamentous network—the red cell cytoskeleton. Unlike all other cells, mammalian red cells only possess a cortical cytoskeleton. The two-dimensional mesh under the lipid bilayer is composed mainly of spectrin, a dimer consisting of α and β subunits, and filamentous actin. The cytoskeleton controls red cell shape and dynamic deformability through anchor linkages with integral membrane proteins, mainly band 3 and glycophorin A (Fig. 13.6). The most important linking proteins are protein 4.1 and ankyrin. Cytoskeleton defects are responsible for some inhe-

Table 13.3 Normal red cell values as the 95% range (mean ± 2 SD). (Data from Dacie, J.V. & Lewis, S.M. (1995) *Practical Haematology*, 8th edn, pp. 12, 17. Churchill Livingstone, London.)

	Men	Women	Children (2–6 years)
Red cell count (×10^{12} L^{-1} blood)	4.5–5.5	3.8–4.8	3.9–5.3
Haemoglobin (g L^{-1} blood)	130–170	120–150	110–140
Haematocrit (packed cell volume)	0.40–0.50	0.36–0.46	0.34–0.40
Mean cell volume (fL)	83–101	83–101	75–87
Mean cell haemoglobin (pg)	27–32	27–32	24–30
Mean cell haemoglobin concentration (g L^{-1} cells)	315–345	315–345	310–370
Reticulocyte count (×10^9 L^{-1} blood)	50–100	50–100	10–100
Reticulocyte count (%)	0.5–2.5	0.5–2.5	0.2–2.0

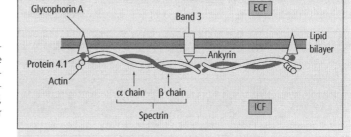

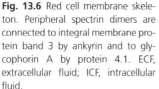

Fig. 13.6 Red cell membrane skeleton. Peripheral spectrin dimers are connected to integral membrane protein band 3 by ankyrin and to glycophorin A by protein 4.1. ECF, extracellular fluid; ICF, intracellular fluid.

rited abnormalities of erythrocyte shape, e.g. hereditary spherocytosis and hereditary elliptocytosis.

The most abundant integral membrane protein within band 3 (Fig. 13.6) is the anion exchanger, with over one million copies per cell. The Na^+ pump (Na^+,K^+–ATPase), with about 400 copies per cell is expressed; and the Ca^{2+} pump (Ca^{2+},Mg^{2+}–ATPase), with about 1000 copies per cell. Carbohydrates occur mainly as glycolipids and glycoproteins on the external surface of the membrane and often have blood-group specificity (e.g. A, B, H antigens; Table 13.5).

Haemoglobin

The red respiratory pigment of the erythrocyte, **haemoglobin**, is composed of four polypeptide chains of the protein globin, each containing a haem molecule. Haem consists of a protoporphyrin ring with a central atom of ferrous iron, which can combine reversibly with a molecule of O_2.

There are four types of globin chains, α, β, γ and δ, which differ in their constituent amino acids. In an adult, 96–98% of the circulating haemoglobin is **haemoglobin A**, the globin of which has two α chains and two β chains. Adults also have small amounts of **haemoglobin A_2** ($\alpha_2\delta_2$) and of **haemoglobin F** ($\alpha_2\gamma_2$), which is the main haemoglobin of the fetus.

The tetrameric structure of haemoglobin allows conformational changes in the molecule, which account for important characteristics of O_2 transport. These are discussed on p. 468.

Red cell metabolism

About 95% of the glucose consumed by red cells is metabolized by anaerobic glycolysis; 5% is used by the pentose–phosphate pathway. The ATP concentration within the red cell is about 1.5 mM and its turnover is about 3 mmol per litre cells per hour. Of this, about 1 mmol per litre cells per hour is consumed by the Na^+ pump to balance the small passive Na^+–K^+ leaks. The glycolytic pathway also maintains a supply of reduced nicotinamide adenine dinucleotide (NADH). This is a coenzyme for a reductase enzyme that helps to maintain the iron of haemoglobin in the ferrous (Fe^{2+}) state. If the iron is oxidized to the ferric (Fe^{3+}) state, the **methaemoglobin** so formed cannot combine reversibly with O_2. Methaemoglobin may also be reduced with the aid of the coenzyme nicotinamide adenine dinucleotide phosphate (NADPH), which is produced by the pentose–phosphate pathway. The reducing power of NADPH is also made available to the cell through its linkage with the tripeptide, **glutathione**. This reducing agent provides protection against the oxidation of sulphydryl groups of enzymes, globin and constituents of the membrane. It also counteracts auto-oxidation of membrane lipids and helps dispose of any hydrogen peroxide that forms.

A side-reaction of the glycolytic pathway in erythrocytes leads to the synthesis of 2,3-bisphosphoglycerate (2,3-BPG) from 1,3-bisphosphoglycerate. The 2,3-BPG combines with haemoglobin to reduce its affinity for O_2, thus promoting delivery of O_2 to the tissues. Conditions causing hypoxia (e.g. high altitude, anaemia) lead to increased synthesis of 2,3-BPG and therefore increased release of O_2 from haemoglobin.

Life-span and breakdown of red cells

Human red cells have programmed senescence, the mechanism of which is still debated. With a life-span of about 120 days in the circulation, a little under 1% of the circulating red cells is destroyed each day and must be replaced by reticulocytes released from the bone marrow. For a man of 70 kg, this turnover of cells amounts to about 2.6 million every second.

As red cells age in the circulation, their volume is slowly reduced by the net loss of KCl and water, becoming more dense. Density fractionation using Percoll or arabinogalactan density gradients is thus routinely used to separate red cell subpopulations of different age, allowing the study of age-related changes. These showed a decline in the activity of glycolytic and other enzymes with cell age. At the end of their lives, probably in response to antigenic changes in the membrane surface, the red cells are removed from the circulation by macrophages in the bone marrow, spleen and liver. Within the macrophage, the red cell is broken down with release and degradation of haemoglobin (Fig. 13.7). The amino acids of globin are returned to the general amino acid pool of the body. The haem groups are broken down by microsomal enzymes, with release of iron to the extracellular protein transferrin and its transport to erythroblasts for insertion into new haem groups (Fig. 13.4), or to iron stores. The remainder of the haem group is converted to **bilirubin** which enters the blood where it is attached to albumin and is carried to the liver. Here the bilirubin is conjugated to glucuronic acid and secreted in the bile. In the intestine bacteria convert the bilirubin into various products which are excreted in the faeces or are absorbed and excreted in the urine or released again into the bile (Fig. 13.7; see also p. 519).

Anaemia

In functional terms, anaemia is a disorder in which a decrease in the amount of circulating haemoglobin reduces the oxygen-carrying capacity of the blood so that this is insufficient to meet the needs of the tissues for oxygen. For clinical purposes, anaemia is defined by a reduction in the concentration of haemoglobin in the blood below the lower limit of the normal range for the age and sex of the patient. A woman is therefore anaemic if her haemoglobin concentration is less than $115 \, g \, L^{-1}$. The corresponding value for men is $130 \, g \, L^{-1}$, and for children aged 1 year it is $105 \, g \, L^{-1}$ (Table 13.3). This way of defining anaemia has obvious limitations. Thus, people may have apparently normal haemoglobin concentrations, which are, nevertheless, suboptimal or pathologically low for them; while others, defined as anaemic, may in fact belong to that part of the population whose haemoglobin concentration is below the lower limit of a 95% range. Interpretation of haemoglobin concentration data may thus require caution. However, anaemias severe enough to cause symptoms are usually associated with unequivocally low concentrations of haemoglobin in the blood.

Causes of anaemia

Anaemia, with a decrease in red cell mass, may arise from one (or more) of three fundamental disturbances: decreased production of red cells, increased destruction of red cells or bleeding. Such disturbances may cause characteristic changes in appearance of circulating erythrocytes, while physiological adjustments occur to maintain oxygenation of the tissues despite the reduced oxygen-carrying capacity of the blood. Decreased production of erythrocytes may be due to a reduction in the rate of proliferation of precursors in the marrow, the **hypoproliferative anaemias**, or may arise from **defective maturation** of red cells, often associated with an abnormal degree of ineffective erythropoiesis.

Reduced proliferation of red cell precursors is commonly caused by deficiency of iron and, in many chronic inflammatory disorders, by an apparent failure of release of iron by macrophages. Decreased output of erythropoietin from diseased kidneys, infiltration of the bone marrow by abnormal cells (e.g. leukaemia), and failure of the mar-

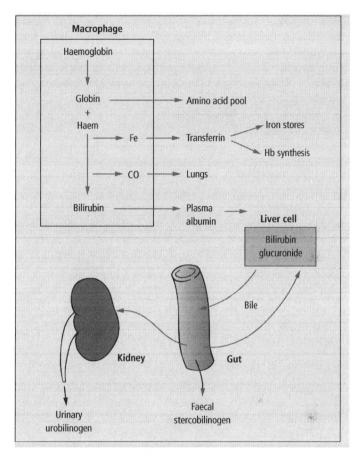

Fig. 13.7 Degradation of haemoglobin (Hb). CO, carbon monoxide.

row due to drugs, toxic chemicals and ionizing radiations also cause anaemia by reducing erythropoiesis. These hypoproliferative anaemias are associated with a blood reticulocyte count that is disproportionately low for the degree of anaemia, and the bone marrow is characteristically hypocellular with depressed erythropoiesis evident.

Abnormalities of maturation may affect nuclear function or synthesis of haemoglobin in erythroblasts. Deficiency of vitamin B_{12}, folate, or both, interferes with DNA synthesis, which leads to megaloblastic erythropoiesis (p. 297). Genetic defects can cause reduced production of globin chains (**thalassaemias**), or variations in the structure of globin chains (**haemoglobinopathies**), with resultant instability of the haemoglobin molecule or abnormal functioning in the transport of oxygen. An increased premature destruction of red cells may arise from an intrinsic defect in the red cell itself (defective synthesis of haemoglobin, enzymes or membrane components), or from extrinsic factors (autoimmune disorders, drugs, infections, etc). In such **haemolytic** anaemias, the life-span of the red cells is reduced and the increased destruction results in a raised output of bilirubin, which may be visible in the tissues as **jaundice** (p. 536). The tissue hypoxia causes increased secretion of erythropoietin, which leads to compensatory erythroid hyperplasia in the bone marrow and a raised blood reticulocyte count.

Among the inherited haemolytic anaemias, **sickle cell anaemia** is one of the most common. It is caused by the homozygous inheritance of the abnormal haemoglobin S. The haemoglobin S gene is prevalent in malaria endemic regions because it confers some protection against cerebral malaria—the most lethal form—caused by *Plasmodium falciparum*. Protection extends even to heterozygous carriers, whose red cells have only about 40% haemoglobin S and are not diseased. The mechanism of protection is still debated. Sickle cell anaemia affects millions throughout the world, particularly people from sub-Saharan Africa or who have ancestors from that region. Haemoglobin S differs from the normal haemoglobin A in a single amino acid, a valine for glutamic acid substitution on the β-chain of haemoglobin. In homozygous patients with 100% haemoglobin S in their red cells, haemoglobin S polymerizes upon deoxygenation in the venous circulation. It forms needle-like projections that deform the red cells into sickle-like shapes. These projections increase the membrane permeability to mono and divalent cations. Permeabilization reverses on reoxygenation, but repeated cycles of polymerization–depolymerization in the circulation lead to a cascade of secondary reactions, which cause profound and variable alterations in the homeostasis of red cells. Critical in this cascade is the participation of two red-cell membrane transporters: a Ca^{2+}-activated K^+-selective channel (the Gardos channel) and a K^+–Cl^- cotransporter. The life-span of sickle cells is dramatically reduced causing anaemia and reticulocytosis. A subpopulation of relatively young red cells becomes profoundly dehydrated and irreversibly sickled (irreversibly sickled cells), predisposing the patients to vaso-occlusion in the microcirculation of different organs, which is responsible for the major symptoms in this disease. Treatment is largely symptomatic; therapies aimed at preventing the formation of dehydrated, irreversibly sickled cells by targeting the transport abnormalities are currently undergoing clinical trials.

Genetic and acquired anomalies may also lead to defective synthesis of haem, with a striking abnormal accumulation of iron in erythroblasts (**sideroblastic anaemias**).

Acute loss of blood and hence of O_2-carrying capacity may result in the medical emergency of hypovolaemic shock (p. 421), but chronic bleeding, especially if it is intermittent, may cause an anaemia to develop very slowly. The anaemia will usually occur only after the iron stores in the body are exhausted (p. 296).

Red cell indices and anaemias

Anaemias may also be classified in terms of the red cell indices—mean cell volume (normocytic, macrocytic or microcytic), mean cell haemoglobin and mean cell haemoglobin concentration (normochromic, hypochromic) (Table 13.3). This classification has the advantage that it immediately suggests a short list of likely disorders and hence any additional tests required. It may also allow identification of an important defect before overt anaemia has developed.

Macrocytic normochromic anaemias are characteristically those associated with megaloblastic erythropoiesis (vitamin B_{12} or folate deficiency) but also rise in alcoholism, liver disease and hypothyroidism. Increased numbers of circulating reticulocytes may also give a macrocytic blood picture. **Microcytic hypochromic** anaemias are most often due to iron deficiency but also occur with thalassaemias and with sideroblastic defects. **Normocytic** and **normochromic** anaemias are commonly secondary to some chronic disorder (e.g. infection, renal failure, rheumatoid arthritis) but also occur in haemolysis, after acute bleeding, in bone marrow failure and as a result of infiltration of the marrow by abnormal cells (e.g. metastatic carcinoma).

Compensatory adjustments in anaemia

Delivery of O_2 from the lungs to the tissues involves a number of steps, of which transport by haemoglobin is only one (Chapter 18). Ventilation, cardiac output, differential control of peripheral resistance to blood flow, and diffusion from the capillaries to cells are other links in the chain. In general, a decrease in effectiveness of any of these components of the O_2-transport system may be counteracted by increased activity of the others. In anaemia, various adjustments occur in order to compensate for the reduced O_2-carrying capacity of the blood so as to maintain oxygenation of the tissues.

As the haemoglobin concentration falls, there is greater deoxygenation of haemoglobin in the capillaries. There is also increased synthesis of 2,3-BPG in the red cells, which promotes deoxygenation of haemoglobin, shifting the oxyhaemoglobin dissociation curve to the right (Fig. 18.27). While the rise in 2,3-BPG allows greater unloading of O_2 from arterial blood, this leaves a smaller venous O_2 content and thus a diminished reserve available for extra demands (e.g. in exercise). The total blood volume is maintained by an increase in plasma volume, despite the decreased red cell mass. There is also a redistribution of the flow of blood away from organs like the kidneys and the skin to more vital areas such as the myocardium, brain and skeletal muscle.

When the blood haemoglobin concentration falls below about $70-80\,g\,L^{-1}$, cardiac output rises, at rest and during exercise. This is due to an increase in both stroke volume and heart rate. A net vasodilation, with more rapid flow of blood with reduced viscosity (because of the decreased red cell mass), gives rise to the characteristic **hyperkinetic** circulation of chronic anaemia.

The extent to which these adjustments allow adaptation to anaemia will depend upon a number of factors, including the severity of the anaemia, its speed of onset and the adequacy of myocardial oxygenation and function.

13.3 The white blood cells

White blood cells defend the body by phagocytosis of foreign organisms and by specific immune responses to non-self invaders. The five types of white cell, which can be identified in stained blood films, develop in the bone marrow under the stimulus of several growth factors. Abnormal white blood cell counts occur in infections, allergies, disorders of the bone marrow and other conditions.

The white cells of the blood form two main groups both with defensive functions: **phagocytes**, which can engulf and destroy bacteria and other foreign matter; and **lymphocytes**, the effector cells of the immune system (p. 306). The phagocytic cells comprise **polymorphonuclear leukocytes**, in which the nucleus is often divided into several lobes, and **monocytes**, the precursors of **macrophages**—phagocytic cells that can be **fixed** or **free** in the tissues. All these phagocytic cells have cytoplasmic granules, which are often lysosomes. The granules of the polymorphonuclear leukocytes react with Romanowsky stains to give characteristic appearances in blood films and this allows the identification of three cell types: neutrophils, eosinophils and basophils, often known collectively as **granulocytes**. Normal ranges of total and differential white cell counts in the blood are listed in Table 13.4.

The **neutrophil** is the most frequently occurring white blood cell in adults. Its cytoplasmic granules are lysosomal in nature and liberate enzymes able to kill bacteria when the granules fuse with **phagosomes** (vacuoles containing bacteria or foreign material taken up by phagocytosis). Neutrophils act as phagocytes in acute inflammation (p. 305).

The granules of the **eosinophil** contain lysosomal enzymes and a protein called **major basic protein**, which has cytotoxic activity against parasites

Table 13.4 Normal white cell counts ($\times 10^9\,L^{-1}$ blood) as the 95% range (mean $\pm$ 2 SD). (Data from Dacie, J.V. & Lewis, S.M. (1995) *Practical Haematology*, 8th edn, pp. 12, 17. Churchill Livingstone, London.)

Cell	Adults	Children (2–6 years)
Neutrophils	2.0–7.0	1.5–8.0
Lymphocytes	1.0–3.0	6.0–9.0
Monocytes	0.2–1.0	0.1–1.0
Eosinophils	0.02–0.5	0.2–1.0
Basophils	0.02–0.1	0.02–0.1
Total	4.0–10.0	5.0–15.0

and may also cause tissue damage. Eosinophils play a role in combating parasitic infestations, in phagocytosing antigen–antibody complexes and in modulating the effects of histamine and leukotrienes in allergic reactions.

The most infrequent white cell in the blood is the **basophil** (Table 13.4). Its granules contain heparin and histamine. There are some similarities between basophils and the mast cells in tissue spaces but the precise relationship is not clear. Both types of cell have membrane receptors for immunoglobulin E (IgE), and the combination of cell and antibody in immediate hypersensitivity reactions (p. 309) leads to release of the contents of the granules.

Monocytes and macrophages contain lysosomal granules. Macrophages have important phagocytic functions and promote stimulation of the immune system by antigens (p. 306).

Most **lymphocytes** in the blood are only a little larger than red cells. They comprise two main groups, **T cells** and **B cells**, which mediate immune reactions triggered by antigens (p. 306).

Granulocyte production and life-span

Granulocytes and monocytes develop in the red bone marrow from a common progenitor. The earliest recognizable granulocyte precursor is the **myeloblast**, which subsequently matures through the stages of **promyelocyte** and **myelocyte** (Fig. 13.2). The specific cytoplasmic granules first appear in the myelocyte and mitosis continues up to the end of this stage. Thereafter, with loss of mitotic capacity, the cells get smaller and there is progressive condensation of the nucleus in the **metamyelocyte** and **band** stages. Nuclear segmentation occurs in the mature granulocyte.

After mitosis, granulocytes spend up to a week maturing further before release to the blood. There are large numbers of metamyelocytes, band forms and mature cells kept in reserve in the marrow. This relative abundance of developing granulocytes is indicated by the ratio of white cell to red cell precursors, the **myeloid to erythroid ratio**. In normal marrow, this varies between 2.5 : 1 and 15 : 1, and a normal marrow stores between 15 and 20

times as many granulocytes as are present in the blood. Control of granulocyte production depends on a number of growth factors (p. 292). Some of these growth factors may be specific for a particular type of developing cell but others appear to act at various points in a number of different cell lines. A number of growth factors have now been made by recombinant DNA technology and one at least is used to accelerate production of neutrophils in patients who have had a bone marrow transplant.

Following release into the blood, neutrophils are present in about equal numbers, either freely circulating or rolling in a marginating pool along the walls of capillaries and venules. These latter cells are not included in a white cell count of blood but there is a rapid and free exchange of cells between the circulating and marginal pools. Neutrophils spend about 10 h in the blood before being lost at random into the tissues. Here they survive for probably 4–5 days before removal by macrophages after they have performed their phagocytic functions or have become senescent.

Eosinophils remain in the circulation longer than neutrophils and show diurnal fluctuations in concentration which are related inversely to the secretion of the hormone cortisol (p. 263). Monocytes are stored to some extent in the marrow and spend 20–40 h in the blood before leaving to become macrophages in the tissues, where they may survive for months or years.

Abnormal white cell counts

An increase in circulating neutrophils, **neutrophil leukocytosis** (neutrophilia), is usually due to increased output from the marrow in response to bacterial infections, to inflammation and necrosis of tissues, or to acute haemorrhage. Very high counts, with precursor marrow cells in the blood, occur in **chronic granulocytic leukaemia**. A neutrophil count below the lower limit of normal, **neutropenia**, can occur due to the action of drugs on the marrow, in severe infections when output of neutrophils may fail to keep pace with demand, and as part of a **pancytopenia**, e.g. in bone marrow failure.

An increased lymphocyte count, **lymphocytosis**, occurs in viral illness, in chronic bacterial infections (e.g. tuberculosis), and commonly in young children as a reaction to infections which produce a neutrophilia in adults. A high lymphocyte count in the middle-aged and elderly is commonly due to **chronic lymphocytic leukaemia**. A reduced lymphocyte count, **lymphopenia**, is uncommon but occurs in severe bone marrow failure, in **acquired immunodeficiency syndrome** (AIDS), and in patients taking immunosuppressive drugs. Raised concentrations of eosinophils, **eosinophilia**, are seen in allergic disorders (e.g. hay fever), parasitic infestations, reactions to drugs and in certain skin diseases (e.g. psoriasis). A **monocytosis** occurs in chronic bacterial infections while a raised basophil count (**basophilia**) is uncommon and is usually an accompaniment of a myeloproliferative disorder such as chronic granulocytic leukaemia.

Acute inflammation

Acute inflammation is the local response of living tissues to injury which may be due, for example, to infection, trauma, extremes of heat and cold, chemical agents, ultraviolet light, ionizing radiation and sometimes to antigen–antibody complexes. Tissue injury is also associated with other local reactions (chronic inflammation, repair and regeneration) and with general reactions (fever and leukocytosis). The **acute inflammatory reaction** is characterized by **local vasodilation** causing redness and heat, and by **increased vascular permeability**, with the consequent increased accumulation of a protein-rich exudate and swelling. These reactions are mediated by a number of substances, such as plasma **kinins** activated in tissues and **histamine** released from mast cells and basophils. Kinins and histamine also stimulate nerve endings in the infected area, producing the sensation of pain. Concomitantly with the exudation of fluid, leukocytes migrate from the circulation into the infected area in response to **chemotaxins** released by microorganisms, by damaged tissues, or as products of complement activation (see below). The cells involved in acute inflammation are **neutrophils** (polymorphs) and **monocytes**, the latter being transformed into **macrophages** on entering the tissues. These cells phagocytose microorganisms and help to remove the tissue debris. The inflammatory exudate facilitates these processes and also serves to dilute noxious agents. The immune system also contributes to inflammation by virtue of:

1 antibacterial and antitoxic antibodies which may be present in the exudate;

2 derivatives of the complement cascade; and

3 the antiviral substance interferon.

The immune system

The immune system, like the inflammatory reaction, deals with foreign invaders but discriminates very precisely between one invader and another. Once learned, its lessons are long remembered.

The relative importance of the immune system is well illustrated by the high mortality accompanying the major immunodeficiency diseases. Immune responses can be distinguished from the inflammatory reaction by virtue of the following characteristics:

1 Specificity—an immune system is tailored to deal with the initiating agent (**antigen**) through specific **antibody** and **cell-mediated** reactions. In contrast, inflammation is non-specific.

2 Memory—a first encounter with an antigen is subsequently remembered, so that second and subsequent encounters with the same antigen provoke a more effective response.

3 Discrimination between self and non-self—the host does not normally react with itself. Indeed, specific immunological non-reactivity (self-tolerance) normally protects the tissues of the host against immunological attack. Thus immune responses are characteristically directed against chemical groupings recognized as foreign.

Antigens

Most antigens are proteins or polysaccharides of M_r above 5000–10 000. Smaller molecules called **haptens** sometimes provoke an immune reaction if they become attached to body proteins or cells (e.g. nickel allergy). Only part of an antigenic molecule, the **antigenic determinant**, reacts specifically with the corresponding antibody. A determinant may be repeated several times on a single antigenic molecule or on a cell. Antigens important in clinical medicine include:

1 parts of the surface membrane of microorganisms;

2 toxic products of microorganisms, e.g. tetanus toxin;

3 parts of the surface membrane of human cells (these antigens are important in blood transfusion and transplantation);

4 substances used therapeutically which sometimes act as haptens giving rise to drug allergies; and

5 plant and animal antigens (e.g. pollen, animal dander, bee venom), which may provoke aberrant (allergic) immune responses.

Proteins from species other than humans will in general be recognized as foreign. The ability to provoke an immune response is not an absolute attribute of a molecule; host factors ultimately determine the extent to which an antigen will be seen as such.

The effector cells of the immune system

Lymphocytes are the main effector cells of the immune system and originate from bone marrow precursor cells. They comprise two main populations: T **lymphocytes** (–80%) and B **lymphocytes** (15–20%). A small population of circulating cells apparently belongs to neither group (**null cells**).

T lymphocytes depend on the thymus for their maturation (hence T cells), while B lymphocytes probably mature in the bone marrow. B lymphocytes were originally identified in birds, in which the bursa of Fabricius (hence B cells) is necessary for their maturation. This organ has no exact mammalian counterpart. While T and B cells are morphologically indistinguishable in routine histological preparations, they differ with respect to:

1 certain cell-surface proteins which can be used as markers in clinical pathology;

2 the nature of their receptors for antigen;

3 their migration patterns and the sites which they occupy in the lymphoid organs; and

4 their functions.

All lymphocytes bear receptors for antigen. In B cells, these are membrane-bound immunoglobulin (antibody) molecules. The T cell receptor is made up of two polypeptide chains and has structural features reminiscent of antibody molecules. Both the T and B cell receptors probably stem from a common ancestral molecule. One T or B lymphocyte and its mitotic progeny (i.e. one lymphocyte **clone**) can respond to only one antigen. The immune system as a whole, however, can cope with a vast array of different antigens. It will thus be apparent that the cells making up the immune system comprise an enormously varied population, which between them carry a huge repertoire of different receptors. An educated guess puts the number of different B cell receptors at 5×10^8 different clones of B cells, each of which reacts with a different antigen. The number of T cell clones is probably of comparable size. Thus the immune system contains lymphocytes bearing complementary (or near-complementary) receptors for virtually all of the foreign antigenic molecules likely to be encountered. 'Holes' in the repertoire are infrequent.

Lymphocyte circulation

Lymphocytes are found in large numbers in the lymph nodes and spleen, and in mucosal lymphoid aggregations in the gastrointestinal and respiratory tracts (e.g. tonsils, Peyer's patches). A substantial proportion of all lymphocytes constantly recirculates between the tissues, the lymph and the blood. If the immune system is to function efficiently, antigens entering the body must make contact reasonably quickly with the lymphocytes that express the complementary receptors. Before the immune system will recognize and respond to it, a new antigen must be displayed on specialized 'antigen-presenting cells'. These comprise **dendritic cells**, which are particularly effective at starting an immune response to a new antigen, and **macrophages**. These cell types are nearly ubiquitous in their distribution. They can pick up antigen

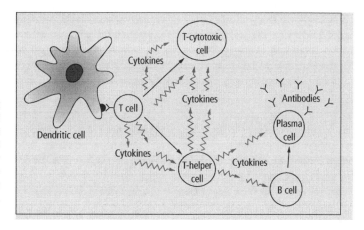

Fig. 13.8 The mechanism of the basic immune response. Antigen presented on dendritic cells activates T cells to produce cytokines. These cause T cells to proliferate and differentiate into T-helper cells and T-cytotoxic cells. Cytokines also help B cells proliferate and differentiate into plasma cells, which secrete antibody.

entering the body, for example through a cut in the skin, and transport it to local lymph nodes. Here they present it on their surface to a stream of circulating lymphocytes (Fig. 13.8). Those lymphocytes bearing receptors specific for the antigen will react with it and will proliferate; those bearing inappropriate receptors will not respond. Effector T lymphocytes can then invade the infected area and help remove the antigen.

T lymphocyte subsets

T cells comprise several subsets, each with its own distinct function, which collectively result in **cell-mediated immunity**. About 80% of the circulating T cells are regulatory, i.e. they facilitate or amplify other T cell or B cell responses (**T-helper cells**), or they dampen down or eliminate the same responses (**T-suppressor cells**). These regulatory mechanisms are still poorly understood. The ratio of helper to suppressor cells in the circulation is about 2:1 and is characteristically reduced in **AIDS**, in which the virus preferentially infects T-helper cells. Because T-helper cells are the first lymphocytes to interact with antigen displayed on macrophages and dendritic cells, they are sometimes referred to as T-helper/inducer cells. T-helper cells can be further divided into two groups: type 1 and type 2 cells. Type 1 cells aid the development of cell-mediated responses effective against intracellular organisms, such as the bacteria that cause tuberculosis. Type 2 cells help in the production of

antibody, which destroys extracellular parasites. Another subset of T cells (**T-effector cells**) subserves two main functions. One group (**cytotoxic T cells**) is able to destroy cells infected with viruses. A second group mediates **delayed-type hypersensitivity** (DTH), an immune response that is important in the defence against those infections in which the causative organisms proliferate intracellularly (e.g. tuberculosis, leprosy), and also in the rejection of foreign tissue grafts. In DTH, the T cells produce several different chemical substances, collectively known as **cytokines** (see below). The term hypersensitivity in DTH implies a pathological reaction. It is, however, with the exception of its extreme variants, a normal response.

Cytokines

Cytokines (previously known as lymphokines) are proteins of low molecular mass that regulate many cellular activities non-specifically (Fig. 13.8). These include:

1 enhancing the inflammatory response and dampening down inflammation;

2 inducing the growth and differentiation of cells of the immune system;

3 influencing whether a cell-mediated immune response or an antibody-mediated response predominates following an infection; and

4 establishing cellular antiviral activity. (One type of cytokine with antiviral activity is interferon.)

A wide variety of cells can transiently synthesize and secrete cytokines. Very small concentrations of cytokines are able to activate cells via receptors present on the cells that produce them (i.e. autocrinally) or on those in close proximity (i.e. paracrinally).

B lymphocytes and antibody production

B cells proliferate on contact with antigen and ultimately develop into **plasma cells**, which synthesize and secrete antibody. While B lymphocytes make up 15–20% of blood lymphocytes, plasma cells are located in lymphoid and other tissues rather than in the circulation. The first encounter with an antigen (the **primary response**) is slow and ineffectual. Antibody levels are low and the reaction takes 10–14 days to reach its peak (Fig. 13.9). The host's memory cells are however primed, with the result that second and subsequent exposures to the same antigen will quickly (within 1–2 days) stimulate the production of high levels of antibody (the **secondary response**).

The antibodies secreted by plasma cells are found predominantly in the γ globulin fraction of plasma, with small quantities in the β globulin fraction (Fig. 13.1). Collectively they are referred to as **immunoglobulins**. The basic monomeric form of all antibody classes consists of four polypeptide chains—two heavy chains and two light chains—held together by disulphide bonds (Fig. 13.10). The immunoglobulins comprise five structural classes of antibody, which subserve different functions. These are named according to their heavy chains, both of which are identical in any one molecule. Thus the immunoglobulin classes IgG, IgA, IgM, IgD and IgE (listed in descending order of their plasma concentrations) are characterized, respectively, by the heavy chains γ, α, μ, δ and ε. There are two types of light chain, κ and λ, both of which are found in all five antibody classes. Within one antibody molecule, however, the two light chains are always the same.

The chemical structure of the antigen-binding site varies from one antibody (and one B cell clone) to another, and forms part of the variable region of the molecule. The structure of the rest of the molecule is relatively constant. It is possible to cleave antibody molecules using papain to give two antigen-binding fragments (Fab fragments) and a crystallizable fragment (Fc fragment), which contains part of the heavy chains. The Fc fragment is responsible for all the biological attributes of antibodies other than antigen binding (e.g. the ability to cross the placenta, to fix to mast cells and to activate the complement cascade). Because

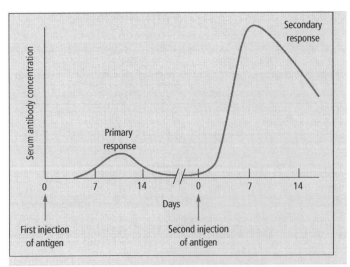

Fig. 13.9 Antibody concentration in serum in response to a first and a second injection of antigen.

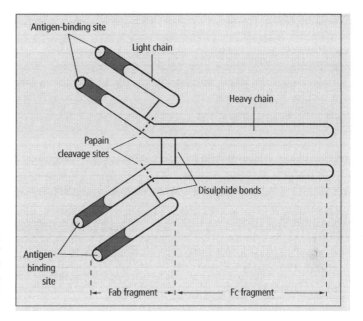

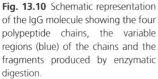

Fig. 13.10 Schematic representation of the IgG molecule showing the four polypeptide chains, the variable regions (blue) of the chains and the fragments produced by enzymatic digestion.

of differences in the structure of the variable region, relative molecular masses for the five different antibody classes given below are approximate.

IgG (M_r 150 000) makes up about 80% of the immunoglobulin in plasma. It is also found in extravascular tissues and can cross the placenta. It is the main antibody synthesized during the secondary response and is of major importance in the defence against micoorganisms and their toxins.

IgM (M_r 900 000) is a pentamer. It is the first immunoglobulin to appear in both phylogeny and ontogeny. It is also the first antibody to be produced in the primary response and the only antibody made by the fetus.

IgA (M_r 160 000) usually exists as a monomer in the plasma and as a dimer in surface secretions (tears, saliva, colostrum, gastrointestinal and bronchial secretions). It provides an important defence mechanism at these sites, particularly against viral infections.

IgD (M_r 185 000) is present mainly on the surface of B lymphocytes where it acts as a receptor for antigen. (A given B cell may have IgD surface receptors while secreting IgM and IgG. Even though the cell produces antibodies of more than one class, the antigen-binding site will be identical in all of them.)

IgE (M_r 200 000) is present at very low concentrations in plasma. It attaches to mast cells and basophils via receptors on the Fc portion of the molecule, i.e. it sensitizes these cells so that they release their granules if the attached antibody combines with antigen. This type of reaction exemplifies type I hypersensitivity, a common example of which is hay fever. IgE levels increase significantly in response to infestation by certain parasites.

Functions of antibodies

The binding of antigen to antibody facilitates the removal of the antigen from the body. In the case of bacteria, antibodies either facilitate phagocytosis of whole organisms or neutralize their toxic products. Antibodies are capable of coating viruses, thereby reducing their pathogenicity. Certain types of antibody, such as IgM and some IgG subclasses, fix (or activate) **complement** on combining with antigen. Complement is a collective term encompassing a series of proteins, which circulate in an inactive precursor form. They are activated sequentially giving rise to the production of several different factors, the functions of which include:

1 increasing vascular permeability;

2 enhancing phagocytosis; and

3 exerting a chemotactic effect towards polymorphs.

Complement is also capable of bringing about lysis of certain bacteria and cells. Complement is activated by IgM and IgG antibody (the **classical pathway**) and in a slightly different fashion by several other substances, e.g. bacterial endotoxin (the **alternative pathway**).

Active and passive immunity

Immunological memory is exploited in prophylactic immunization, which aims to provoke a primary response using vaccines (organisms or their toxic products treated to render them non-pathogenic). This is an instance of **active immunity** as the antibodies are made by the host's own cells. A subsequent encounter with the corresponding live organisms or their toxic products evokes a secondary response, which will prevent or significantly attenuate the associated disease. Memory is a function of modified T and B cells but the nature of the underlying changes is still uncertain. Its duration varies with the nature of the antigen and it can be life-long for certain diseases. It is, for example, very uncommon to get measles twice.

It is possible to transfer antibodies from one person to another or even from animals to humans. Immunity gained in this way is referred to as **passive immunity**. Antibodies transferred in the maternal milk provide significant protection to breast-fed infants (the antibodies are not extensively degraded in the gut at this age). Antiserum may also be useful as a stop-gap measure; for example, human serum containing anti-hepatitis A antibodies is sometimes given to short-term travellers to countries where the hygiene is poor. Passive immunity has a short duration of a few weeks at best. Animal serum is prone to cause hypersensitivity reactions and is now seldom used in clinical practice.

Tissue transplantation and the major histocompatibility complex

An individual will reject tissue or organ grafts from a genetically non-identical member of the same species. The cell-surface proteins that account for these individual differences are called **histocompatibility** (or **transplantation**) **antigens**, and they are both numerous and complex. The most obtrusive of these antigens in transplant surgery belong to a genetic system known as the **major histocompatibility complex** (MHC), which in humans is called the **human leukocyte antigen** (HLA) **system**. The MHC, which is present in all higher species, is a recognition system that controls a variety of cell–cell reactions. It plays a crucial part in the interaction between T and B cells, and also between antigen-presenting cells and T cells. Susceptibility to a variety of human diseases can be correlated with the HLA antigenic make-up.

Abnormalities of the immune response

Many disorders of the immune system have been described. Broadly these fall into three groups.

1 Immunodeficiencies affecting one or other component of the immune system. AIDS is the best publicized and now the commonest, but there are many others. The prevention and treatment of graft rejection involves the administration of immunosuppressive drugs (e.g. azathioprine and cyclosporin) and some measure of immunodeficiency is the price of a successful transplant. Immunodeficiency of varying severity also complicates other conditions, e.g. uraemia and severe burns.

2 Aberrant or excessive function of the immune system. In hypersensitivity (which occurs in several forms, one of which is allergy) the immune response to extraneous antigens (i.e. from outside the body) is harmful to the host. In autoimmune diseases the immune system reacts against the host's own tissues, e.g. in **Graves' disease** against the thyroid-stimulating hormone receptor of the thyroid gland and in **myasthenia gravis** against acetylcholine receptors in skeletal muscle.

3 Neoplasms (cancers) arising in cells of the immune system. All lymphocytes can be triggered to proliferate in the uncontrolled fashion that characterizes cancer. The overproduction of one cell type at the expense of the others will sooner or later result in immunodeficiency. In **multiple myeloma** there is excessive synthesis of a single **aberrant** immunoglobulin arising from a malignant change in a single plasma cell and this **monoclonal antibody** appears in the serum and in some cases in the urine. Characteristically, the levels of the normal immunoglobulins are markedly reduced in myeloma, resulting in increased susceptibility to infection.

13.4 Blood groups

Blood groups are systems of genetically determined **antigenic** substances on the membranes of red cells, e.g. the ABO and Rhesus blood group systems. If red cells with a particular antigen are mixed with the corresponding antibody, the red cells can clump together or **agglutinate**, a phenomenon that forms the basis of blood grouping tests. If the combination of red cells and antibodies occurs in the body, the reaction can lead to dangerous breakdown of red cells within the circulation (**intravascular haemolysis**) or outside it due to phagocytosis by macrophages (**extravascular haemolysis**).

If a patient receiving a blood transfusion has antibodies in the plasma which react with the transfused red cells, potentially lethal haemolysis may follow. The aim of the strict **cross-matching** procedures used in blood banks is to ensure that such **incompatible** transfusions do not occur. During pregnancy, following leakage of fetal red cells across the placenta into maternal blood, a woman may be stimulated to produce antibodies to an antigen on the fetal red cells if her own erythrocytes lack this antigen. This may occur if her lymphocytes have been sensitized to the antigen in a previous pregnancy. The maternal antibodies may cross the placenta and react with fetal red cells, causing them to be destroyed. This haemolytic anaemia, and its consequences, may be severe enough to cause death of the fetus or to lead to complications after birth (**haemolytic disease of the newborn**).

Blood group antigens and genes

The antigens on red cells that define blood groups are genetically determined. When it is shown that a set of red cell antigens is inherited independently of others, these antigens are said to form a particular **blood group system**. In people of European origin, there are, at present, 15 well-defined blood group systems. Antigens in some of these systems are shown in Table 13.5.

The genes determining blood group antigens are carried on pairs of autosomal chromosomes, except in the case of the Xg system, in which the gene concerned is on the X chromosome. The genes of blood group systems generally behave as codominants, so that if a person has a particular gene, the corresponding antigen can be detected on the red cells. In such cases the genetic constitution of a person for the blood group system concerned, the **genotype**, can be determined directly from the recognizable characteristics the genes produce in the red cells, the **phenotype**. However, genes of some blood group systems have no detectable effect on the red cells. These are **amorphic** genes (amorphs). When such genes are present, it may not be possible to determine a person's genotype directly from the phenotype but it may be possible to work it out by study of phenotypes in the family.

In those blood group systems that have been investigated, the genes have been found to control synthesis of enzymes which modify the composition of the antigens, which are glycoproteins or glycolipids on the red cell membrane.

Blood group antibodies

Blood group antibodies are of two kinds — naturally occurring and immune. Naturally occurring antibodies are those found in the blood of people who have not been exposed to the red cell antigens concerned (Table 13.5). The most common are those of the ABO system, which occur regularly in people whose own red cells lack the

Table 13.5 Examples of antigens and antibodies in blood group systems.

System	Antigens	Antibodies	Antibody type
ABO	A, B, H	Anti-A, anti-B	N
Rhesus	C, D, E, c, e	Anti-C, -D, -E, -c, -e,	I
MNS	M, N, S, s	Anti-M, -N, -S	N
P	P, P_1	Anti-P_1	N
Lutheran	Lu^a, Lu^b	Anti-Lu^a	N, I
Lewis	Le^a, Le^b	Anti-Le^a	N
Kell	K, k	Anti-K	I
Duffy	Fy^a, Fy^b	Anti-Fy^a	I
I	I, i	Anti-I	N

I, immune; N, naturally occurring.

corresponding antigens. Naturally occurring antibodies are usually IgM in type and, probably because of their large size, they cannot cross the placenta and thus cannot cause haemolytic disease of the newborn.

Immune blood group antibodies arise as the result of an immune response to red cell antigens not normally possessed by an individual but acquired by blood transfusion or by transplacental passage of fetal red cells during pregnancy. Thus most antibodies of the Rhesus, Kell and Duffy systems (Table 13.5) are formed in this way. Immune antibodies are most often IgG in type, although IgM antibodies also occur, often early, in an immune response. The IgG antibodies can cross the placenta and can thus cause haemolytic disease of the newborn.

IgG antibodies are often **incomplete**, i.e. they fail to agglutinate red cells having the corresponding antigens when the cells are suspended in physiological saline. This is because the IgG molecule, in contrast to IgM (**complete antibody**), is too short to bridge the gap between adjacent red cells kept apart by a net negative surface charge. Agglutination will occur if these electrostatic repulsive forces between the red cells are reduced, e.g. by treating the cells with enzymes to remove charged groups from the membrane. Incomplete antibodies or complement (p. 309) attached to red cells can also be detected by the **antiglobulin test** (Coombs test).

ABO blood group system

The four main groups (phenotypes) of the ABO system, **A**, **B**, **AB** and **O**, are defined by the presence or absence of two red cell antigens, A and B (Table 13.6). Either antigen may be present on the cells (group A or group B), both antigens may be present (group AB) or neither (group O). In addition, the naturally occurring antibodies, anti-A and anti-B, are present in the serum if the red cells lack the corresponding antigens (Table 13.6).

The A and B antigens are determined by the allelomorphic genes *A* and *B*. These genes, together with an amorphic third gene, *O*, are inherited as a pair—one from each parent. There are thus six genotypes but only four phenotypes (Table 13.6). The gene frequencies are not equal and, in people of European origin, groups O and A are much more common than B and AB (Table 13.6). Different phenotypic frequencies are found in other races. In some populations of Australian aborigines, for example, the groups B and AB do not occur.

Rhesus blood group system

The five main antigens of the Rhesus system are known in Fisher's notation as **C**, **c**, **D**, **E** and **e**. According to Fisher's theory, these antigens are determined by three pairs of allelic genes: *C* and *c*, *D* and *d*, *E* and *e* (Table 13.7). These genes are inherited in

Table 13.6 ABO blood group system. Frequencies (UK) are approximate.

Phenotype	Genotype	Antigen on cells	Antibody in serum	Frequency (%)
A	AA, AO	A	Anti-B	42
B	BB, BO	B	Anti-A	8
AB	AB	A, B	None	3
O	OO	None*	Anti-A, anti-B	47

* Almost always, red cells have H antigen, with maximal amount on group O cells.

Table 13.7 Rhesus blood group system. Frequencies (UK) are approximate.

Phenotype	Most common genotype		Frequency of genotype (%)
	Fisher notation	**Short notation**	
CcDee	CDe/cde	R_1r	32
CCDee	CDe/CDe	R_1R_1	17
ccee	cde/cde	rr	15
CcDEe	CDe/cDE	R_1R_2	14
ccDEe	cDE/cde	R_2r	13
ccDEE	cDE/cDE	R_2R_2	3
Others			6

sets of three, one set from each parent, and the *d* gene is amorphic.

The term rhesus-positive is sometimes used for a person whose red cells have the D antigen, and rhesus-negative for a person whose red cells lack it. However, in transfusion practice, it is usual to reserve the term rhesus-negative for persons of genotype *cde/cde*, whose red cells lack the antigens C, D and E.

Naturally occurring rhesus antibodies are very rare, e.g. some forms of anti-E. Immune antibodies are common following sensitization by transfusion or by pregnancy. Anti-D has been responsible for many problems and causes haemolytic transfusion reactions and haemolytic disease of the newborn, often of a severe degree. Fortunately, this latter disorder, due to anti-D, can now be avoided if, after transplacental leakage of fetal red cells into the maternal circulation (e.g. during parturition), anti-D immunoglobulin is injected into the mother. This will prevent her lymphocytes being sensitized by the fetal red cell D antigen. Transfusion reactions

and haemolytic disease of the newborn are sometimes caused by antibodies with other rhesus specificities, e.g. anti-c and anti-E.

Other blood group systems are occasionally implicated in transfusion reactions and haemolytic disease of the newborn, e.g. the immune antibodies anti-Fy^a and anti-K (Table 13.5). However, such reactions are usually of much less clinical importance than those due to the ABO and Rhesus systems.

Blood transfusion

Blood for transfusion can be kept for several weeks if it is collected from donors under aseptic conditions into sterile plastic packs containing a suitable preservative solution, and it is stored at 4°C. A commonly used preservative, citrate–phosphate–dextrose (CPD) solution, provides citrate as anticoagulant and glucose (dextrose) as metabolic substrate for the red cells. Adequate numbers (i.e. not less than 70%) of red cells remain viable after transfusion when previously stored in CPD solution for 3–4 weeks at 4°C. Adding adenine to the solution can increase this period to 5 weeks.

During storage at 4°C, the red cells show a progressive decrease in content of adenosine triphosphate (ATP) and 2,3-BPG. The low temperature inhibits the Na^+–K^+ pump, and the cells gradually lose K^+ to the surrounding plasma and gain Na^+ from it. The concentration of K^+ in the plasma may reach values as high as $30\,mmol\,L^{-1}$ after storage of blood for 4 weeks. The pH of the plasma also decreases with time of storage and its concentration of ammonia rises. These changes can make stored blood dangerous for transfusion in certain patients, e.g. those with renal or hepatic failure. Some red cells become spherocytic, with loss of deformability. These effects may be irreversible and after transfusion the abnormal red cells are destroyed very rapidly by macrophages in the spleen and elsewhere. Other constituents of blood do not withstand prolonged storage. Granulocytes begin to lose their phagocytic capacity within 6h of collection and become functionally inert after 24h. Platelets lose their haemostatic effect (p. 317) within 48h at 4°C, while the labile coagulation factors, V and VIII (p. 321), also rapidly deteriorate in chilled blood.

Before donated blood is made available for issue from a blood bank, the ABO and rhesus groups of the cells are determined and commonly the serum is screened for atypical antibodies. Serological tests are also done for syphilis, hepatitis and human immunodeficiency virus (HIV). Before transfusion, the ABO and rhesus groups of the patient's red cells are determined, the serum is checked for unexpected antibodies and red cells from the donor are tested against the patient's serum by **cross-matching** tests (compatibility tests). These cross-matching tests are essential for checking that there has been no error in ABO grouping of donor and recipient, and for ensuring that the recipient's serum does not contain naturally occurring or immune antibodies active against the donor's cells.

Transfusion of whole blood is sometimes necessary but, over recent years, the use of cell-separator machines and large-scale production of plasma constituents have made it increasingly possible to transfuse specific components of blood which the patient lacks. Thus **red cell concentrates**, often resuspended in a small volume of electrolyte solution, are used to restore the haemoglobin concentration in an anaemic patient in whom the plasma volume may already be expanded. **Platelet concentrates** are of use in patients with severe thrombocytopenia (p. 324). A variety of plasma fractions is also available to supply coagulation factors, e.g. **cryoprecipitate**, which is rich in factor VIII and fibrinogen, and for expanding plasma volume, e.g. **stable plasma protein solution**. A useful source of antibodies against common viruses is **pooled normal immunoglobulin** and various specific immunoglobulins are also available, e.g. anti-D and antibodies against tetanus, hepatitis B and diphtheria.

However much care is taken in cross-matching and administering blood, transfusion carries definite risks of unpleasant or even fatal complications. Major red cell incompatibility can lead to lethal intravascular haemolysis or delayed extravascular breakdown of donor cells. Transfusion of blood contaminated with bacteria can cause profound shock with hyperpyrexia, while allergic reactions to transfused white cells, platelets and plasma proteins can also be severe. Circulatory overload, air embolism and changes in plasma electrolyte concentrations (e.g. hyperkalaemia) may occur and there may be direct transmission of disease, e.g. HIV and cytomegalovirus infections, hepatitis and malaria.

13.5 Haemostasis

Haemostasis is the process by which bleeding from an injured blood vessel is arrested or reduced. Similar mechanisms appear to confine blood to the cardiovascular system by keeping vessels free of leaks, while other agents maintain the fluidity of the blood.

A haemostatic defect, if it is severe enough, can cause a **bleeding disorder** and activation of haemostasis within the circulatory system can lead to the formation of a solid mass of blood constituents, a **thrombus**, within an intact blood vessel. In arteries, thrombosis can cause **ischaemia**—reduction or cessation of the supply of blood to a tissue—and this can lead to death of cells (**necrosis**), with areas of ischaemic necrosis (**infarcts**) often seriously, or fatally, impairing the function of an organ (e.g. myocardial infarction). In veins, such as the deep veins of the leg or the veins of the pelvis, fragmentation and onward movement of thrombi (**embolism**) can also have fatal consequences (e.g. pulmonary embolism).

Haemostasis involves interlocking reactions of blood vessels, platelets and the coagulation system (Fig. 13.11). The **haemostatic response to injury** comprises two main phases. In the **primary** phase, reactions of blood vessels and platelets promote slowing of flow and formation of an aggregate of platelets at the site of injury. In the **secondary** phase, activation of coagulation by tissue factor released from damaged cells and by contact of plasma with disrupted vascular surfaces leads to the formation of **fibrin**, which stabilizes the platelet mass to yield a **haemostatic plug**.

Reactions of blood vessels

Many blood vessels respond to trauma by **vasoconstriction** and this reduces the rate of bleeding.

Capillaries are probably not able to contract but their endothelial cells seem able to adhere to one another so as to seal small gaps. Contraction of smooth muscle in larger vessels, such as arterioles and venules, occurs promptly after injury as a result of depolarization of smooth-muscle cells. Contraction is also mediated by local reflexes, utilizing **thromboxane A$_2$**, and possibly **serotonin** released by activated platelets, and also by vasoconstrictor substances liberated from vascular endothelium. Intense vasoconstriction of large arteries in avulsion injuries can sometimes produce surprisingly effective, although temporary, haemostasis.

Vascular damage also promotes haemostasis if the endothelial lining of vessels is lost or disrupted. When injury removes endothelium, exposure of blood to subendothelial constituents of a vascular wall, particularly collagen, allows adhesion of platelets to the damaged area and activation of the **intrinsic** pathway of coagulation, which is catalysed by phospholipid in platelet membranes. Damaged endothelial cells also release **tissue factor**, which triggers the **extrinsic** pathway of coagulation, and **von Willebrand factor**, which is necessary for platelet adhesion.

While endothelial damage activates haemostasis, a normal intact endothelium can limit

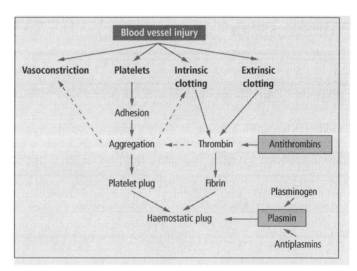

Fig. 13.11 Summary of normal haemostasis.

haemostatic reactions. The luminal surface of intact endothelium has a coating, about 50 nm thick, of **glycosaminoglycans**. These are polysaccharides made by endothelial cells and the main one, **heparan sulphate**, may act like the anticoagulant, heparin, in accelerating inactivation of coagulation factors by a plasma protein, **antithrombin III** (p. 322). **Protein C**, another inactivator of coagulation factors, is also activated by an endothelial component (p. 322). The endothelial glycosaminoglycans are strongly negatively charged and are thought to repel platelets, the surfaces of which are also negatively charged. Platelets may also be prevented from aggregating on normal vascular walls by **prostacyclin**, a prostaglandin synthesized by endothelial cells. Endothelium also liberates **tissue plasminogen activator**. This stimulates generation of the protease **plasmin**, which can lyse fibrin. When these various antihaemostatic actions of endothelium are impaired by vascular injury, the balance will swing towards the haemostatic reactions generated by exposure of blood to subendothelial tissue.

Platelets

Platelets are cytoplasmic fragments, without a nucleus, which circulate as biconvex discs, 2–4 μm in diameter, 0.6–1.2 μm in thickness, and with a volume of 6–9 fL. The normal platelet count is $150–400 \times 10^9\ L^{-1}$ of blood. Platelets are derived from megakaryocytes in the bone marrow (see Fig. 13.2) and survive in the circulation for 8–10 days. At any one time, up to a third of the platelets released from the marrow may be sequestered in the spleen.

Electron microscopy reveals structural components of platelets important for their haemostatic functions (Fig. 13.12). The plasma membrane is associated with glycoproteins, which are receptors for agents activating platelets. The membrane also contains phospholipids, which provide a catalytic surface for coagulation (**platelet factor 3**) and yield **arachidonic acid** for synthesis of prostaglandins. Just under the plasma membrane is a circumferential band of **microtubules**, which probably helps maintain the discoid shape of the

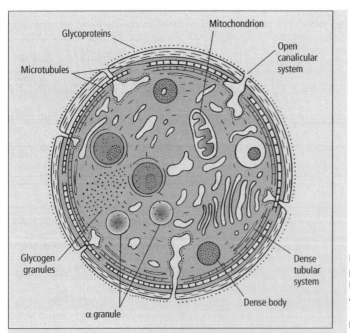

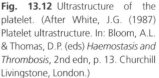

Fig. **13.12** Ultrastructure of the platelet. (After White, J.G. (1987) Platelet ultrastructure. In: Bloom, A.L. & Thomas, D.P. (eds) *Haemostasis and Thrombosis*, 2nd edn, p. 13. Churchill Livingstone, London.)

unactivated platelet. Extensive invaginations of the plasma membrane, the **open canalicular system**, increase the reactive surface area of the platelet and provide a route to the exterior for substances released from granules in the cytoplasm. A **dense tubular system**, probably analogous to the sarcoplasmic reticulum of skeletal muscle, stores Ca^{2+} ions, which are released into the cytoplasm when platelets are activated.

The cytoplasm of platelets contains contractile filaments of **actin** and **myosin**, which enable activated platelets to change their shape. There are various organelles. **Dense bodies** store adenosine diphosphate (ADP), 5-hydroxytryptamine (serotonin) and Ca^{2+}. The **α granules** contain a number of proteins including fibrinogen, von Willebrand factor, coagulation factor V, heparin-neutralizing factor (platelet factor 4), β thromboglobulin, thrombospondin and platelet-derived growth factor. **Lysosomes**, **mitochondria** and **glycogen granules** are also present.

Haemostatic reactions

Platelets take part in a sequence of actions in haemostasis (Fig. 13.13). After damage to the endothelium of a blood vessel, platelets adhere to subendothelial collagen fibres. Adhesion depends upon **von Willebrand factor**, part of the coagulation–factor VIII complex. This protein is thought to bind to collagen and to a glycoprotein (Ib) receptor in the platelet membrane. The adhering platelets then change shape from smooth discs to spiny spheres, with many projecting filopodia (spines). The loss of discoid shape is thought to be due to depolymerization of the microtubules, while formation of the filopodia probably results from polymerization of actin.

The sequence may stop at this stage but usually activation by collagen goes on to trigger the **release reaction**, a Ca^{2+}-dependent step in which the contents of the platelet granules are secreted to the outside of the platelet. Thromboxane A_2 released

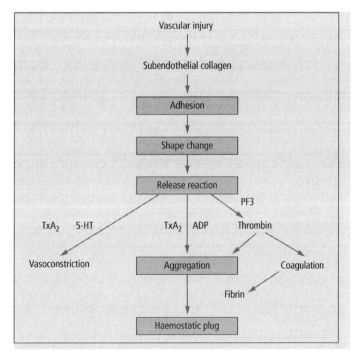

Fig. 13.13 Haemostatic reactions of platelets. ADP, adenosine diphosphate; 5-HT, 5-hydroxytryptamine (serotonin); PF3, platelet factor 3; TxA_2, thromboxane A_2.

in this way, and to some extent serotonin, reinforce local vasoconstriction, while ADP and thromboxane A_2 cause more platelets to become attached to those already adhering, so that a clump forms. This process of **aggregation** depends upon Ca^{2+} and also upon fibrinogen, which is thought to link the platelets together by attaching to glycoprotein receptors (IIb and IIIa). At this point aggregation is reversible.

During these events, platelets also act as catalysts of coagulation, with local generation of thrombin and conversion of fibrinogen to fibrin. Negatively charged phospholipids become exposed on the plasma membrane of the platelets. These phospholipids act as catalytic sites to which complexes of the vitamin K-dependent coagulation factors are bound by Ca^{2+} bridges in optimal orientation for the generation of factor Xa and thrombin (p. 320).

Thrombin causes further aggregation of platelets, which is irreversible (platelet fusion), and this effect may be mediated by thrombospondin from the α granules, which stabilizes the links of fibrinogen between platelets. Local production of fibrin reinforces the platelet aggregates. Eventually the mass of platelets and fibrin is compacted to form the definitive **haemostatic plug** (Fig. 13.13) by the action of actin and myosin filaments, causing contraction of the platelets. A similar phenomenon can be seen as **clot retraction** in freshly collected blood allowed to coagulate in a test tube.

Prostaglandin synthesis and actions

An important mediator of the haemostatic reactions of platelets is thromboxane A_2, which is formed from the unsaturated fatty acid, **arachidonic acid** (Fig. 13.14). A phospholipase (A_2), activated by agents such as collagen and thrombin, releases arachidonic acid from phospholipids in the plasma membrane of the platelet. Arachidonic acid is then converted by cyclo-oxygenase to the unstable prostaglandins (PG), PGG_2 and PGH_2, and these are transformed to thromboxane A_2 by a synthase enzyme. Thromboxane A_2 is very unstable, with a half-life of 30 s, and it spontaneously breaks down to an inactive product, thromboxane B_2. Thromboxane A_2 is a powerful vasoconstrictor, it induces the release reaction and is one of the

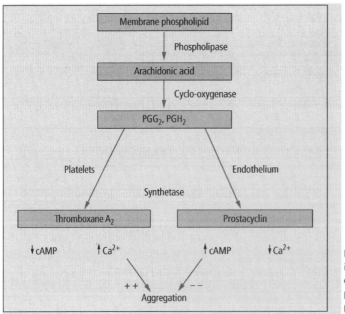

Fig. 13.14 Prostaglandin metabolism in platelets and endothelial cells. cAMP, cyclic adenosine monophosphate; PGG_2, prostaglandin G_2; PGH_2, prostaglandin H_2.

most potent natural platelet aggregators known. The mode of action of thromboxane A_2 appears to involve inhibition of adenylate cyclase, with a decrease in the concentration of the second messenger cyclic adenosine monophosphate (cAMP) (p. 26) and a resultant rise in the concentration of free Ca^{2+} in the cytoplasm of the platelet.

A similar synthetic pathway produces prostaglandins in the endothelial cells (Fig. 13.14) but PGH_2 is converted to **prostacyclin**—a vasodilator and potent **inhibitor** of platelet aggregation. This inhibitory effect seems to depend on stimulation of adenylate cyclase, with an increase in platelet cAMP and a fall in the concentration of Ca^{2+} in the cytoplasm. Prostacyclin may help to prevent deposition of platelets on normal endothelium but the total amount produced per day probably allows only partial control of platelets in this respect. However, release of prostacyclin by endothelium near an area of vascular damage may prevent unlimited accretion of a platelet plug.

Other actions of platelets

Platelets appear to take part in the process of **repair** after vascular injury. **Platelet-derived growth fac-** tor is mitogenic for smooth muscle, fibroblasts and glial cells. It is probably also chemotactic for neutrophils and macrophages and may be involved in the development of atherosclerosis.

Blood coagulation

The coagulation system consists of co-factors and a series of zymogens (proenzymes), which sequentially activate one another, leading to the formation of a fibrin clot at a site of vascular injury. The coagulation factors (Table 13.8) are mostly globulins, which are made by the liver and circulate in plasma at low concentrations. Most are known by capital Roman numerals, although the first four are usually referred to by name. The active forms of the zymogens are serine proteases, which activate the next factor in the sequence by splitting a limited number of specific peptide bonds to uncover the active enzymic site containing serine. The chain of proteolytic reactions in the coagulation system produces a **cascade** effect with amplification and acceleration at each step, so that even though the initiating stimulus may have been trivial, there is eventually an explosive production of large amounts of fibrin at the site of injury. The

Table 13.8 Coagulation factors.

Factor	Name	Approx. plasma concentration $(mg\,L^{-1})$	Function
I	Fibrinogen	3000	Fibrin polymer unit
II*	Prothrombin	0100	Protease
III	Tissue factor	—	Co-factor
IV	Calcium	0100 (2.5 mmol L^{-1})	Co-factor
V	Proaccelerin	0010	Co-factor
VII*	Proconvertin	0000.5	Protease
VIII	Antihaemophilic factor, VIII: C	0000.1	Co-factor
IX*	Christmas factor	0005	Protease
X*	Stuart–Prower factor	0010	Protease
XI	Plasma thromboplastin antecedent	0005	Protease
XII	Hageman factor	0040	Protease
XIII	Fibrin-stabilizing factor	0010	Transamidase
—	High molecular weight kininogen (Fitzgerald factor)	0080	Co-factor
—	Prekallikrein (Fletcher factor)	0035	Protease

* Hepatic synthesis requires vitamin K.

sequences of amino acids around the active sites and the mode of action of the coagulation enzymes are very similar to those of the pancreatic serine proteases—trypsin, chymotrypsin and elastase. These enzymes probably all have a common evolutionary origin.

The end-stage of blood coagulation (Fig. 13.15) is conversion of the soluble plasma protein, **fibrinogen** (factor I) into insoluble **fibrin** by the protease, **thrombin** (factor IIa).

Fibrinogen consists of three pairs of polypeptide chains—α, β and γ. Thrombin splits arginyl–glycine bonds near the N-terminus of each α and β chain to form **fibrin monomer** and two pairs of small peptides, fibrinopeptides A and B. Fibrin monomer molecules spontaneously polymerize to form a weak gel held together by electrostatic bonds. Thrombin activates factor XIII and, by transamidation in the presence of Ca^{2+}, this enzyme (XIIIa) causes strong peptide bonds to form between glutamine and lysine residues of the chains in the fibrin polymer, converting it to the insoluble, stable fibrin clot.

Prothrombin is converted to thrombin by sequential cleavage of two peptide bonds in the prothrombin molecule by activated factor X, in the presence of Ca^{2+} and platelet phospholipid, and with factor V as co-factor (Fig. 13.15).

By itself, factor Xa generates thrombin slowly but the reaction is about 10^5 times faster when factor Xa is bound by Ca^{2+} to the phospholipid surfaces of platelets, together with factor V and prothrombin.

The co-factor activity of factor V is initiated by splitting of peptide bonds in the molecule by thrombin, which thus has an autocatalytic action on its own production. This effect is limited, however, because thrombin also triggers inactivation of factor V by protein C (p. 322).

Intrinsic and extrinsic coagulation systems

Activation of factor X is the culmination of preceding enzyme reactions in two pathways, the **intrinsic** and **extrinsic** systems (Fig. 13.15). The

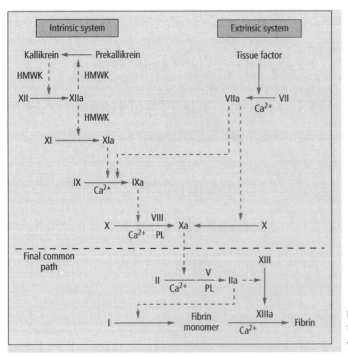

Fig. 13.15 The intrinsic, extrinsic and final common pathways of blood coagulation. PL, platelet phospholipid.

components of the intrinsic pathway are already present in circulating blood; the extrinsic pathway requires, in addition, **tissue factor** (thromboplastin), which is released by damaged cells.

The intrinsic system is activated when plasma comes into contact with constituents of subendothelial tissues, e.g. collagen fibrils or negatively charged, 'foreign' surfaces such as glass or particles of kaolin. Three zymogens—factor XII, factor XI and prekallikrein (Fletcher factor)—and one co-factor—high molecular weight kininogen (HMWK)—are involved in this phase of **contact activation**.

The first stage (Fig. 13.15) is reciprocal proteolytic activation of factor XII and prekallikrein, in which factor XIIa, in the presence of HMWK, converts prekallikrein to kallikrein. Kallikrein, in the presence of HMWK, then activates factor XII. With HMWK as co-factor, factor XIIa then converts factor XI to its active form. It is uncertain what triggers this cyclic activation of factor XII and prekallikrein. Binding of factor XII to foreign surfaces may cause a conformational change in the molecule, which could either expose the proteolytic site able to activate prekallikrein or make factor XII susceptible to a low level of protease activity in prekallikrein.

The next reaction in the intrinsic pathway is activation of factor IX in two proteolytic steps by factor XIa in the presence of Ca^{2+}. Factor IXa then activates factor X in a complex formed with factor VIII as co-factor, and with Ca^{2+} binding the reactants together on the phospholipid matrix of the platelet membrane. Thrombin acts on factor VIII, as it does on factor V, to increase the reactivity of the co-factor and eventually to cause its inactivation through the protein C system and by direct proteolysis.

Factor X may also be activated by the extrinsic pathway. Here, a complex formed of factor VII, tissue factor (III) and Ca^{2+} directly activates factor X (Fig. 13.15). Tissue factor is a lipoprotein found in microsomal preparations of various tissues and on the membrane of injured endothelial cells. The extrinsic pathway shows positive feedback with a reciprocating activating cycle between factor Xa and the activated form of factor VII.

The idea of separate intrinsic and extrinsic pathways leading to activation of factor X is useful as a basis for laboratory tests but from a functional point of view the distinction is probably artificial since there are cross-links between the pathways. Thus the factor VII–tissue factor complex directly activates factor IX (Fig. 13.15), and a product of the activation of factor XII can generate VIIa. Although the physiological importance of these reactions is uncertain, they may indicate why both intrinsic and extrinsic systems are necessary for normal haemostasis. Moreover, it is also known that platelets can directly activate factor XI without the intervention of factor XII, HMWK or prekallikrein. This may explain why people with a deficiency of these three coagulation factors do not have a bleeding tendency, whereas patients deficient in factor XI do.

The coagulation factors

The plasma protein coagulation factors fall into three main groups. The **contact factors** (XII, XI, prekallikrein and HMWK) are stable in blood or plasma stored at 4°C, do not need Ca^{2+} for activation to serine proteases, and are also concerned in pathways other than coagulation (see note below). The **vitamin K-dependent** factors (II, VII, IX, X) require vitamin K for their synthesis and Ca^{2+} for their activation, are stable in plasma kept at 4°C and, except for prothrombin, are not consumed in coagulation and consequently are present in serum. The **fibrinogen group** are those coagulation factors that react with thrombin (fibrinogen, factors V, VIII and XIII), and they are all consumed or inactivated during coagulation. Factors V and VIII rapidly lose their activity in blood or plasma stored at 4°C and special blood products must be used for transfusing these factors. The concentrations of the fibrinogen group of plasma proteins increase in pregnancy, in women taking the contraceptive pill and in inflammatory states.

The contact factors XIIa, and kallikrein with HMWK, can activate the fibrinolytic system (p. 323) and HMWK is both a co-factor for the activation of prekallikrein and a substrate for kallikrein.

Kallikrein splits off from HMWK the nonapeptide, **bradykinin**, one of a group of **kinins**, which increase vascular permeability, cause smooth muscle to contract and generate chemotactic activity in leukocytes. In the case of the vitamin K-dependent coagulation factors, vitamin K is needed for a final post-ribosomal step in their synthesis, in which an extra carboxyl group is added to glutamate residues to form γ-carboxyglutamic acid side-chains. These carboxyl groups allow the coagulation factors to bind to platelet phospholipid by Ca^{2+} bridges.

Factor VIII in the blood is a complex of two proteins. Factor VIII:C is the coagulation co-factor and its activity is deficient in patients with haemophilia A. Factor VIII:C is a single-chain glycoprotein (M_r 330 000), which is made in the liver, and possibly in other tissues, under the control of a gene on the X chromosome. It has been synthesized by recombinant DNA techniques and is available for treating haemophilia A.

The other part of the factor VIII complex is von Willebrand factor (VIII:WF), which is required for the adhesion of platelets to collagen and also acts as a carrier for VIII:C. This factor derives from a monomer of M_r 250 000, and circulates as a population of multimers (M_r 500 000 to more than 10^6). The von Willebrand factor is synthesized by endothelial cells and by megakaryocytes under the control of a gene on autosomal chromosome 13. This factor is deficient or defective in patients with von Willebrand's disease. It is not known how or where the two components of factor VIII become associated.

Inhibitors of coagulation

Thrombin is a very potent enzyme: there is potentially enough thrombin in 10 mL of blood to coagulate all the circulating plasma in an adult in less than 20s at 37°C. Various inhibiting agents limit the action of thrombin.

Phagocytic cells in the liver, and elsewhere, remove particulate thromboplastins from blood and hepatocytes can degrade activated coagulation factors (e.g. IXa, Xa, XIa). Flow of blood past an area of injury dilutes activated intermediates of coagulation and disperses loose aggregates of platelets.

These actions limit the generation of thrombin. Thrombin is also removed from the blood during coagulation by adsorption of fibrin. This process, which is called **antithrombin I**, inactivates only small amounts of thrombin. More important inhibitors are certain plasma proteins, particularly **antithrombin III** and **protein C** (Fig. 13.16).

Antithrombin III is a single-chain glycoprotein, which reacts on a mole-to-mole basis with thrombin to form an irreversible complex in which both molecules are inactivated. Antithrombin III also inactivates factor Xa and the other serine proteases in the intrinsic pathway (IXa, XIa and XIIa). Two other proteins, $α_2$-**macroglobulin** and $α_1$-**antitrypsin**, also contribute to the antithrombin effect of plasma.

Thrombin is also bound by a specific receptor on endothelial cells, **thrombomodulin**. The result of this interaction is conversion of circulating protein C to its active form, protein Ca (Fig. 13.16). Protein Ca is a serine protease which, in the presence of phospholipid, Ca^{2+} and a co-factor, **protein S**, inactivates factors V and VII and thus limits the generation of thrombin. Proteins C and S require vitamin K for their synthesis in the liver and protein Ca also enhances fibrinolysis. Protein Ca is itself inactivated by a specific inhibitor in plasma.

Anticoagulants

Ca^{2+} ions are needed at a number of steps in the coagulation pathways (Fig. 13.15) and agents that reduce the Ca^{2+} concentration keep the blood fluid *in vitro*. Ethylenediamine tetra-acetic acid (EDTA) as the sodium or potassium salt, and sodium oxalate, are used for this purpose; while trisodium citrate is the anticoagulant constituent of various solutions used for preserving blood for transfusion.

Heparin is a naturally occurring glycosaminoglycan, which is used therapeutically as an anticoagulant *in vivo* when rapid onset of action is desired. **Warfarin** and similar drugs are also used as anticoagulants *in vivo*.

Heparin acts by binding to antithrombin III, thereby inducing in the molecule a conformational change, which greatly accelerates inactiva-

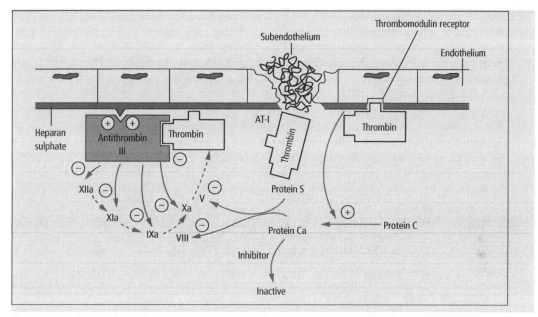

Fig. 13.16 Inactivation of coagulation by antithrombins and the protein C system. AT-I, anti-thrombin I.

tion of factor Xa in particular, but also of thrombin. Thrombin is also inactivated to a small extent by the circulating glycoprotein, **heparin co-factor II**. Heparin accelerates this reaction.

Coumarin–indanedione drugs, like warfarin, interfere with the action of vitamin K and their anticoagulant effect takes time to develop. By depleting the amount of functional vitamin K in the liver, they prevent formation of the γ-carboxyglutamate residues in factors II, VII, IX and X. This effectively renders the proteins functionally inactive.

Fibrinolysis

During the repair of blood vessels and healing of wounds, fibrin deposited in haemostatic plugs and in extravascular sites is removed by the **fibrinolytic system**. Fibrin is broken down to soluble fragments (fibrin degradation products) by a serine protease, **plasmin**. Plasmin, a two-chain polypeptide, is derived by cleavage of a single peptide bond in plasminogen, a single-chain β globulin in the plasma; this proteolytic reaction is brought about by **plasminogen activators**.

There are extrinsic plasminogen activators in many tissues, in endothelium and in various body fluids, including urine (**urokinase**), tears and saliva. Intrinsic plasminogen activator activity arises in the blood itself and is generated by the coagulation factors involved in contact activation (factor XII, kallikrein and HMWK). The importance of this form of activator is probably slight since physiological fibrinolysis seems to be due largely to release of **tissue plasminogen activator** from endothelial cells. This activator has now been synthesized by recombinant DNA techniques and is being used to treat coronary thrombosis.

Plasmin seems able to lyse fibrin selectively because plasminogen binds avidly to fibrin as the polymer forms. Tissue plasminogen activator—also incorporated into the fibrin as it forms, or diffusing in later from adjacent damaged tissue—lets plasmin be generated in close association with its natural substrate—fibrin. As the fibrin in a haemostatic plug is laid down, it is thus provided with an enzyme system for its subsequent dissolution.

While fibrin is the physiological substrate for plasmin, this protease will also attack other proteins, especially fibrinogen, factor V and factor

VIII. This non-specific proteolysis is normally prevented, since any free plasmin in the blood is rapidly inactivated by irreversible binding to α_2-antiplasmin, a circulating glycoprotein. Control of the activation of plasminogen is provided by **plasminogen-activator inhibitor 1**. This is released by endothelial cells and rapidly inactivates tissue plasminogen activator.

Small amounts of plasminogen activator can be detected in venous blood and this seems to originate from endothelium of capillaries and venules in the microcirculation. Flow of blood through these vessels may at times be sluggish, and slowly flowing blood coagulates easily. A continuous slow release of plasminogen activator and the subsequent formation of plasmin may therefore be important for maintaining the fluidity of blood in small vessels. Increase in the level of circulating plasminogen activator occurs in exercise, acute stress and in response to adrenaline.

Bleeding disorders

People with haemostatic defects typically suffer from two kinds of bleeding: they bleed for an abnormally long time after injury and they bleed spontaneously, without preceding trauma. In defects of platelets and small blood vessels, certain features of this bleeding differ from those found in disorders of coagulation. Thus **purpura**, i.e. multiple small bruises and haemorrhagic spots (petechiae) in the skin, and bleeding from mucosal surfaces, are characteristic of the spontaneous bleeding seen with platelet and vascular defects. Severe coagulation defects are typically associated with single, spreading bleeds in deep tissues or joints. The responses to mild and moderate trauma also tend to differ in these two groups of haemostatic disorders.

Purpuras due to acquired vascular defects may be benign local phenomena, e.g. simple easy bruising and senile purpura, or may be more generalized haemorrhagic lesions associated with, for example, severe infections, hypersensitivity reactions (e.g. Henoch–Schönlein syndrome) and drug allergies. Inherited malformations of small vessels (heredi-

tary haemorrhagic telangiectasia) and defective perivascular connective tissue (e.g. scurvy) can also cause troublesome bleeding. A low platelet count and **thrombocytopenic purpura** can arise from decreased production of platelets by the bone marrow, because of drugs, ionizing radiations, viral infections, failure of the marrow or infiltration of it by abnormal cells, e.g. in leukaemia. Thrombocytopenia may also be due to increased destruction of platelets by immune reactions, as in immune thrombocytopenic purpura, after viral infections (e.g. measles) and as an allergic response to drugs. Purpura can also occur in people with normal numbers of circulating platelets but with functional defects, e.g. failure of aggregation in thrombasthenia.

Inherited deficiencies of coagulation factors are rare but may be severe. They usually involve only one factor (e.g. deficiency of factor VIII:C in haemophilia A). In von Willebrand's disease, in addition to a deficiency of factor VIII:C, there is also an inherited lack of von Willebrand factor (VIII:WF) leading to defective adhesion of platelets and bleeding typical of that seen with platelet defects. Acquired disorders of coagulation factors are due usually to multiple deficiencies, commonly of the vitamin K-dependent factors because of lack of vitamin K. Since this vitamin is fat-soluble, deficiency of it and defective vitamin K-dependent coagulation factors can arise in disorders impairing absorption of fats. Similar effects can also occur in liver disease, in premature babies and during treatment with anticoagulants like warfarin (an overdose of which often causes bleeding). Disease of the liver can also be associated with other haemostatic abnormalities, including thrombocytopenia, reduced synthesis of fibrinogen and increased fibrinolytic activity.

Diffuse intravascular thrombosis (disseminated intravascular coagulation) can arise because of release of procoagulant material (e.g. amniotic fluid) into the circulation or because of widespread endothelial damage (e.g. severe bacterial infections). There may be such gross depletion of coagulation factors and platelets that generalized bleeding occurs.

Tests of haemostatic function

Certain simple screening tests are useful for assessing haemostatic function quickly. These are a platelet count, examination of a blood film, a bleeding time and tests of coagulation.

A **platelet count** will expose a thrombocytopenia; examination of a **blood film** will often confirm a **low platelet count** and may reveal its cause, e.g. leukaemia. The **bleeding time**, the time taken for cessation of bleeding from small punctures in the skin (made by a standard technique), is an index of the integrity of platelets. In people with a normal platelet count, a prolonged bleeding time would suggest defective platelet function or von Willebrand's disease.

Two simple coagulation tests are used to monitor the extrinsic and intrinsic pathways. The **pro-thrombin time** (PT) tests the extrinsic system and the final common path (Fig. 13.15) by measuring the time taken for a sample of citrated plasma to coagulate when tissue factor and Ca^{2+} are added. If a test plasma takes longer to coagulate than a known normal plasma, this suggests deficiency (or inhibition) of one or more of the factors VII, X, V, II and I. The ratio of the prothrombin time of a test plasma to a normal plasma can now be standardized among different laboratories in terms of a reference thromboplastin as the international normalized ratio (INR).

In the **partial thromboplastin time with kaolin** (PTTK), the intrinsic system of a sample of citrated plasma is activated by incubating it with kaolin for several minutes, then substitutes for platelet phospholipid and Ca^{2+} are added. If the test sample takes longer to coagulate than a control sample, this indicates deficiency (or inhibition) of one or more of the factors XII, XI, IX, VIII, X, V, II and I. The combined results of the two tests, PT and PTTK, will usually indicate if a coagulation defect is present and will suggest the likely possible defect(s), depending on whether either or neither test, or both, give abnormal results.

If thrombin and Ca^{2+} are added to a sample of citrated plasma, the time taken for the plasma to coagulate, the **thrombin time**, is a useful test for rapidly assessing the concentration and reactivity of fibrinogen.

Chapter 14

Introduction to the Cardiovascular System

'. . . and when I had a long time considered with myself how great abundance of blood was passed through, and in how short time that transmission was done. . . . I began to bethink myself if it might not have a circular motion. . . .' William Harvey, De Moto Cordis, 1648; from the first English translation of the Latin text.

The cardiovascular system, comprising the heart and circulation, is the body's transport system and is central to the integration and maintenance of body function. It carries oxygen and nutrients to the tissues and removes carbon dioxide and non-volatile by-products of metabolism. Preservation of a stable chemical and physical environment in the body is dependent on the circulation of blood through the lungs where respiratory exchange takes place, and through organs, such as the gastrointestinal tract, kidneys and liver, that extract and process nutrients and remove by-products of metabolism. The cardiovascular system also plays an important role in the active regulation of body function and maintenance of the body's defences. Hormones are secreted into the circulation and distributed throughout the body where they act on specific target organs. Blood also carries the factors required for haemostasis and tissue repair, as well as the effector cells and antibodies that coordinate immune system responses.

The purpose of this chapter is to provide an overview of the cardiovascular system and to iden-

tify the fundamental biophysical principles that underlie its function. Selection pressure has ensured that almost all aspects of the cardiovascular system have evolved in an optimal fashion to meet a wide range of demands. A systematic understanding of the demands imposed on the cardiovascular system and the way in which its structure and function have adapted to meet these requirements provide an obvious and satisfying way of organizing knowledge on the subject. We will approach the topic on this basis.

14.1 Organization of the cardiovascular system

The organization of the cardiovascular system is represented in Fig. 14.1. The cardiovascular system is subdivided into **systemic** and **pulmonary** circulations, and the heart consists of separate pumps that serve these two circulations. Deoxygenated blood, which returns to the right heart via the systemic veins, is pumped into the pulmonary circulation where respiratory gas exchange takes place. Oxygenated blood from the lungs flows into the left heart through the pulmonary veins and is then pumped into the aorta, which supplies the systemic arteries. Cardiac pumping is a pulsatile process. The heart generates maximum pressures of around 120 mm Hg in the major systemic arteries and around 25 mm Hg in the pulmonary artery.

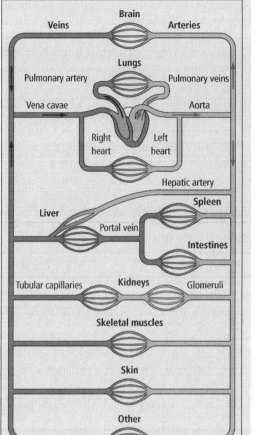

Veins Brain Arteries
Lungs
Pulmonary artery Pulmonary veins
Vena cavae Aorta
Right heart Left heart
Hepatic artery
Spleen
Liver
Portal vein
Intestines
Tubular capillaries Kidneys Glomeruli
Skeletal muscles
Skin
Other

Fig. 14.1 Schematic representation of the cardiovascular system. The right heart, pulmonary circulation and left heart are in series. The arrangement of the vascular supply to the spleen (splenic circulation), gastrointestinal tract (mesenteric circulation) and liver (hepatic circulation) is more complex than for other organ systems. Splenic and mesenteric circulations are in parallel and the outflow from both is routed to the liver via the portal vein. The liver also receives direct arterial supply from the hepatic artery.

Table 14.1 Distribution of blood flow within the systemic circulation at rest and in moderately vigorous exercise. Note that maximum cardiac output varies between individuals, dependent on age, fitness, nutritional status and training.

	Rest		Exercise	
	L min⁻¹	%	L min⁻¹	%
Cardiac output	5.8	100	20	100
Brain	0.75	13	0.75	4
Heart	0.25	4	0.85	4
Gut	1.5	26	0.6	3
Kidney	1.0	17	0.5	3
Skeletal muscle	1.2	21	15	75
Skin	0.5	7	1.95	10
Other	0.6	10	0.35	2

The systemic circulation is a set of parallel vascular circuits, each receiving blood via the arteries and discharging its outflow into the veins. In Fig. 14.1, brain (cerebral), kidney (renal), skeletal muscle, skin (cutaneous) and 'other' circulations are represented as single lumped compartments. This is a simplification, as the vascular beds supplying skeletal muscle and skin in particular, are widely distributed throughout the body.

A consequence of the organization of the cardiovascular system is that each of the parallel vascular circuits of the systemic circulation competes for blood supply. At rest, the **cardiac output** for a typical adult human is 5 to 6 L min⁻¹ and this is distributed among the various organ systems, as shown in Table 14.1. With exercise, the distribution pattern changes markedly. Cardiac output increases substantially and blood is directed preferentially to exercising skeletal muscle, to the skin and to the heart. Table 14.1 indicates that blood flow to skeletal muscle, around 1.2 L min⁻¹ at rest, can exceed 15 L min⁻¹ in exercise.

Blood flow to the heart increases four-fold from around 250 mL min⁻¹ to more than 850 mL min⁻¹, while blood flow to the brain remains remarkably constant at around 750 mL min⁻¹. On the other hand, blood flow to the liver, spleen, GI tract and kidneys decreases, both as a proportion of cardiac output and absolutely. There is tight linkage between the increase in blood flow and increased oxygen consumption during exercise, and it appears that the mechanisms operating to regulate the distribution of blood flow are to ensure that it is routed to tissues with an immediate requirement for metabolic support, at the expense of organ systems that can tolerate reduced blood flow in the short-term.

The distribution of blood flow in the systemic circulation both at rest and in exercise is determined by simple physical principles, and it is informative to study these a little more fully. The energy required to deliver blood throughout the circulation is imparted to it by the heart and, in particular, by the pressures which the heart generates. (The total energy per unit volume in a fluid is the sum of potential and kinetic energy. The pressure in a fluid is a form of potential energy. More detail is provided in Chapter 16, which deals with haemodynamics.) As blood flows through the circulation, energy is dissipated and pressure falls. Under conditions of steady flow, it can be shown that the pressure drop across a vascular circuit is related to the rate at which blood flows through it and this relationship defines the resistance presented to blood flow by the vascular segment. This is expressed as:

$$\Delta P = R\dot{Q}$$

where ΔP is the pressure gradient, $\dot{Q}$ is blood flow and R is vascular resistance, which can be rearranged as:

$$\dot{Q} = \Delta P / R$$

Thus for a given pressure gradient, an increase in vascular resistance will reduce blood flow and vice versa. The relatively high pressures that the heart

generates in the aorta ensure that blood flow can be routed as required to any of the parallel vascular circuits, which make up the systemic circulation. Moreover, if input pressure is maintained, then blood flow to any systemic vascular circuit can be controlled by adjusting its resistance. Thus the design of the circulation may be equated with a domestic plumbing system. High-pressure supply is necessary if we wish to maintain flow in the shower when a tap elsewhere in the house is switched on. Because all the blood from the right heart passes through the lungs, it is not necessary to generate pressures in the pulmonary circulation as high as those in the systemic circulation.

Characteristics of the heart

The heart has four chambers. Blood from the systemic circulation enters the right heart via the superior and inferior vena cavae and passes through the right atrium into the right ventricle. Likewise, blood from the lungs enters the left heart through the pulmonary veins and passes through the left atrium into the left ventricle. Unidirectional flow of blood through the heart is ensured by the inlet and outlet valves, which are located in the atrioventricular (AV) plane between atria and ventricles (see Fig. 14.2).

The heart beats automatically, independent of external input from the central nervous system. Blood is pumped into pulmonary and systemic cir-

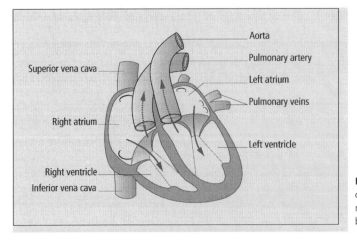

Superior vena cava

Right atrium

Right ventricle
Inferior vena cava

Aorta
Pulmonary artery
Left atrium
Pulmonary veins

Left ventricle

Fig. 14.2 A schematic representation of the heart and great vessels. The arrows indicate the normal direction of blood flow.

culations during **systole**, as a result of coordinated contraction of the cardiac muscle in right and left ventricles. The thick walled left ventricle has a much greater muscle mass than the right ventricle, reflecting the difference in the maximum pressures generated in the systemic and pulmonary circulations. When ventricular pressures rise during systole the closed inlet valves prevent blood from flowing back through the atria into the veins. Likewise, closure of the pulmonary and aortic valves prevents reflux of blood into the ventricles at the end of systole.

The ventricles fill during **diastole**, when they are relaxed. The atria play an important role in this process. Downward movement of the AV valve plane during ventricular systole draws blood into the compliant atrial chambers and this is transferred rapidly into the ventricles, when the valve plane recoils early in diastole. In mid-diastole, both atria and ventricles fill with blood returning from the veins. Finally, the atria contract in late diastole. This produces a modest boost of the volume in the ventricles and also contributes to smooth closure of the inlet valves immediately prior to ventricular contraction.

The human heart is an extraordinarily robust and efficient pump, which completes around 10^{11} cycles in the average human lifetime. Cardiac output is the product of stroke volume (the volume pumped per contraction) and heart rate (the frequency of contraction). Both heart rate and the vigour of contraction are subject to external modulation by the autonomic nervous system and by circulating hormones such as adrenaline and noradrenaline. In the normal heart, around 60% of the blood stored in the left ventricle at the end of diastole is ejected during systole, but the ejection fraction may rise to 80% in exercise.

Of particular importance to the regulation of cardiovascular function, is the intrinsic coupling between cardiac filling and cardiac output. This was first observed by Otto Frank in 1895, and was described more systematically by Ernest Starling in 1914. They found that increasing the filling of the cardiac chambers during diastole increased ventricular output in systole. We know now that the Frank–Starling mechanism is a result of the unique arrangement and properties of cardiac muscles in left and right ventricles. This mechanism is necessary to maintain stable function in the cardiovascular system. It ensures that there is balance between right and left hearts, and that blood does not accumulate either in the systemic veins or in the lungs. Both can happen in congestive heart failure, when the sensitive balance between filling and output is disrupted.

Finally, the heart also functions as an endocrine organ, releasing atrial natriuretic peptide (ANP) and brain natriuretic peptide (BNP) into the circulation in response to abnormal pressure and volume loading. A localized renin–angiotensin system in the heart is also stimulated by altered mechanical loading.

Characteristics of the vascular circuit

Blood is delivered to the vascular bed of an organ or tissue region by a relatively small number of large arteries. Uniform distribution of blood flow to the tissues involves progressive vascular bifurcation, in which a parent vessel gives rise to many vessels of smaller cross-sectional dimension. This process continues through progressive vessel generations until the **microcirculation** is reached. Exchange between blood and tissues takes place mainly in the microcirculation. Collection of blood and its return to the large veins that carry blood back to the heart mirrors the distribution process. Key anatomic features of the different classes of blood vessel in a typical systemic vascular bed are shown in Fig. 14.3.

Blood vessels are lined with endothelial cells. This inner layer provides a barrier between circulating blood and the vessel wall, but also releases substances, such as nitric oxide, endothelin and prostaglandins, which play an important role in the regulation of vascular function. The blood vessel wall consists of smooth muscle cells, elastic fibres (elastin) and connective tissue, of which the most important component is collagen. Vascular smooth muscle cells maintain a slowly varying background level of contraction. An increase in contractile activity will cause **vasoconstriction** (reduction of vessel cross-sectional dimensions),

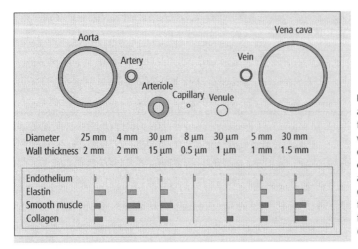

Fig. 14.3 Cross-sectional dimensions and principal structural components for different classes of blood vessel within a typical systemic vascular circuit. Aorta, artery, vein and vena cava are approximately to scale. The arteriole, capillary and venule are rendered in a common scale that magnifies them considerably. (Redrawn from Burton, A.C. *Biophysics of the Circulation.*)

while relaxation will result in **vasodilation**. Elastin enables the blood vessel to expand if the pressure difference across the vessel wall is increased, while collagen reinforces the blood vessel wall and limits expansion.

The important aspects of the vascular structure, as represented in Fig. 14.3, are summarized below:

1 The aorta and large arteries have a relatively high proportion of elastin in their vessel walls and for this reason are sometimes referred to as elastic arteries.

2 The walls of arterioles are thick relative to their internal diameter and contain a high proportion of vascular smooth muscle.

3 The cross-sectional dimensions of the capillaries are comparable to those of the red blood cell and the capillary wall consists of a single layer of endothelial cells.

4 **Postcapillary** vessels have a smaller proportion of vascular smooth muscle than **precapillary** vessels of comparable size.

Vascular anatomy reflects the specialized functions served by different organs and tissues and there are variations in the generic structures outlined above. For instance, specific regions of the skin have a high density of shunt vessels or **arterio–venous anastomoses** that bypass the capillaries. Arterio–venous anastomoses are found primarily in the skin of hands, feet and face. These anastomoses have greater internal diameter than capillaries and provide an exchange surface for

heat transfer between blood and the external environment. As a further example, blood flow in the kidney is routed through glomerular capillaries where it is filtered. The blood vessels on either side of the glomerular capillaries have thick muscular walls and for this reason are identified as **afferent** and **efferent** arterioles (see Fig. 14.1).

Pressure, cross-sectional area, velocity and blood volume in the vascular system

Pressure, cross-sectional area, average velocity of blood flow and blood volume in the blood vessels of the systemic circulation can be related to their structure.

The approximate distribution of pressures across the systemic circulation are given in Fig. 14.4. Because the heart pumps intermittently, pressure is markedly pulsatile throughout much of the precapillary circuit. The blood ejected by the left ventricle in systole is initially stored in the aorta and large arteries, which expand during systole and recoil during diastole thus producing a more even discharge of blood toward the periphery than would otherwise be the case. In a healthy young adult at rest, pressures in the aorta rise to a maximum value around 120 mmHg in systole and fall to around 80 mmHg at the end of diastole. The pressure pulse is progressively damped, and blood pressure in the microcirculation is relatively steady. Mean pressure (around 95 mmHg in the

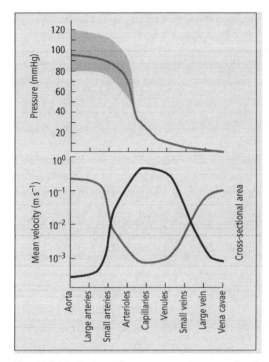

Fig. 14.4 Distributions of pressure, vessel cross-sectional area and mean velocity for different classes of blood vessel in a typical systemic vascular circuit. Mean pressures and the range of pulsatile pressure variation are shown in the upper panel. Total cross-sectional area (black line) and mean blood flow velocity (blue line) are given in the lower panel. Both cross-sectional area and mean velocity are presented on logarithmic scales. Cross-sectional area is in arbitrary units.

are referred to as **precapillary resistance** vessels. Small changes in the cross-sectional dimensions of these vessels produce large changes in vascular resistance and can markedly alter the distribution of blood flow to the microcirculation. The high proportion of vascular smooth muscle in the walls of these vessels is consistent with their role in regulating vascular resistance and regional blood flow. Finally, it is evident that postcapillary vessels present only modest resistance to blood flow at rest.

The mean velocity of blood flow through each class of blood vessels in a vascular circuit is inversely related to the total cross-sectional area of those vessels (see Fig. 14.4). Total cross-sectional area increases substantially with each new generation of precapillary vessels. It is greatest for the capillaries and then decreases progressively for subsequent generations of postcapillary vessels. (The cross-sectional area of an individual capillary is much less than that of an individual arteriole. However, because there are many more capillaries than arterioles, their total cross-sectional area is much greater.) As a result, the velocity at which blood flows through the capillaries (and the venules) is very slow indeed. Mean velocity in postcapillary vessels is less than in precapillary vessels of comparable generation. At rest, the mean velocity of blood flow in the vena cavae is around $0.1\,\text{m}\,\text{s}^{-1}$ compared with $0.2\,\text{m}\,\text{s}^{-1}$ in the aorta. The diameters of superior and inferior vena cavae are similar to the aorta and their total cross-sectional area is therefore twice that of the aorta.

Total blood volume is 5–6 L and 4–5 L in men and women, respectively. The distribution of the blood volume throughout the cardiovascular system is represented in Fig. 14.5.

The heart and pulmonary circulation jointly constitute about 18% of total blood volume. Despite their large cross-sectional area, the capillaries contain only a small fraction of total blood volume (around 5%). Surprisingly, more blood is stored in the aorta and large arteries than in the capillaries. Nearly 60% of the blood volume is stored in the systemic veins, with the largest proportion of this in the venules and small veins. The systemic veins are therefore the main reservoir for blood in the cardiovascular system. They are referred to as

aorta) changes little across the large arteries, but falls sharply through the small arteries and arterioles. On average, pressure falls from around 30 mmHg at the arterial end of the capillary to near 15 mmHg at the venous end of the capillary. Pressure then drops progressively across the postcapillary vascular network.

The pressure drop across the blood vessels in a vascular circuit reflects the total resistance that they present to blood flow. The large arteries, which distribute blood to the organs and tissues, contribute almost no resistance to blood flow indicating that energy losses in these vessels are negligible. At rest, most of the resistance to blood flow occurs in the small arteries and arterioles, which

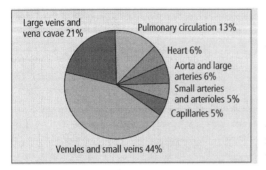

Fig. 14.5 The distribution of total blood volume across the different compartments of the cardiovascular system. Note that 65% of blood volume is stored in the systemic veins.

capacitance vessels and their storage function is essential in maintaining steady venous return to the heart.

Exchange in the microcirculation

The exchange of substances between blood and tissue takes place in the microcirculation, principally across the capillary wall. The capillaries are bathed in interstitial fluid, but are in very close contact with the cells and tissues that they supply. There are two main pathways for exchange: diffusive transport of solutes and exchange of fluids by bulk transport.

Diffusive transport of solutes is driven by the concentration gradient of the solute across the capillary wall and by its permeability to the solute. Diffusion provides a particularly efficient mechanism for transporting substances over dimensions of the order 1 to 10 μm. The microcirculation is superbly adapted to maximize transport via diffusion; diffusion distances are small and the capillary wall is thin and highly permeable to solutes of low molecular weight. As a result, respiratory gases, nutrients and by-products of metabolism all pass freely between blood and tissue fluids. Effective diffusive transport is also aided by the slow velocity with which blood passes through the capillaries. This ensures that the exchange of respiratory gases along the capillary wall occurs swiftly and is complete.

The exchange of fluids by bulk transport occurs much more slowly than diffusion. Fluid pressures are greater in the capillaries than in the surrounding interstitial space, and this favours water movement from the blood into the interstitial space. However, it is essential that the capillaries retain fluid so that blood volume is preserved. This is achieved by the relative impermeability of the capillaries to plasma proteins. Although there is some protein in the tissue fluid, the concentration of proteins in plasma is greater. As a result, there is a net osmotic pressure gradient that favours movement of fluid from the interstitial space into the blood stream. Thus the net fluid movement across the capillary wall is determined by the balance between **filtration** and **absorption**, which are driven by the hydrostatic pressure gradient and the colloid osmotic pressure gradients across the capillary wall, respectively. Under normal circumstances, filtration and absorption are closely matched with a small net outward fluid movement—less than 0.025% of total blood flow. This fluid is returned to the venous system through the lymphatic circulation, together with plasma proteins that have leaked from the capillaries. (The lymphatics are a closed-ended network of highly permeable lymph capillaries that drain into larger lymph collection vessels.)

Two final points should be noted here. First, some properties of capillaries are specific to the organ or tissue under consideration. For instance, the tight coupling of capillary endothelial cells in many regions of the brain prevents the transfer of circulating angiotensin II and catecholamines to brain tissue. Second, the fact that water moves between plasma and interstitial space means that the maintenance of blood volume is intimately linked with the regulation of extracellular fluid volume.

14.2 Regulation of cardiovascular function

The cardiovascular system has the capacity to function in an inherently stable fashion in the absence of active external control. For instance, anaesthetized patients undergoing surgery can maintain stable cardiovascular function for long periods, even though neural and humoral mechanisms known to regulate the cardiovascular system are suppressed. In this section, we will consider the basis of the intrinsic regulation of cardiovascular function and how it is modified in the face of external demands on the system.

Intrinsic regulation

While the function of the heart and circulation are profoundly affected by autonomic nervous system activity and circulating hormones, such as adrenaline, noradrenaline and angiotensin II, both also have the capacity to operate with a high degree of autonomy. In the absence of external influences, blood flow to many systemic vascular beds is matched to metabolic requirements, and remains relatively constant in the medium-term, despite changes in arterial pressure. This phenomenon is called **autoregulation** and provides evidence that local factors play a role in adjusting the distribution of blood flow in the circulation. Local mechanisms are most influential (and extrinsic regulation has least impact) in the coronary and cerebral circulations, where continuous maintenance of blood flow is critical for survival.

The direct linkage between cardiac filling and output is an example of an intrinsic mechanism that operates in the heart. We have already stated that the Frank–Starling mechanism is central to the function of the cardiovascular system as a whole, because it ensures that blood does not accumulate in the systemic veins or in the lungs. However, this balance also depends on the affects of both heart and circulation on venous return. To a reasonable approximation, the pressures in small veins and venules may be seen as driving blood back to the heart, but an increase in the average pressures in the cardiac chambers during diastole will reduce venous return and vice versa. The heart and circulation form a closed system, and when venous return exceeds cardiac output then cardiac filling is increased and diastolic pressures in the heart are elevated. As a result, cardiac output is boosted and venous return falls. The cardiovascular system therefore operates around an inherently

stable level of cardiac filling at which cardiac output matches venous return. This equilibrium setting can be altered by changes in both cardiac and vascular function. For instance, in the absence of compensatory neuro–humoral adjustments, loss of blood volume will reduce the peripheral venous pressures that drive venous return, and both cardiac filling and cardiac output will fall. Thus, there is considerable emphasis on preservation of circulating volumes and replacement of fluid losses in surgery.

Extrinsic regulation

We have argued above that the organization of the cardiovascular system and the intrinsic linkage between venous return, cardiac filling and cardiac output ensure that the cardiovascular system behaves in a stable and predictable manner when external neural and humoral factors that affect the heart and circulation do not change. However, maintenance of body function and coordination of programmed cardiovascular responses requires active control that can override these intrinsic regulatory mechanisms. Extrinsic control of cardiovascular function has much in common with the control of complex, multi-input, technological processes. An array of different sensors monitor the status of the cardiovascular 'plant', and this information is relayed back to the central nervous system, which adjusts hormone levels and autonomic nervous system activity to correct any deviation from the target operating state.

The reflex mechanisms that buffer short-term variation in systemic arterial pressure provide a straightforward example of the way in which this negative feedback control operates. An acute fall in systemic arterial pressure will lead to reduced firing of stretch receptors located close to the left heart at the arch of the aorta, and in the carotid arteries. The resultant neuro–humoral response is coordinated in the central nervous system at the level of the brainstem. Vascular resistance is increased and venous return is enhanced, and hence contraction of the heart becomes more vigorous and cardiac output rises. As a result of these adjustments, systemic arterial pressure is restored.

Regulation of cardiovascular function requires the control of many variables in addition to systemic arterial pressure. For instance, stretch receptors in the cardiac chambers provide information on the extent of cardiac filling and are sensitive to altered venous return. These so-called 'low pressure' receptors play an important role in the regulation of blood volume and extracellular fluid volume. Finally, specialized receptors that sense blood chemistry and body temperature, among other things, give rise to neuro–humoral responses that affect cardiovascular function.

The coordinated cardiovascular responses to exercise outlined at the beginning of this chapter provides an excellent example of a higher level of regulation, in which intrinsic and extrinsic regulation mechanisms are modified to produce an integrated response to an external challenge. Matching changes in both cardiac pumping capacity and venous return are required to produce the marked increases in cardiac output observed in vigorous exercise. Sympathetic nervous system activity increases, parasympathetic activity is reduced and circulating levels of adrenaline and noradrenaline are elevated. As a result, the cardiac output that can be achieved at a given level of cardiac filling may be increased by a factor of four or five. In addition, there is widespread venous constriction, which increases venous return at all levels of cardiac filling. The altered neuro–humoral drive increases precapillary resistance in renal, hepatic, mesenteric and splenic circulations enabling blood flow to be redirected to exercising skeletal muscle, the heart and the cutaneous circulation. These integrated cardiovascular responses involve inputs from higher brain centres such as the cortex and hypothalamus, which reset the control mechanisms operative at rest. This ensures that blood flow and oxygen delivery in the cardiovascular system are maximized and that both are utilized in a way that optimizes exercise performance.

Chapter 15

Cardiovascular System—The Heart

15.1 Introduction

The heart is an electrically controlled and chemically driven mechanical pressure-suction pump. The electrical control signals and emerging mechanical activity are generated in the heart itself (i.e. it beats rhythmically in the absence of external stimulation even after isolation or transplantation), and the underlying processes are modulated by extra-cardiac parameters.

Regulation, by definition, consists of feed-forward and feedback information pathways, whose combination gives rise to a regulatory loop. The intra-cardiac electro-mechanical regulatory loop consists of a feed-forward pathway that links cardiac electrical excitation to mechanical activity via excitation–contraction coupling (ECC), and a mechano–electric feedback pathway (MEF; see Fig. 15.1). This regulatory loop is affected by higher-order neuro-hormonal control, and is subject to modulation by extra-cardiac physical factors, such as the mechanical environment of the heart, temperature, or external electrical stimulation.

All essential components and mechanisms of the intra-cardiac mechano–electric regulatory loop are present at the level of the heart's basic functional unit—the cardiomyocyte. Cardiomyocytes are structurally and functionally integrated into a highly coordinated tissue network, and they show regionally varying functional properties. They underlie such specialized functions as cardiac

pacemaking (rhythmic generation of electrical excitation that drives the heartbeat), conduction of excitation, and contraction. The following sections will review essential aspects of cardiac structure, address in detail the electrical and mechanical processes that give rise to the heartbeat, and describe their dynamic interaction during the cardiac cycle.

15.2 Cardiac structure

Functional gross anatomy

The four-chambered heart contains several functionally relevant sites of specialized electro-mechanical function. In mechanical terms, the right and left atria serve as a reservoir for ventricular blood filling and, via their own contractile activity, contribute 10–15% to ventricular filling. The right and left ventricles form the actual pump of the circulatory system. Electrically specialized tissue includes: the sino-atrial (SA) node in the dorsal wall of the right atrium, where the primary pacemaker cells of the heart are located; the atrio-ventricular (AV) node, which forms the only conducting passage through a connective tissue layer separating the atria from the ventricles; and additional fast conduction pathways between AV node and ventricular myocardium, which support uniform electrical activation of the ventricular muscle mass. Blood flow through the heart is directed by a dual system of ventricular inlet (AV valves) and outlet valves (pulmonary and aortic

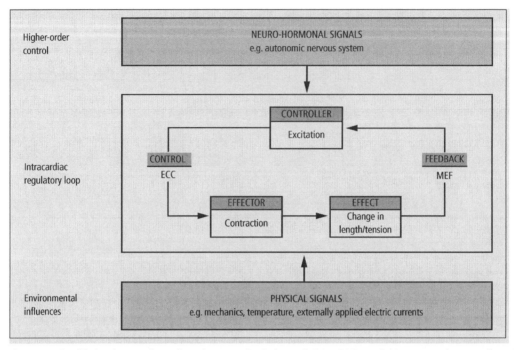

Fig. 15.1 Simplified scheme of cardiac electro-mechanical regulation. ECC, excitation–contraction coupling; MEF, mechano–electric feedback.

valves), which prevent back-flow into preceding sections of the circulatory system during the cycle of ventricular contraction and relaxation.

The heart consists of four chambers: the **right atrium** receives venous blood from the systemic circulation via the upper and lower 'hollow' veins (**superior** and **inferior vena cava**, respectively) and delivers it to the **right ventricle**; the **left atrium** receives blood from the pulmonary circulation (via four pulmonary veins) and conveys it to the **left ventricle** (see Fig. 14.2). The aperture between each atrium and its corresponding ventricle is guarded by an **AV valve**. The right AV valve has three cusps (the **tricuspid valve**) and the left AV valve has two cusps (the **bicuspid** or **mitral valve**). Attached to the free margins of these valves are tendinous cords (**chordae tendineae**), which project from specialized ventricular muscle bundles known as **papillary muscles**. The exits from the right ventricle into the pulmonary artery and from the left ventricle into the aorta are guarded by the

pulmonary and aortic **semilunar valves**, respectively. Rings of connective tissue, the **AV rings**, separate the atria from the ventricles. The AV rings act as a fibrous skeleton for the origin and insertion of atrial and ventricular muscle, and for the attachment of heart valves. They also insulate electrical activity in atria and ventricles.

In order for the heart to function as a pump, its chambers must be filled with sufficient amounts of blood before each contraction. Venous blood return from the **systemic circulation** to the heart is principally driven by three mechanisms: **peripheral vein compression**; the **respiratory pump**; and the **cardiac suction pump**. Peripheral vein compression is afforded by skeletal muscle activity (and, to a lesser extent, by the lateral pulse-wave transmitted to the veins from adjacent arteries), which, in the presence of competent semi-lunar valves in the veins, pushes venous blood into vessel segments that are closer to the heart. The respiratory pump causes alternating pressure gradients between abdomen and thorax that favour venous return during inspiration (while the opposite effect during expiration is limited by the presence of semi-lunar valves in the veins), thereby causing a positive net-contribution to venous blood return to the heart. The most relevant driving force for right atrial filling is afforded by active ventricular contraction (ventricular systole), which shifts the **AV border** 'downwards' in the direction of the cardiac **apex**. Since the AV valves are closed at this time, this shift draws blood from the **venae cavae** and pulmonary veins into the atria (cardiac suction pump effect; Fig. 15.2—note atrial volume increase between frames 1 and 3). Venous return from the **pulmonary circulation** is additionally helped by the residual pressure of right ventricular contrac-

tions, which (in contrast to the systemic circulation) provides a significant remaining driving force for filling of the left side of the heart (in contrast, contributions from vein compression and the respiratory pump are less pertinent). Upon ventricular relaxation (ventricular diastole), the AV border moves back towards the **base** of the heart, this time with open AV valves, thereby encompassing a large proportion of the blood volume previously drawn into the atria (Fig. 15.2, frame 4). Refilling of ventricles to about 85% of **end-diastolic volume** is obtained passively via this mechanism (and very early during ventricular relaxation), while the remainder is achieved by atrial contraction (at the very end of ventricular diastole).

Active cardiac contraction is initiated by

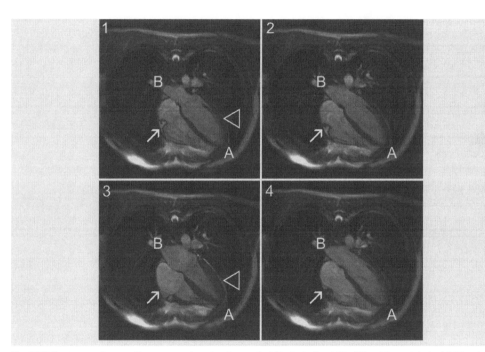

Fig. 15.2 Sequence of magnetic resonance imaging frames that illustrate the shift of the atrio-ventricular (AV) border during the cardiac cycle in a healthy man. Note that both the apex (A) and the base of the heart (B) remain almost stationary, and that the overall volume occupied by the heart shows little change. Slanted arrow indicates right AV border position just prior to ventricular contraction (frame 1); open arrow-head highlights increase in left ventricular wall thickness during contraction (compare frames 1 and 3). Note: magnetic resonance imaging techniques are based on the interaction of the nuclear magnetic moment (consequence of the intrinsic spin, for example of hydrogen nuclei in tissue water) with a controlled external magnetic field, resulting in a macroscopic magnetization that can be measured with dedicated detectors (radio-frequency coils). This can be used to non-invasively provide information about structure, function and metabolic activity of living tissue. (Fig. courtesy of Francis, J. and Robson, M., University of Oxford Centre for Clinical Magnetic Resonance Research.)

electrical excitation, which originates in the heart's own pacemaker tissue—the **SA node**—located in the right atrium. The pacemaker tissue generates rhythmic waves of electrical excitation that spread through the atria and then, via the **AV node** and specialized conduction pathways, to both ventricles. As the spread of this electrical signal determines the sequence of active mechanical contraction, atrial systole precedes ventricular systole. Atrial contraction increases ventricular volume to its end-diastolic levels, just before ventricular contraction starts. Once ventricular pressure exceeds atrial pressure, the AV valves close, thereby preventing back-flow of blood into the atria. Papillary muscles also contract during ventricular systole, tensing the **chordae tendineae** that prevent AV valves from opening backwards into the atria. Continued contraction of the ventricles raises the ventricular pressure above that in the downstream vessels, opening the pulmonary and aortic valves. Blood is then ejected from the right ventricle at low pressure into the pulmonary circulation, and from the left ventricle at high pressure into the systemic circulation.

Upon termination of active ventricular contraction, ventricular pressures drop below those in the downstream vessels. This causes the pulmonary and aortic valves to close, terminating blood ejection and preventing reflux of blood back into the ventricles. Further ventricular relaxation reduces ventricular pressures below atrial pressures, and shifts the AV border back towards the base of the heart. AV valves then open and the ventricles refill with blood, as described above.

Myocardial tissue organization

Cardiac muscle tissue (myocardium) is a heterogeneous structure containing cardiomyocytes, connective tissue, neurones, and a great number of blood vessels with endothelial and smooth muscle cells. Cardiomyocytes are electrically coupled by gap junctions—proteins that form channels interconnecting the interior of neighbouring cells.

The magnitude of pressure generated by each heart chamber during contraction correlates with the thickness of the **myocardium** forming its muscle wall (Fig. 15.2). Atrial myocardium is thin, whilst ventricular myocardium is thick (especially in the left ventricle, which generates the highest pressures). The inner surface of the cardiac chambers is lined with **endocardium**, which is essentially a continuation of the endothelium that makes up the inside of blood vessels. The outer surface of the myocardium is covered with mesothelial tissue, called **epicardium**. Enclosing the heart is a thin fibrous sac (the **pericardium**), which is lined by a parietal layer of mesothelium. The pericardium is relatively stiff and limits excessive acute enlargement of the heart. The **pericardial space** between the epicardium and pericardium contains just enough interstitial fluid to act as a lubricant to allow movement of the cardiac surface relative to the pericardium.

Cardiomyocytes form the bulk of myocardium, but they are exceeded in number by smaller connective tissue cells, such as **fibroblasts**. Indeed, every cardiomyocyte borders to one or more fibroblast in the heart (Fig. 15.3). Cardiomyocytes show little, if any, proliferative potential in the adult mammalian heart, therefore growth of cardiac muscle is achieved either by an increase in cardiomyocyte cell dimensions (hypertrophy), or via invasion/replacement of muscle cells by connective tissue (fibrosis, scarring).

Cardiomyocytes are cross-striated and—just like in skeletal muscle—this striation is a consequence of the regular sarcomeric arrangement of contractile proteins. These are 'in register' even between neighbouring myocardial cells. Cardiomyocytes are shorter than most skeletal muscle cells (about 150–200 μm compared to several millimetres or even centimetres), narrower (15–20 μm compared to 40 μm), and they have more mitochondria (which, in contrast to skeletal muscle, are located not only underneath the sarcolemma, but also in strands between contractile proteins). Cardiomyocytes have no neuro-muscular junctions. They abut end-to-end (and, to a lesser extent, side-to-side), where they are electrically coupled via protein channels (connexins) that form low-conductance electrical communication pathways (**gap junctions**); therefore the response to a nor-

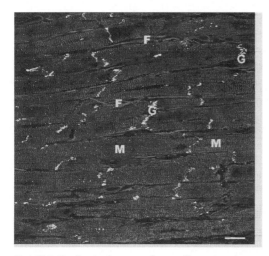

Fig. 15.3 Confocal microscopy image, illustrating tissue architecture in mammalian myocardium. Heart muscle consists of cardiomyocyte layers (pale cross-striated cells, M) that are interconnected by gap junctions (brightly labelled disks between myocytes, G) and interspersed with fibroblasts (thin solidly stained cell strands, F). Scale bar 20 μm. Note: confocal microscopy is a laser-based scanning technique of fluorescent dyes in biological samples, where both dye-excitation and observation of emitted light are focused at exactly the same point (hence con-focal, from *cum*—Latin for 'with' or 'together'), which allows 'optical slicing' of mechanically intact tissue (up to a certain depth, in cardiac tissue usually <0.2 mm). (Fig. courtesy of Camelliti, P., University of Oxford, Department of Physiology, Anatomy and Genetics.)

mal cycle of electrical excitation is 'all-or-nothing' at the myocardial level (i.e. all cardiomyocytes are stimulated during each heartbeat).

The apposition of one cardiac cell with another coincides with the location of sarcomeric Z lines and contains electron-dense **intercalated discs** (Fig. 15.4). Within these discs, **desmosomes** provide sites of mechanical adhesion between cardiac cells and ensure that the tension developed by one cell is transmitted to the next.

The myocardium is furthermore characterized by a very dense network of capillaries that are fed from **coronary arteries** that originate from the aorta, just downstream of the aortic valve. Venous return from this system is either to the **sinus venosus** in the right atrium, or through **Thebesian veins** directly into both ventricles.

The cardiomyocyte

Cardiomyocytes—the basic functional units of the heart—are usually poly-nucleated and show very clear cross-striation. They are excitable cells that respond to an electrical stimulus by mechanical contraction.

Cardiomyocyte contractile proteins are arranged in sarcomeres with their characteristic cross-striation pattern, formed by the sequence of myosin-rich **anisotropic** (A) and actin filament-only **isotropic** (I) bands (see Fig. 5.1). The centre of each I band is marked by a Z line (Z from 'zwischen'—German for 'in-between'), and provides the anchor plane for actin filaments that extend to both sides of most Z lines (except at cell ends). The distance between two neighbouring Z lines is referred to as the sarcomere length (~1.85 μm in isolated, i.e. mechanically unloaded cardiomyocytes at rest, compared to >2.0 μm in skeletal muscle). The centre of the A band is characterized by an M line (M from 'mittel'—German for 'middle') where myosin fibres are spatially coordinated.

In comparison with skeletal muscle, cardiomyocytes have a less extensive **sarcoplasmic reticulum** (SR). Their **transverse (T) tubular system** is, where present (i.e. in ventricular, but not in atrial cardiomyocytes), more voluminous (i.e. has larger diameters) than in skeletal muscle, and is located at the Z line (rather than the A–I junction, Fig. 15.5). T tubules form intimate connections with the SR that are of high importance to cardiac ECC (see Fig. 15.20).

Cardiac gap junctions

Transport between adjacent cells can be either by a combination of diffusion and exo-/endocytosis through cell membranes, or via gap junctions. These channel-like structures provide direct links between the interior of neighbouring cells and allow passage of ions and small molecules up to a molecular weight of 1 kDa—equivalent to the mass of 1000 hydrogen atoms, i.e. including substances such as adenosine tri-phosphate (ATP). All cardiac myocytes are interconnected into a 'functional syncytium' by gap junctions, which underlie the fast spread of electrical signals though the

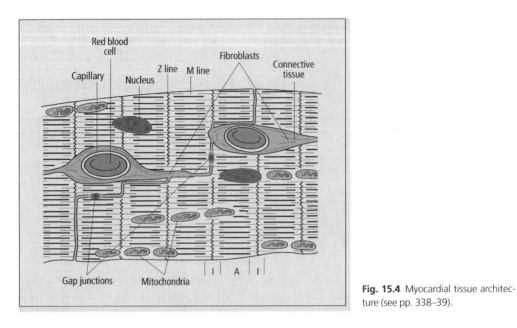

Fig. 15.4 Myocardial tissue architecture (see pp. 338–39).

cardiac muscle and the coordinated electro-mechanical activity of the heart.

Gap junctions form by docking of two hemi-channels, one each in the membrane of neighbouring cells, to form a direct pathway between the interiors of the two cells (see Fig. 2.3). Each hemi-channel (**connexon**) is formed by six **connexin** molecules. Connexins (Cx) are classed by their molecular weight, and Cx43 is the protein involved in forming the majority of cardiac gap junctions in the working myocardium. Other connexins, including Cx40 and Cx45, are found in pacemaker tissue or the cardiac conduction system, and some connect non-myocytes in the heart.

Connexin specificity underlies the selective coupling of cardiac cells, so that electrical impulses are first spread throughout the cardiac conduction system, before they invade ventricular working myocardium. Their dissimilar electrical conductance (highest for Cx40, followed by Cx43 and Cx45) also contributes to differences in the speed of action potential (AP) propagation in different regions of the heart, and pathological changes in connexin expression or distribution may have significant negative effects on cardiac activity.

15.3 Electrical properties of the heart

The heart is able to beat rhythmically in isolation, i.e. without nervous input. The wave of electrical excitation that causes cardiac contraction is initiated in the pacemaker cells of the SA node in the right atrium, and is transmitted through the heart along specialized cardiomyocytes that form fast-conducting pathways. In contrast to working myocardium, pacemaker cells have no stable resting membrane potential. They spontaneously depolarize to a threshold, at which an AP is generated. Cardiac AP are of significantly longer duration than those observed in nerve or skeletal muscle, and there is considerable overlap in time between the AP and active contraction. For this reason, cardiac contractions cannot summate, and tetanic contractions do not occur. Pacemaker firing rate, and therefore heart rate, is increased by sympathetic and decreased by parasympathetic nerve activity. The autonomic nervous system also influences conduction velocity through the heart, myocardial excitability, and contraction. The electrocardiogram (ECG)—comprising the P wave and the QRS complex that reflect atrial and ventricular depolarization, respectively, and the T wave that reflects ventricular repolarization—is the clinically most relevant tool for monitoring cardiac electrical activity. The

ECG can reveal abnormalities in cardiac excitation and conduction patterns, and is of great diagnostic importance.

Origin and spread of electrical excitation

A denervated (isolated or transplanted) heart, maintained appropriately, continues to beat in an orderly sequence of atrial and ventricular contraction (systole) and relaxation/rest (diastole). This mechanical activity is caused by the regular spread of excitation, originating in cardiac pacemaker cells and conducted via gap junctions to the whole myocardium.

The pacemaker region with the highest intrinsic rate, and hence the **primary pacemaker**, is the **SA node**. This is a small tissue area, located in the dorsal wall of the right atrium between the entrances of superior and inferior **venae cavae** (Fig. 15.6). In the absence of nervous control, the SA node initiates AP at a rate of 90–100 beats min^{-1} (bpm). This rate is reduced by the dominant vagal activity in healthy individuals to 60–70 bpm at rest.

Lower-order pacemaker tissue (composed of cells whose *in situ* pacemaking rates are slower than those of the SA node) include the **AV node** (intrinsic beating rate about 40–50 bpm), **bundle of His** (30–40 bpm), and **Purkinje fibres** (20–30 bpm). Pacemaker cells are cardiomyocytes, and as such

they possess visible (although less prominent than in working myocardium) sarcomeric structures. A common property of all pacemaker cells is their **spontaneous diastolic depolarization**, i.e. the absence of a stable diastolic membrane potential between subsequent cycles of excitation.

AP propagation (spread of excitation) from one cell to the next is via gap junctions. Electrical excitation, initiated in the SA node (primary pacemaker), invades the atrial myocardium and travels from one atrial cell to the next (regionally aided by well-aligned muscle strands of low electrical resistance) throughout both atria and towards the AV node. The AV node is the sole pathway for AV conduction through the fibrous tissue layer that separates atria and ventricles. Conduction through the AV node is slow (0.05 m s^{-1}) compared to atrial or ventricular muscle (0.5–1.0 m s^{-1}). This effectively delays AP transmission from atria to ventricles by about 0.1 s at resting heart rates. As a consequence, atrial excitation finishes at about the time that ventricular excitation begins (Fig. 15.6).

Lower-order pacemaker centres are in direct electrical contact to each other, and provide a **specialized conduction pathway** that assists in the fast and orderly spread of cardiac excitation to the whole of the ventricular myocardium (Fig. 15.6). From the AV node, the AP swiftly

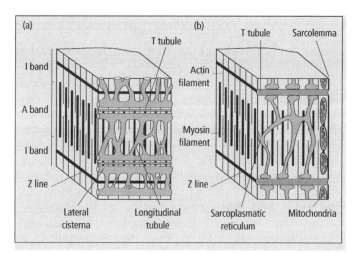

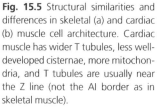

Fig. 15.5 Structural similarities and differences in skeletal (a) and cardiac (b) muscle cell architecture. Cardiac muscle has wider T tubules, less well-developed cisternae, more mitochondria, and T tubules are usually near the Z line (not the AI border as in skeletal muscle).

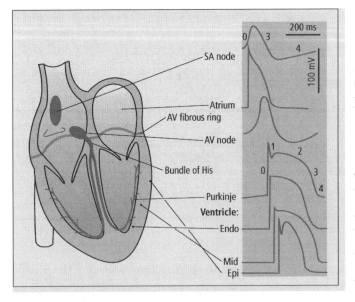

Fig. 15.6 Location of sino-atrial (SA) node and specialized conduction pathways, and the shape, duration and sequence of cardiac action potentials (AP) in different regions of the heart. Delays in excitation are caused by the anatomical sequence of depolarization and by regional differences in conduction velocities. Note that ventricular AP have different duration, causing repolarization to occur roughly in an inverse sequence to the spread of excitation. Numerals above AP curves indicate upstroke (0), early partial repolarization (1), plateau (2), full repolarization (3) and diastolic membrane potential (4). AV, atrioventricular.

travels down the ventricular septum in the **bundle of His** ($1\,\mathrm{m\,s^{-1}}$) and then along the right and left bundle branches to enter the **Purkinje network**, which ramifies throughout the ventricles. The Purkinje network has very high conduction velocities ($5\,\mathrm{m\,s^{-1}}$) and delivers excitation to the subendocardial layers of both ventricles with minimal delay. From there, excitation travels, as in the atria, from one working cardiomyocyte to the next, via gap junctions. Since the innermost layers of both ventricles are excited with little difference in time, excitation reaches all parts of both ventricles in a well-coordinated manner, causing them to depolarize and consequently contract, almost simultaneously.

Characteristics of cardiac transmembrane potentials

Cardiac cells can be divided into pacemaking cells that show spontaneous diastolic depolarization, and working cardiomyocytes that have a stable diastolic membrane potential. All cardiomyocytes are excitable, i.e. when depolarized to threshold they generate an AP. Characteristics of an AP, such as maximum diastolic potential, AP shape, and AP duration, vary in different *regions of the heart and underlie the well-orchestrated electrical activity of the heart.*

Pacemaker cells

Pacemaker cells are characterized by their intrinsic ability to reach threshold for AP generation, i.e. 'to beat', in the absence of an external trigger (Fig. 15.7). Pacemaking is therefore an intrinsic property of the heart, although the rate at which pacemaker AP are generated is affected by external influences, such as autonomic nervous input, or the mechanical environment and temperature (Fig. 15.1).

Pacemaker cell membrane potentials are characterized by a **maximum diastolic potential (MDP)**—the most negative point reached during a cycle. From the MDP, **spontaneous diastolic depolarization** slowly shifts the membrane towards the AP **threshold** potential. The MDP is least negative in SA node cells (−45 mV to −55 mV), followed by AV node cells (−50 mV to −65 mV), and it becomes increasingly more negative further down the cardiac conduction system until it is indistinguishable from working cardiomyocytes (−80 mV to −90 mV). In contrast, the slope of spontaneous

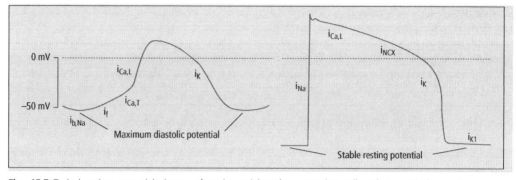

Fig. 15.7 Typical action potential shapes of a sino-atrial node pacemaker cell and a ventricular cardiomyocyte. Key underlying ion currents are labelled and explained in the text.

diastolic depolarization is greatest in SA node cells. Therefore, threshold for AP generation is reached fastest in SA node, making it the pacemaker from which each normal heartbeat originates. The AP propagates from SA node through the atria and arrives at the AV node well before the intrinsic diastolic depolarization of AV node cells would reach threshold. Thus, under normal conditions, the AP that occurs in the AV node is initiated by the AP conducted from the SA node.

Pacemaker cell spontaneous diastolic depolarization is caused by a reduction in repolarizing currents in the presence of sustained or increasing depolarizing currents. This natural oscillator involves negative feedback via voltage sensitive currents such as a depolarization-activated (but itself repolarizing) potassium current (i_K), and a hyperpolarization-activated (but itself depolarizing) mixed sodium–potassium 'funny' current (i_f). Additional contributors to spontaneous diastolic depolarization are the sodium background current ($i_{b,Na}$), as well as the transient calcium current ($i_{Ca,T}$) and, possibly, current via the electrogenic sodium–calcium exchanger (i_{NCX}; when near-membrane calcium is elevated, the exchanger extrudes one Ca^{2+} ion from the cell in exchange for import of three Na^+ ions, thereby generating a net inward flux of one positive charge per cycle).

Once threshold is reached, an AP is generated. The upstroke of SA node pacemaker AP is carried almost exclusively by the long-lasting calcium current ($i_{Ca,L}$) in man. Lower-order pacemaker cells show an increasingly prominent contribution of the fast sodium current (i_{Na}) to their AP upstroke (in atrial and ventricular working cardiomyocytes, AP upstroke is carried by i_{Na} only), which is evident from increasingly fast AP upstroke velocities as one moves 'down' the cardiac conduction system (Fig. 15.6).

SA node pacemaker AP reach a peak at about 20 mV, and repolarize slowly without formation of a plateau potential. Repolarization ensues as a consequence of a reduction in depolarizing currents (both i_f and $i_{Ca,L}$ are inactivated by positive potentials) and an increase in repolarizing currents (i_K becomes activated at positive potentials), until the membrane potential returns to MDP and the next cycle resumes.

Thus, cardiac pacemaking is the result of the interplay of several ion currents and it cannot be attributed solely to a single mechanism. This multitude of pacemaking mechanisms provides a solid functional reserve that ensures stability of this vital function, and a foundation for multiple regulatory pathways that affect heart rate (see Fig. 15.10).

Working cardiomyocytes

The bulk volume of atrial and ventricular myocardium is occupied by working cardiomyocytes. Their diastolic potential is stable at about −80 mV to −90 mV. These cells do not generate an AP unless stimulated. The physiological trigger event is depolarization, conducted via gap junctions, that is associated with the approach of an AP through neighbouring cells.

The stable resting membrane potential is caused by the lack in i_f in working myocardium, and by the existence of a potassium conductance that shows different activation properties, compared to i_K in pacemaker cells, in that it is hyperpolarization-activated and hyperpolarizing (i_{K1}). This is an example of a 'self-enforcing', or positive, feedback. It ensures that small depolarizing background currents, such as i_{bNa}, will merely shift the resting membrane potential from the equilibrium potential for potassium (–96 mV) to slightly more positive levels, but not trigger AP outside the normal sequence of cardiac activation.

Upon externally-induced depolarization to AP threshold, fast sodium channels open and i_{Na} causes swift depolarization. This is further aided by the depolarization-induced inactivation of i_{K1}. The AP reaches a peak of +40 mV within about 1 ms, after which time i_{Na} channels close abruptly. The AP then shows brief decline, followed by the AP plateau (Fig. 15.7). The net transmembrane current, flowing during the plateau, is very low indeed. It is initially carried by $i_{Ca,L}$ (which triggers ECC, see p. 361), and subsequently by i_{NCX} (which extrudes one Ca^{2+} ion in exchange for influx of three Na^+ ions, thereby providing an inward current for as long as the cytosolic free calcium concentration, $[Ca^{2+}]_i$, is elevated). This link between $[Ca^{2+}]_i$ (which determines mechanical activity) and AP plateau maintenance (which is a key factor in setting overall AP duration) is crucial in understanding how the duration of the cardiac AP may match active mechanical contraction (thereby preventing summation or tetanic contractions of cardiac muscle).

Once $[Ca^{2+}]_i$, and consequently i_{NCX}, begin to decline, the membrane repolarizes into the potential range where i_K (the 'pacemaker cell' potassium current) activates, leading to increasingly swift repolarization of the cell. Upon return towards near-resting membrane potential levels, i_K inactivates in exchange for i_{K1}, and the cardiomyocyte is quiescent again until further stimulation.

AP mechanisms are similar in atrial and ventricular cardiomyocytes, although there are differences in AP time course caused by differences in the extent to which individual currents are expressed (and by additional ion currents that will not be discussed in detail here). Atrial cardiomyocytes tend to have shorter AP duration, a less obvious plateau, and less steep late repolarization (Fig. 15.6).

Temporal relationship between electrical and mechanical events

Cardiac electrical and mechanical activity are closely coupled. The AP upstroke initiates the events involved in ECC, which, in turn, contribute to AP plateau maintenance. This renders cardiomyocytes insensitive to additional stimulation and prevents summation of cardiac contractions.

When measured from the AP upstroke, there is a latency of about 10 ms before cardiomyocytes start to contract (Fig. 15.8), compared to about 2 ms in skeletal muscle (see Fig. 5.9). This is due to differences in ECC, primarily related to the need, in cardiomyocytes, for influx of external calcium (carried by $i_{Ca,L}$) to trigger large-scale calcium release from the SR (calcium-induced calcium release; CICR) (see p. 361). Peak contraction occurs during the late AP plateau, and relaxation overlaps with, or extends slightly beyond, cardiomyocyte repolarization.

Thus, cardiomyocyte electrical and mechanical activity overlap considerably in time (in contrast to skeletal muscle where the short-lasting AP is virtually over before contraction even begins). As a consequence, cardiac contractile force may not be graded by temporal summation (as seen in skeletal muscle; see Fig. 5.9), and myocardium does not show tetanic contractions. Equally, there is no spatial summation (characteristic for skeletal muscle and based on stimulation of increasing numbers of individual fibres in a muscle), as myocardium has no neuro-muscular junctions and responds to stimulation in an all-or-nothing fashion. In contrast to skeletal muscle, cardiac contractility is adjusted via changes in cellular calcium handling, as discussed on p. 362.

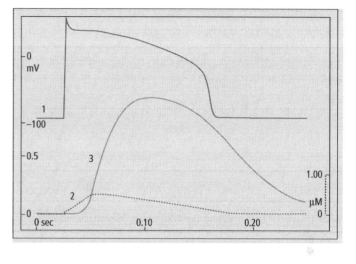

Fig. 15.8 Temporal interrelation of ventricular action potentials (1); intracellular calcium concentration $[Ca_i^{2+}]$ (2); and contraction (3).

From the AP upstroke, during the subsequent plateau, and until repolarization to about −20 mV, cardiomyocytes are **inexcitable** (Fig. 15.9). This is called the **absolute refractory period** (ARP; about 250 ms during an AP of 300 ms duration) and is a consequence of the voltage-sensitivity of fast sodium channels carrying i_{Na}. This current is required for the AP upstroke in working myocardium and, as described on p. 344, inactivates within about 1 ms. Channels remain inactivated (and the cell is absolutely refractory) until the membrane returns to a potential below −20 mV. During further repolarization towards resting membrane potential levels, i_{Na} channels start to recover from inactivation, and cardiomyocytes progressively regain excitability. They are then said to be in the **relative refractory period** (RRP; about 50 ms in the given example). During the ARP, no AP can be triggered (even by very large stimuli); while in the RRP, a strong stimulus can elicit a curtailed AP with reduced upstroke velocity and amplitude (as recovery of i_{Na} channels from inactivation is still incomplete), and shortened duration (as calcium entry via $i_{Ca,L}$ is equally still diminished by voltage-dependent inactivation).

The prolonged cardiac refractory period effectively limits the rate at which the heart can beat. Combined with the absence of tetanic contractions, this is a pre-requirement for cyclic contraction and relaxation (note: ventricular filling occurs during early ventricular relaxation and determines the volume available for ejection during the subsequent beat). Furthermore, since the ARP extends beyond the time taken for AP conduction through the atria and ventricles, recycling of excitation in the muscular network is not seen in the normal heart.

Extra-cardiac effects on origin and conduction of electrical activity

SA node pacemaking rate and conduction of excitation are acutely affected by higher-order neuro-hormonal control mechanisms, and by environmental factors, such as mechanics, temperature, or external electrical stimulation (Fig. 15.1).

Neuro-hormonal control

Higher-order neuro-hormonal control affects the heart via the autonomic nervous system. Innervation of the heart is both via **sympathetic** and **parasympathetic** nerves, which have opposite effects on cardiac electro-mechanical activity. Effects of sympathetic nerve activation are: positive **chronotropy** (increasing heart rate; from *chronos*—Greek for 'time', and *trepein*—Greek for 'to turn' or 'change'); positive **inotropy** (increasing force of contraction; from *inos*—Greek for [muscle] 'fibre'); positive **dromotropy** (increasing speed of

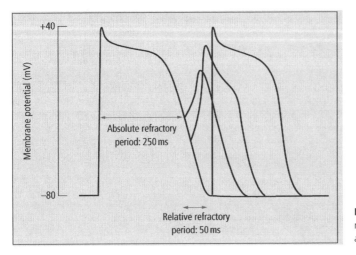

Fig. 15.9 Absolute and relative refractory periods of the ventricular action potential.

conduction; from *dromos*—Greek for 'course' or 'progression'); and positive **bathmotropy** (increasing excitability; from bathmos—Greek for 'step' or 'threshold'). Parasympathetic activation reduces all four parameters, which are described as negative chronotropic, negative inotropic, negative dromotropic and negative bathmotropic responses.

At rest, parasympathetic activity dominates. Since the parasympathetic fibres project to the heart in the **vagus nerve** (cranial nerve X), their normal activity is often referred to as **vagal tone**. Intense parasympathetic activity can actually stop the pacemaker of the heart for a brief period. Normally, a low heart rate (**bradycardia**, from *bradys*—Greek for 'slow', and *kardia*—Greek for 'heart'), for example during sleep, is due to an increase in parasympathetic discharge and a decrease in, or even absence of, cardiac sympathetic stimulation. With physical or emotional stress, sympathetic activity increases, and parasympathetic activity is reduced. This leads to increased pacemaking rate, faster conduction and excitation of working myocardium, and stronger contractions. During severe exercise (or in acute anxiety), heart rate may increase in humans up to about 200 bpm (**tachycardia**, from *tachys*—Greek for 'rapid').

Acceleration of heart rate can principally be achieved in three ways: by increasing the rate of spontaneous diastolic depolarization; by shifting the MDP to more depolarized potentials; or by moving the threshold for AP generation towards more negative potentials. In all three cases, the time taken to depolarize a pacemaker cell from MDP to AP threshold is reduced (Fig. 15.10).

Catecholamines bind to **β-adrenoceptors** (mainly of the β_1 receptor subtype in the heart, whereas β_2 receptors dominate in tracheal and vascular musculature. There are two catecholamines: **noradrenaline**, the transmitter substance of postganglionic **sympathetic** fibres, and **adrenaline**, the hormone released in response to increased sympathetic activity from the medulla of the adrenal gland—a triangular endocrine gland positioned on top of each kidney which may itself be considered as a large 'postganglionic' catecholamine release site. (The term 'adrenaline' stems from *ad*—Latin for 'near', and *renes*—Latin for 'kidneys'; in the US better known as **epinephrine**, from *epi*—Greek for 'upon', and *nephros*—Greek for kidney.) In the SA node, catecholamines enhance both i_f and $i_{Ca,L}$. This increases the rate of diastolic depolarization and moves threshold for AP generation towards more negative potentials, causing a positive chronotropic response. Catecholamines increase $i_{Ca,L}$ also in atrial and ventricular working cardiomyocytes, leading to a positive ionotropic response.

Acetylcholine (the transmitter released by

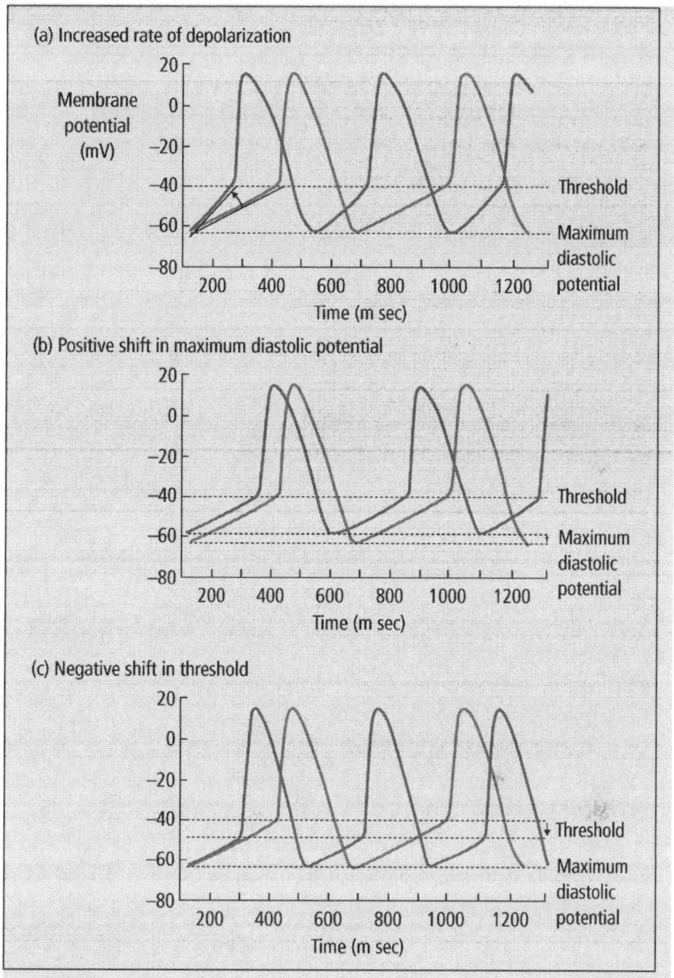

Fig. 15.10 Three principal mechanisms that may increase sino-atrial (SA) node pacemaker rate (control, light blue; intervention, dark blue). (a) Increased rate of diastolic depolarization brings membrane faster to threshold for AP generation. (b) Shift of the maximum diastolic potential towards less negative potentials decreases time to threshold, even at unchanged rate of diastolic depolarization. (c) Shift of threshold towards more negative potentials reduces time to threshold, even if diastolic depolarization rate and maximum diastolic potential were unaffected.

parasympathetic fibres), in contrast, binds to **muscarinic cholinoceptors** (mainly the M_2 receptor subtype in the heart, one of five subtypes located throughout the body) and acts via inverse effects on all three electrophysiological mechanisms described above to slow heart rate. In SA node cells, acetylcholine decreases i_f (reducing the rate of diastolic depolarization), increases an acetylcholine-sensitive potassium current (thereby shifting MDP towards more negative potentials), and reduces $i_{Ca,L}$ (thereby shifting threshold towards more positive potentials and reducing AP upstroke velocity). Together, these effects lead to a negative chronotropic response. Acetylcholine has similar effects on AV node cells, causing a slowing in conduction velocity and an increase in AV conduction delay (negative dromotropic effect). In working cardiomyocytes, the acetylcholine-induced increase in potassium currents reduces their excitability (negative bathmotropic effect), and the acetylcholine-reduced $i_{Ca,L}$ lowers contractility (negative inotropic effect).

Environmental influences

The cardiac mechanical environment has direct effects on heart rate and force of contraction. Stretch of the SA node will tend to increase beating rate (**Bainbridge effect**), both via a reflex pathway and via local mechanisms, such as stretch-activated ion channels that depolarize MDP and increase the rate of diastolic depolarization. Stretch also increases the contractility of working myocardium (see **Frank-Starling effect**, p. 363). This combination of chronotropic and inotropic responses to stretch allows the heart to adjust the number of contractions per unit of time, and the volume pumped on each beat, to match cardiac output to venous return.

Pacemaker rate and contractility are also sensitive to temperature changes (hypothermia, fever). In humans, SA node pacemaker rate increases by approximately 10 bpm per degree centigrade increase in body temperature; in contrast, contractility is increased by cooling. Here, the two effects are not additive to each other, but act in a compensatory fashion to a stimulus of patho-physiological relevance.

Dysfunction of SA node pacemaking or electrical conduction are frequently corrected by implantation of electronic circuitry, to electrically pace or synchronize contractions. Since the introduction of cardiac pacemakers in the 1950s, devices have been miniaturized and equipped with advanced rhythm recognition software, so that they can even be used as implantable defibrillators in high-risk patient populations.

Electrocardiogram

*The synchronized activity of the cardiac chambers gives rise to electrical potential differences that can be recorded from the body surface. This signal can be amplified and recorded as an **electrocardiogram** (**ECG**). The ECG provides information on heart rate and rhythm, electrical conduction, cardiac position, and it can be used to diagnose and roughly localize pathological disturbances, such as myocardial ischaemia and infarction.*

Characteristics of the ECG

The body surface potential differences recorded by ECG arise as a consequence of current flow at the interface of electrically excited and non-excited myocardium within either the atria or the ventricles (as the atria are electrically isolated from the ventricles by the AV fibrous ring, potential differences between atria and ventricles cause no deflection on the ECG). Cardiac chambers that are either wholly resting, or wholly excited, do not give rise to surface potential differences, and the ECG shows an **isoelectric line** (0 mV).

Notable interfaces between excited and resting tissue, whose projection can be determined at the body surface, occur in the atria during the spread of excitation from SA node through the atrial muscle and towards the AV node, in the ventricles during the spread of excitation from the ventricular septum towards the whole ventricular muscle mass, and during ventricular repolarization (Fig. 15.11). Atrial repolarization does not produce a detectable ECG signal (it occurs during ventricular excitation which gives rise to much larger ECG deflections).

The amplitude and distribution of body surface potential differences depends on the direction and amplitude of the current flow between excited and non-excited tissue. The net current at any point in time can be described by a vector that changes direction and amplitude, as waves of excitation or repolarization travel through the cardiac muscle (Fig. 15.11). During each cardiac cycle, the tip of this vector describes three loops in space, and its projections onto any plane can be visualized as a **vector cardiogram** (VCG; Fig. 15.12).

The frontal projection of the summary ECG vector lies in the same body plane as the standard recording points introduced by Einthoven (right hand, left hand, left foot—forming 'Einthoven's triangle'). In this recording configuration, the ECG examines body surface potential differences as right arm → left arm (lead I), right arm → left foot (lead II), and left arm → left foot (lead III). ECG recordings obtained with any of these lead configurations are, in essence, projections of the two-dimensional VCG loop onto a single edge of the triangle (Fig. 15.13). If one would move a pen up and down along one edge of the triangle to follow the position of the VCG vector tip projection onto that very edge, and at the same time pull the

Fig. 15.11 Direction and amplitude of net current flow (see arrows in first, third and fifth frames) at the interface between excited and non-excited tissue during one cardiac cycle. From top left to bottom right: (1) atrial excitation wave; (2) atrio-ventricular conduction (potential differences too small to matter); (3) ventricular excitation wave; (4) ventricular excitation plateau (no potential difference); (5) ventricular repolarization wave; (6) full repolarization (no potential difference). Note that, similar to a wave that travels up on a beach and then back, waves of ventricular excitation and repolarization largely travel in opposite directions (caused by the shorter action potential (AP) durations in sub-epicardial layers of myocardium; see Fig. 15.6).

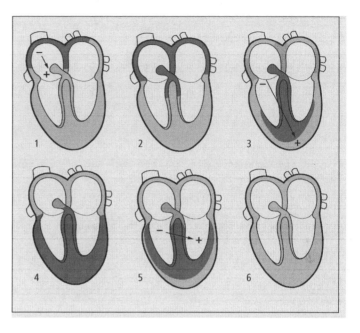

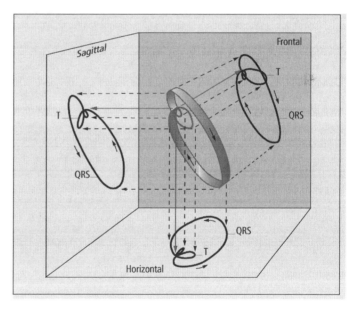

Fig. 15.12 Cardiac electrical vector projections during one electrical cycle. For an explanation see text. (Adapted from Schmidt, R. F. & Thews, G. (1985) *Physiologie des Menschen*, 22nd edn. p. 408. Springer-Verlag, Berlin, Heidelberg, New York.)

recording paper underneath the pen with a constant speed (direction opposite to the 'time' arrow in Fig. 15.13), one would obtain the ECG recording used in clinical practice.

The actual pattern of the ECG varies depending on the position of the electrodes on the body surface, but principal components indicative of atrial and ventricular excitation, as well as of ventricular repolarization, are evident in all recording lead configurations. A typical lead II ECG has five

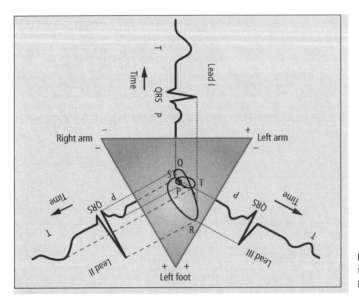

Fig. 15.13 Projection of frontal vector cardiogram onto the edges of the Einthoven triangle (for detail see text).

distinct peaks: P, Q, R, S and T (Fig. 15.14). The **P wave** is produced by the spread of electrical activity during atrial depolarization. The **QRS complex** is produced by the wave of ventricular depolarization, and the **T wave** by ventricular repolarization. Since ventricular repolarization is less well synchronized than ventricular depolarization, the T wave is longer in duration and smaller in amplitude than the QRS complex.

Depending on the electrode position, the QRS complex may have three, two or sometimes only one component (see Figs 15.13 and 15.15). If the first deflection from the isoelectric line after the P wave is negative (by convention downwards), it is called a Q wave; if positive, it is called an R wave, and if the deflection following the R wave falls below the isoelectric line, it is called an S wave. Also, the T wave may consist of one or two deflections (see lead III in Fig. 15.13).

At any given electrode, the polarity of the voltage change plotted on the ECG depends on the nature of the electrical wave that is spreading through the myocardium (either depolarization or repolarization), and the direction in which this wave is moving relative to the electrode. If a depolarization wave is travelling towards a positive electrode (see polarity signs indicated for each lead at

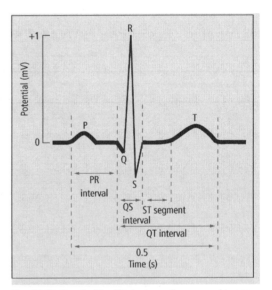

Fig. 15.14 Standard lead II electrocardiogram and important time intervals (for detail see text).

the corners of the Einthoven triangle in Fig. 15.13), a positive ECG deflection is recorded; if a depolarization wave is travelling away from the positive electrode, a negative ECG change occurs. Repolarization waves show an inverse relation between di-

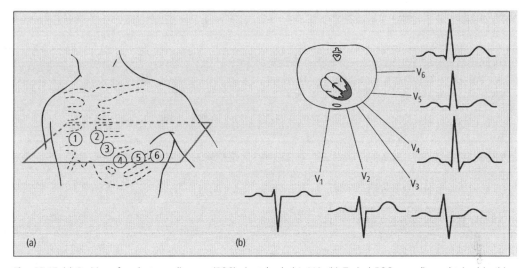

Fig. 15.15 (a) Positions for electrocardiogram (ECG) chest leads (V_1–V_6). (b) Typical ECG recordings obtained in this configuration (for detail see text).

rection of travel and polarity of the ECG deflection. Since the direction of repolarization of the ventricles is largely inverse to that of the excitation wave front, both R and T wave tend to show the same polarity in most ECG recordings.

In addition to the ECG peaks, a number of time intervals are frequently determined (Fig. 15.14). The **PR interval** is the time required for excitation to spread from SA node through the atria, AV node and bundle of His, and it is measured from the onset of the P wave to the beginning of the QRS complex. The **QS interval** is the time required for excitation to spread through the ventricles and denotes the duration of the QRS complex. The **QT interval** is a measure of the maximum duration of ventricular depolarization, and lasts from the onset of the QRS complex to the end of the T wave. The **ST segment** during which all ventricular cardiomyocytes are at plateau potential lasts from the end of the QRS complex to the onset of the T wave and is, in healthy myocardium, isoelectric.

Common ECG recording configurations

The **standard limb leads I, II and III** are obtained as bipolar recordings between any two corners of the Einthoven triangle (left hand, right hand, left foot), with a fourth electrode on the right foot acting as an earth. For **augmented limb leads**, unipolar recordings are obtained, using one of the three corners of the Einthoven triangle as an active (positive) electrode, while the remaining two are electrically connected to form the indifferent (negative) electrode (again with the right foot earthed). When the active electrode is the right arm, left arm or left foot, the augmented lead is designated aVR, aVL or aVF, respectively (with aV standing for 'augmented voltage').

Chest leads are obtained as unipolar recordings with an active electrode in one of six positions on the thorax (Fig. 15.15). The indifferent electrode consists of right arm, left arm, and left foot, electrically connected together (the right foot is again earthed). Lead V_1 is placed over the fourth right intercostal space near the sternum; V_2 is in a similar position to the left of the sternum; V_3 is further to the left midway between V_2 and V_4; V_4 is over the left fifth intercostal space in the mid-clavicular line; and V_5 and V_6 are in the same transverse plane as V_4 but in the anterior axillary line and mid-axillary line, respectively. Chest leads give larger ECG deflections than limb leads and allow a better spatial correlation with underlying myocardial regions.

Intraoesophageal leads and additional leads located on the **right chest** (V_r leads) or the **left back** (V_7–V_9) are sometimes used for differential diagnosis, for example to locate ischaemic foci or infarcts.

Mean electrical axis and transition point

The direction of the electrical vector at any point in time is the electrical axis of the heart at that instant. The **mean electrical axis** is defined as the frontal projection of the largest vector during ventricular depolarization. It can be established by triangulating any two of the R wave amplitudes in the standard limb leads (Fig. 15.16). In the given example, the mean electrical axis is about +65° (measured clockwise from left horizontal; see 0 deg line in Fig. 15.16). The normal range is anywhere between –30° (i.e. above left horizontal) and +90° (i.e. vertical). Tall, thin people with a narrow thorax tend to have a more vertical orientation of the heart (and hence a more vertical mean electrical axis). Hypertrophy of the left ventricle shifts the electrical axis to the left (i.e. to lower angle values), termed left axis deviation, while hypertrophy of the right ventricle produces right axis deviation.

The chest lead that gives equal-amplitude R and S waves, usually V_3 or V_4 (see Fig. 15.15), overlies the anterior projection of the inter-ventricular septum and is said to mark the **transition point**. Rotation of the heart about its longitudinal axis shifts the transition point (right or left shift). Transition point location depends on body build and also shifts with hypertrophy of one ventricle.

Cardiac arrhythmias

*One clinical use of the ECG is the diagnosis of cardiac rhythm disturbances, or **arrhythmias** (see Fig. 15.17 for some typical examples). One of the most common causes of arrhythmias is ischaemic heart disease—an inadequate blood supply to the myocardium, often produced by narrowing or blockage of the heart's coronary arteries.*

An arrhythmia is the manifestation of distur-

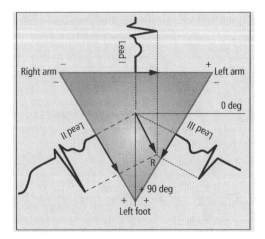

Fig. 15.16 Establishment of mean electrical axis (for detail see text).

bances in the initiation or propagation of one or more AP. Any heartbeat that is triggered by an AP that arises outside the normal pacemaking tissue is called an **ectopic beat** (from *ek*—Greek for 'out of', and *topos*—Greek for 'place'). Every human experiences ectopic beats, and in the overwhelming majority of cases these have no adverse consequences.

Arrhythmias arising from changed SA node pacemaker activity cause more sustained changes to beating rate. The small physiological changes in SA node beating rate, which occur in the rhythm of respiration, are termed **respiratory sinus arrhythmia**. Respiratory sinus arrhythmia is characterized by an increase in SA node beating rate during inspiration, and a decrease during expiration. It serves as a fitting illustration of extra-cardiac modulation of heart rate (Fig. 15.1), both by higher nervous control (more than 95% of respiratory sinus arrhythmia at resting heart rate is caused by respiration-related fluctuations in vagal tone), and by the mechanical environment (non-neural mechanisms dominate respiratory sinus arrhythmia during peak physical activity, and are its sole cause in heart transplant recipients).

Pathologies of SA node structure and function may lead to cessation of pacemaking or of AP conduction towards atrial tissue. This can cause car-

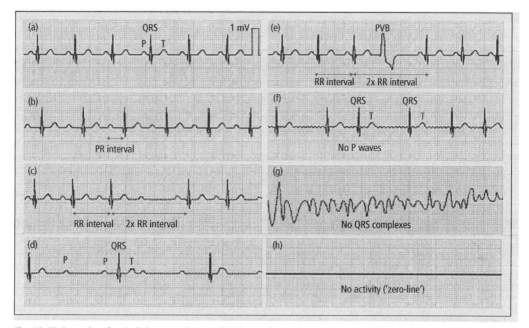

Fig. 15.17 Examples of typical electrocardiogram (ECG) recordings. (a) Normal ECG with standard sequence of P, QRS and T waves (see also Fig. 15.14), and 1 mV calibration signal at the right. (b) Slowed atrio-ventricular (AV) conduction prolongs the PR interval which, at a duration of >0.2 s (equivalent to one 5 mm block on the ECG paper; see note below) is referred to as first-degree heart block. (c) Progressive delay in AV conduction may cause a 'dropped beat' (second-degree heart block), where a P wave is not followed by ventricular excitation, roughly doubling the RR interval timing. (d) Complete failure of AV conduction (third-degree heart block) is accompanied by a loss of temporal relation between atrial (P waves) and ventricular excitation (QRS complexes), usually causing reduced ventricular beating rates. (e) Ectopic excitation of ventricular tissue may give rise to a premature ventricular beat (PVB) which, in the absence of any arrhythmia-sustaining substrate, does not usually have any clinically relevant consequences. (f) In atrial fibrillation, the lack of an ordered cycle of atrial excitation and repolarization leads to disappearance of the P wave. (g) Ventricular fibrillation can be identified by the lack of discernible ventricular complexes (no QRS), and is lethal within minutes unless treated. (h) Complete asystole is characterized by zero electrical (and mechanical) activity. Note: ECG recording paper is traditionally divided into 5 × 5 blocks of 1 mm squares. Vertically, the amplitude of ten squares usually corresponds to the calibration voltage of 1 mV, while horizontally, one square corresponds to 0.04 s (at the standard paper speed 25 mm s^{-1}).

diac standstill, called **asystole**. Unless lower-order pacemaker centres start to introduce rhythmic ventricular contractions at reduced rate, this is a serious condition that is incompatible with life. Heart rates of less than 60 bpm are called **bradycardia**, while non-physiologically increased beating rates are termed **tachycardia** (see p. 346). Both have negative consequences for **cardiac output**, defined as the volume of blood pumped during one minute. Cardiac output is calculated as the product of heart rate (number of beats per minute) and stroke volume (volume pumped per beat).

In bradycardic states, the heart rate is too low to sustain sufficient cardiac output (except in endurance-trained athletes with above-average stroke volumes), whereas in tachycardic conditions there may be too little time for ventricular filling, which impedes stroke volume.

Atrial tachycardias (beating rates up to 220 bpm) carry the additional risk that they may deteriorate into **atrial flutter** (up to 350 bpm) or **atrial fibrillation** (de-synchronized atrial excitation waves and lack of coordinated force development of the atrial myocardium as a whole). As AV node conduction is sufficiently slow, atrial rates exceeding about 200 bpm will not normally be conducted to the ventricles. Atrial fibrillation, despite leading to a lack of effective atrial contraction, is not incompatible with life, as the majority of ventricular filling occurs passively upon ventricular relaxation (see p. 337). Nonetheless, atrial fibrillation reduces an individual's exercise tolerance and carries significant risks, such as the potential to cause ventricular rhythm disturbances. It may also give rise to formation of blood clots in insufficiently agitated atrial blood volumes (in particular inside the atrial appendages), which, if mobilized, may lead to sudden death from pulmonary or cerebral embolism.

Ventricular tachycardia may originate as a result of repetitive firing of ectopic AP, and/or of **re-entry** of excitation. Re-entrant waves of excitation are not normally encountered, as the ventricular tissue that is excited last tends to repolarize first (see Figs 15.6 and 15.11). In pathological conditions, circular waves may develop in the ventricles, giving rise to a re-entry pathway of excitation that is wholly sustained in the ventricular myocardium. This may deteriorate into **ventricular fibrillation**, where individual tissue segments and cells contract and relax asynchronously, so that there is no coordinated contraction and, hence, no efficient cardiac pump action. This condition is incompatible with life and requires immediate life support (cardiac compressions) and emergency resuscitation measures by medically qualified personnel (such as application of electrical defibrillation shocks or pre-cordial fist thumps; both are in essence environmental effects on cardiac activity, used to restore normal cardiac activity; Fig. 15.1).

In addition to pathological pacemaking, ectopic excitation, and re-entry, heart rhythm disturbances may arise from malfunction in the cardiac conduction system. The AV node is particularly susceptible to electrophysiological changes that may decrease the speed of AP conduction. A pathological increase in the interval between atrial and ventricular depolarization (PR interval >0.2 s) is called **first-degree heart block**. If atrial AP reach the AV node while still refractory from the preced-

ing cycle of excitation, only some of the atrial impulses will be conducted to the ventricle, a condition that is termed **second-degree heart block**. Complete failure of AV conduction is termed **third-degree heart block**. The atria then beat at the rhythm dictated by the SA node, while lower-order pacemaker tissue initiates ventricular excitation at rates of 20–40 bpm.

All of the above rhythm disturbances can be identified on the basis of their corresponding ECG changes (Fig. 15.17). Non-physiological SA node beating rates that are conducted to the whole heart show a typical ECG pattern (with consecutive P, QRS and T waves), with increased (bradycardia) or decreased (tachycardia) intervals between two subsequent P or R waves. Slowed AV conduction increases the PQ interval, while disturbed function of the bundle of His or the Purkinje network reduces the normal synchronicity of ventricular excitation and leads to a widening (and possibly deformation) of the QRS complex. Dissociation of atrial and ventricular excitation can be established by comparing the frequency and interrelation of P and R waves, and atrial or ventricular fibrillation give rise to irregular changes in the corresponding ECG waves. In addition, the presence of ischaemic foci or other areas of disturbed electrical activity can be identified by shifts in the ST segment away from the isopotential line (caused by the absence of a true isopotential state, even during full ventricular excitation, as the pathologically disturbed tissue will be at different membrane potentials than the normal myocardium).

15.4 The cardiac cycle and heart sounds

Each heartbeat involves a complex sequence of both electrical and mechanical processes. These can be monitored in patients by various techniques, such as recording the ECG, blood pressure, and heart sounds. In order to interpret these recordings, it is essential to understand the temporal interrelation of ECG, ventricular volume changes, as well as venous, atrial, ventricular and arterial pressures during the cardiac cycle.

Basic forms of contraction

Contractile properties of muscles can be examined by length–tension curves, as described previously for skeletal muscle (see Fig. 5.7). Muscles have viscous and elastic elements that, when stretched, generate a passive tension (or passive force), which increases with their new length.

If during an active contraction the muscle remains at the same length, the contraction is referred to as **isometric** (or **isovolumetric** if the volume inside a cardiac chamber does not change). In isometric contractions **active tension** plus **passive tension** comprise the **total tension** measured during the contraction. When a muscle shortens while lifting a set weight (load), the contraction occurs with a constant force and is referred to as **isotonic**. The speed at which a muscle shortens is load-dependent. Maximum speed is available at zero load and, as load increases to the maximum that a muscle can move, speed approaches zero (shortening speed is zero in isometric contraction).

Length–tension curves are essentially the one-dimensional equivalents of three-dimensional events in the whole heart, described by volume–pressure curves. Passive tension in cardiac muscle before contraction depends on end-diastolic volume loading, or **preload**. The external load against which the muscle shortens (in the heart, this is the pressure in the arteries leaving each ventricle) is the **afterload**. During a cycle of contraction and relaxation, the muscle will initially develop sufficient isometric tension to match this load and then shorten, thereby shifting the load. For the left ventricle, aortic pressure is the afterload; the ventricle will first develop sufficient isovolumetric tension, and hence ventricular pressure, to match diastolic pressure in the aorta, and will then increase pressure further while opening the aortic valve and ejecting blood. In muscle strip experiments, afterload is usually a fixed weight that needs to be lifted, so that muscle shortening will be isotonic. In the heart, ejection of blood from the ventricles occurs by contracting against a varying afterload (as aortic pressure changes from its diastolic low level to the systolic peak pressure; see segment C to D in Fig. 15.18), and such a con-

traction is referred to as **auxotonic**. Figure 15.18 illustrates, on the same timescale, the ECG, left ventricular volume, changes in blood pressure inside the left atrium, left ventricle and aorta, and the heart sounds that can be recorded during one complete cardiac cycle. It is useful to review these parameters and their dynamic interaction in a step-by-step fashion.

The contractile cycle step-by-step

Atrial contraction: the start of systole

The cardiac cycle consists of an orderly sequence of atrial and ventricular excitation, contraction and relaxation, which normally begins with the generation of an SA node pacemaker AP. This causes atrial excitation, which is identifiable by the P wave in the ECG (Fig. 15.18). Conduction delays cause the start of contraction in the left atrium to trail that of the right by a few milliseconds. Atrial contraction leads to an increase in atrial pressure (**a wave** on the atrial pressure curve). As the AV valves are already open at this point of the cardiac cycle, atrial pressure increases by a very small amount only. More noticeable is the increase in ventricular volume (the 'atrial kick'), which contributes about 10–15% to the end-diastolic ventricular volume (see p. 337). The functional relevance of this contribution at resting heart rates is debated, as even in the absence of organized atrial contraction (for example in people suffering from atrial fibrillation) the heart can function normally for years. Atrial contribution is thought to become more important with an increase in heart rate (e.g. during exercise or emotional stress; pp. 346–47), when the overall duration of diastole shortens to an extent that passive filling of the ventricles is incomplete, and the atrial contribution to ventricular filling increases in order to maintain performance.

Start of ventricular contraction: closure of AV valves and 1st heart sound

After excitation of the atria, the AP passes slowly through the AV node and travels in an apical direction via the bundle of His towards the Purkinje

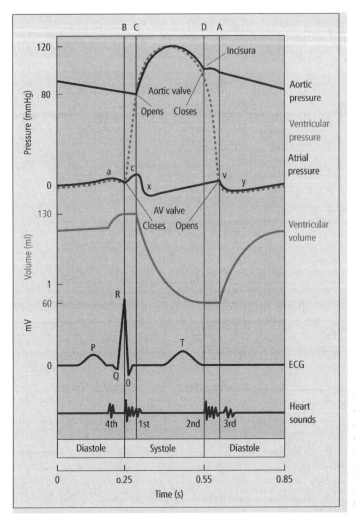

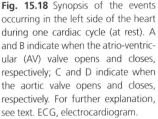

Fig. 15.18 Synopsis of the events occurring in the left side of the heart during one cardiac cycle (at rest). A and B indicate when the atrio-ventricular (AV) valve opens and closes, respectively; C and D indicate when the aortic valve opens and closes, respectively. For further explanation, see text. ECG, electrocardiogram.

network. This conduction delay separates the onset of atrial and ventricular contraction. Near-synchronous depolarization of the ventricle is brought about by the fast spread of excitation in the Purkinje network (now left ventricular activation precedes right), and is indicated by the QRS complex of the ECG. Contraction of the ventricular muscle commences soon after the onset of ventricular excitation, and ventricular pressure starts to rise. As soon as ventricular pressure rises, it exceeds atrial pressure and the AV valves (bi- and tricuspid valves, p. 336) close. Because of the fast rise in ventricular pressure, the closure of valves is

quite rapid, and with a stethoscope, the vibration caused by this abrupt closure can be heard as a low-pitched sound—the **1st heart sound**. This sound is prolonged by vibrations in the ventricular wall caused by the same rapid rise in ventricular pressure. As long as the pressure in the aorta (pulmonary artery for the right side of the heart) is higher than in the left (right) ventricle, the aortic (pulmonary artery) valve remains closed. Since the AV valves are closed as well, the blood in the ventricles has nowhere to go, and pressure rises in the absence of any change in ventricular volume. This is named the **isovolumetric** phase of ventricular contraction (see period from B to C in Fig. 15.18). In the diagram a small rise in atrial pressure can also be observed during this phase (**c wave** on the atrial pressure curve). This is due to the high pressure in the ventricles, which causes the leaves of the closed AV valves to bulge towards the atria (they are held in place at their base by the AV fibrous ring, and kept shut at their free margins by **chordae tendineae** attached to the papillary muscles; see p. 338).

Peak ventricular contraction: opening of ventricular outflow valves, ventricular ejection, and atrial re-filling

Once ventricular pressure exceeds that in the aorta (pulmonary artery), the ventricular outflow valves open, and ejection of blood from the ventricles starts. Although depolarization of the right ventricle (and hence mechanical activation) lags behind that of the left, the blood pressure in the pulmonary artery is much lower than in the aorta (8 mmHg compared to 80 mmHg), causing the pulmonary valve to open first. Contraction of the ventricular muscle at this point is still faster than the ventricle can empty, so pressure continues to rise until it peaks at about 120 mmHg in the left ventricle (80 mmHg for the right ventricle). Due to the opening of the aortic and pulmonary valves, the pressure in the aorta and pulmonary artery rises to the same level as in the corresponding ventricle. The walls of arteries are elastic, and an increase in pressure causes distension of the vessel, increasing its capacity and thereby supporting rapid ejection of blood from the ventricles. As the ventricles eject blood, they will shorten and pull the AV border in an apical direction (see Fig. 15.2). Given that the position of base and apex of the heart are fairly stable *in vivo*, this movement stretches the atria and leads to a rapid drop in atrial pressure, often to negative values (**x wave** on the atrial pressure curve). This is a key mechanism underlying return of venous blood to the heart and causes atrial filling in preparation for the next cycle of contraction. During this phase of the contraction the T wave in the ECG develops, indicating that repolarization of the ventricles has started.

End of ventricular contraction: closure of the ventricular outflow valves, 2nd heart sound

Towards the end of the T wave, in late systole, the ventricular muscle starts to relax and ventricular pressure drops. The momentum of the outflowing blood allows the ejection to continue beyond the point where ventricular pressure drops just below aortic (pulmonary artery) pressure. The maintained high pressure in the arteries leading away from the heart (in particular in the aorta) is caused by the elastic distension of the arterial vessel wall earlier during contraction. As the walls start to recoil, they provide a maintained driving force for blood flow throughout diastole. The progressive reduction in ventricular pressure eventually causes the direction of the blood flow to reverse briefly. This retrograde flow results in immediate closure of the aortic (and pulmonary) valves, and is linked to a transient drop in aortic pressure, called **incisura** (from *incidere* — Latin for 'to cut into'; Fig. 15.18). During this period the **2nd heart sound** (a shorter and higher-pitched sound than the first) is heard. This results from the vibration generated by closure of aortic and pulmonary valves. The sound is often split, especially during inspiration, because the aortic valve closes slightly before the pulmonary valve. The volume contained in each ventricle at the end of ejection is called the **end-systolic volume**; it is about 60 mL when standing. As end-diastolic volume was 130 mL, about 70 mL (the **stroke volume**) has been ejected in systole (see Table 15.1 for an overview of key haemodynamic values). The proportion of the end-diastolic volume that is ejected (i.e. stroke volume/end-diastolic volume) is the **ejection fraction**, which is a measure of cardiac contractile efficiency, and should be 0.55–0.75 in healthy individuals (i.e. during each beat the normal heart ejects between just over half, and three-quarters, of its end-diastolic volume).

Early ventricular relaxation: isovolumetric phase

In early diastole all valves are closed, so no blood

Table 15.1 Representative cardiac variables at rest and during maximum exercise for non-athletes and endurance-trained athletes. EDV, end-diastolic volume; ESV, end-systolic volume.

	Cardiac output (L min⁻¹)	Heart rate (bpm)	Stroke volume (mL)	EDV (mL)	ESV (mL)
Non-athlete					
Rest	5	70	70	130	60
Severe exercise	20	200	100	130	30
Trained athlete					
Rest	5	40	120	200	80
Severe exercise	36	200	170	200	30

can enter or leave the ventricles. This period of ventricular relaxation with rapidly falling ventricular pressure is called the **isovolumetric phase** of ventricular relaxation (see period from D to A in Fig. 15.18). Throughout systole, the atrial pressure has gradually increased from below zero and, by the end of isovolumetric ventricular relaxation, it reaches a peak (**v wave** on atrial pressure curve) of about 5 mmHg in the left atrium (2 mmHg in the right atrium). This gradual increase in atrial pressure results from blood from the veins accumulating in the atria against closed AV valves, while the AV border is moving back towards the base of the heart into its resting position.

Full relaxation: opening of AV valves, rapid ventricular filling, and 3rd heart sound

Slightly later in diastole, when ventricular pressures have dropped just below those in the atria, the AV valves re-open. Ventricular pressure may even drop to negative levels, as ventricles had shortened to below their resting length and are now recoiling into their fully relaxed shape. As the AV border continues to move back to its normal position, the ventricular walls shift over the blood previously drawn into the atria. This causes rapid ventricular filling by an essentially passive process. As the former atrial blood is being encompassed by the ventricles, atrial pressure follows that of the ventricles and falls (**y wave**, or y-descend, on the

atrial pressure curve). This rapid filling of the ventricles sets up vibrations sometimes detectable as a **3rd heart sound**.

Inter-systolic pause: waiting for the next atrial contraction

After the initial decline in early diastole, atrial and ventricular pressures gradually increase during mid-diastole. This is a passive process and results from continued venous blood return to the heart, which, at that time, is being aided by peripheral vein compression and the respiratory pump (see p. 336). Ventricular filling progresses very slowly (against the closed aortic and pulmonary valves). This period has traditionally been regarded as one of complete atrial and ventricular rest, called **diastasis** (from *dia*—Greek for 'throughout', and *statsis*—Greek for 'being stationary'). It coincides with the period of time during which the pressure gradient between coronary vessel origin (just downstream of the aortic valves) and ventricular myocardium (mainly determined by ventricular pressure) is largest, giving rise to peak flow rates through the vessels of the heart, replenishing the tissue with oxygen and nutrients. Any increase in heart rate occurs predominantly at the expense of diastasis duration (overall duration of systole changes much less than that of diastole). In this context, the rapid initial filling of the ventricles early in diastole is important as it ensures near-complete replenishment of ventricular volume by passive means. Throughout diastole, the aortic pressure gradually declines from its post-systolic level just after the incisura (about 110 mmHg at rest) to the diastolic minimum (near 80 mmHg at rest). Blood pressure in the arteries remains elevated due to both the continuing elastic recoil of aortic walls (stretched during the previous systole) and the resistance to flow downstream. The diastolic decline in arterial pressure is caused by the blood flows from the aorta into the rest of the vascular system.

Additional parameters during the cardiac cycle

Abnormal heart sounds

A **4th heart sound** can sometimes be heard just before the 1st heart sound, if vibrations are set up during late ventricular filling by atrial contraction. These vibrations may occur when atrial pressure is high, or when the ventricle is stiff (as in ventricular hypertrophy).

Other abnormal heart sounds, called **murmurs**, may occur at any stage of the cardiac cycle and some (but not all) have a pathological basis. When blood passes through a narrowed orifice, or regurgitates back into a chamber, its flow becomes turbulent, usually generating a murmur. Pathological narrowing of a valve's orifice is referred to as **stenosis** (from *stenos*—Greek for 'narrow'). Stenosis of an AV valve results in turbulent flow during ventricular filling (**diastolic murmur**), while stenosis of the aortic or pulmonary valves causes turbulent flow during ventricular ejection into the aorta or pulmonary artery (**systolic murmur**). If a valve is incompetent and fails to close properly, backflow of blood occurs. Incompetent AV valves allow regurgitation of blood into the atria during ventricular contraction (**systolic murmur**), while incompetent aortic or pulmonary valves permit regurgitation of blood when ventricles are relaxed (**diastolic murmur**). Defects in the inter-atrial or inter-ventricular septum also cause systolic murmurs, while in patients with **persistent ductus arteriosus** (a fetal connection between the aorta and the pulmonary artery that normally closes upon resumption of spontaneous respiration after deliv-

ery) a **continuous murmur** can be noticed throughout the cardiac cycle. In addition to frequency, character, duration and timing of murmurs, the site on the chest wall where they are loudest, provide diagnostic clues to the underlying abnormality.

Korotkoff sounds

The **Korotkoff sounds** refer to the noises that arise in the context of opening and closure of a blood vessel (usually the brachial artery), compressed by an external inflatable cuff. This technique, introduced over a century ago, allows non-invasive assessment of peak systolic and diastolic blood pressures. The working principle is such that a stethoscope, placed in the cubital fossa, should not normally yield any pulse-related sounds. If a cuff is placed upstream of this area and inflated to a pressure that exceeds maximum systolic pressure, the brachial artery is occluded and no sounds are heard either. The appearance of a pulse-related sound during slow reduction in cuff pressure indicates the point at which arterial pressure exceeds the external compression pressure. This sound is caused by the turbulent blood flow in the brachial artery during temporary re-opening of the vessel by peak systolic pressure, and the corresponding cuff pressure is taken to indicate peak systolic pressure. Upon further gradual reduction in cuff pressure, there are continued 'thumping' pulse-related sounds. Once cuff pressure drops to within 10 mmHg of diastolic pressure levels, the sound becomes muted and, upon progression of cuff pressure below diastolic pressure, it disappears completely, providing an indication of diastolic arterial pressure. Modern patient monitoring techniques increasingly use automated systems for arterial pressure determination, but the basic measurement technique is often based on the same acoustic principle.

Jugular venous pulse

It is often wrongly assumed that **venous return** from the systemic circulation to the right atrium is driven chiefly by the kinetic energy imparted on the blood during left ventricular ejection (for mechanisms of venous return, see pp. 335–36). In fact, once the blood has passed through the capillaries of the systemic circulation, no pressure oscillations that would be related to systole and diastole are discernible (see Fig. 14.4). Nonetheless, clear venous pressure fluctuations reappear in the large veins leading to the right atrium. An example of this phenomenon is the **jugular venous pulse** (pressure oscillations in the large veins of the neck; Fig. 15.19).

These fluctuations are transmitted 'backwards' from the right atrium, to which the jugular veins are linked via the superior **vena cava** (there are no valves separating these veins from intra-atrial pressure changes). Peaks and troughs in jugular vein pulse therefore occur with a slight delay in time relative to the atrial peaks (a, c, x, v and y, see Fig. 15.18), and are largely caused by the same mechanisms (the pressure pulse transmitted from the adjacent carotid artery during peak systole makes an additional contribution to the jugular c wave).

The relative amplitudes of jugular venous pressure are variable, because the return of venous blood from the systemic circulation to the heart is affected by respiratory pressure fluctuation (pp. 335–36), which occur at a lower rate than the heartbeat. Nonetheless, the shape and magnitude of jugular venous pressure can convey information about the presence of cardiac arrhythmias, or right atrial pressure abnormalities such as can be caused

by stenosis or incompetence of the **tricuspid valve**.

15.5 Contractile properties of cardiac muscle

Although basic principles of contraction and relaxation are similar in skeletal and cardiac muscle, there are a number of important differences. In both muscles, calcium is the mediator between electrical and mechanical activity. In the heart, AP are generated intrinsically by pacemaker cells, while skeletal muscle requires external nerve impulses to selectively activate the individual fibres that participate in muscle contraction. The heart functions as one unit where all muscle cells participate in AP conduction and subsequent contraction on every heartbeat (functional syncytium), whereas the heterogeneous and electrically independent fibres in skeletal muscle are selectively recruited to modulate contractile activity. Furthermore, in cardiac muscle every AP triggers a full contraction followed by relaxation (twitch-like contraction), while in skeletal muscle intracellular calcium, and hence force and duration of contraction, are adjusted by AP train frequency. Thus, the heart lacks the typical mechanisms utilized in skeletal muscle to grade force of contraction. Nonetheless, cardiac output can vary greatly, in an untrained adult from 5 L min^{-1} at rest, to 20 L min^{-1} during maximum exercise — a four-fold increase. In order to understand the mechanisms underlying changes in mechanical performance of cardiac muscle, it is essential to identify the sequence of events involved in cardiac ECC, and to highlight how

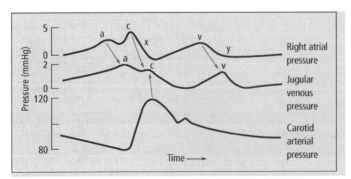

Fig. 15.19 Temporal relationship between blood pressures in the right atrium, jugular veins, and carotid arteries. See Fig. 15.18 for interrelation to other haemodynamic parameters and electrocardiogram/heart sounds.

this is affected by higher-order control mechanisms and by physical signals from the cardiac environment (Fig. 15.1).

Cardiac excitation contraction coupling

Cardiac ECC is the sequence of events that occur at the cellular level and link electrical excitation to changes in cytosolic calcium concentration ($[Ca^{2+}]_i$) which, in turn, governs the process of mechanical contraction and relaxation. In contrast to skeletal muscle, the rise in $[Ca^{2+}]_i$ in cardiac muscle is caused by entry into the cytosol of calcium from extracellular and intracellular compartments. Activation of the contractile process starts in the heart with an initial influx of external calcium which, in turn, triggers release of more calcium from the SR. Relaxation requires both re-uptake of calcium into the SR and extrusion to the cell exterior. At steady-state, influx of trigger calcium and extrusion to the outside must match each other on a beat-by-beat basis, as otherwise there would be a net-gain (or loss) of calcium by the cell. The balancing of calcium influx, SR-release, re-uptake and extrusion is, therefore, the main mechanism of adjusting cardiac cell calcium content and, hence, force generating capacity at any given sarcomere length.

Calcium currents and calcium-induced calcium release

Calcium enters cardiac myocytes via $i_{Ca,L}$ (activated by AP-induced membrane depolarization) and via i_{NCX} (activated by the sodium-influx associated with the AP upstroke, which is extruded in exchange for calcium).

The proteins that carry $i_{Ca,L}$ and i_{NCX} are located in the sarcolemma at the cell surface and, more prominently, in the T tubular invaginations of the sarcolemma (see Fig. 15.5). In addition to contributing to the overall rise in $[Ca^{2+}]_i$, calcium influx via the L type calcium channels is also essential in causing **calcium-induced calcium release** (CICR) from the SR. Some L type calcium channels are positioned in very close proximity to the SR calcium-release channels (often referred to as ryanodine receptors, or RyR, as they were first characterized using ryanodine, a drug that blocks this channel). In contrast to skeletal muscle, where a conformational change in the L type calcium channel protein (there referred to as the dihydropyridine receptor, DHP; pp. 103–104) causes RyR channels to open, cardiac RyR are activated by the actual influx of trigger-calcium carried by $i_{Ca,L}$.

The calcium concentration gradient between the SR-inside and the cytosol is very steep (1 mM in the SR compared to 100 nM in the cytosol—a 10 000-fold difference). Opening of the SR calcium-release channels (RyR) thus results in a high calcium flux. This CICR is an example of a powerful positive feedback system, leading to a very rapid increase in $[Ca^{2+}]_i$ during an AP. The combined action of i_{NCX}, $i_{Ca,L}$ and CICR from the SR combine to increase $[Ca^{2+}]_i$ from its low diastolic levels to 1–2 μM within a few milliseconds (see grey arrows in Fig. 15.20).

Calcium re-uptake and extrusion

At steady-state, the cellular calcium balance is stable. Calcium released from the SR during one contraction is pumped back upon relaxation, while an amount equal to that 'gained' from the outside during CICR is extruded.

Re-uptake of calcium into the SR is via an ATP-consuming calcium pump (the **Sarco-(Endo-)plasmic Reticulum Calcium ATPase**; SERCA). This pump removes the bulk of the calcium from the cytosol. SERCA is located mainly in the longitudinal SR between T tubules (see Fig. 15.5), and less so in the cisternae that lie alongside T tubular membrane invaginations. The spatial separation between the calcium uptake and release sites is thought to potentially reduce the concentration step against which SERCA has to pump calcium back into the SR (although this would require active transport cascades between sub-compartments inside the SR, the presence of which is debated). Once in the SR, calcium moves towards the release site in the cisternae to be available for release in subsequent cardiac cycles.

Calcium extrusion from the cell back into the extracellular space is via sodium–calcium

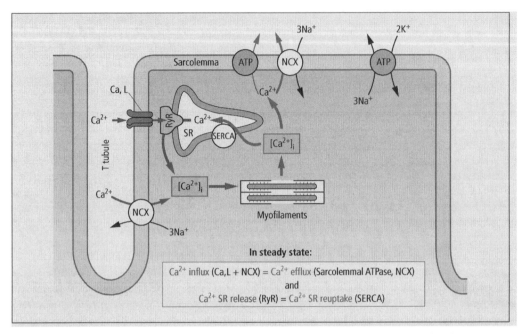

Sarcolemma
ATP
NCX
ATP
3Na⁺
2K⁺
Ca, L
Ca²⁺
Ca²⁺
3Na⁺
Ca²⁺
RyR
Ca²⁺
SR
SERCA
[Ca²⁺]ᵢ
T tubule
Ca²⁺
[Ca²⁺]ᵢ
NCX
Myofilaments
3Na⁺

Fig. 15.20 Excitation–contraction coupling mechanisms. For explanation, see text. ATP, adenosine triphosphate; Ca, L, L-type calcium channel; NCX, sodium-calcium exchanger; SR, sarcoplasmic reticulum; RyR, ryanodine receptor; SERCA, sarco-(endo-)plasmic reticulum calcium ATPase. (Adapted from Bers, D. M. (2001) Excitation-Contraction Coupling and Cardiac Contractile Force, 2nd edn, p. 40. Kluwer Academic Publishers, Dordrecht, Boston, London.)

exchange and an ATP-consuming calcium pump (calcium ATPase) in the plasmalemma (see blue arrows in Fig. 15.20).

Beta-adrenergic regulation of calcium handling

In a steady-state, the amount of calcium entering a cardiomyocyte during activation, and the amount of calcium being extruded during relaxation are in equilibrium. Any change in this equilibrium (such as via changes in calcium influx via $i_{Ca,L}$, alterations in sodium–calcium exchanger activity, or SERCA pump rates) will affect $[Ca^{2+}]_i$ during the cardiac cycle and, hence, directly alter contractile force. The most profound, physiologically relevant way of changing all of these factors at once is by β-adrenergic stimulation.

The pathway starts with the binding of **catecholamines** (circulating adrenaline, or noradrenaline from intracardiac nerve endings) to

β-adrenoceptors. These receptors are coupled to G proteins (short for guanidine nucleotide binding proteins; a family of proteins involved in cell signalling mechanisms which involve guanidine di- and triphosphate), which, via complex signalling cascades, increase the phosphorylation state of both the $i_{Ca,L}$ channel and the SR calcium-release channel, RyR. This increases the open times of both channels and raises the amount of trigger-calcium and the gain of CICR, thus increasing $[Ca^{2+}]_i$. In addition, phospholamdan will be phosphorylated. **Phospholamdan** inhibits SERCA and phosphorylation removes this inhibitory effect, thereby supporting more rapid re-uptake of calcium into the SR. This not only increases SR calcium load (at the expense of calcium extrusion to the cell exterior), but it also speeds-up relaxation. This is important since β-adrenergic activation is normally accompanied by elevated heart rates, when diastolic duration (and hence time available for filling of cardiac chambers) is reduced. Last, but not least, catecholamine effects reduce the calcium sensitivity of contractile proteins (via phosphorylation of **troponin I**, which reduces the calcium sensitivity of **troponin C**; see p. 364); this again promotes fast muscle relaxation.

Importance of calcium homeostasis

Although changing calcium levels is a very powerful tool for altering the contractile status of cardiac muscle, it is mainly used for short-term adaptation, e.g. in exercise. Calcium plays crucial roles in many signalling pathways, and elevated calcium levels can be detrimental to cell function. Naturally occurring proteases, for example, are activated by high $[Ca^{2+}]_i$, increasing protein turnover. High calcium levels are also associated with higher levels of programmed cell death (apoptosis—the 'dropping out'; from *apo*—Greek for 'away from', and *ptosis*—Greek for 'drop'). Since turnover of cardiac myocyte proteins is normally very finely balanced (and proliferation, i.e. generation of new cardiomyocytes, is thought to be absent in the adult mammalian heart), this is an undesirable situation. In addition, elevated $[Ca^{2+}]_i$ can also impair muscle relaxation during diastole. This may increase wall stiffness and affect diastolic filling, which would impede cardiac adaptation to high workloads.

Mechanical modulation of contractility

Stretching of cardiac muscle within physiological limits (for example by increasing venous blood return) will raise the force of its contraction, even at unchanged cytosolic $[Ca^{2+}]_i$ levels. This behaviour had been discov- ered in the mid-19*th* *century, and it was studied extensively by Otto Frank and Ernest Starling, after whom it is named—the Frank–Starling relation. Even though whole-organ expressions of length-dependent activation had been observed over 150 years ago, the underlying molecular mechanisms are still the subject of intensive research and debate.*

Frank–Starling relation of the heart

Physiologists of the late 19th century were well aware of the fact that '... *a strong heart that is filled with blood empties itself more or less completely, in other words, (filling of the heart with blood) changes the extent of contractile power*' (from Carl Ludwig's Physiology textbook of 1852). This ability of the heart to respond to increased venous blood return by raising stroke volume (Fig. 15.21) is essential, both for the matching of input and output on either side of the heart, but equally for ensuring that both sides pump the same amount of blood over any length of time (failure to do so would cause blood-pooling in either the pulmonary or systemic circulation).

Length-dependent activation of cardiac muscle

The process by which cardiac muscle preparations respond to an acute increase in preload (see p. 355) is called **length-dependent activation**. In skeletal muscle, similar behaviour is related to the variable extent of overlap between thin (actin) and thick (myosin) filaments in sarcomeres held at different lengths (Fig. 5.6). Initially thought to be similar in

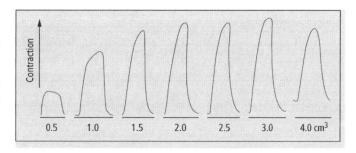

Fig. 15.21 Stretch-induced increase in cardiac contractility, elicited by increasing left ventricular filling. Contraction amplitudes point upwards; note that excessive filling (far right) reduces contraction amplitude. (After Starling & Patterson (1914) *J Physiol*, **48**, 357–79.)

the heart, it is now understood that filament overlap cannot satisfactorily explain length-dependent activation in the heart. Cardiac sarcomeres operate over a much narrower range (about 1.6–2.2 μm, compared to 1.5–3.6 μm in skeletal muscle); their length-dependent activation is much steeper than that seen in skeletal muscle; and the higher passive stiffness of myocardium prevents it from actually being stretched to the significantly reduced levels of filament overlap seen during extreme stretch of skeletal muscle. Instead, length-dependent activation in cardiac muscle is caused by mechanisms that either increase the availability of cross-bridge binding sites, or the ease with which cross-bridges may form.

The first effect is thought to be largely brought about by a stretch-induced increase in the calcium affinity of **troponin C**, a regulatory protein on the thin filament whose activation shifts the position of **tropomyosin** to unblock binding sites for cross-bridge formation (Fig. 15.22). The stretch-induced increase in calcium affinity of troponin C therefore allows more effective activation of myofilaments at low calcium concentrations, and gives rise to earlier activation and higher forces at a given $[Ca^{2+}]_i$.

A second set of mechanisms is based on so-called **cooperativity effects**, where conformational changes at one binding site affect the ease with which cross-bridges may form at neighbouring locations. Thus, calcium-induced activation of the troponin C–tropomyosin complex at one binding site causes conformational changes in the thin filament that are not restricted to that site. Instead, the tropomyosin shift is partially transmitted to neighbouring binding sites, and this aids the calcium-induced conformational changes at further troponin C sites (Fig. 15.22, bottom right panel). Similarly, the binding of cross-bridges is cooperative; one cross-bridge binding to actin will pull actin and myosin filaments somewhat closer, facilitating the formation of cross-bridges at neighbouring sites. The cross-bridge formation also moves the blocking tropomyosin chain further away from the binding sites, again facilitating formation of further cross-bridges downstream. The cooperativity of both mechanisms explains the steep length dependent curve. A 5%

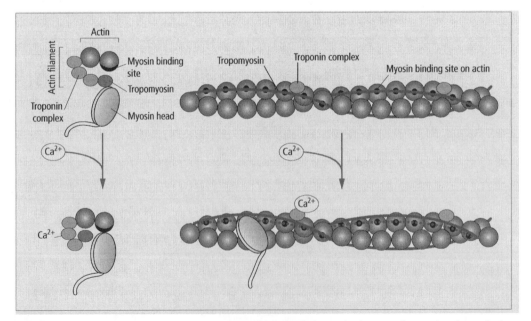

Fig. 15.22 Calcium binding to troponin C causes a configurational change in the troponin complex that pulls the tropomyosin chain away from cross-bridge binding sites on actin (left, cross-section; right, lateral view).

increase in sarcomere length, from 2.0 to 2.1 µm, can lead to a two- to three-fold increase in active myocardial force generation.

Although readily observed in mechanical experiments on individual myocytes or cardiac muscle strips, the mechanisms that increase troponin C calcium sensitivity and foster cross-bridge formation are still poorly understood. Current thinking is that titin, a giant protein that spans the entire half-sarcomere, from Z line to M line, might play a major role. Titin links the thin filament anchor point in the Z line to the end of thick filaments, and then runs along the thick filament all the way up to the M line in the middle of the sarcomere (Fig. 15.23). Therefore, titin mechanically interconnects half-sarcomeres, and it is well-situated to be a length sensor. The proportion of titin that crosses from thin to thick filament functions as a passive spring which, given its slightly slanted orientation, will give rise to a radial force that pulls thick and thin filaments closer together upon stretch (see bottom panel of Fig. 15.23). Such a reduction in inter-filament spacing would also be expected from the understanding that the volume of the contractile machinery during stretch remains unchanged, so that lateral dimensions must be reduced upon axial sarcomere elongation. Reduced inter-filament spacing favours cross-bridge formation and, thus, enhances contractility. Further research is directed at identifying the precise mechanisms and the balance of their individual contribution to length-dependent activation of cardiac contractile activity.

The working heart

The work of the heart can be illustrated by monitoring the dynamic changes in pressure and volume that occur during a heartbeat. These work-loops provide insight into important aspects of cardiac mechanical performance, and help illustrate mechanisms of auto-regulation.

Equilibrium curves

For every cavity volume, each cardiac chamber has a minimum passive pressure that it develops when fully relaxed, and a maximum active pressure, generated during isovolumic contraction. These values can be obtained experimentally by filling a heart to a given volume (**preload**), measuring the passive pressure generated by the volume injection in the resting cardiac chamber, and then triggering the heart to contract against a closed outflow tube (infinite **afterload**) to establish the isovolumetric pressure maximum. By repeating these measurements at different volumes, one can obtain two of three equilibrium curves in a pressure-volume diagram (Fig. 15.24); the lowermost curve describes passive tension, and the uppermost — isovolumetric maxima.

From any given preload, one may equally trigger

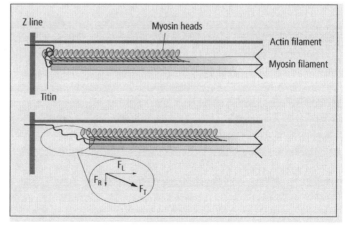

Fig. 15.23 The structural arrangement of titin, linking actin filament and myosin at an angle (see circle in lower panel and force component labeled F_T), gives rise to a large longitudinal (F_L) and a smaller radial force component (F_R) when sarcomeres are lengthened (bottom). This radial force is understood to support reduction in inter-filament lattice spacing during stretch.

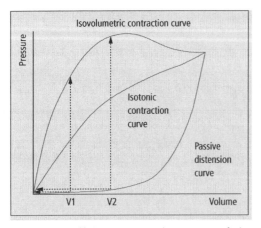

Fig. 15.24 Equilibrium pressure–volume curves of the heart.

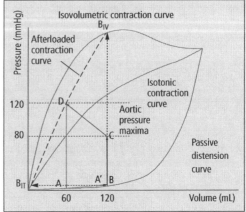

Fig. 15.25 Work-loop representation of the left ventricular pressure–volume changes. Labels A–D match those in Fig. 15.18; see text for detail.

contraction against a constant afterload that matches the passively generated tension of the ventricle (simply by connecting the outflow tract to an overflow, the height of which is adjusted to exactly the passive tension level at any given volume). This gives rise to the third equilibrium curve, denoting isotonic maxima. This curve is located between the isovolumetric maxima and the passive distension minima.

The term 'equilibrium curves' implies existence of a universally-stable relationship between cardiac volumes and pressures. This is not the case (β-adrenergic stimulation, for example, affects passive and active mechanical properties of the heart), so these curves are representative only for a given contractile status of the heart. The steep rise of the isovolumetric contraction maxima in the first half of the curve reflects length-dependent activation of myocardium, and the heart tends to normally operate on this part of the curve. Passive tension is rather small in this range, and only starts to rise steeply at higher volumes. Passive tension is due to the mechanical properties of intracellular titin and the extracellular collagen matrix of the heart. The contribution of titin is dominant in the physiological range, while the very steep rise in passive tension upon excess distension is caused by the collagen matrix which prevents overstretching of myocardium.

Work-loops

During a normal cardiac cycle, the heart changes modes of contraction, including isovolumetric contraction, auxotonic ejection, isovolumetric relaxation, and near-isotonic filling (see section 15.4 and Fig. 15.18). The pressure–volume relation of a heartbeat can be plotted, utilizing the previously identified equilibrium curves.

Atrial contraction (segment A' → B in Fig. 15.25) will initiate the cardiac cycle and load the ventricle, at modest pressure, with the final 10–15% of its end-diastolic volume (130 mL; point B). Ventricular contraction is initially isovolumetric, so that pressure rises without change in volume (segment B → C in Fig. 15.25; see also Fig. 15.18). Once ventricular pressure reaches blood pressure in the aorta (80 mmHg), the aortic valve opens and the heart starts to eject blood. Both pressure and volume change during this auxotonic contraction (segment C → D; the linear connection between points C and D is a simplification, as the pressure maximum is normally reached before the end of ejection, see Fig. 15.18). Point D is defined as the maximum pressure observed during ejection (120 mmHg) and lies on the afterloaded contractions curve, a connection between the projections from the end-diastolic point B onto both isovolumetric and isotonic maxima curves (points B_{IV} and B_{IT}, respectively). Upon relaxation, the aortic valve closes again and ventricular relaxation results in a rapid drop in pressure without volume change (isovolumetric relaxation, segment D → A). Once ventricular pressure reaches that in the atrium, AV valves open, and the ventricle rapidly fills to about 85% of its end-diastolic volume with very little change in pressure (segment A → A′), until the next atrial contraction occurs. Connecting all points A–D, one obtains the cardiac work-loop; the area within this loop represents the external work performed by the heart during the given cardiac cycle.

Integrated function: responses to acute changes in pressure and volume

Work-loop representations can be used to illustrate the regulation of cardiac performance, for example during changes in inotropic state by β-adrenergic stimulation, or during haemodynamic alterations (representing higher-order control and environmental effects on the heart).

If, for example, venous return is increased for one single beat by the volume Δ1 (e.g. during a change in posture), end-diastolic volume shifts on the passive distension curve to point B* (Fig. 15.26). Projecting from B* to the isovolumetric

maxima and isotonic contraction curves (points B^*_{IV} and B^*_{IT}, respectively), one can establish the position of the new afterloaded contractions curve applicable to this preload. Assuming that everything else remained unchanged, isovolumetric contraction will end at the same aortic pressure level (80 mmHg; point C*) and turn into auxotonic ejection towards the intersection of the systolic pressure (120 mmHg) with the new afterloaded contractions curve (point D*). Isovolumetric relaxation will yield a new point A*, from which ventricular re-filling will resume. It can be seen that, in the absence of any changes in contractile status, the additional volume in the ventricle remaining *after* one single heartbeat (Δ2) is significantly smaller that the original volume disturbance (Δ1). Thus, the ventricle responds to increased filling with an increase in blood ejection on the very next beat. Within a few cycles, the ventricle either adjusts to a new steady-state (if venous return remains elevated), or returns to its original work-loop (if filling normalizes). This response occurs independently of any external control, and it underlies the adjustment of ventricular ejection to venous return on either side of the heart, as well as the matching of left and right ventricular output.

In contrast, β-adrenergic stimulation, for example during exercise, will increase the contractile state of the myocardium, most notably by shifting the isovolumetric maxima curve to higher pressure levels (Fig. 15.27). This will shift the afterloaded contractions curve to the left and allow the ventricle to either create a larger peak-systolic pressure (point D^) while maintaining end-diastolic volume (point A), or to increase ventricular ejection (points D^^ and A^^) at maintained systolic pressure levels. Normal adaptation to exercise will be somewhere between these two extremes, and it is notable, therefore, that the heart tends to work at overall smaller volumes and with a higher ejection fraction during physical activity. This illustrates that the effects of autonomic tone can overwrite Frank–Starling responses, which would require larger volumes for peak pressure generation and would be energetically less efficient. Note that the extent to which pressure–volume loops in the human heart are preload-dependent and, hence,

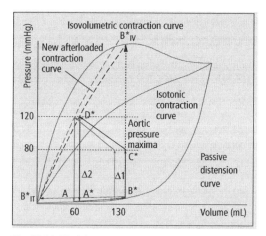

Fig. 15.26 Work-loop response to a temporary increase in ventricular filling. (See text for details.)

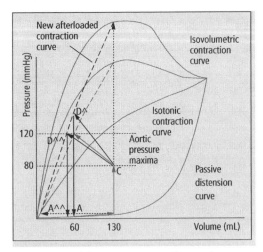

Fig. 15.27 Work-loop response to an increase in contractility. For detail see p. 367.

the applicability of the Frank–Starling Law, are debated.

Mechanical implications of chamber geometry

The heart is a three-dimensional structure, and it is important to understand the implications this has on cardiac mechanical performance, both on a beat-by-beat basis, and for more slowly occurring changes, such as with growth or hypertrophy of the heart. Much research into cardiac physiology is conducted on isolated cells or tissue strips—essentially 'linear' preparations for which length-tension characteristics can be established. Cardiac activity at the organ level is determined by volume–pressure work, and it is important to interrelate tension within the cardiac wall to pressure inside cardiac cavities, a relation that is governed by the Law of Laplace.

Law of Laplace

The law of Laplace describes the relation between wall stress and cavity pressure in a closed hollow sphere. Such a sphere can be viewed as a simplified representation of cardiac chambers, where wall stress is equivalent to the sum of active and passive forces within the myocardium, and cavity pressure is the blood pressure inside that chamber.

Wall stress is defined as force per unit cross-sectional area of the wall ($T = F(2\pi ru)^{-1}$; where T is tension, F is force, $2\pi r$ is the mean circumference of the wall, and u its thickness). Cavity pressure is force per unit surface area ($P = F(\pi r^2)^{-1}$; where P is the pressure difference between inside and outside of the chamber, which is usually simplified by assuming zero pressure on the outside so that cavity pressure is blood pressure in that chamber, and πr^2 is the cross-sectional area of a sphere). Laplace highlighted that when the two forces are in equilibrium ($F_T = F_P$, or $T2\pi ru = P\pi r^2$), then the resulting equation can be resolved for tension $\left(T = \dfrac{Pr}{2u} \right)$ or pressure $\left(P = \dfrac{T \cdot 2u}{r} \right)$.

From the latter Laplace equation, it can be seen that cavity pressure is inversely proportional to the radius: if the radius is reduced and tension within the wall stays constant, pressure will go up (Fig. 15.28). At the same time, the cavity pressure that can be developed is proportional to wall thickness, so a thicker heart muscle will normally be able to generate higher blood pressures.

The law of Laplace provides interesting insight into mechanical loading effects on cardiac performance, in particular if seen in the context of length-dependent activation of cardiomyocyte contractility (pp. 363–65). Thus, the rise in ventricular pressure during the ejection phase (C to D in Fig. 15.18) occurs despite a gradual reduction in cardiomyocyte length, which will reverse length-dependent activation and reduce contractility. However, the radius of cardiac chambers gets smaller during ejection, and the wall thicker, so that additional ventricular pressure is generated for the same (or even reduced) tension in the ventricular wall. In contrast, when there is an increase in end-diastolic volume, cardiac muscle will need to contract more forcefully (i.e. generate higher wall tension) in order to produce the same systolic pressures. Within the normal range of fluctuations, this occurs on a beat-by-beat basis via length-dependent activation of cardiomyocyte contractility. When increased preloads are more frequent

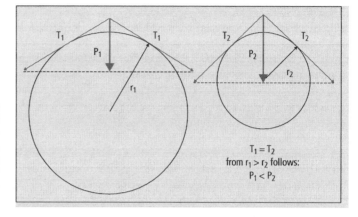

Fig. 15.28 The effect of radius on how wall tension (T) can be translated into effective cavity pressure (P), illustrated by vector analysis of the forces. Equal tension in the material forming the sphere will create a larger 'inward' force component, and hence pressure, at a smaller radius (r).

and pronounced (say during endurance training), the normal heart will adapt and normalize wall stress by an increase in wall thickness (see Cardiac growth, below). If an increase in cardiac dimensions occurs as a consequence of a pre-existing pathology, however, the interrelation between the two mechanisms may be disturbed, and in fact give rise to more serious disturbances of cardiac function (see Pathological hypertrophy, p. 370).

Cardiac growth

Cardiac growth is a complex process, influenced by circulating and locally produced growth factors, of which the **renin–angiotensin system** is most relevant. The heart contains significant amounts of angiotensin converting enzyme (ACE), which breaks up angiotensin into a number of subfragments, including angiotensin II, one of the most potent growth factors for the heart.

The main growth period of the heart occurs in early human development; it continues, at slower rate, through childhood. A few weeks after birth, the human heart contains about $2–3 \times 10^9$ cardiomyocytes, and a roughly matching number of connective tissue cells. From there on, cardiomyocyte numbers remain relatively stable, while the connective tissue cell count doubles within the first two months. This is caused by a difference in proliferative potential, which is maintained in cardiac connective tissue, but absent in cardiac muscle cells of the developed mammalian heart. It has

been proposed that circulating stem cells may differentiate into additional cardiomyocytes, although the physiological relevance of this process is being questioned. Each cardiomyocyte in the heart is in close proximity to a blood capillary. As the numbers of cardiac muscle cells change little after early post-natal development, the number of blood vessels also stays relatively constant. Any disease affecting blood vessel numbers or their blood transport capacity may lead to irreversible cell death from myocardial ischaemia (insufficient blood supply; from *ischein*—Greek for 'to restrain', and *haima*—Greek for 'blood'). Re-growth of blood vessels is possible, but usually the time taken is too long for cardiomyocytes to survive the period of reduced perfusion.

Body growth is paralleled by an increase in blood volume. The increased blood volume results in increased venous return, and thus increased volume loading of the heart. This causes chronically increased wall stress which, via mechanisms including activation of the renin–angiotensin system, leads to further cardiac growth through changes in cardiomyocyte geometry, not numbers.

Growth of cardiomyocytes will, in part, be in an axial direction, adding sarcomeres in series with existing ones. This adaptation increases overall muscle length and allows cardiac chambers to accommodate a larger blood volume, without increasing individual sarcomere lengths outside the normal range. This mechanism alone would offer only inadequate adaptation, as an increase in chamber dimensions in the absence of wall thickening would reduce cavity pressure, even at maintained myocardial contractility (see Law of Laplace, above). In reality, myocyte growth is also accompanied by myofibril addition in parallel to existing sarcomeres. This increases the contractile capacity of individual myocytes and, as a result of wall thickening, aids translation of wall stress into cavity pressure generation.

Even the adult heart still shows plasticity. A good example is the so-called athlete's heart (Fig. 15.29). There are two types of adaptation, **eccentric hypertrophy** and **concentric hypertrophy**, which are usually most pronounced in the ventricles. Eccentric hypertrophy is characterized by an increase in inner and outer diameter of the ventricle, and accompanied by a marked increase in end-diastolic volume (usually seen in endurance athletes whose hearts adapt to largely increased blood volume transport requirements). Concentric hypertrophy may also show an increase in the outer diameter, but the inner diameter is either unchanged or even reduced, due to a more pronounced increase in wall thickness (often seen with static exercise train-ing, such as weightlifting, where the heart adapts to an increased demand in peak blood pressure generation). These compensatory responses seen in athletes are reversible in principle. When athletes retire, their heart geometry tends to return towards a more normal size, provided the athlete follows a suitable de-training programme.

Pathological hypertrophy

Volume or pressure overload also occur due to pathologic causes, such as stenosis or incompetence of heart valves (see Abnormal heart sounds, p. 359). Aortic or mitral regurgitation, for example, will lead to chronic ventricular volume overload and often result in eccentric hypertrophy. Aortic or mitral stenosis, in contrast, will increase resistance to ventricular blood ejection and result in chronic pressure overload which may cause concentric hypertrophy.

Chronically increased blood pressure levels (hypertension) may also lead to ventricular pressure overload and hypertrophy. To a certain extent, this is an expression of 'proper' compensatory response mechanisms, where the hypertrophy at least initially compensates for the pathologic disorder. The intrinsic compensatory capacity may be exceeded, however, when the heart is not able to adjust to a maintained increase in mechanical demand. This may be the case when continued hypertrophic remodelling and increased peak pressures cause valve insufficiency, or when the underlying pathologies worsen. The continued growth stimulus will then cause the heart to progressively enlarge (dilate). This may give rise to **dilated cardiomyopathy**. In this condition, individual cardiomyocytes can have grown to more than twice the length of those found in normal myocardium. The heart then seems like a big bag, and can be more than double its normal size. Developed peak pressure is low, and the ejection fraction (p. 358) can drop to 0.1 or less. This impaired pressure development is not so much caused by pathologies of the cardiac muscle itself: at the myocyte level contraction can be near-normal. However, the extreme dilation impairs translation of wall tension into sufficient cavity pressure (see Law

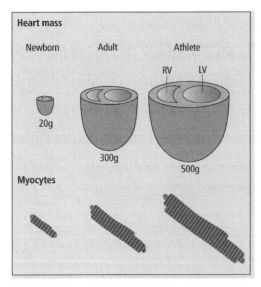

Fig. 15.29 Changes in cardiac dimensions and geometry during development. Note that the number of cardiomyocytes remains constant, while length and width of individual muscle cells increases. RV, right ventricle; LV, left ventricle.

of Laplace and Fig. 15.28). In addition, wall stress remains high, even during diastole, so that blood flow through the coronary system is impaired (see pp. 358–59). That is contrasted by a higher oxygen demand in the dilated heart, which turns the pathology into a vicious circle.

This circle may be broken by implantation of a cardiac assist device that pumps blood from the enlarged ventricle into the systemic circulation. Initially developed as a 'bridge to transplantation', it has been observed that the mechanical removal of hypertrophic growth stimuli may, in fact, allow 'reverse remodelling' of the tissue, and at least partial normalization of cardiac function (observed when the cardiac assist device is turned off). Whether this may offer a 'bridge to recovery' in some patients is currently being investigated.

Among the possible pharmacological interventions, application of ACE inhibitors has become particularly promising. When hypertrophy is diagnosed due to hypertension or valve insufficiencies, patients are placed on these drugs to specifically inhibit the effects of the renin–angiotensin system on cardiac growth.

Chapter 16

Vascular System

The vessels forming the vascular system comprise a luminal monolayer of endothelial cells in contact with the blood, surrounded by a variable number of layers of circumferentially aligned smooth muscle. In arteries and arterioles, the extent of smooth muscle contraction, or tone, is modulated by factors released from the endothelium, by transmitters released from a plexus of perivascular autonomic (predominantly sympathetic) nerves and by locally released metabolites and autacoids. Changes in muscle tone translate to a change in vessel diameter, altering the resistance to intraluminal blood flow and, as a consequence, the blood pressure and blood distribution through the various tissues and organs of the body. The capillaries, which lack smooth muscle, then provide a large surface area for the exchange of oxygen and carbon dioxide and for the movement of water and solutes. Veins provide a distensible low resistance, high capacity control on venous return to the heart, regulated by autonomic sympathetic nerves, hormones and autacoids.

Haemodynamic concepts, which underlie the development of blood pressure and flow, and associated interactions with vessels of the vascular system, are key to understanding the physiology of the cardiovascular system. Ejection of blood from the heart, or cardiac output (see Chapter 15), into a vascular system that presents a variable resistance to blood flow enables the generation of variable pressures, described by adapting Ohm's Law ($V = I \times R$) such that

$$\text{Blood pressure} = \text{cardiac output} \times \text{total peripheral resistance}$$

However, for blood to flow it is the gradient of pressure across the cardiovascular system which is critical.

16.1 Haemodynamics of blood flow

Relationship between pressure and flow of blood

The rate of blood flow (volume per unit of time) through a vessel depends absolutely on the pressure gradient from one end to the other, and the resistance encountered. In an idealized system, fluid flows along the lumen of a rigid tube from a higher to a lower hydrostatic pressure, such that the **rate of flow** ($\dot{V}$, volume/unit of time) is directly proportional to the **hydrostatic pressure gradient** (ΔP) (Table 16.1, equation 1). In the vascular system, blood pressure (force/unit area) is usually expressed in mmHg, although other units may be used (1 mmHg ~1.36 cmH$_2$O ~133 Pa).

Resistance

Resistance (R) to flow is determined by the vessel dimensions (radius and length) and blood

Table 16.1 Haemodynamic relationships.

1. Flow	Blood Flow $(\dot{V}) = \Delta$ Pressure (P)/Resistance (R)	Adaptation of Ohm's Law
2. Resistance to flow	$Resistance\ (R) = \dfrac{8 \cdot \text{Visocity}\ (\eta) \cdot \text{length}\ (l)}{\pi \cdot \text{Vessel radius}\ (r)^4}$	
3. Hagen–Poiseuille equation	$\dot{V} = \dfrac{\Delta P \pi r^4}{8 \eta l}$	Combination of 1 and 2
4. Velocity	$\text{Blood velocity}\ (v) = \dfrac{\dot{V}}{\pi r^2}$	
5. Bernoulli's equation	Total fluid energy $(E) =$ Kinetic energy $(0.5\rho v^2)$ + potential energy (P) and gravitational potential energy (ρgh)	Relate fluid density (ρ) to velocity (v), gravity (g) and height (h)
6. Law of Laplace	$P_t = \dfrac{Tu}{r}$	Relates blood vessel transmural pressure (P_t) to wall tension (T) thickness (u) and radius (r)

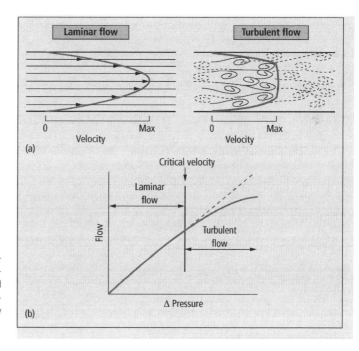

Fig. 16.1 (a) Velocity profiles of laminar and turbulent flow. (b) Relationship between pressure gradient and flow rate (or velocity) and the transition from laminar to turbulent flow once a critical velocity is reached.

viscosity. It results from the **friction** (viscous forces) between the molecules or particles of the fluid as they move, and from the friction between this fluid and the walls of the vessel. As a result, an infinitesimally thin layer of fluid in contact with the wall does not move, whilst the next layer moves slowly and so forth with the most axial (central) stream moving at the fastest rate. Such layered or **laminar flow**, parallel to the axis of the vessel, thus has a **parabolic velocity profile** (see Fig. 16.1). At higher velocity, laminar flow is disrupted and flow becomes turbulent. The concept of viscosity (η) of a fluid expresses the fact that adjacent layers interact rather than slip with infinite ease over one another. The greater the viscosity of a fluid the greater the resistance to flow.

Since friction is greatest between the fluid and the vessel wall, vessel **length** (l) and **radius** (r) affect the resistance to flow. The longer the vessel or the smaller its radius, the greater the resistance offered. This relationship is summarized in Table 16.1, equation 2. Resistance is affected most by changes in radius; a two-fold decrease in radius causing a 16-fold increase in resistance. As blood vessel length and blood viscosity are relatively constant, flow can be increased only by increasing radius or pressure gradient, or both. Only the arterioles can achieve marked changes in radii and alter resistance; a change in flow through other types of blood vessel requires a change in the pressure gradient.

If $\dot{V}$ and ΔP are in units of $\mathrm{L\,min^{-1}}$ and mmHg, respectively, then calculated values of resistance have the units $\mathrm{mmHg\,L^{-1}\,min^{-1}}$. Introducing the resistance term into the Ohm's law equation gives the **Hagen–Poiseuille equation** (Table 16.1, equation 3). The Hagen–Poiseuille equation also indicates that, at a constant flow, an increase in an arteriolar radius will result in a decrease in the pressure gradient along it (see p. 387). This may de-

crease the pressure upstream (arteries) and increase the pressure downstream (capillaries).

Resistance is influenced by blood vessel orientation: vessels lie in series and in parallel

In the vascular system, it is important to consider not only an individual vessel but also the entire network. When the vessels are arranged **in series**, the total resistance to flow through all the vessels in a network is the sum of all the individual resistances. In contrast, when vessels are arranged **in parallel**, the reciprocal of the total resistance is the sum of all the reciprocals of the individual resistances (Fig.16.2). So with vessels in parallel the total resistance presented is considerably smaller than the resistance of each individual vessel. In general, arteries, arterioles, capillaries, venules and veins lie in series with respect to one another. However, the vascular supply to the various organs and the vessels within any organ, e.g. capillaries, are arranged in parallel.

For tubes in series, provided they are not branched, application of the Poiseuille equation reveals that the same volume/unit of time ($\dot{V}$) will flow sequentially from one tube to the next with a pressure gradient along each tube that is inversely

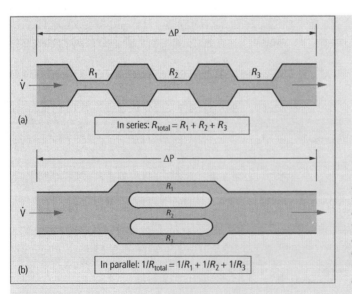

Fig. 16.2 (a) Resistances (R_1, R_2, R_3) arranged in series. Addition of a fourth resistance in series would increase the total resistance. (b) Resistances arranged in parallel. Addition of a fourth resistance in parallel would decrease the total resistance. (The resistance of the connecting tubes is assumed to be negligible.)

related to the fourth power of the radius. Thus, the narrower the tube, the greater the pressure drop as fluid flows through it. As the velocity equation indicates (Table 16.1, equation 4), the velocity will be highest in the narrowest tube.

When tubes are *in parallel*, if $\dot{V}$ is the same as in the series example above and if total cross-sectional area is the same as the feeder tube, the combined resistance of the parallel tubes and the pressure gradient along them will be smaller than in the series example. Furthermore, the pressure gradient across each of the parallel tubes will be the same and the flow through each tube will be directly proportional to the fourth power of the radius.

As the flow of blood through each parallel vessel will be different, the velocity in each is derived by substituting from the Hagen–Poiseuille equation for $\dot{V}$ in the velocity equation. Thus, velocity = $\Delta Pr^2/8\eta l$ and, in each individual parallel vessel, velocity will be directly proportional to the square of its radius. So the narrower the vessel, the slower the blood flow velocity.

If a network of parallel vessels provide an increase in total cross-sectional area, as occurs in a capillary network, the mean linear velocity through them will be slower.

Velocity of blood flow

Blood flows at a **mean linear velocity** (v, distance/unit of time), which is proportional to the **rate of flow** ($\dot{V}$) through a vessel and inversely proportional to the **cross-sectional area** (πr^2). Thus, for a given $\dot{V}$, the narrower the vessel the smaller is its cross-sectional area and the faster the velocity of flow through it.

Fluid energy

Flowing fluid such as blood has three forms of energy—kinetic, potential and gravitational. As described by **Bernoulli's equation**, the **total fluid energy** (E) per unit volume (in $kg\,m^{-1}\,s^{-2}$) in a fluid moving in a horizontal vessel is the sum of its **kinetic energy** and **potential energy**. Kinetic energy is dependent on the fluid's density (ρ, in $kg\,m^{-3}$) and the square of the mean linear velocity

(v, in $m\,s^{-1}$) such that kinetic energy is equal to $0.5\rho v^2$. Potential energy (P) is the (hydrostatic) pressure (mmHg converted to $kg\,m^{-1}\,s^{-2}$) at a particular point along the length of the vessel.

If blood suddenly flows from a narrower vessel into a much wider vessel, the large decrease in velocity which results causes a large decrease in kinetic energy. However, as there will be little change in total energy, there is an increase in the hydrostatic pressure (referred to here as **lateral pressure**) in the wider vessel. This becomes important in the cardiovascular system whenever there is a pathological dilation (**aneurysm**) in a vessel.

If the fluid is moving in a vertical vessel, which is the case in the majority of blood vessels when the body is upright, the total fluid energy in Bernoulli's equation is now the sum of the kinetic energy ($0.5\rho v^2$), the potential energy due to hydrostatic pressure (P) and the **gravitational potential energy**. This relationship is described in Table 16.1, equation 5, in which gravitational potential energy equals ρgh where ρ is the density, g the acceleration due to gravity and h the height above (+) or below (–) the heart, the site of energy generation. In an applied sense, this means that blood which is pumped above the level of the heart has a positive gravitational potential energy, while its hydrostatic pressure potential energy decreases by an amount related to the height above the heart (see p. 418). The converse occurs below the heart. Hence the change in gravitational potential energy is equal but opposite to the change in hydrostatic pressure potential energy. It follows that the total fluid energy of blood in a particular vessel is the same whether the vessel is aligned horizontally or vertically.

Deviations from predicted blood flows

The Hagen–Poiseuille equation was formulated for the laminar flow of a homogeneous fluid with constant viscosity through a rigid unbranched tube. These characteristics are of course not typical of the vascular system and blood flow is not always laminar. Under certain conditions, flow can become **turbulent**. Turbulent flow is characterized by eddies of fluid moving not only parallel to the overall direction of flow but also across it and counter to it. The result is a flattening of the velocity profile (Fig. 16.1). When turbulence occurs, the volume flow becomes proportional to the square root of the pressure gradient. In other words, for turbulent flow the pressure gradient must increase four-fold to generate a doubling of flow. Turbulence always occurs transiently in the aorta or pulmonary artery during early systole. It can occur in large arteries if the velocity is high and exceeds a critical value of about $40\,cm\,s^{-1}$ (e.g. during extreme forms of exercise). If blood viscosity is low (e.g. in severe anaemia) or there are pathological irregularities of the vascular wall (sclerosis), turbulence occurs at a lower critical velocity. The noise of turbulent blood flow can often be heard with a stethoscope.

Note also that in arteries, because of the rhythmic ejection of blood by the heart, laminar flow is also **pulsatile** and, because of the rhythmic pausing of the heart, the velocity profile is flat rather than parabolic, which effectively lowers the mean velocity.

Blood is not a homogeneous liquid of a constant viscosity

Blood is made up of both cells and plasma; the former, in particular the red blood cells, providing most of the viscosity. When blood flow is established (i.e. laminar), a greater proportion of the cells travel in the axial (central) stream. So a greater proportion of the less viscous plasma is present near to the vessel wall (which flattens the parabolic velocity profile). Axial streaming is more evident as velocity increases, and therefore the **effective viscosity** of blood is less at high velocities and greater at low velocities. At low velocities, red blood cells aggregate into rouleaux, which causes even larger increases in effective viscosity.

Low blood velocities can occur even in large vessels under pathological conditions, such as heart failure or distal to a pathological obstruction of a blood vessel lumen. The resulting rouleaux formation and consequential increase in effective viscosity will serve to reduce the blood velocity still further.

As the velocity of blood flow through arterioles and capillaries is low, it would be expected that the effective viscosity would be high. However, this is not the case because of an unexplained phenomenon in which the effective viscosity of any fluid suspension decreases considerably with decreasing tube radius, when flow is through tubes with a radius of less than $100\,\mu m$ (**Fahraeus–Lindqvist** effect).

The effective viscosity of capillary blood is also decreased because erythrocytes travel through these vessels in single file, a phenomenon referred to as **plug flow**. Furthermore, the effective viscosity of blood in the capillaries depends on the **deformability** of the erythrocytes as they are often larger than the capillaries they traverse. In sickle-cell anaemia, the desaturated haemoglobin can become crystalline which reduces considerably erythrocyte deformability.

Depending on the degree of severity, blood viscosity is decreased in all types of anaemia (p. 302). In contrast, blood viscosity is increased in hyperproteinaemia and if the haematocrit increases, as it does for example at high altitude (p. 491). In these situations, the heart has to do more work to maintain normal blood flow.

Blood vessels are not rigid tubes

When intraluminal pressure increases, vessels are **passively stretched** to a variable extent. This effect is most marked in systemic veins and in all pulmonary vessels. The passive increase in vessel radius allows a disproportionate increase in blood flow as intraluminal pressure increases (Fig. 16.3). Passive changes in radius caused in this way will result in deviations of pressure–flow relationships from values predicted by the Hagen–Poiseuille equation.

In small blood vessels, especially systemic arterioles, the pressure–flow curves do not pass through the origin but intersect at a positive pressure (normally about $20\,mmHg$ for an arteriole) called the **critical closing pressure** (Fig. 16.3). Below this pressure, flow will cease. The cause of this phenomenon is unknown, but in arterioles the critical closing pressure alters depending on the radius; it

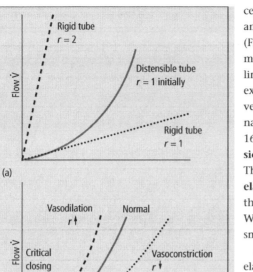

(a)

(b)

Fig. 16.3 Pressure–flow relationships (a) in rigid tubes of two different radii and in a distensible tube, and (b) in cutaneous arterioles as a function of arteriolar radius; note the critical closing pressure.

increases when arterioles constrict and decreases when they dilate.

In pathological situations, e.g. in shock, the pressure generated by the heart may not be sufficient to exceed the critical closing pressure of a vessel. The consequence is that blood flow to an organ will be severely compromised. Furthermore, concurrent reflex sympathetic constriction of arterioles during shock, in an attempt to maintain arterial blood pressure, may actually raise the critical closing pressure and thus reduce blood flow still further.

Elastance, compliance and capacitance

The ability of blood vessels to distend reflects their structure. All blood vessels are lined by a monolayer of endothelial cells and, with the ex-

ception of capillaries, they also contain varying amounts of elastin, collagen and smooth muscle (Fig. 16.4). Elastin, and to some extent smooth muscle, allow the vessel to stretch while collagen limits the extent of stretching. These effects can be examined by taking an isolated segment of a blood vessel tied at both ends and determining the luminal pressure generated at various volumes (Fig. 16.5). As the vessel is stretched it exerts **elastic tension**, which serves to raise the luminal pressure. The elastic properties are described by the term **elastance** ($\Delta P/\Delta V$), whereas the distensibility of the vessel is expressed as the **compliance** ($\Delta V/\Delta P$). When the wall is easy to stretch, its elastance is small and its compliance large.

Arteries, including the aorta have a moderate elastance and compliance over a normal range of physiological pressures. However, at pressures higher than 200 mmHg they become overfilled and their walls become rather rigid and incompliant. With ageing, the major arteries become infiltrated with fibrous tissue and therefore at all pressures they become less distensible, i.e. stiffer. The smallest arteries, the arterioles, and the capillaries, contain little or no elastin. As a result, these vessels have a low distensibility and are therefore relatively rigid.

Veins contain less elastin than arteries (Fig. 16.4) so that with high intraluminal volumes where the wall is stretched (Fig. 16.5) a vein is very stiff. However, below this range, veins are very distensible because the cross-sectional profile changes from the flattened ellipse of low volumes to the circular shape of higher volumes. The ability of veins markedly to increase their volume at low pressures explains their high **capacitance**. Use of the term capacitance in the cardiovascular system is sometimes interchanged with the term compliance. Venous compliance, and hence venous capacity, is decreased by sympathetic nerve activity, reflecting the action of the transmitter noradrenaline on smooth muscle α-adrenoreceptors.

Over the range of normal physiological pressures and volumes, arteries are about 10-fold (systemic) and two-fold (pulmonary) less distensible than systemic and pulmonary veins.

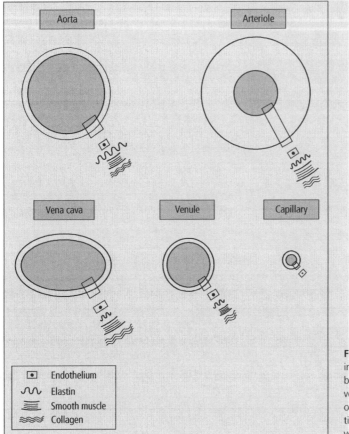

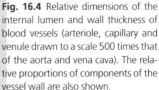

Fig. 16.4 Relative dimensions of the internal lumen and wall thickness of blood vessels (arteriole, capillary and venule drawn to a scale 500 times that of the aorta and vena cava). The relative proportions of components of the vessel wall are also shown.

Blood vessels and the law of Laplace

Strictly speaking, in Fig. 16.5 one should consider the **transmural pressure**, P_t (i.e. the pressure on the inside minus the pressure on the outside of the wall), rather than the luminal pressure. An elastic tube will distend if the inside pressure is higher and collapse if the outside pressure is higher. Within the body, the outside pressure is the hydrostatic pressure of the interstitium and usually has a mean value close to zero (p. 394). Thus, a change in the transmural pressure will alter the radius (r) of a vessel and as a result affects the total circumferential wall tension. For hollow open-ended cylinders, as opposed to spherical organs like the heart, there is only one radius of curvature, u is the thickness of the wall and T is the **passive wall tension** per unit

cross-sectional area of the wall. The total circumferential wall tension ($\pi r u T$) at equilibrium is counterbalanced by the total pressure in the lumen ($\pi r^2 P_t$) as described by the **law of Laplace** (Table 16.1, equation 6).

The tension in the wall of a blood vessel, therefore, depends on the radius, thickness of the wall and the transmural pressure. For a given transmural pressure, the tension in the wall is greater the larger the radius and the thinner the wall. The vessel's radius and wall thickness are appropriate for the transmural pressure to which the vessel is usually subjected (Table 16.2). As a consequence, capillaries that have a small radius and low transmural pressure only require a thin wall to sustain the lesser tension. On the other hand, an artery with a larger radius and high pressure will have a higher tension and a need for a thicker wall. As venous pressures are low, the thick wall of a vein is not related to a high transmural pressure but to the presence of the elastin and smooth muscle required for changing venous compliance.

When a particular vessel is subjected to an increase in transmural pressure, its distensibility (Fig. 16.5) will result in an increase in the radius and a decrease in the wall thickness leading to increased wall tension. On passive stretching, the elastin, collagen and smooth muscle withstand these increased tensions but only within the physiological range of transmural pressures; beyond this, the wall will tear.

When an area of an arterial wall becomes weakened (for example by arteriosclerosis) it becomes more distensible, resulting in a bulge or aneurysm. The increasing radius and progressive wall thinning of this bulge will result in higher tension (law of Laplace) in an already weakened region. Furthermore, the slower velocity of flowing blood at this point will result in a greater lateral pressure on the wall (from the Bernoulli equation). These changes all predispose to rupture the wall of the artery at the disease site.

In arterioles and smaller veins, which contain sufficient smooth muscle to decrease the radius of the vessel by contracting, a reduction in radius and increase in wall thickness reduce the resulting passive wall stress (law of Laplace). Thus, the active tension generated by contraction of the smooth muscle will not elevate the total tension as much as expected and the resultant effect of raising transmural pressure on total tension is dampened.

Integrated haemodynamics across the vascular system

All the variables already considered for blood vessels in series and in parallel need also to be set in the context of the complete vascular system

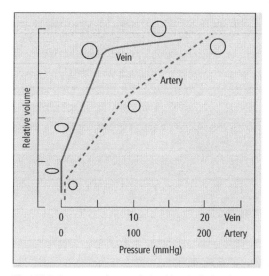

Fig. 16.5 Pressure–volume relationships in isolated segments of a vein and artery.

Table 16.2 Passive wall tension and wall stress in blood vessels expressed in $N\,m^{-1}$ ($T = P_t r$) and in $kN\,m^{-2}$ ($T = P_t r/u$), respectively.

			WALL TENSION/STRESS IN BLOOD VESSELS			
			Transmural pressure		**Wall tension**	**Wall stress**
Vessel	**Internal radius**	**Wall thickness**	**(mmHg)**	**(kPa)**	**$(N\,m^{-1})$**	**$(kN\,m^{-2})$**
Aorta	13 mm	2.0 mm	100	13.3	173	86.7
Artery	2 mm	1.0 mm	85	11.3	23	22.7
Arteriole	15 μm	20 μm	65	8.7	0.13	6.5
Capillary	4 μm	1 μm	25	3.3	0.01	13.3
Venule	15 μm	2 μm	15	2.0	0.03	15.0
Vein	2 mm	0.5 mm	10	1.3	2.7	5.3
Vena cava	15 mm	1.5 mm	5	0.7	10	6.7

(Fig. 16.6). Parallel branching of the blood vessels as the vascular system spreads from the heart means that there is a rise in the **cross-sectional area**, which is greatest in the capillaries.

The **percentage of total blood volume** accommodated in each set of vessels is determined by the cross-sectional area and the length of individual vessels. Total blood volume is about 5–6 L and 4–5 L in average men and women, respectively. In the supine position at rest, about 75% of this blood volume is contained in the systemic circuit, about 8% in the heart and about 16% in the pulmonary circuit. The volume in the heart and pulmonary circuit is referred to as the **central blood volume**. The aorta and systemic arteries contain about 12% of the blood but there is only about 3% in the systemic arterioles and about 6% in the systemic capillaries, because despite the very large total cross-sectional area they represent, the capillaries are very short (~1 mm). Most of the blood (about 55%) is accommodated within the systemic venous system, indicating its importance as a **blood reservoir**. In the pulmonary circuit, about 5% of the total blood volume is in the arterial system, 3% in the capillaries and 8% in the veins.

Standing at rest (p. 418), the cross-sectional areas are slightly different. As a consequence, about 6% of the total blood volume is in the heart and about 9% in the pulmonary circuit, resulting in an increase to about 65% in the systemic venous system. During exercise a greater proportion of blood is in the capillaries, venules and, to a lesser extent, the arterioles of skeletal muscle, as well as in the heart and in the pulmonary circuit. The proportion in the systemic venous system is reduced correspondingly.

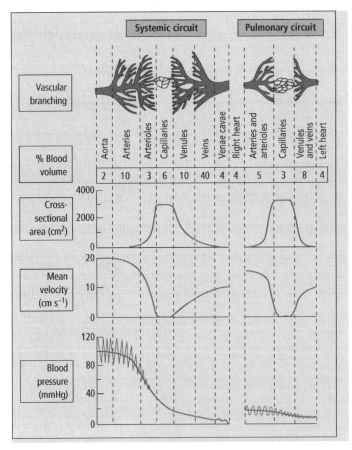

Fig. 16.6 Relationships between percentage blood volume, total cross-sectional area, mean velocity and blood pressure in the systemic and pulmonary circuits at rest in the supine position.

The **velocity** in a particular type of vessel will be the volume flow rate divided by the total cross-sectional area. Flow is pulsatile in the aorta and arteries, hence the velocity varies above and below a mean of about $20\,\mathrm{cm\,s^{-1}}$ (Fig. 16.6). Flow becomes non-pulsatile part-way through the arterioles and is very slow ($0.05\,\mathrm{cm\,s^{-1}}$), relatively, within the capillaries. This low velocity is necessary to allow sufficient time for adequate diffusion between blood and cells across the capillary wall. By the time blood reaches the venae cavae, the mean velocity has increased to about $10\,\mathrm{cm\,s^{-1}}$, less than the $20\,\mathrm{cm\,s^{-1}}$ within the aorta, because the total cross-sectional area is about twice that of the aorta.

During exercise, increases in cardiac output can cause up to a five-fold increase in velocity in the arteries and veins but in the capillaries of skeletal muscle a concomitant increase in cross-sectional area means there is little increase in velocity.

In the systemic circuit at rest, the pulsatile nature of blood pressure in the aorta and arteries results in a systolic peak of about $120\,\mathrm{mmHg}$ and a diastolic trough of about $80\,\mathrm{mmHg}$ in a healthy young adult (see Fig. 16.6). Since pressure is related to volume flow and resistance (Poiseuille's equation), the drop in mean pressure along each set of vessels will indicate their relative resistance to flow. Because of the relatively large radii of the aorta and large arteries, these vessels offer very little resistance to flow and the mean pressure drop along them is small, i.e. only from ~100 to $\sim95\,\mathrm{mmHg}$. As the arteries get narrower, the pressure drop becomes bigger (from 95 to $75\,\mathrm{mmHg}$). The greatest resistance and hence the largest fall in pressure (from 75 to $35\,\mathrm{mmHg}$) occurs along the arterioles and here there is a progressive transition from pulsatile to non-pulsatile pressure. Despite the even smaller radii of the capillaries, their total resistance is only about half that of the arterioles, so the pressure drop is smaller (from 35 to $15\,\mathrm{mmHg}$). The relatively smaller total resistance of the capillaries is a result of their vast parallel network.

The pressure fall across the venous system is small (15 to $1\text{–}2\,\mathrm{mmHg}$) because, although veins and arteries are of a similar size, the veins are more numerous and arranged in parallel. In the large veins, the blood pressure becomes slightly pulsatile

from the action of the right atrium and pulsations in nearby arteries (Fig. 16.6). So at rest, the aorta and arteries constitute about 25% of the total resistance to blood flow in the systemic circuit, the arterioles about 40%, the capillaries about 20% and the venous system overall only about 15%. The combined resistance to flow of all the parallel vascular beds of the systemic circuit is termed the **total peripheral resistance**. With a total pressure drop of $\sim100\,\mathrm{mmHg}$ from aorta to right atrium, and a cardiac output of $\sim6\,\mathrm{L\,min^{-1}}$, this resistance amounts to $\sim17\,\mathrm{mmHg\,L^{-1}\,min^{-1}}$. In the pulmonary circuit, with a total pressure gradient of $\sim10\,\mathrm{mmHg}$, **pulmonary resistance** is $\sim1.7\,\mathrm{mmHg\,L^{-1}\,min^{-1}}$.

All the pressures given in Fig. 16.6 are for the supine position, when all the vessels are at the level of the heart. When the body is upright, these pressures are affected by gravity; pressures and resistances within the pulmonary circuit are considered on p. 410.

During exercise, the profiles in Fig. 16.6 will change, because the increased force of ventricular contraction and consequent increase in cardiac output will elevate the mean arterial blood pressure (p. 619). There is also an increase in the radii of arterioles supplying skeletal muscle. This increase dominates the systemic response, resulting in a decrease in total systemic arteriolar resistance. In the working muscle, the smaller drop in pressure along its arterioles will elevate mean pressure in the downstream capillaries and veins.

16.2 Characteristics of the systemic arterial circulation

The aorta and large arteries are highly elastic, and as a result they are stretched during systole and recoil in diastole. These changes convert the intermittent flow of blood from the heart into a continuous pulsatile flow through the vessels. The maximum and minimum pressure attained in the main arteries is referred to as the systolic and diastolic blood pressure, respectively. These pressures can be measured with a sphygmomanometer, and are determined to varying degrees by the pumping of the heart, arterial distensibility and the

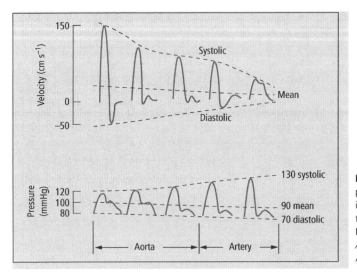

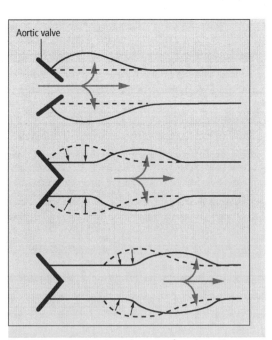

Fig. 16.7 Changes in velocity (flow pulse) and in pressure (pressure pulse) in the arterial system at increasing distances away from the heart. (After McDonald, D.A. (1974) *Blood Flow in Arteries*, 2nd edn, p. 271. Edward Arnold, London.)

resistance of blood vessels, particularly the down-stream arterioles.

Blood enters the aorta at high velocity, so flow tends to be turbulent. As it enters only during systole, flow, velocity and pressure are pulsatile (see Figs. 16.6 and 16.7). Aortic flow and velocity reach a peak early in systole, because two-thirds of the stroke volume is ejected from the heart during the first third of systole. However, the peak of the blood pressure pulse occurs slightly later due to the elastic stretch of the aorta (Fig. 16.7).

The aorta stretches in systole to accommodate about 50% of the stroke volume whilst the other 50% flows on into the peripheral vessels (Fig. 16.8). During diastole the stretched area elastically recoils, propelling the accommodated blood on to the next arterial segment which stretches as it fills, and so on. When elastin in the artery wall is stretched, the kinetic energy of liquid motion is converted into potential energy. When the elastin recoils it converts potential energy back to kinetic energy. This effect prevents pressure in the aorta from dropping to zero, and causes it to fall only gradually (to a minimum of about 80 mmHg). Maintaining a relatively high pressure during diastole ensures that the blood accommodated in systole is propelled out to the periphery during diastole. Elastic recoil thus converts the intermit-

Fig. 16.8 Progression along the aorta of an alternating sequence of elastic stretching, accommodating about 50% of the stroke volume, followed by elastic recoil propelling blood to the next segment. Blue arrows indicate direction of blood movement; black arrows indicate direction of elastic recoil.

tent flow of blood from the heart into a continuous, albeit pulsatile, flow through the arterial system.

The forward movement of blood itself (**flow pulse**) has a mean velocity of about $20\,cm\,s^{-1}$ in the aorta, decreasing to about $15\,cm\,s^{-1}$ in a small artery (Fig. 16.6). In comparison, the **pressure pulse** (pulse wave) is transmitted through the column of blood and along the walls of the arteries at a very high mean velocity. This velocity is about $4\,m\,s^{-1}$ in the aorta, and increases to about $12\,m\,s^{-1}$ in small arteries. The velocity of this pressure pulse is higher:

1 the less viscous the blood;
2 the greater the mean blood pressure;
3 the more rigid or thicker the vessel wall; and
4 the smaller the lumen radius.

With increasing age, the walls of the arteries become stiffer, which results in an increased pulse-wave velocity. A similar effect occurs in hypertension, when, arterial walls are overstretched.

The velocity, and therefore the amplitude of the flow pulse decreases with increasing distance from the heart due to branching of the arteries and increasing cross-sectional area (Fig. 16.7). In contrast, the velocity and amplitude of the pressure pulse increases. First, the diastolic pressure decreases as a result of the loss of energy from the pulse wave due to alternating transfer between kinetic and potential energy. Second, the systolic pressure increases as a result of complex fluid dynamics. The latter includes the reflection of energy back towards the heart due to the decreased elasticity of the smaller arteries and from reflections at branching points. Such factors also dampen the sharp incisura of the aortic pressure wave and convert it to the smaller **dicrotic notch** and the distinct **dicrotic wave** (Figs 16.7 and 16.9).

Clinically, these arterial pressure pulses can be felt, giving information not only about heart rate and its regularity, but also about stroke volume and arterial distensibility. The tension or hardness of the pulse reflects the pulse pressure. More precise information about the shape of the pulse is provided using electromechanical transducers placed on the skin over an artery.

Measuring arterial blood pressure

The maximum to which arterial pressure rises is called the **systolic blood pressure** (at rest the range is 100–140 mmHg at 20 years of age) and the minimum to which it falls is the **diastolic blood pressure** (range 50–90 mmHg). With increasing age both diastolic and, in particular, systolic pressure increase; the latter is due to loss of arterial elasticity. The difference between systolic and diastolic pressure is the **pulse pressure**.

The **mean arterial blood pressure** is not simply the average of the systolic and diastolic pressure. This is because systole occupies a smaller proportion of the cardiac cycle than diastole (see Fig. 15.18). Mean blood pressure is therefore calculated by integrating pressure against time (Fig. 16.9). In the aorta, the mean arterial blood pressure (about 100 mmHg) is approximately the arithmetic mean of the systolic and diastolic pressure or, expressed another way, the diastolic pressure plus half the pulse pressure. In a peripheral artery, which has a different pressure–time contour, it is approximately the diastolic pressure plus one-third of the pulse pressure (about 95 mmHg).

The systolic and diastolic arterial blood pressures can be measured directly by inserting a liquid-filled catheter into the appropriate artery and recording with a pressure transducer. Clinically, this is routinely not practical and pressure is measured indirectly with a **sphygmomanometer** (Fig. 16.10). This comprises an inflatable rubber cuff, covered by a layer of non-distensible fabric, which is usually wrapped around the upper arm at the level of the heart and connected to a mercury manometer. The cuff pressure is increased by pumping air in, and then reduced by releasing the air through a needle valve. During this procedure, a stethoscope is placed distal to the cuff and over the brachial artery in the antecubital fossa. Inflating the cuff to a pressure higher than the expected systolic pressure compresses the brachial artery so no blood flows through it. When the cuff pressure is slowly reduced, the degree of arterial compression progressively decreases and varying sounds (**Korotkoff sounds**) audible with the stethoscope result from intermittent and turbulent blood flow through the

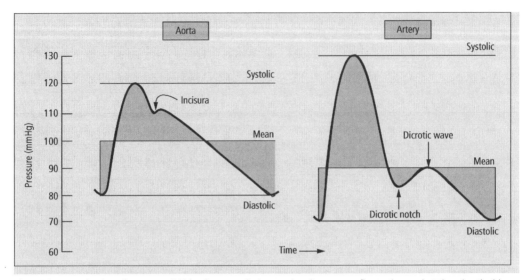
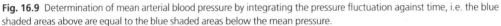

Fig. 16.9 Determination of mean arterial blood pressure by integrating the pressure fluctuation against time, i.e. the blue shaded areas above are equal to the blue shaded areas below the mean pressure.

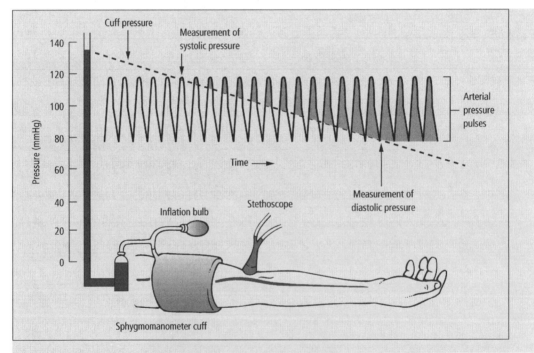

Fig. 16.10 Use of sphygmomanometer and stethoscope to measure indirectly systolic and diastolic pressure at the appearance and disappearance, respectively, of the Korotkoff sounds. (After Rushmer, R.F. (1970) *Cardiovascular Dynamics*, 3rd edn, p. 155. WB Saunders, Philadelphia.)

artery. Four phases of sound followed by a fifth phase of silence can be distinguished as follows:

1 When the cuff pressure falls just below the systolic pressure, a clear, but often faint, tapping sound suddenly appears in phase with each cardiac contraction. The tapping sound is produced by the transient and turbulent blood flow through the artery during the peak of each systole. The systolic pressure is defined as the cuff pressure at which the tapping sound is first heard. During the next ~15 mmHg fall in the cuff pressure, the tapping sound becomes louder (phase I).

2 In the following ~20 mmHg fall, the sound becomes quieter with a murmuring quality (phase II) and may suddenly disappear in the latter part of this phase (the auscultatory gap).

3 In the next ~5 mmHg fall in cuff pressure, the sound of the murmuring becomes very loud and thumping (phase III).

4 In the following ~5 mmHg fall, the sound becomes muffled and rapidly grows fainter (phase IV).

5 Finally, the sound disappears (phase V). When blood flow velocity is high, for example in exercise, the start of phases IV and V may be separated by 40 mmHg or more. The start of phase IV (muffling) and of phase V (disappearance) are used to measure diastolic pressure. The diastolic pressure is usually defined as the cuff pressure at which muffling, not disappearance, occurs, although this probably slightly overestimates diastolic pressure. However, if there is an obvious difference at rest between these, both values are reported.

Determinants of arterial blood pressure

The prime parameters of arterial blood pressure—mean, systolic and diastolic—are determined by cardiac output and total peripheral resistance (Chapter 17). However, at a secondary level **systolic pressure** is modified mainly by changes in ejection velocity and, to a lesser extent, stroke volume, while **diastolic pressure** is modified mainly by changes in total peripheral resistance and the time available for blood to leave the arteries, i.e. the duration of diastole, which decreases as heart rate increases.

Systolic pressure is seen to increase (Fig. 16.11) when there is:

1 an increase in diastolic pressure of the previous pulse;

2 an increase in stroke volume;

3 an increase in ejection velocity (without a change in stroke volume); or

4 a decrease in aortic or arterial distensibility.

Diastolic pressure is seen to increase when there is:

1 an increase in the systolic pressure of that particular pulse;

2 a decrease in ejection velocity;

3 an increase in aortic or arterial distensibility;

4 an increase in heart rate; or

5 an increase in total peripheral resistance.

16.3 Circulation through systemic arterioles

Because of the small diameter and the large surface area they present, arterioles are the site of greatest resistance to blood flow in the vascular system. Vessel diameter is controlled through contraction or relaxation of the smooth muscle in the arteriolar wall (vasoconstriction or vasodilatation). Resulting changes in resistance alter both the amount of blood flowing through the arterioles and the upstream arterial and downstream capillary pressures. Arteriolar calibre, and hence blood flow, is altered intrinsically by changes in wall stretch, the elaboration of tissue metabolites and the local release of chemicals (autacoids). Extrinsic control is exerted by hormones and the autonomic nervous system, in both cases mainly due to sympathetic nerve activity.

At rest, arterioles constitute about 40% of the total peripheral vascular resistance in the body. Classically, arterioles are considered to be the smallest arteries, with a single layer of smooth muscle surrounding the endothelium. They represent the site of the largest fall in blood pressure (Figs 16.6 and 16.12) and the site at which resistance is altered most. As already mentioned (Chapter 14) contraction of the vascular smooth muscle in their walls (**vasoconstriction**) decreases arteriolar radius, thereby increasing resistance. As a

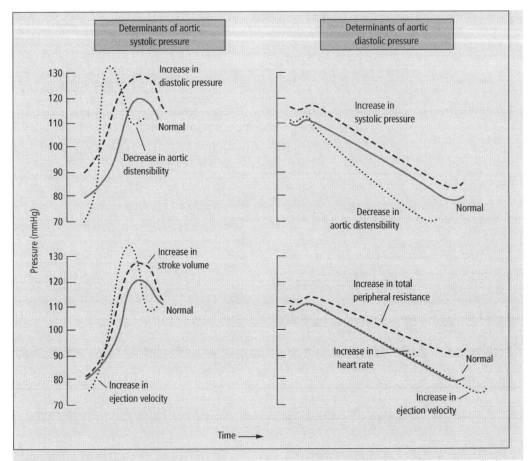

Fig. 16.11 Determinants of systolic and diastolic pressure in the aorta. The effect of each factor is shown when all other factors are held constant.

consequence, there is a decrease in blood flow through the arterioles and a larger than usual fall in blood pressure because the upstream arterial pressure is elevated and downstream capillary pressure is reduced (Fig. 16.12). Converse changes follow relaxation of the smooth muscle (**vasodilatation**).

Smooth muscle cells in the arterioles spontaneously develop contraction or 'tone' in response to intraluminal pressure (**myogenic** contraction/tone), which varies in extent in different parts of the vascular system. For example, myogenic tone is lower in arterioles supplying the gut compared to vessels within cardiac muscle. Myogenic tone appears mainly due to the arterial wall tension, in-

creasing tension somehow causing smooth muscle depolarization and a consequent opening of voltage-dependent calcium channels; Ca^{2+} influx follows and thus muscle contraction. Superimposed on top of myogenic tone is the effect of activity in **sympathetic nerves** and circulating hormones and/or local humoral agents (autacoids) and metabolites. Sympathetic nerves are normally tonically active, thus providing a background degree of vasoconstriction, which together with the spontaneous myogenic tone and contraction caused by circulating or local humoral agents is referred to as **vasomotor tone**. Its extent at any moment varies from organ to organ and influences the proportion of the cardiac output that each

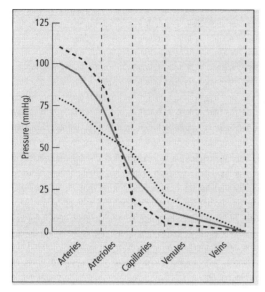

Fig. 16.12 Blood pressure profile in the vessels: control conditions (blue line), after vasoconstriction (dashed line) and after vasodilation (dotted line).

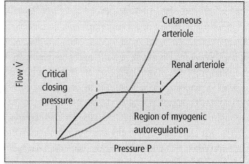

Fig. 16.13 Pressure–flow relationships in arterioles which do (renal) and do not (cutaneous) exhibit autoregulation.

receives. For example, at rest the vasomotor tone is high in arterioles of skeletal muscle and low in those of the gut, kidney and skin. The higher the vasomotor tone in a person at rest, the greater the increase in blood flow during maximal vasodilatation.

Intrinsic control of arteriolar blood flow

Many organs, especially those with a small degree of neurogenic control, exhibit the phenomenon of **autoregulation** of blood flow; that is, regardless of large changes in perfusion pressure the blood flow to these organs remains remarkably constant (Fig. 16.13). The mechanism underlying autoregulation remains uncertain—both the intrinsic response of arteriolar smooth muscle to stretch (myogenic) or local metabolites have been suggested, but both mechanisms may operate to varying degrees in different tissues.

Myogenic autoregulation

In key organs such as the brain, kidney and heart the ability of the smooth muscle of arterioles spon-

taneously to contract when, as described by the law of Laplace, the arteriolar wall tension is passively increased by an increase in blood pressure, is of critical importance. The reduction in radius caused by the contraction matches the increase in perfusion pressure such that (Poiseuille equation) there is no change in blood flow over a certain range of pressure. Conversely the arterioles relax when the pressure decreases and thus maintain flow. This is referred to as **myogenic autoregulation** of blood flow (Fig. 16.13). It means blood flow to a specific organ is independent of variations in arterial blood pressure, at least over a physiological range. Myogenic autoregulation is also present to varying degrees in the gut, skeletal musculature and skin but in these beds it is subject to more dominant influences, for example from autonomic nerves in the skin and local metabolites in the gut (see also Chapters 14 and 17).

The skin and gut have an additional series of specialized arteries, particularly prominent in the former, the **arteriovenous anastomes**. These provide low resistance pathways which when they are open enable blood to shunt or bypass the capillary network in the skin. These vessels are densely innervated by sympathetic constrictor nerves and appear not to be influenced by local metabolites. The net result is that they are controlled closely by reflex activation or inhibition of these nerves, facilitating the redistribution of blood away from the skin during situations of raised sympathetic activity.

Metabolic regulation or active hyperaemia

All organs need to receive variable blood flow, in proportion to their metabolic requirements. During increased metabolism there is a local decrease in the partial pressure of O_2 (Po_2), an increase in the partial pressure of CO_2 (Pco_2) with an associated increase in H^+ concentration in the interstitial fluid. These changes cause the smooth muscle to relax to a degree that reflects the magnitude of the increased metabolism and ensures an increase in flow with little (or no) change in perfusion pressure. This is called **metabolic regulation** (or active hyperaemia). Increases in local temperature and in the local concentrations of other metabolites (such as adenosine triphosphate (ATP), adenosine diphosphate (ADP), adenosine monophosphate (AMP), adenosine, inorganic phosphate, lactate and pyruvate, as well as increases in K^+ concentration and interstitial osmolarity of exercising skeletal musculature) can also contribute to vasodilatation. Metabolic regulation is well developed in the skeletal musculature, heart and brain, but, in other organs and to some extent also in skeletal muscle, it can be overriden by extrinsic nervous control of arteriolar diameter.

Metabolic regulation may contribute to the overall phenomenon of autoregulation illustrated in Fig. 16.13, inasmuch as an increase in pressure increases blood flow, and in the face of constant metabolism this increase will lower tissue metabolites, so contributing to vasoconstriction.

When the blood supply to an organ is temporarily obstructed (for a period of seconds up to a few minutes), restoring the supply is accompanied by a larger than expected increase in blood flow (**reactive hyperaemia**). The increase depends on the duration of the obstruction and the metabolic rate of the organ over the period of obstruction. Vasodilator metabolites that accumulate during the obstruction contribute to this reactive hyperaemia.

When an increase in Pco_2 (hypercapnia) or decrease in Po_2 (hypoxia) occurs throughout the body (for example, when breathing or gaseous exchange is impaired) then all the systemic arterioles will dilate. The fall in mean arterial blood pressure and the arterial hypercapnia and hypoxia elicit various cardiovascular reflexes (e.g. baroreceptor, chemoreceptor; Chapter 17), which will oppose the local drive to vasodilatation.

Usually, small changes in the metabolism of an organ can be satisfied by local metabolic regulation, without affecting significantly the total peripheral resistance. However if the metabolism of the organ increases markedly there will be a fall in total peripheral resistance. The resultant initial fall in mean arterial blood pressure will then elicit cardiovascular reflexes (p. 404) to increase cardiac output and restrict the blood flow to other organs in order to maintain the overall mean arterial blood pressure.

Humoral control

In addition to tissue metabolites, other chemicals released locally within an organ also affect blood flow. Agents that act as local hormones, or paracrine agents, are described as **autacoids**. The definition of an autacoid is not restrictive, and agents which act in this way may also act as transmitters in other parts of the body, e.g histamine and serotonin (5-HT).

The sweat and salivary glands, and the gastrointestinal mucosa, produce not only their exocrine secretions but also an enzyme, kallikrein. This enzyme converts plasma kininogens into active **kinins**, such as kallidin and **bradykinin**, which have marked vasodilator effects in the glands as well as locally within the skin or gut. The kinins are inactivated locally by other tissue enzymes. During inflammatory or allergic reactions, or tissue damage, kinins are also liberated from tissues and the vasodilator **histamine** is released from basophils and mast cells (p. 304). Inflammatory responses are also modulated by vasoconstricting **leukotrienes** released from leukocytes (p. 315). When a blood vessel is cut, **serotonin** and the prostaglandin derivative **thromboxane** A_2 are released from activated platelets and cause direct smooth muscle vasoconstriction and platelet aggregation, which together serve to limit blood loss. The latter is additionally amplified by the release of ATP from platelets.

A key autacoid influence on the diameter of blood vessels, including arterioles, originates in the monolayer of endothelial cells. These cells were long thought to be simply a passive barrier, separating the flowing blood from sub-intimal aggregatory surfaces. However, they also provide an active regulation of artery/arteriolar diameter through the synthesis and release of a number of agents or factors. These are predominately dilator in nature but can include at least one potent constrictor factor, endothelin. A key endothelium-derived dilator agent released in arteries is **nitric oxide**, which before its identification was referred to as an **endothelium-derived relaxing factor** (EDRF). Nitric oxide (NO) is continuously synthesized (by the constitutive enzyme NO synthase) and released by endothelial cells in both arteries and arterioles. Release can be stimulated by the shear stress, or viscous drag, which follows an increase in blood flow in arteries, but it is not clear if a similar response occurs in arterioles. However, other autacoids, such as bradykinin, ADP and substance P can stimulate the endothelium to release dilators, including nitric oxide. Although nitric oxide is released from arterioles, its contribution as a dilator influence appears not to be as great as in the larger arteries upstream, with other less well-defined dilator influences predominant in the arterioles. These include **endothelium-derived hyperpolarizing factor** (EDHF), which dilates by hyperpolarizing the smooth muscle and reducing Ca^{2+} entry (due to opening of voltage-sensitive Ca^{2+} channels). EDHF has not been identified, but in the smaller arteries it may be due to passive spread of hyperpolarization from the endothelial cells to the smooth muscle via gap junctions, as well as diffusible factors. There also appears to be some variation in the endothelium-derived factors released between vascular beds, for example the arachidonic acid derivative **prostacyclin (PGI$_2$)** seems to contribute to vasodilatation in the coronary circulation but is less active elsewhere. What is clear, is that the dilator influence of the endothelium is disrupted in disease states which impinge on the vasculature, i.e. diabetes.

Vascular (and endocardial) endothelial cells also release a potent vasoconstrictor **endothelin** (ET-1) in response to various chemical and physical stress factors such as thrombin, hypoxia and mechanical stretch.

Recently, the endothelium has been suggested to be the conduction pathway underlying the phenomenon of **spreading vasodilatation**. This describes the ascent of dilatation from the microcirculation through arteries of increasing size to the feed arteries of skeletal muscle. It means local dilators, generated by muscle contraction, can evoke distant 'upstream' dilatation and thus increase the supply of O_2 and nutrients by increasing blood flow. The mechanism responsible is not clear, but it requires cell-cell coupling through gap-junctions to enable a signal to pass up through walls of the different size arterioles and arteries, against the direction of blood flow.

Extrinsic control of arteriolar blood flow

Nervous control

In organs with a resting level of sympathetic nerve-evoked vasomotor tone, an increase in **sympathetic** nerve firing to arterioles causes further vasoconstriction whilst a decrease in discharge rate results in passive vasodilatation. The sympathetic neurotransmitter **noradrenaline** is responsible, and acts powerfully on α_1-**adrenoceptors** on the plasma membrane of vascular smooth muscle cells to cause contraction. Arterioles of the skin, gut, skeletal musculature and kidneys have a dense sympathetic innervation, whereas those of the brain and heart are more sparsely innervated.

Noradrenaline also acts on the β_2-adrenoceptors of vascular smooth muscle, the activation of these receptors leading to relaxation. However, unlike with adrenaline this effect of noradrenaline is very weak, and the strong α_1-mediated constrictions are normally dominant.

The vasoconstriction resulting from a certain level of sympathetic discharge is considerably greater in the skin, kidney and gut than in skeletal muscle. Thus, the blood flow to the skin, kidney and gut can be restricted, favouring blood flow to other organs. This sympathetic pathway is controlled by cardiovascular centres in the brainstem, and operates as part of the baroreceptor reflex, to regulate mean arterial blood pressure (Chapter 17).

A special system of sympathetic nerves controlled from the motor cortex and hypothalamus (p. 415) innervates arterioles of the skeletal musculature. It releases acetylcholine at postganglionic nerve endings, which results in arteriolar vasodilatation. The action of acetylcholine is mediated by muscarinc receptors, although it is not clear where they are located. Endothelial cells almost uniformly do contain these receptors and stimulation with acetylcholine leads to the release of the dilator NO. However, it is not clear if this is the pathway to dilatation in skeletal muscle arterioles, which may in part reflect inhibition of the tonic firing of 'classic' sympathetic nerves. The **sympathetic cholinergic pathway** is usually silent, in contrast to the tonically active sympathetic nerves. These nerves are activated during emotional reactions of alarm, rage or fear and during the initial phase of exercise, and they may have a large part to play in the rapid drop in blood pressure, which leads to syncope. In humans, sweat glands are also innervated by sympathetic–cholinergic nerves, and activation stimulates both sweating and an associated increase in local blood flow. Although, in addition, part of this response is mediated by a non-cholinergic, non-adrenergic effect (see below).

Although vasodilatation in most tissues is brought about by a reduction in sympathetic nerve activity, some vascular beds are innervated by **parasympathetic** vasodilator nerves. The extent of parasympathetic innervation of the vascular system is extremely limited when compared to the sympathetic branch of the autonomic nervous system. But parasympathetic nerves do supply some of the cerebral and coronary arteries, and blood vessels in the erectile tissue of the external genitalia. Dilatation in the salivary glands, exocrine pancreas, and in the gastric and colonic mucosa, is also influenced by parasympathetic nerves. Along with acetylcholine, vasoactive intestinal polypeptide (VIP) seems to act as a co-transmitter following release from the parasympathetic nerves. In addition, there is a distinct population of

postganglionic autonomic nerves to discrete vascular beds that do not use either noradrenaline or acetylcholine as a neurotransmitter. These nerves are referred to as non-cholinergic, non-adrenergic or **NANC nerves**. They appear to be particularly involved in initiating vasodilatation in the gut and in the genitalia. A number of putative neurotransmitters have been suggested to contribute to vasodilatation, and in the latter, release of nitric oxide from NANC nerves appears to play a crucial role in the dilatation that leads to erection of the penis.

Hormonal control

The chromaffin cells in the adrenal medulla continuously secrete **adrenaline** together with a small amount of noradrenaline. The level of secretion by the adrenal medulla is proportional to its sympathetic input, which is mainly under the immediate control of the hypothalamus (Chapter 11). Adrenaline can activate both α_1-**adrenoceptors** and β_2-**adrenoceptors** on vascular smooth muscle cells, and to a similar extent. Activation of each receptor type results in either vasoconstriction or vasodilatation, respectively. The net arteriolar response of a particular organ to adrenaline therefore depends on the relative densities of α_1- and β_2-receptors. The density of β_2-receptors is higher than α_1-receptors in the heart and skeletal musculature. Thus, during exercise the increased release of adrenaline contributes to the increased blood flow to the heart and skeletal musculature, whilst decreasing blood flow to the skin, gut and kidney where the density of α_1-receptors is greater and vasoconstriction to both circulating adrenaline and nerve-released noradrenaline predominates. Across the cardiovascular system, it was thought that β_1-adrenoceptors were restricted to cardiac muscle and β_2-adrenoceptors to vascular smooth muscle. However, it is becoming clear that this was an oversimplification, and both β_1- and β_2-adrenoceptors are found within systemic blood vessels, stimulation in both cases leading to vasodilatation.

The hormones **angiotensin II** and **antidiuretic hormone** (ADH/vasopressin) are powerful vasoconstrictors, while **atrial natriuretic peptide** decreases the sensitivity of vascular smooth muscle to these and other vasoconstrictor substances. Physiologically, these hormones appear to be concerned primarily with the control of blood volume and thus the long-term maintenance of a normal arterial blood pressure (Chapters 11 and 21).

14.4 Circulation through systemic capillaries

Precapillary sphincters and arterioles control how much blood passes (at a slow velocity) through a capillary. Capillary walls provide a large surface area for the diffusion of substances between blood and interstitial fluid surrounding cells. Diffusion is by far the most important process for exchange of gases, solutes and water across the capillary wall. The capillary wall is, however, somewhat leaky and allows a little water, and solutes smaller than M_r 70000, to move by bulk flow. Some capillaries are less permeable because of tight junctions between endothelial cells; others are more permeable because of fenestrations made up of fused-vesicle channels spanning the endothelial cells. The amount of fluid leaving a capillary by bulk flow depends on the permeability and surface area of its wall and the hydrostatic and osmotic pressure gradients between the blood and interstitial fluid. The hydrostatic pressure gradient results in ultrafiltration of fluid from the capillary while osmotic pressure gradients normally promote reabsorption of fluid; in most tissues there is on balance a slight excess of ultrafiltration—the Starling equilibrium.

The entrance of an arteriole (or a metarteriole, see below), leading into the vast network of capillaries of the body, is regulated by a ring of smooth muscle—the **precapillary sphincter** (Fig. 16.14). These sphincters exhibit **myogenic rhythmicity**, resulting in intermittent and variable flow rates through any individual capillary. The direction of flow may change in some capillaries depending on both their location within the capillary bed and the degree of constriction of nearby sphincters. This can be observed visually, for instance, in the capillary bed of the rabbit's ear. The net degree of constriction or dilation of the sphincters is controlled by **metabolic regulation**. For example, at any one moment in resting skeletal muscle about 10% of the capillaries are open and the remainder contain blood that is stationary (these capillaries may even be completely empty). Blood may bypass the capillaries by flowing through the **metarterioles**. These specialized vessels represent **thoroughfare channels** and contain, in contrast to the capillaries, some scattered smooth muscle

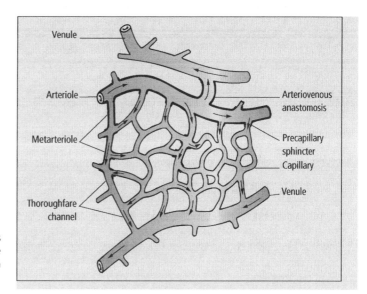

Fig. 16.14 A capillary network and its associated vessels. Thick walls denote considerable amounts of smooth muscle.

(Fig. 16.14). In the skin and gut, short, relatively large-diameter vessels called **arteriovenous anastomoses** can additionally act as shunts between arterioles and venules (Fig. 16.14). They have thick walls of smooth muscle controlled by sympathetic nerves acting on α_1-adrenoceptors to shut the anastomoses. Both the metarterioles and the arteriovenous anastomoses contrast with capillaries, which comprise only a monolayer of endothelial cells on a basement membrane, and cannot contract nor distend.

The major characteristics of capillary beds have already been considered (Fig. 16.6): a parallel arrangement of these narrow (4 μm radius) and short (~1 mm long) vessels; their contribution (~20%) to the resting total peripheral resistance; the blood pressure drop along them; the absence of pulsatile flow; their vast cross-sectional area; the low velocity of flow in the capillary bed; and the low flow rate through an individual capillary.

It is important to remember that the blood flow and pressure in the capillaries are determined by the arterioles (Fig. 16.12). Under resting conditions, only about 25% of the capillaries are open at any one time, giving a total capillary cross-sectional area of about 3000 cm^2. Since the average length of a capillary is about 0.1 cm and the velocity of capillary blood flow at rest is 0.05 cm s^{-1}, blood will take about 2 s to traverse the length of a capillary. When a tissue increases its metabolic rate, more of its capillaries open and the total cross-sectional area is increased. As upstream arteriolar vasodilatation increases the pressure gradient (ΔP) across each individual capillary, the velocity of blood flow through each capillary (the capillary radius does not change) will also increase (velocity is proportional to ΔPr^2). The **transit time** through a capillary is, however, rarely shorter than 1 s which is still sufficient to allow adequate **diffusion** (Chapter 1) of gases and nutrients across the capillary wall. The vast network of capillaries also provides a **large surface area** for exchange with the tissue cells, with a **short diffusion distance** (no more than 50 μm) between blood and cells. The area increases and the distance decreases whenever more capillaries are open.

Structure of capillary walls

The wall of the capillaries is composed of a single layer of endothelial cells about 1 μm in thickness. In contrast to the plasma membrane of cells (Chapter 1), the capillary wall in most tissues is leaky, allowing substances of M_r less than about 70 000 to cross. These substances include practically all the solutes in the plasma except for the plasma proteins. But capillary permeability does differ in different tissues, for example in the liver proteins pass through to a greater extent than elsewhere, while in brain, movement of water-soluble solutes is markedly reduced. These differences reflect the regional organization of the capillary wall. In liver, obvious spaces between adjacent endothelial cells can be seen in electron micrographs, whereas in most brain capillaries adjacent endothelial cells are held firmly together by **tight junctions** which restrict water and solute movement and comprise a **blood–brain barrier** (Chapter 3). In some specialized capillaries in the gut and kidney (renal glomerulus) exchange of solutes is facilitated by **fenestrations**—areas within the endothelial cells where little or no cytoplasm separates the plasma membranes on the two surfaces of the cell. Endothelial cells generally contain large numbers of cytoplasmic vesicles; fenestrations are formed by fusion of vesicles to bridge the cytoplasm of a cell. In most vascular beds, adjacent endothelial cells are attached to each other at their margins, though the attachment offers relatively little resistance to solute exchange. Furthermore, a continuous **basement membrane** encircles the periluminal surface of all capillaries, providing additional support to the endothelial cells.

It is now realized that the plasma membranes of endothelial cells, like those of epithelial cells (Chapter 1), contain a variety of specific pathways through which ions and other water-soluble solutes can be transported between blood and interstitial fluid. In brain capillaries, because of the tightness of the junctions holding adjacent cells together, the cellular pathway provides the dominant route for transendothelial movements of water-soluble solutes. However, in other capillary beds much of the exchange of these solutes and of water occurs by diffusion between the cells (paracellular pathway). Proteins and other macromolecules may also be transported across endothelial cells by a process of transcytosis (Chapter 1). In contrast, lipid-soluble substances, including O_2 and CO_2, diffuse passively across the plasma membranes of the endothelial cells.

Ultrafiltration and reabsorption of fluid across capillary walls

It must be emphasized that passive diffusional movements are responsible for virtually all the exchange of gases, solutes and water between capillaries and surrounding interstitial fluid. However for solutes and water, such exchange requires a relatively permeable capillary wall. At the same time, in order to drive blood through the systemic circulation a relatively high hydrostatic pressure is required. As a consequence of these two factors, it is inevitable that some fluid will be moved by **bulk flow** from capillaries to the interstitial fluid, a process called ultrafiltration. To maintain the circulating blood volume, this fluid must be returned by bulk flow to the circulation. This is achieved mostly by reabsorption back into the capillary by osmosis, with the remainder returned to the venous circulation by the lymphatic system. So, effectively, the direction and the amount of fluid that moves across the wall of the capillaries is determined by the algebraic sum of the hydrostatic and the osmotic pressure across the capillary wall.

Colloid osmotic pressure

As the structure of the capillary wall allows free permeability to water and to solutes of M_r less than 70000, small molecules diffuse through the capillary wall and achieve equal concentrations on both sides. Thus, they make no contribution to the effective osmotic pressure. As plasma proteins with M_r greater than *circa* 70000 cannot normally cross the capillary wall (i.e. proteins with a reflection coefficient $\sigma = 1$ are reflected; σ for water = 0; everything else lies between 0 and 1), they generate an **effective osmotic pressure**. Since plasma proteins

are large enough to be classed as colloids, this effective osmotic pressure is known as the **plasma colloid osmotic pressure** (or plasma oncotic pressure). Although the oncotic pressure is low (~25 mmHg; see below) compared to the total osmotic pressure of the plasma (~5800 mmHg) it is very important, because it is generated by proteins unable, by and large, to cross the capillary wall. This is in contrast to the electrolytes, which determine the majority of the osmotic pressure.

Proteins are present in plasma at a concentration of about $1 \, mmol \, L^{-1}$ of plasma, whereas the protein concentration in the interstitial fluid is much lower ($0.1–0.33 \, mmol \, L^{-1}$) depending on the tissue. The most important protein contributing to the oncotic pressure is albumin, which at M_r 69000 is borderline, in terms of its potential ability to cross the capillary membrane. However, some does enter the interstitial fluid and contributes to the interstitial oncotic pressure. Albumin is important for two main reasons. First, the plasma concentration is high, i.e. it is present at twice the concentration of the much larger globulins. Second, at physiological pH it can bind both cations (mainly Na^+) and to a lesser extent, anions (mainly Cl^-). As albumin is effectively trapped within the vascular compartment and thus impermeant, it therefore influences the distribution of the permeant electrolytes, i.e. it exerts a **Gibbs–Donnan Effect**.

With these points in mind, if the interstitial protein concentration is close to zero, the concentration difference for protein represents an effective osmotic pressure for plasma of 16 mmHg (calculated using the van't Hoff equation, Chapter 1). The **Gibbs–Donnan Effect** causes an uneven distribution of small ions with a small excess (Donnan excess of about $0.5 \, mmol \, L^{-1}$) inside the capillary. The excess contributes a further 9 mmHg to the effective osmotic pressure of plasma. Hence the total plasma colloid osmotic pressure is 25 mmHg—first measured by the British physiologist, Ernest Starling.

Starling equilibrium

Starling realized that the plasma colloid osmotic pressure was very important because at 25 mmHg it lay between the blood pressure in the arterioles and the venules. The blood pressure (hydrostatic pressure) at the arteriolar end of a capillary is about 32 mmHg and at the venular end about 15 mmHg. Hydrostatic pressure in the interstitial fluid varies from place to place, but on average it is a few mmHg below atmospheric, say about –2 mmHg. The net hydrostatic pressure gradient between the blood and interstitial fluid (ΔP) forces fluid out of the capillaries by **ultrafiltration** and this force is greater at the arteriolar than the venular end of capillaries (Fig. 16.15). Ultrafiltration is opposed by **osmosis**, which draws fluid into the capillaries, the effective osmotic force being due to the colloid component (as opposed to permeant electrolytes) and represented by the difference in colloid osmotic pressure between plasma and interstitial fluid ($\Delta \pi$). (In the figure, interstitial colloid osmotic pressure has been assumed to be zero; in fact, it is about 2–8 mmHg depending on the tissue.) The key to enabling reabsorption to occur, is that the

osmotic force remains constant along the length of the capillary. At the arteriolar end, the net difference between hydrostatic and osmotic forces results in ultrafiltration with fluid leaving the capillary, while at the venular end, the hydrostatic pressure has decreased so the net difference causes reabsorption, with fluid returning to the capillary. This balancing of ultrafiltration and osmosis is referred to as the **Starling equilibrium**. The equilibrium is not complete, as there is slightly more ultrafiltration than osmosis (Fig. 16.15). The small amount of fluid lost into the interstitial space is then drained by the **lymphatic system**.

In some capillary beds, blood perfusion is intermittent and ultrafiltration when capillary blood pressure is high is balanced by osmosis when capillary blood pressure is low. In particular organs, special conditions exist in the capillary beds. For example, in the glomeruli of the kidneys capillary blood pressure is high and there is only ultrafiltration (Chapter 20). In the alveolar capillaries of

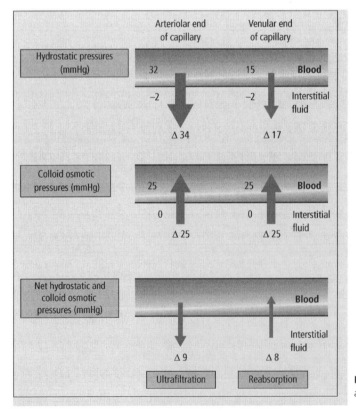

Fig. 16.15 The Starling equilibrium across the capillary.

the lungs, blood pressure is below the colloid osmotic pressure, hence there is only osmosis which ensures liquid does not accumulate in the alveoli. In the liver, the interstitial fluid outside the capillaries is rich in protein and a very small capillary hydrostatic pressure is almost balanced by an equally small difference in colloid osmotic pressure.

Alterations in capillary blood pressure and in the colloid osmotic pressure of either plasma or interstitial fluid will alter the extent of ultrafiltration or reabsorption. Net flow of fluid per unit time (J_v) across capillary walls is also affected by the number of capillaries that are open, which determines the surface area (A), and by the hydraulic conductivity (L_p), which is a measure of the ease with which water flows across ($J_v = AL_p(\Delta P - \Delta \pi)$), see p. 16; a positive value for J_v indicates ultrafiltration). Thus J_v increases in the skeletal musculature during exercise because ΔP increases and more capillaries are open. L_p and hence J_v are increased by substances such as histamine, bradykinin and substance P.

Excess ultrafiltration (Fig. 16.16) occurs when there is:

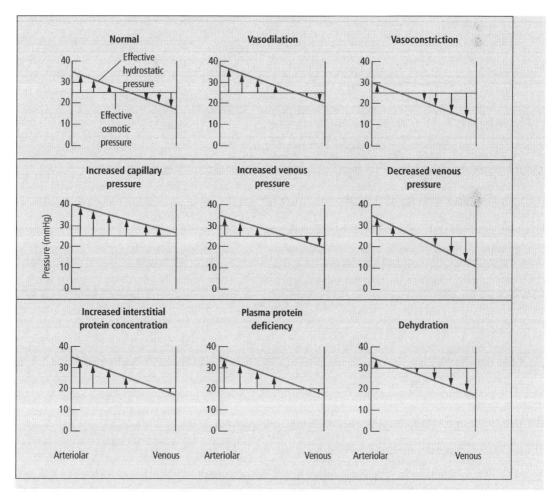

Fig. 16.16 The balance of ultrafiltration (↑) and reabsorption (↓) of fluid across the capillary walls under various conditions. Effective hydrostatic pressure is the difference in hydrostatic pressure between capillary blood and interstitial fluid; effective osmotic pressure is the difference in colloid pressure between capillary blood and interstitial fluid. The fall in blood pressure from arteriole to vein for each condition is kept constant for simplicity (cf. Fig. 16.12).

1 arteriolar vasodilatation;

2 an elevated capillary pressure (e.g. caused by venous obstruction or chronic right heart failure);

3 an elevated venous blood pressure (i.e. in the lower limbs in the erect posture);

4 an increase in interstitial protein concentration (due to an increase in protein permeability of the capillaries in inflammatory or allergic reactions); and

5 a decrease in plasma colloid osmotic pressure (e.g. plasma protein deficiency).

An excess of reabsorption will result mainly from:

1 arteriolar vasoconstriction;

2 a decreased venous blood pressure; and

3 dehydration, which when severe, will increase the protein concentration in plasma more than in interstitial fluid.

Moderate amounts of fluid produced by capillary ultrafiltration are normally removed by the lymphatic system. If ultrafiltration is excessive, the volume of interstitial fluid increases. When clinically detectable this is called **oedema**. Oedema can be local to an organ (localized) or widespread (generalized). However, excessive oedema is usually limited by the distensibility of the organ concerned.

After a haemorrhage p. 420, fluid reabsorption into the capillaries increases because capillary blood pressure is reduced by the haemorrhage itself and because of reflex arteriolar vasoconstriction. The resulting fluid movement helps acutely to restore the blood volume by drawing on the reservoir of the interstitial fluid. The Starling equilibrium thus provides a rapid and automatic control of the constancy of circulating plasma volume at the expense of shrinkage (or expansion) of the interstitial fluid.

16.5 Characteristics of the lymphatic system

Plasma proteins that leak out of the capillaries and fluid that is not reabsorbed back into the capillaries at the venous end are returned to the circulatory system via the lymphatic vessels.

The lymphatic system consists of a network of blind-ending **lymph capillaries** lying in the interstitial space near blood capillaries. The walls of lymph and blood capillaries are similar, except that the spaces between endothelial cells in lymph capillaries are larger, making them readily permeable to protein and fluid. Lymph capillaries collect into thin-walled **lymph vessels**, which eventually empty on the right side of the thorax via the **lymphatic duct** and on the left via the **thoracic duct** into the subclavian veins of the circulatory system. **Lymph** is composed of fluid (**plasma**) and cells called **lymphocytes** (Chapter 13), many of which are stored in **lymph nodes** found in the larger lymph vessels.

The **functions** of the lymphatic system are to return to the cardiovascular system the excess interstitial fluid that has resulted from more capillary ultrafiltration than reabsorption, and any **protein** that has leaked across the capillary wall. It also acts as a pathway for the **absorption of fats** from the gut (Chapter 19) and, by virtue of its lymph nodes and lymphocytes, is involved in **immune responses** (p. 306).

Because of lymph flow, the **Starling equilibrium** should be restated as follows (with approximate values for a 70-kg adult):

$$\text{Ultrafiltration} = \text{Reabsorption} + \text{Lymph flow}$$
$$20\,\text{L day}^{-1} \qquad 16\text{--}18\,\text{L day}^{-1} \quad 4\text{--}2\,\text{L day}^{-1}$$

Since the cardiac output amounts to at least $8000\,\text{L day}^{-1}$ in an adult man, or say $4000\,\text{L day}^{-1}$ of blood plasma, then the 20 L of fluid passing through the blood capillary walls by ultrafiltration is less than 0.5% of blood plasma volume flowing per day. Hence, these bulk movements of fluid through the blood capillary walls are of little importance for the exchange of nutrients, O_2 and CO_2, which as already explained, move predominantly by diffusion. Furthermore, the daily exchange of water across the capillaries by diffusion amount to $80\,000\,\text{L}$, which is 4000 times the rate of ultrafiltration.

Lymph flow is sluggish and occurs at a rate of $2\text{--}4\,\text{L day}^{-1}$. The pressure gradient driving this flow is dependent on the upstream pressure—the interstitial hydrostatic pressure—the magnitude of which depends on the amount of excess interstitial fluid and the distensibility of the interstitial space. The downstream hydrostatic pressure in the thoracic duct is negative because of its intrathoracic location. Lymph flow is aided by **myogenic** rhythmic contractions of **smooth muscle** in the walls of lymph vessels, retrograde flow being prevented by **lymphatic valves** similar to those found in veins. During exercise, the rate of ultrafiltration from capillaries in skeletal muscle increases, and the increased lymph flow required is aided by compression, due to the rhythmic contraction of skeletal muscle around the lymph vessels. Similarly, increased contraction of gut muscle increases lymphatic return from the intestine, and rhythmic alterations in lymphatic transmural pressure resulting from the cardiac and respiratory cycles will aid lymphatic return from the heart and lungs, respectively.

16.6 Characteristics of the systemic venous circulation

The venous system has a large capacity, which, because it is also distensible, can be altered passively by changes in transmural pressure. Venous capacity is also controlled by the degree of venoconstriction with hormones, autacoids and changes in sympathetic nerve activity. Venous return is determined primarily by the gradient between **mean systemic filling pressure** (MSFP) and right atrial pressure. Venous return is also influenced by the suction effect of the heart, by intrathoracic pressure changes accompanying breathing and by skeletal muscle contractions, all of which rely on the presence of valves within the veins.

Several characteristics of the venous system have already been described (Fig. 16.6), namely the moderately large cross-sectional area, the fact that the veins accommodate 55% of the blood volume when the body is supine, the moderate venous velocity, the contribution of ~15% to the total peripheral resistance, the resulting small pressure gradient (from 15 to 1–2 mmHg) and the small pressure pulses (a, c and v waves) in the largest veins. Two important characteristics of the venous system which require further discussion are the venous pressure gradient, which will determine **venous return** to the right atrium, and venous distensibility, which influences the **venous capacity** to accommodate blood, a factor which also affects venous return.

Alterations in venous capacity

The distensibility of the venous system allows variable amounts of blood to be accommodated passively with little detectable change in venous pressure (Fig. 16.5). It also means that an increased or decreased transmural pressure will result in the passive distension or collapse of the veins.

Smooth muscle in the walls of the venous system (Fig. 16.4) has α_1-**adrenoceptors** innervated by the **sympathetic system**. There is normally some degree of tonic sympathetic discharge causing some constriction or **venomotor tone**. An increase in sympathetic nerve activity will cause **venoconstriction**, which reduces the **capacity** of the venous system by reducing distensibility. Because of the relatively large radii of vessels in the venous system, venoconstriction has little effect on venous resistance or the overall total peripheral resistance. Conversely, a decrease in sympathetic nerve activity to the veins results in **venodilatation** and an increase in venous capacity. Venoconstriction occurs as part of the reflex responses coordinated by cardiovascular centres in the medulla, for example to haemorrhage and to exercise. An increase in the circulating hormones **adrenaline** and **angiotensin II** will also cause venoconstriction.

Determinants of venous return

As the circulatory system is a closed circuit, the venous return, in all but moment-to-moment fluctuations, must equal the cardiac output. As explained previously, the magnitude of blood flow depends on the pressure gradient from the left ventricle to the right atrium and on the resistance encountered in the blood vessels (Poiseuille equation). Venous return can be greater or smaller than cardiac output but only for a short time.

Primary determinant of venous return

The right atrial filling pressure is the pressure difference between MSFP and mean right atrial pressure. Quite simply, the greater the pressure difference the greater the venous return.

MSFP was defined by Guyton in the 1950s, as the weighted average of the pressures in all portions of the systemic circulation; the weighting is in proportion to the volume capacity of the vessel. It is also the static blood pressure, the pressure prevailing throughout the systemic circulation when the heart is suddenly arrested experimentally and rapid equilibration of pressures in arterial and venous circuits occurs. The MSFP is usually about 7 mmHg. An alternative term for MSFP is mean circulatory pressure.

For a given venous capacity, MSFP increases when the blood volume is expanded. For a given total blood volume, MSFP increases when the venous blood is compressed by venoconstriction (or, in other words, when the venous capacity is decreased). Arteriolar vasoconstriction will not alter MSFP because the arterioles only contain 3% of the total blood volume. MSFP and venous return are considered further on p. 399. Note that MSFP can increase to a maximum of about 20 mmHg and the minimum MSFP can be close to zero.

Mean right atrial pressure is often referred to as **central venous pressure** and is about 1 mmHg. The filling of the external jugular vein, which can be observed visually (pp. 418–19), is used clinically as a measure of central venous pressure. It is elevated slightly either when blood volume is increased or when a person adopts a supine as opposed to a standing posture. It can be elevated appreciably during right heart failure (Chapter 17).

Secondary factors influencing venous return
Suction effect of the heart

During each cardiac cycle, the right atrial pressure fluctuates and the associated decreases in pressure, which is often to negative values, are called the x and y descents (see Chapter 15). They are caused respectively by the downward movement of the atrioventricular (AV) ring (early systole) and the rapid filling of the ventricle after the AV valve opens (early diastole). It is these decreases in atrial pressure that constitute the so-called **suction effect of the heart**. This effect aids venous return, an influence which increases during increased cardiac activity. Note, however, that at negative atrial pressures there is a limit to the possible increase in venous return, because the venae cavae collapse at the point of entry into the chest.

Respiratory venous pump

Venous return is assisted by the actions of breathing on intrathoracic and abdominal veins, the so-called **respiratory venous pump**. Flow in the venae cavae increases during inspiration and falls during expiration. The effect of the respiratory pump on venous return is enhanced whenever the depth of breathing increases, for instance during exercise.

The intrathoracic (or intrapleural pressure) is subatmospheric, and for the small tidal volume which occurs under resting conditions is about –5 mmHg at the end of inspiration and about –3 mmHg at the end of expiration (Chapter 18). Since veins have distensible walls, these fluctuations in transmural pressure in the thorax cause dilation of intrathoracic veins during inspiration, and compression during expiration. At the same time, the descent of the diaphragm during inspiration will raise intra-abdominal pressure and compress the abdominal veins; the converse occurring during expiration. These influences are together referred to as the respiratory pump. Within certain limits, this effect aids venous return as the relative dilation of intrathoracic veins during inspiration will decrease their resistance to flow and cause some movement of blood towards the heart from the abdominal veins or upper extremities. Compression of abdominal veins, which can occur during both inspiration and expiration, also propels blood towards the heart, since valves in the limb veins prevent retrograde flow. **Venous valves** are thin cup-like structures, whose cusps obstruct the lumen and ensure unidirectional flow at the threat of any retrograde flow. Values are found mainly in limb veins, although a few valves, which are not very effective are also present in abdominal and thoracic veins.

Flow in the venae cavae can decrease markedly during forced expirations, coughing or the Valsalva manoeuvre (p. 447), as a result of compression of both abdominal and intrathoracic veins. If venous return is excessively impeded fainting can result.

Since the heart and intrathoracic vessels have a lower pressure during inspiration, the venous return towards the right atrium from the extrathoracic veins will increase during inspiration. The resulting increase in right ventricular output will in turn increase the arterial flow into the pulmonary vessels and potentially the pulmonary venous flow into the left atrium. However, because the expansion of the lungs in inspiration increases the capacity of the pulmonary veins and arteries, the pulmonary pressure, i.e. the filling pressure of the left heart, may not increase until expiration reduces the lung volume. This explains why the preload of the right ventricle is higher in inspiration, and the preload of the left ventricle is higher in early expiration.

Skeletal muscle venous pump

During exercise a further mechanism, the **skeletal muscle venous pump**, aids venous return. The exercise must not be a sustained contraction but one of alternating contraction and relaxation. The contraction of skeletal muscle alters the transmural pressure of the veins within it and compresses them. This propels blood towards the heart, because the venous valves prevent retrograde flow. When skeletal muscle relaxes, the veins are dilated by inflow but only from below, as again the venous valves prevent retrograde flow. The further advantages of this pump in the upright posture will be considered later (Chapter 17).

16.7 Relationship between cardiac output, venous return and atrial pressure

On average, cardiac output and venous return are equal. The graphical relationship of these to atrial pressure is called the cardiac function curve and

vascular function curve, respectively. These graphs allow visualization of the effects of changes in myocardial contractility, vasomotor tone, blood volume or venous capacity on cardiac output and venous return.

Separate consideration of the control of cardiac output (in particular of stroke volume; Chapter 17) and of venous return can be combined in a graphical approach designed by Guyton in the 1950s. These graphs represent only steady-state responses and not momentary changes, so their use requires some simplification of concepts and abstraction of ideas.

Cardiac function curve

The relationships between pressures generated in the left ventricle and its volume are described in Chapter 15. Also, on p. 363 it was stated that cardiac output (at a constant heart rate) is proportional to stroke volume and that mean atrial pressure is directly related to end-diastolic volume. The relationship between cardiac output and mean right atrial pressure is referred to as the **cardiac function curve** (Fig. 16.17a). The operating point A moves up the 'normal' curve when venous return increases, since this results in a larger end-diastolic volume and hence a higher mean atrial pressure. Conversely, A moves down the normal curve when venous return decreases. A new, steeper curve describes the influence of increased sympathetic nerve stimulation on the ventricular muscle (i.e. an increase in myocardial contractility, or positive inotropic effect). A flatter curve describes a decrease in myocardial contractility. A steeper curve also occurs (Fig. 16.17b) if there is a decrease in arteriolar resistance (i.e. vasodilatation), since this reduces the afterload on the heart and effectively allows a larger stroke volume for a particular end-diastolic volume. Conversely, a flatter curve will result during vasoconstriction.

Vascular function curve

The equivalent relationship between venous return and mean right atrial pressure is referred to as

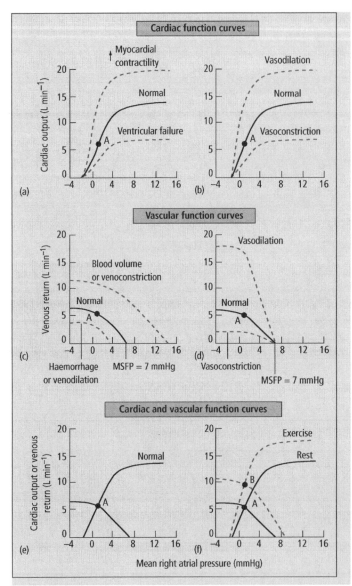

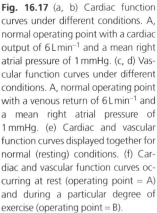

Fig. 16.17 (a, b) Cardiac function curves under different conditions. A, normal operating point with a cardiac output of $6 \, L \, min^{-1}$ and a mean right atrial pressure of 1 mmHg. (c, d) Vascular function curves under different conditions. A, normal operating point with a venous return of $6 \, L \, min^{-1}$ and a mean right atrial pressure of 1 mmHg. (e) Cardiac and vascular function curves displayed together for normal (resting) conditions. (f) Cardiac and vascular function curves occurring at rest (operating point = A) and during a particular degree of exercise (operating point = B).

the systemic **vascular function curve** (Fig. 16.17c). The shape of this curve reflects the fact that, as right atrial pressure increases, venous return is opposed. However, as stated earlier there is a limit to the possible increase in venous return because the venae cavae collapse at the point of entry into the chest at negative atrial pressures. The operating point A moves up or down the 'normal' curve as venous return increases or decreases,

respectively. At a venous return of zero, the atrial pressure in this graph is +7 mmHg. This is the static pressure prevailing throughout the systemic circulation when the circulation has stopped long enough for the pressures to equalize. (It is also the MSFP, which was defined on p. 398.) The vascular function curve is shifted upward in a parallel manner (Fig. 16.17c) whenever there is an increase in blood volume or during venoconstriction. This indicates an increase in MSFP. The converse occurs during haemorrhage or venodilation. A decrease in arteriolar resistance (vasodilatation) increases blood flow and causes a steeper curve (Fig. 16.17d) but does not alter the MSFP; vasoconstriction flattens the curve.

Cardiac and vascular function curves

When these function curves are displayed together, the operating point A is the point of intersection (Fig. 16.17e). During exercise, the new cardiac function curve is steeper because of increased myocardial contractility and the reduced afterload due to vasodilatation (Fig. 16.17f). The vascular function curve in exercise is steeper, due to vasodilatation, and shifted upwards with a higher MSFP, due to venoconstriction. Thus, the operating point in exercise is at B. These curves will be used again in Chapter 17 to demonstrate the sequence of events occurring during haemorrhage and cardiac failure.

Cardiovascular Regulation, Regional Circulation and Circulatory Adjustments

17.1 Integrated regulation of the cardiovascular system

Short-term regulation of the cardiovascular system is concerned with rapid alterations in cardiac output ($\dot{Q}$) and vascular resistance to meet the requirements of individual organs while at the same time maintaining arterial blood pressure. The arterial blood pressure is regulated around a set-point which varies according to the behavioural state. Long-term regulation maintains a constant blood volume and the correct balance of water between the blood and interstitial fluid. Baroreceptors continuously monitor arterial blood pressure and atrial stretch receptors monitor the heart's end-diastolic blood volume. These sensory inputs and those from other receptors are integrated by the cardiovascular centres. These centres are found predominantly in the medulla oblongata and in other specific areas between the cerebral cortex and spinal cord. Central integration alters not only autonomic nervous activity to the heart, arterioles and veins but also the production of hormones such as adrenaline and antidiuretic hormone.

The relationship $\dot{V} = \Delta P/R$, used on p. 373 with respect to flow through a single vessel, also applies to the systemic circuit as a whole, so that:

$$\text{Cardiac output } (\dot{Q}) = \frac{\text{MABP} - \text{mean right atrial blood pressure}}{\text{TPR}}$$

where MABP is the mean arterial blood pressure, and TPR is the total peripheral resistance (i.e. resistance of the entire systemic circulation). Since the mean right atrial pressure is close to zero, this equation can be condensed to:

$$\dot{Q} = \frac{\text{MABP}}{\text{TPR}}$$

Cardiac output ($\dot{Q}$) is the product of heart rate and stroke volume. **Heart rate** is altered by parasympathetic and sympathetic nerves and by circulating adrenaline (p. 261). **Stroke volume** is determined by end-diastolic volume (intrinsic control, Starling's law of the heart; p. 363) and is altered by sympathetic activity and circulating adrenaline (extrinsic control; p. 367). In addition, end-diastolic volume and therefore stroke volume are altered by changes in venous capacity (p. 397) occurring either passively, or by adrenaline and sympathetic activity (p. 397).

TPR is controlled by intrinsic autoregulation and by sympathetic nerves and circulating hormones (especially adrenaline, noradrenaline, angiotensin II and antidiuretic hormone, pp. 387 and 389). There is no direct control of **MABP**; it is determined entirely by $\dot{Q}$ and TPR. Thus:

$$\text{MABP} = \dot{Q} \times \text{TPR}$$

MABP is monitored by sensory receptors. Information from these receptors is integrated by cardiovascular centres in the central nervous system, which reflexly control $\dot{Q}$ and TPR by efferent activity in autonomic nerves to the heart and blood vessels. This autonomic control interacts with the intrinsic mechanisms operating simultaneously in the heart and vessels.

Short-term regulation of the cardiovascular system is concerned with the rapid adjustments of these three variables, $\dot{Q}$, TPR and MABP. Compensatory changes occur or start to occur within seconds following perturbations induced, for example, by a change in posture, the onset of exercise or a haemorrhage.

Arterial baroreceptor reflexes

Characteristics of baroreceptors

The receptors which monitor MABP are called arterial baroreceptors. They are located in the wall of the aortic arch and in the carotid sinus, an enlarged part of the internal carotid artery just after it arises from the common carotid artery (Fig. 17.1). Baroreceptor nerve endings (both free and encapsulated) are embedded in the outer (adventitial) layer of the arterial wall, which contains some elastic tissue. The sensory axons from the aortic baroreceptors travel in the vagus nerve and those from the carotid baroreceptors travel in the glossopharyngeal nerve. More than half of the baroreceptor axons are unmyelinated. Information from these receptors is relayed to the cardiovascular centres.

An increase in transmural pressure, usually brought about by an increase in arterial blood pressure, stretches the arterial wall and stimulates the baroreceptors. At normal MABP some baroreceptor afferents are tonically active, as shown by streams of action potentials recorded from their axons. The mean frequency of these action potentials changes in response to changes in MABP and, in addition, as the pressure gets higher, more afferents are recruited. Total baroreceptor activity is graded over the blood pressure range of approximately 50–180 mmHg. Baroreceptor activity depends not only on the level of MABP, but also on the magnitude of the pulse pressure (i.e. the difference between systolic and diastolic pressures). The continuous monitoring of MABP by the baroreceptors permits adjustment of $\dot{Q}$ and TPR, via the autonomic efferent nerves, such that the MABP is regulated close to its set-point at any particular time.

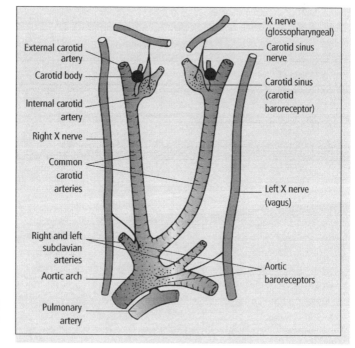

External carotid artery

Carotid body

Internal carotid artery

Right X nerve

Common carotid arteries

Right and left subclavian arteries

Aortic arch

Pulmonary artery

IX nerve (glossopharyngeal)

Carotid sinus nerve

Carotid sinus (carotid baroreceptor)

Left X nerve (vagus)

Aortic baroreceptors

Fig. 17.1 Location of the aortic and carotid baroreceptors and their sensory nerves.

Baroreceptor reflex

An increase in MABP (caused, for instance, by a sudden change in posture from standing to lying down; p. 418) will increase baroreceptor activity. The reflex changes initiated are as follows:

1 an increase in parasympathetic, and a decrease in sympathetic, discharge to the sinoatrial node causing a decrease in heart rate;

2 a decrease in sympathetic discharge to ventricular muscle causing a decrease in contractility and hence a reduction in stroke volume;

3 a decrease in sympathetic discharge to the veins, causing an increased venous compliance and capacity, and hence a reduced end-diastolic volume and subsequent stroke volume; and

4 a decrease in sympathetic discharge to the arterioles, causing a decrease in TPR. The arteriolar vasodilation is greatest in the splanchnic area, modest in skeletal musculature and least in the kidneys.

Steps 1–3 will reduce $\dot{Q}$ and all of steps 1–4 take only a few seconds to occur. The vasodilation in step 4 also results in a greater capillary pressure which if sustained over periods of several minutes or longer leads to an increased ultrafiltration across the capillary wall and hence to some reduction in blood volume. These reflex reductions in $\dot{Q}$ and TPR will decrease MABP and oppose the initial elevation, thus **restoring MABP to or towards normal**.

A decrease in MABP initiates the converse changes. In addition, a large decrease in baroreceptor activity, for example after a haemorrhage, stimulates breathing (p. 482), the secretion of adrenaline (p. 420) and antidiuretic hormone (p. 420) and activates the renin–angiotensin–aldosterone system via increased sympathetic activity to the kidney (p. 575). Adrenaline accelerates the heart and antidiuretic hormone augments the vasoconstriction.

The baroreceptor reflexes adjust the balance between $\dot{Q}$, TPR and MABP whenever there is a small change in the metabolism of an organ. If one organ increases its metabolism, dilation of its arterioles by local metabolic regulation rapidly increases its blood flow. This local vasodilation will slightly decrease the TPR and hence the MABP. The smallest decrease in MABP will be detected by the baroreceptors and will result in a reflex increase in $\dot{Q}$ and, to some extent, an increased vasoconstriction in all other organs, except the heart and brain. Thus, within a few seconds, the final decrease in TPR will be minimized and the extra blood flow required by that organ will be supplied by reducing blood flow to some of the other organs and by increasing the total blood flow. At the same time the decrease in MABP will be very small or even undetectable.

The set-point at which MABP is regulated by the baroreceptor reflex depends upon inputs from other peripheral receptors (e.g. arterial chemoreceptors, cardiac receptors or receptors in skeletal muscle that are activated during exercise) and also inputs from higher centres in the brain. Thus, the set-point varies depending upon such factors as the level of activity or arousal. For example, the set-point increases during exercise and acute stress, and decreases during sleep.

Reflexes intiated by cardiac stretch receptors

Atrial stretch receptors

Stretch receptors are found in the walls of the atria, mainly at their junctions with the venae cavae and pulmonary veins. Collectively they are referred to as **atrial stretch receptors**. Their afferent fibres are myelinated and unmyelinated and travel in the **vagus** to the cardiovascular centres. Atrial stretch receptors are stimulated by the stretch resulting from an increase in **atrial (central venous) pressure**. Because the atria are very distensible, an increase in volume of the atria considerably stretches their walls with only a small increase in pressure. The atrial stretch receptors are thus low-pressure receptors, which, in effect, monitor atrial blood volume (**atrial blood volume receptors**).

Atrial receptors are often categorized as atrial A and atrial B receptors because two distinct types of activity are seen in their afferent nerves. Atrial A receptors respond most strongly to atrial contraction, while atrial B receptors respond most strongly to atrial filling.

Atrial receptor reflexes

A sustained increase in blood volume reflexly initiates an increase in parasympathetic and a decrease in sympathetic activity. This complements the reflex adjustments initiated by the baroreceptors, which will also be stimulated by the increase in MABP that usually accompanies an increase in blood volume. These reflex changes together result in a decrease in $\dot{Q}$ and TPR, an increase in venous capacity and an excess of ultrafiltration across the capillary wall. Thus MABP and blood volume decrease towards normal and the excess fluid is temporarily accommodated in the interstitial fluid.

Atrial receptors and hormone release

Whereas increased stimulation of atrial receptors reflexly alters autonomic activity, decreased stimulation affects also the release of certain hormones. When atrial receptor stimulation is reduced, there is a decrease in parasympathetic activity and an increase in sympathetic activity, in particular to the renal arterioles. This decreases renal blood flow and hence glomerular filtration rate, which reduces urinary **sodium excretion**, and increases the release of **renin** by the juxtaglomerular cells of the kidney (p. 574). The rise in plasma renin increases the concentration of circulating **angiotensin II** that:

1 causes further vasoconstriction and hence increases TPR;

2 stimulates the release of **aldosterone** from the adrenal cortex, which increases reabsorption of sodium;

3 stimulates **thirst**; and

4 increases the secretion of **antidiuretic hormone** from the posterior pituitary, which not only reduces urinary loss of water but also contributes to systemic vasoconstriction.

In addition, the atrial and baroreceptor afferents relay to the hypothalamus and, in response to the reduced sensory input, stimulate thirst and release of antidiuretic hormone (pp. 248 and 572). Thus

the urinary loss of water and salt is restricted and decreases in blood volume are minimized.

These effects of renin, angiotensin II, aldosterone and antidiuretic hormone take from minutes to hours to develop. This **long-term regulation** of blood volume and hence of mean systemic filling pressure (p. 397) and MABP clearly involves the endocrine, renal and cardiovascular systems. It not only compensates for the decreased blood volume of a **haemorrhage** but also operates at all times to maintain **total body water** and the **correct distribution of extracellular fluid** between the interstitium and the blood.

Other cardiac receptors

1 There are stretch receptors located in the **ventricle** (predominantly the left) that have afferents (mainly myelinated) in the vagus. They normally increase their discharge at the same time as ventricular pressure increases. When their average discharge increases they cause reflex bradycardia and vasodilation in parallel with the baroreceptor reflex.

2 Vagal receptors with unmyelinated axons are also present, predominantly in the left ventricle. These can be stimulated experimentally by various chemicals (e.g. veratridine and nicotine) causing reflex bradycardia, vasodilation and depression of breathing (**Bezold–Jarisch reflex**). It is thought that prostaglandins, serotonin, bradykinin and the accumulation of metabolites, as in myocardial ischaemia, are the natural stimuli for this inhibitory reflex.

3 Afferent fibres from all regions of the heart travel with sympathetic nerves (so-called **sympathetic afferents**) and are also stimulated by the above chemicals and myocardial ischaemia. However, the reflex in this case is excitatory and thus tachycardia, vasoconstriction, increased breathing and angina (p. 422) result.

Atrial natriuretic peptide

The hormones renin, angiotensin II, aldosterone and antidiuretic hormone act to increase extracellular fluid volume but a recently discovered family of peptides, **atrial natriuretic peptide** (ANP), can decrease effective circulating plasma volume. The physiological role of ANP is, however, not established. It is known that ANP is released from secretory granules of the atria in response to atrial stretch—this could be caused physiologically by an increased blood volume. In very high doses (outside the normal physiological range) ANP causes arteriolar vasodilation and also venodilation by decreasing the sensitivity of vascular smooth muscle to vasoconstrictor substances such as noradrenaline and angiotensin II. In the kidney it increases glomerular filtration rate and inhibits tubular Na^+ reabsorption, leading to increased urinary loss of water (diuresis) and sodium (natriuresis). ANP also decreases the release of antidiuretic hormone and renin/aldosterone, which may contribute to the diuresis and natriuresis, respectively.

Reflexes initiated by other receptors

Input from the receptors described below also affect cardiovascular function.

1 Nasal receptors (p. 483) when stimulated by irritants result in bradycardia and vasoconstriction with variable changes in MABP. Stimulation by water causes a cessation of breathing, bradycardia and vasoconstriction in all but the heart and brain, leading to an increase in both TPR and MABP (this is the diving reflex which is well developed in diving mammals).

2 Laryngeal and **tracheal receptors** that cause the cough reflex (p. 483) also produce marked bradycardia and increases in TPR and MABP.

3 Pulmonary C receptors (also known as **juxtacapillary (J) receptors**) in the alveoli of the lung (p. 483) are stimulated by pulmonary oedema. This causes not only rapid, shallow breathing but also a decrease in heart rate, TPR and MABP. The bronchial C receptors in the airways have no known cardiovascular reflex.

4 Lung stretch receptors (p. 483) in the lower airways are stimulated by an increase in tidal volume and not only help to determine the pattern of breathing but also cause an increase in heart rate and a decrease in TPR. The accelerated heart rate

during inspiration (**sinus arrhythmia**) is partially due to this reflex. In contrast, lung irritant receptors of the lower airways have no known reflex effects on the cardiovascular system.

5 Peripheral or **arterial chemoreceptors** (p. 485) in the carotid and aortic bodies are stimulated primarily by low O_2 (hypoxia), and to a lesser extent by high CO_2 (hypercapnia) and acidosis. Stimulation of these receptors causes a reflex decrease in heart rate and an increase in TPR and MABP, together with increased secretion of antidiuretic hormone.

Stimulation of the peripheral chemoreceptors normally results in an increase in ventilation, which at the same time stimulates the lung stretch receptors. Thus the bradycardia from the carotid body reflex can be demonstrated only during a breath-hold when the dominant tachycardia from the lung reflex is prevented. The increase in TPR and MABP from the chemoreceptor reflex is also tempered by local systemic vasodilation and by severe hypoxia or acidosis decreasing myocardial contractility.

6 Central chemoreceptors (p. 486) near the ventral surface of the medulla oblongata are stimulated by hypercapnia and reflexly increase heart rate, TPR and MABP. Most of the increase in TPR and MABP is opposed by local systemic vasodilation and by the accompanying increase in ventilation, stimulating the lung stretch receptors.

7 Limb muscle chemoreceptors (metaboloreceptors or ergoreceptors) with thin unmyelinated (group IV) afferents are stimulated by metabolites, notably H^+ and K^+ ions, released during exercise (p. 618) to cause increases in $\dot{Q}$, TPR, MABP and ventilation.

8 Limb muscle stretch receptors with thin myelinated afferents (group III) are stimulated by movement during exercise (p. 619) and also cause increases in $\dot{Q}$, TPR, MABP and ventilation.

9 Peripheral and **central temperature receptors** (p. 607) during an elevated body temperature reflexly cause an increase in $\dot{Q}$, and possibly in MABP, and a decrease in TPR with preferential vasodilation in the skin.

10 Pain receptors (also called nociceptors, p. 227) usually initiate increases in heart rate, TPR and

MABP if the pain arises from receptors on the surface of the body. If pain receptors in the viscera or within skeletal muscles are stimulated, however, signalling 'deep pain', then a reflex decrease in heart rate, TPR and MABP can be evoked.

Cardiovascular centres

Early studies identified widespread regions in the lower brainstem which, when electrically stimulated, evoked increases in MABP and HR. This led to the view that central neurones controlling cardiovascular function are diffusely distributed throughout the lower brainstem. Studies in the 1970s and 1980s, however, using microinjections of drugs that selectively excite or inhibit neuronal cell bodies revealed that central neurones controlling the sympathetic outflow to the cardiovascular system are located in discrete regions. In particular, there are several discrete groups of neurones, located in the rostral ventrolateral medulla (RVLM), medullary raphe nuclei, ventrolateral pons and in the paraventricular nucleus in the hypothalamus that project directly to the sympathetic preganglionic neurones in the spinal cord; they are therefore referred to as **sympathetic premotor neurones**. In addition, there are other neurones at all levels of the brain, including the midbrain, cerebellum, hypothalamus, limbic system and cortex, which project directly or indirectly to the sympathetic premotor neurones or to cardiac vagal preganglionic neurones. These neurones contribute to the control of the autonomic outflow to the heart and blood vessels, both in response to inputs from peripheral receptors and as part of co-ordinated physiological responses associated with different behaviours.

Spinal cord

The preganglionc sympathetic neurones supplying the arterioles, veins, myocardial muscle and the sinoatrial node are found in the **intermediolateral cell** column of the spinal cord (Fig. 17.2). It must be appreciated that sympathetic activation is not *en masse*; control of one organ can occur independently of another. Furthermore, sympathetic tone to the vessels is greater than to the heart. The intermediolateral cell column is controlled by three areas in the medulla but it is capable of some independent cardiovascular integration, predominantly some of the reflexes connected with pain and peripheral temperature.

Medulla oblongata

Information from most of the relevant receptors is transmitted in the vagus or glossopharyngeal nerve; their afferents synapse in the **nucleus of the tractus solitarius** of the medulla oblongata (Fig. 17.2) before reaching the main integrating areas. There is also an excitatory pathway within the medulla from the nucleus of the tractus solitarius to vagal preganglionic parasympathetic neurones, which provides marked inhibitory tone to the sinoatrial node. These parasympathetic neurones emanate mainly from the **nucleus ambiguus** and to a lesser extent from the dorsal motor nucleus of the vagus (Fig. 17.2).

The sympathetic premotor neurones in the RVLM (Fig. 17.2) play a critical role in the tonic and reflex control of sympathetic vasomotor activity. They are the major source of the tonic excitatory drive that maintains the resting activity of sympathetic preganglionic vasomotor neurones, which in turn maintains resting MABP. They are also an essential component of the central pathways mediating the baroreceptor reflex. As shown in Fig. 17.2, baroreceptor primary afferent inputs terminate in the nucleus of the tractus solitarius, and synapse there with interneurones, which in turn project to and excite interneurones in the caudal ventrolateral medulla, which in turn project to and inhibit RVLM sympathetic premotor neurones, via γ-aminobutyric acid (GABA) receptors. In addition, RVLM sympathetic premotor neurones receive a variety of other excitatory and inhibitory inputs, arising from peripheral receptors as well as higher brain centres. Thus, in addition to the baroreceptor reflex, RVLM sympathetic premotor neurones are a crucial component of the central pathways mediating cardiovascular responses to inputs from arterial chemoreceptors, cardiac receptors, pain receptors, etc. as well as the cardiovascular changes

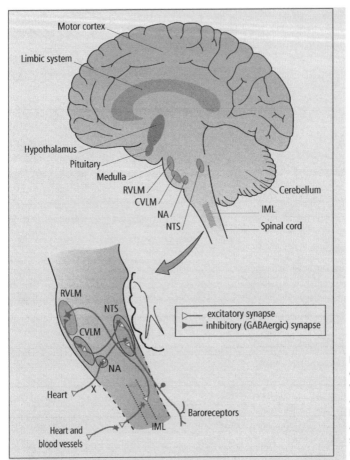

Fig. 17.2 Location in the brain of the cardiovascular centres. CVLM, caudal ventrolateral medulla; GABA, γ-aminobutyric acid; IML, intermediolateral cell column; NA, nucleus ambiguus; NTS, nucleus of the tractus solitarius; RVLM, rostral ventrolateral medulla; X, vagus nerve.

associated with more generalized physiological responses during exercise, alerting reactions or other behaviours. Finally, apart from synaptic inputs, RVLM sympathetic premotor neurones can be directly excited by severe local hypoxia caused by brain ischaemia (reduced blood flow; **central nervous system ischaemic** or **Cushing response**).

There are also sympathetic premotor neurones in the **raphe nucleus**, located in the ventral medulla near the midline. These neurones do not participate in the normal reflex control of sympathetic outflow by inputs from baroreceptors and other peripheral receptors; instead, they appear to be activated mainly via descending inputs from the midbrain, hypothalamus and other forebrain regions, in response to acute stress, such as an alerting stimulus or cold stress. In particular, skin vasoconstriction and tachycardia that are evoked by alerting reactions and cold stress is mediated largely via sympathetic premotor neurones in the raphe.

Cerebellum

The **cerebellum** helps coordinate the cardiovascular response to exercise. Its fastigial nuclei and vermal cortex receive medullary projections from the nucleus of the tractus solitarius and the lateral reticular nucleus; the latter is an extra relay for some of the input from limb muscle afferents. In exercise, the cerebellum contributes to excitation of sympathetic premotor neurones in the RVLM.

Hypothalamus

The hypothalamus contains neurones that regulate the cardiovascular system as part of integrated responses associated with many different behaviours, including defensive behaviour, temperature regulation, sexual activity, eating and drinking. The precise organization of the neural centres that subserve these responses are not well understood, but some details are now emerging. In particular, neurones in the dorsomedial hypothalamic nucleus and immediately surrounding regions (an area which is sometimes referred to as the 'hypothalamic defence area') are activated during acute psychological stress, and this results in increases in heart rate, $\dot{Q}$ and MABP, together with vasoconstriction in all organs except the heart, brain and skeletal musculature. These cardiovascular effects are also accompanied by other responses, including increases in respiration, pupillary dilation and behavioural changes. The descending pathways from the **dorsomedial hypothalamic nucleus** mediating the cardiovascular changes associated with defensive behaviour include synapses with medullary sympathetic premotor neurones, in both the RVLM and raphe.

The hypothalamic **paraventricular nucleus**, which is located anterior or rostral to the dorsomedial hypothalamic nucleus, also contains neurones that regulate the sympathetic outflow, both via direct connections to the spinal cord and indirectly via the RVLM. The paraventricular sympathoexcitatory neurones do not appear to participate in the short-term reflex control of the circulation, but instead regulate sympathetic activity in response to longer-term challenges, such as during fever or in response to alterations in fluid and electrolyte balance. There is also evidence that these neurones are activated in pathological states such as congestive heart failure and at least some types of hypertension, and that this contributes to the sympathetic over-activity associated with these conditions.

A separate subset of neurones within the paraventricular nucleus, together with neurones in the hypothalamic supraoptic nucleus synthesize antidiuretic hormone (vasopressin), and release vasopressin via their projections to the posterior pituitary (p. 248) in response to excitation of local osmoreceptors, stimulation of arterial chemoreceptors and depressed activity from atrial stretch receptors and arterial baroreceptors.

The **temperature-regulating centre** is also in the hypothalamus (p. 610). During heat stress, it receives peripheral and central thermoreceptor input and increases $\dot{Q}$, causes vasoconstriction in all organs except the heart and brain, and dilates the blood vessels of the skin (p. 611). The consequent large blood flow through the skin increases heat loss and thus aids in the maintenance of a normal body temperature. The final decrease in TPR and MABP caused by vasodilation in the skin depends on the degree of vasoconstriction elsewhere and the magnitude of the increase in $\dot{Q}$.

Limbic system

The **limbic system** integrates many emotional and behavioural reflexes (p. 59) and, via the hypothalamus, can elicit different responses, including the pressor and sympathoexcitatory response triggered by an alerting stimulus, or a depressor and sympathoinhibitory response (vasovagal response) which can be triggered by emotional shock or deep pain.

Motor cortex

In exercise the **motor cortex** gives rise to a central command (p. 621), which is relayed via centres in the hypothalamus and medulla, leading to an increase in heart rate and in sympathetic vasomotor activity.

Respiratory centres

The dorsal inspiratory cells of the **respiratory centres** (p. 482) in the medulla have an inhibitory effect on the cardiac vagal motor neurones in the nucleus ambiguus. This results in the tachycardia that usually accompanies inspiration (**sinus arrhythmia**).

17.2 Characteristics of blood circulation through different organs

The entire cardiac output flows through the pulmonary circuit, the alveolar capillaries of which subserve gas exchange with the external environment. Each of the organs supplied by the systemic circulation receives a different fraction of the resting cardiac output according to its mass, metabolic activity and how much extra blood flow it requires to satisfy its role in acquiring or disposing of nutrients, waste products, electrolytes or heat. The balance of the mechanisms controlling blood flow to each organ therefore varies—in some organs metabolic regulation and myogenic autoregulation are dominant; in others nervous control takes precedence. In most circumstances flow to the brain and heart is protected at the expense of the other systemic organs.

Pulmonary circulation

Resistance and pressure

The pulmonary vessels have thinner, more compliant walls and are shorter in length and larger in diameter than the equivalent vessels in the systemic circuit. The entire cardiac output flows through the pulmonary circuit, the resistance of which is about a tenth that of the systemic circuit (p. 381). In the pulmonary artery, the systolic, diastolic and mean pressures at rest are about 25, 8 and 15 mmHg, respectively, and the pressure declines gradually to about 10 mmHg in the capillaries and to a mean of about 5 mmHg in the left atrium (see Fig. 16.6). Thus, in contrast to the systemic circulation, the arterial and venous parts of the pulmonary circulation contribute equally to the total pulmonary resistance. Since the pulmonary resistance is so low, flow remains pulsatile throughout, although the amplitude decreases as blood flows through the pulmonary vessels (see Fig. 16.6).

Capillaries

Pulmonary arteries deliver, from the rest of the body, systemic venous blood (which is low in O_2 and high in CO_2) to the pulmonary capillaries for exchange of gases between blood and alveolar air (p. 429); the oxygenated blood leaving in the pulmonary veins becomes the systemic arterial blood. The vast network of pulmonary capillaries in the alveolar walls provides the large surface area required for gas exchanges between the alveolar air and pulmonary blood (p. 429). The total cross-sectional area of the pulmonary capillaries, and hence the velocity of capillary flow, is similar to that of the systemic circuit (see Fig. 16.6). However, since the pulmonary capillaries are shorter, the transit time through each capillary at rest is about 1 s rather than 2 s. During severe exercise, there is about a five-fold increase in cardiac output and hence in pulmonary blood flow. This is associated with an increase in mean pulmonary arterial pressure, which opens up lung capillaries that at rest were unperfused, thus increasing their total cross-sectional area but by only 1.5 times. Hence, the velocity of flow through the pulmonary capillary increases considerably and the transit time can be as little as 0.3 s. Although this will impede diffusion of gases, it is not normally the limiting factor in the supply of O_2 during exercise, at least at sea level (p. 456).

Capacity

In the erect posture about 9% of the blood volume is in the pulmonary circuit. Since both pulmonary arterioles and veins are very compliant, the pulmonary circuit accommodates about 16% of the total blood volume in the supine position (see Fig. 16.6). Pulmonary blood volume also increases passively in exercise, generalized systemic vasoconstriction, left heart failure or mitral stenosis, and decreases passively in generalized systemic vasodilation and haemorrhage. Thus the pulmonary circulation functions as a blood reservoir (the **pulmonary reservoir**).

The compliant pulmonary vessels are also subjected to variations in transmural pressure induced by the fluctuating intrapleural pressure of ventilation. Thus their volume increases during inspiration and decreases during expiration. Powerful expiration or positive pressure breathing can markedly reduce pulmonary (and cardiac) blood volume and pulmonary flow, as well as impeding systemic venous return.

The effect of gravity in the erect posture (p. 418), and the low pressure and high distensibility of the pulmonary circuit, results in less, or even intermittent, flow to the apex of the lung relative to the base. The consequence of this for gas exchange and the total ventilation/perfusion ratio of the lung is considered on p. 466.

Although pulmonary arterioles and veins are well supplied with sympathetic vasoconstrictor and parasympathetic vasodilator fibres, the roles of these nerves are not clear. However, stimulation of the sympathetic system and administration of adrenaline can decrease the pulmonary blood volume by as much as 30%.

Hypoxic vasoconstriction

Neither myogenic autoregulation nor metabolic regulation is demonstrable in the pulmonary circuit. In fact, the response of pulmonary arterioles to local hypoxia, hypercapnia and acidity is the opposite of that of systemic arterioles. **Hypoxia** is the more potent of the three stimuli. In poorly ventilated regions of the lung, where alveolar O_2 is low and CO_2 is high, local pulmonary **vasoconstriction** diverts blood flow to better ventilated areas. This improves gas exchange by helping to equalize the regional ventilation/perfusion ratios in the lung. However, this hypoxic vasoconstriction has the disadvantage that during the hypoxia associated with high altitude or chronic obstructive lung disease, all pulmonary arterioles are affected. The resultant increase in pulmonary resistance increases pressure in the right ventricle and pulmonary artery (pulmonary hypertension).

Ultrafiltration/reabsorption balance

Since it is essential for gas exchange that the alveoli do not accumulate liquid, the pulmonary circuit is accompanied by a lymphatic system more extensive than in any other organ. Furthermore, the normal colloid osmotic pressure of the plasma

(25 mmHg) is greater than the difference in hydrostatic pressure between capillary (10 mmHg) and alveolar interstitium (−4 mmHg; pp. 394–95) and favours reabsorption of fluid across the entire length of the capillary. However, accumulation of fluid in the alveoli (pulmonary oedema) may occur and lead to dyspnoea (breathlessness; p. 483) when the left atrial pressure is increased during left ventricular failure or mitral stenosis or when the pulmonary vascular pressures increase during severe exercise.

Bronchial circulation

The metabolic needs of the airways (trachea to bronchioles) are met by blood delivered from the aorta through the **bronchial arteries**. This bronchial circulation constitutes only about 1% of the total cardiac output. Some venous drainage (about 25%) is via **bronchial veins** into the superior vena cava but the remaining 75% enters the **pulmonary veins**. There are also direct connections between the bronchial and pulmonary capillaries. This intermingling of the two circulations results in a very small degree of desaturation of the oxygenated pulmonary venous blood (p. 462).

Coronary circulation

Right and left **coronary arteries** branching from the aorta supply the arterioles and capillaries of the myocardium. Venous drainage is via the **coronary sinus** (75%) and **anterior cardiac vein** (20%) which both empty into the right atrium. Some venous blood drains directly via **Thebesian veins** and small venules into all heart chambers. Venous blood entering the left side of the heart in this manner will cause a small reduction in the O_2 content of systemic arterial blood (p. 462).

Metabolism and control of blood flow

Since the heart at rest receives about 5% of the cardiac output and has a very high O_2 consumption relative to its mass (Table 17.1), the coronary

Table 17.1 Blood flow, oxygen consumption, arteriovenous (AV) O_2 difference and vascular resistance of tissues at rest.

Organ	Weight (kg)	Blood flow (L min⁻¹)	Oxygen consumption (mL min⁻¹)	AV O_2 difference (mL L⁻¹)	Absolute resistance (mmHg L⁻¹ min)	Specific resistance (mmHg L⁻¹ min kg tissue wt)
Heart	0.3	0.25	30	120	400	120
Brain	1.5	0.75	45	60	133	200
Skin	5.0	0.50	10	25	200	1000
Skeletal muscle	30.0	1.20	55	60	83	2490
Gut	2.8	1.40	55	40	71	200
Kidney	0.3	1.10	20	15	91	27
Other	30.0	0.60	35	50	167	5010
Total	70.0	5.80	250	45	17	1190

venous O_2 content is low and there is thus a very large arteriovenous O_2 difference. In contrast to other active organs, during increased cardiac activity there is little further decrease in its venous O_2 content and the increased demand for O_2 is satisfied mainly by a large increase (up to four-fold) in coronary blood flow. This is a prime example of **metabolic regulation**. Hypoxia and adenosine are more potent coronary vasodilators than an increase in P_{CO_2} or blood acidity.

Coronary arterioles also exhibit autoregulation such that coronary flow at rest is constant in the pressure range of 60–180 mmHg. (The important pressure here is aortic diastolic pressure; see below.) Such autoregulation is due to a combination of myogenic and metabolic mechanisms (p. 387).

Although the smooth muscle of the coronary arterioles receives both sympathetic and parasympathetic innervation and contains α_1-adrenoceptors (mediating vasoconstriction) and muscarinic cholinoceptors (mediating vasodilation), the importance of these pathways is not clear. Any neurally induced vasoconstriction occurring during increased sympathetic stimulation is overridden by the metabolic vasodilation resulting from the simultaneous increase in cardiac activity. Similarly, during increased parasympathetic stimulation, any neurally induced vasodilation will tend to be overridden by the metabolic vasoconstriction. Note that adrenaline acting on β_2-adrenoceptors causes coronary vasodilation.

Coronary artery compression and blood flow

Much of the resistance of the heart's vascular bed (Table 17.1) is due to the compression of the blood vessels during cardiac contraction. In systole, the peak pressure is about 120 mmHg in the aorta, coronary arteries and left ventricle and about 25 mmHg in the right ventricle (Fig. 17.3). Within the myocardial wall, contracting muscle will cause the intramyocardial pressures to be higher, particularly during the isovolumetric contraction phase. Thus, in systole, the coronary vessels of the left ventricle are compressed and flow in the left coronary artery is markedly reduced, whereas in the right ventricle the transmural pressure of the coronary arteries is reduced from 120 to only 95 mmHg and the right coronary flow is hardly affected. In diastole, the pressure in the coronary arteries falls to about 80 mmHg whilst that in both ventricles is close to 0 mmHg. Hence there is no compression of blood vessels in diastole. Left coronary arterial flow is therefore intermittent, ceasing and even reversing in early systole, and right coronary arterial flow is pulsatile, being slightly greater in systole than in diastole. Venous flow through the coronary sinus into the right atrium is greatest during the compression of systole and subsides during diastole.

Since coronary vessels are compressed during systole and since at rest diastole occupies about two-thirds of the cardiac cycle, about 85% of the

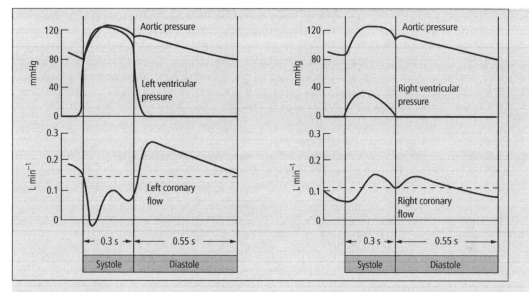

Fig. 17.3 Left and right coronary arterial flow in relation to aortic and ventricular pressures during a cardiac cycle of 70 beats min⁻¹.

left and 70% of the right coronary flow occurs during diastole (Fig. 17.3). (Note that as the left ventricle is the bigger, left coronary arterial flow is about 60% of the total flow.) As about 80% of the total coronary arterial flow occurs during diastole, a pressure somewhat nearer the **aortic diastolic pressure**, not the MABP, becomes the primary determinant of the pressure gradient for coronary flow. With tachycardia, which reduces the period of diastole considerably, and with increased myocardial contractility, a greater proportion of the coronary resistance arises from compression and coronary arterial flow is impeded for shorter but more frequent intervals.

Cerebral circulation

The soft tissue of the brain, with its pial surface covered by a highly vascular arachnoid membrane and a tough dura mater, is encased in a rigid skull (p. 52). From the **vertebral** and **internal carotid arteries** are derived the arteries of the brain which, until they branch and penetrate the brain, lie close to the pia amongst the trabeculae in the subarachnoid space (Fig. 3.21). Venules drain into the superficial veins of the pia which in turn drain either into the **venous sinuses** in the dura before entering the internal jugular veins or into the **vertebral veins** of the spinal cord and thence to the external jugular veins. Unlike other capillaries (p. 392), those of the brain (except in the circumventricular organs) are relatively impermeable to most substances except fat-soluble drugs, glucose, O_2 and CO_2. This impermeability is referred to as the **blood–brain barrier** and its significance is considered on p. 59.

Cerebrospinal fluid (CSF) fills the four ventricles and subarachnoid space of the brain (see Fig. 3.21). It is formed from plasma by brain capillaries, in particular those in the **choroid plexuses**, and is reabsorbed from the subarachnoid space through the **arachnoid villi** into the venous sinuses of the dura (Fig. 3.21). There is no lymphatic system in the brain; its drainage function is taken over by the CSF.

Cerebral blood flow and its control

The brain receives about 13% of the cardiac output, has a moderately resistant vascular bed, a fairly

413

high O_2 consumption and a large arteriovenous O_2 difference (Table 17.1). **Cerebral blood flow** (CBF) remains remarkably constant at 0.75 L min^{-1} (see Table 14.1) over a wide range of bodily activities.

Although the cerebral arterioles are innervated by the sympathetic and parasympathetic nervous systems, the autonomic nerves appear to have little physiological effect on CBF. In contrast, **myogenic autoregulation** and **metabolic regulation** are important mechanisms. Both mechanisms help to maintain CBF remarkably constant in the MABP range of about 50–150 mmHg, while the latter alters local blood flow to maintain a constant supply of O_2 to individual regions of the brain according to their level of activity.

CBF is also affected when partial pressures of O_2 and CO_2 change throughout the body. Between the normal arterial Po_2 of 100 mmHg and a hypoxia of 50 mmHg Po_2, there is little increase in CBF. Below 50 mmHg Po_2, the cerebral arterioles are sensitive to the vasodilating effects of hypoxia and CBF increases about two-fold as Po_2 decreases from 50 to 25 mmHg. However, the cerebral arterioles are much more sensitive to the slightest increase or decrease in arterial Pco_2 and acidity. Considerable vasodilation occurs when Pco_2 is elevated (40–100 mmHg, hypercapnia) and considerable vasoconstriction occurs when Pco_2 is reduced (40–20 mmHg, hypocapnia). Within such limits, a doubling or halving of Pco_2 results in about a two-fold change in CBF. The **dizziness** felt after excessive hyperventilation is the result of the reduced CBF, which accompanies the resultant lowered Pco_2 (hypocapnia). Since a reduced O_2 supply is usually accompanied by an increase in arterial Pco_2 and acidity (except at high altitude), the CBF is regulated by hypercapnia rather than hypoxia, to maintain a constant O_2 supply.

Intracranial pressure

Since liquid is essentially incompressible, the volume of blood, brain tissue and CSF within the rigid cranium must be constant (the **Monro–Kellie doctrine**). An increase in CSF volume caused by insufficient reabsorption of CSF or a blockage in its normal route of flow will thus increase intracranial pressure and compress cerebral vessels and reduce CBF. The consequent hypoxia and hypercapnia will directly stimulate vasomotor sympathetic activity from the cardiovascular centres (p. 407) and the resultant rise in MABP, coupled with local cerebral vasodilation, will tend to restore CBF. At the same time, the rise in MABP will reflexly decrease heart rate via the baroreceptors. These reflex responses to an increased intracranial pressure are called the **Cushing response**. There is obviously a limit to the increase in MABP that can be evoked by the Cushing response, and if intracranial pressure exceeds this (as in severe hydrocephalus), then CBF ceases.

A further consequence of the Monro–Kellie doctrine is that increases in cerebral blood pressure caused by **gravity** (p. 417) during a head-stand, together with any tendency to an increase in cerebral venous volume, are transmitted to the CSF such that intracranial pressure also increases. Thus little change occurs in the transmural pressure and cerebral venous return decreases only slightly. Conversely, in the erect posture, the decreases in cerebral blood pressure are compensated for by a corresponding fall in intracranial pressure. Furthermore, the major cerebral veins do not collapse because they are held open by their association with the dura.

Cutaneous circulation

At rest the skin receives about 8% of the cardiac output through its moderately resistant vascular bed. Since it has a very low O_2 consumption, the arteriovenous O_2 difference is also small (Table 17.1). The skin has an extensive superficial network of arterioles, capillaries and venules and an extensive **deep plexus of veins**. The latter may contain up to 1.5 L of blood.

Control of cutaneous blood flow and volume

The arterioles and veins are richly innervated with **sympathetic** fibres acting predominantly via α_1-**adrenoceptors**, and hence the vascular resistance

and capacitance of the skin can be altered by reflexes integrated by the cardiovascular centres. For
instance, during hypotension, haemorrhage or exercise that does not generate a heat load, the blood
flow to the skin can be restricted, making it feel
cold, and the accompanying venoconstriction mobilizes, for the rest of the body, a sizeable volume of
blood from the deep venous plexus of the skin. Cutaneous tissue, to a much greater extent than other
tissues, can tolerate such a reduced blood flow by
reducing its O_2 consumption proportionately.
Metabolic regulation is therefore considered to be
poorly developed in the skin (unless the blood flow
has been reduced for some time). Note also that
skin arterioles are incapable of myogenic autoregulation (see Fig. 16.13).

The sympathetic pathway to cutaneous vessels,
controlled by centres in the hypothalamus and
other forebrain regions, is also responsible for
blushing or pallor during the **emotions** of embar-
rassment or fear, respectively.

Sympathetic control for temperature regulation

In the skin of the hands, feet and face (particularly
the ears, nose and lips), there are also large numbers of **arteriovenous anastomoses** (see Fig.
16.14). These are vessels about 50 μm in diameter
with thick walls of smooth muscle, which contain
α_1-**adrenoceptors** activated by sympathetic fibres.
When **body temperature** increases, sympathetic
activity to the skin decreases under the control of
the hypothalamus (p. 409) resulting in vasodilation, particularly of these arteriovenous anastomoses. This vasodilation is enhanced by
bradykinin, which is released by sweat glands due
to hypothalamic activation of the cholinergic sympathetic fibres to the glands. The decrease in total
peripheral resistance results in a fall in MABP and
the resultant baroreceptor reflex causes a corresponding increase in cardiac output. The massive
increase in skin blood flow is accommodated mainly within the arteriovenous anastomoses and the
venous plexuses, which together provide a large
area for heat exchange between the blood, skin and
external environment. Thus the temperature of

the body is regulated (p. 604) to a large extent by
the amount of blood flowing through the skin
which, from the thermoneutral state, can increase
about 30-fold in heat stress and decrease about 10-
fold in cold stress.

During prolonged exposure to the cold, skin
vasoconstriction changes to vasodilation which
produces a ruddy complexion on a cold day.
This vasodilation is not sympathetically mediated,
but is believed to be caused by **metabolic
regulation**, which overrides sympathetic control,
and by damaged skin cells eliciting an axon–
axonal reflex (see below). **Frostbite** (skin necrosis)
occurs when the skin becomes so cold that the
tissue freezes.

The triple response

In the skin, the reactions of blood vessels can easily be observed. A pointed object drawn lightly over
the skin causes the area of contact rapidly to become pale (the **white reaction**). The mechanical
stimulation is thought to initiate local contraction
of venules or precapillary sphincters. Greater pressure will cause the skin to become red (the **red reaction**), followed by a diffuse mottled reddening
around the area of injury (the **flare**) and then a
local swelling (the **wheal**). The latter three reactions comprise the so-called **triple response**. The
red reaction probably results from the damaged
cells of the skin releasing substances like histamine, which rapidly cause a local vasodilation or
venodilation. The flare results from the mechanical stimulation of nociceptive sensory endings of
C fibres causing antidromic conduction in axon
branches (axon–axonal reflex) that release substance P, which vasodilates nearby arterioles
and causes local mast cells to release histamine.
The wheal results from an increase in permeability of capillaries induced by histamine and substance P, with a consequent increase in interstitial
fluid.

Skeletal muscle circulation

Skeletal muscle receives at rest about 20% of the
cardiac output through a highly resistant vascular

bed, the tone of which is controlled by **myogenic autoregulation** and by **sympathetic** activity predominantly affecting α_1-adrenoceptors. Because of the large mass of skeletal muscle (about 50% of body weight but about 90% of the total cellular mass), even at rest skeletal muscle accounts for about 20% of the body's O_2 consumption (Table 17.1). Its large mass is also why skeletal musculature is an important contributor to overall vasoconstriction during reflexes initiated, for example, by hypotension or haemorrhage. In contrast to splanchnic and cutaneous veins, the veins in skeletal musculature are almost devoid of sympathetic nerve endings and so cannot alter neurogenically their venous capacity and be part of the blood reservoir.

During maximal exercise skeletal musculature receives, due to vasodilation, about 90% of the cardiac output and accounts for about 90% of the total O_2 consumption (p. 618). The vasodilation in skeletal muscles during established exercise results mainly from **metabolic regulation**. The vasodilation resulting from adrenaline acting on β_2-**adrenoceptors** also contributes, especially at the beginning of exercise.

In rhythmic exercise, blood flow in the muscles concerned can cease during the contraction phase but because of the accumulation of metabolites it is then augmented during the relaxation phase. In non-rhythmic exercise, especially that involving static contractions (isometric exercise), blood flow can cease entirely, thus limiting the duration of such exercise.

Splanchnic circulation

The splanchnic area receives through a low-resistance vascular bed about 25% of the cardiac output at rest (Table 17.1). A number of arterial branches from the **abdominal aorta** supply the stomach, intestine, pancreas and spleen, which are drained by the **hepatic portal vein** into the liver. The liver receives about 75% of its blood from this source, the remainder coming from the **hepatic artery**. Blood from the liver drains via **hepatic veins** into the inferior vena cava.

Blood flow to the liver

In the splanchnic and hepatic arteries, the mean blood pressure is about 90 mmHg whilst in the portal and hepatic veins it is about 10 and 5 mmHg, respectively. The hepatic venous pressure is low because the hepatic arterioles are highly constricted due to an **intense vasomotor tone** from sympathetic fibres acting via α_1-adrenoceptors. Consequently blood enters the large sinusoidal liver capillaries at a pressure less than 10 mmHg. This vasoconstriction and hence the proportion of the blood flow to the liver from the hepatic artery are further controlled by metabolic regulation and myogenic autoregulation. When the liver is more active, or there is a decrease in portal flow, **metabolic regulation** of hepatic arterioles causes the hepatic artery to supply up to 50% of the hepatic blood flow. Conversely, when the pressure and therefore flow in the portal system increase, the pressure is also raised (retrogradely via the capillaries) in hepatic arterioles which constrict through **myogenic autoregulation** to reduce hepatic arterial flow.

Note that the low hydrostatic pressure in the capillaries of the liver is matched by the high interstitial colloid osmotic pressure generated by the proteins which are being manufactured by the liver for the plasma. Hence the Starling forces for ultrafiltration and reabsorption across the capillary wall remain in balance (p. 395).

Blood flow to the gut

The arrangement of the blood vessels in the gut is described in Chapter 19. Splanchnic blood flow is adjusted to the degree of activity in the smooth muscle layers by **metabolic regulation**, and in the mucosal and submucosal layers by increased glandular activity releasing **bradykinin**, which causes local vasodilation.

Splanchnic contribution to control of MABP

The α_1-**adrenoceptors** in the splanchnic arterioles and veins mediate vaso- and venoconstriction in response to the generalized increase in sympathetic activity and adrenaline secretion that occurs, for instance, during exercise, hypotension and haemorrhage. This serves to counteract a fall in MABP and to redistribute blood to other more essential regions. Furthermore, the reduction in **splanchnic venous capacity** can make about 300 mL of blood available to the rest of the body. Venous reservoirs of blood are also found in the spleen of some animals (for example, the dog) but not in humans. However, since prolonged splanchnic vasoconstriction would lead to cell damage in the gut, accumulation of metabolites will eventually override some of the vasoconstriction.

Renal circulation

Because its role is to filter blood plasma and maintain electrolyte and water balance, the kidneys receive through a very-low-resistance vascular bed about 20% of the cardiac output (Table 17.1). Its blood supply and blood pressures are described on p. 540. The arterioles of the isolated kidney exhibit well-developed **myogenic autoregulation** such that renal perfusion is maintained constant at MABP between 80 and 180 mmHg (see Fig. 20.4). Thus the renal functions of filtering plasma and regulating electrolyte and water balance are independent of fluctuations in blood pressure. However, this myogenic autoregulation can be overridden by sympathetic activity, and via adrenaline acting on α_1-**adrenoceptors** in the kidney arterioles. Normally there is little sympathetic tone but, during exercise, hypotension, haemorrhage, systemic hypoxia and systemic hypercapnia, the renal arterioles participate in the vasoconstriction that ensures maintenance of an adequate MABP. Furthermore, during exercise or heat stress, renal vasoconstriction helps to compensate for the vasodilation in skeletal musculature and skin. (For renal blood flow changes in exercise, see Chapter 24.) Metabolic regulation in the renal circulation is poor and hence, when intense reflex sympathetic vasoconstriction occurs, the kidneys are vulnerable to damage (e.g. **tubular necrosis**).

17.3 Cardiovascular adjustments in health and disease

The cardiovascular system has to adjust to the demands imposed by alterations in posture, thermal stress (p. 604) and exercise (p. 618). When standing, the effects of gravity cause an increase or decrease in hydrostatic pressures within the blood vessels below and above the heart, respectively. This has no effect on the energy gradients for blood flow but, at sites below the level of the heart, increases primarily the volume capacity of the veins and the amount of capillary ultrafiltration. Reflex mechanisms and the skeletal muscle venous pump counteract these problems. The cardiovascular system and its regulating mechanisms also compensate for the abnormalities induced by haemorrhage, hypotension, hypertension and cardiac failure.

Effects of posture

In Fig. 15.18 the pressures and volumes in the heart are described for the standing posture, whilst in Fig. 17.4 these variables in the vascular system are for the supine position. A change in posture alters the hydrostatic pressures in the blood vessels, with resultant effects on transmural pressures and, in particular, on venous capacity. This in turn affects where the blood is distributed and, in particular, the size of the end-diastolic volume of the heart.

Hydrostatic pressure

In the supine or prone posture, all blood vessels are approximately at the level of the heart and the mean blood pressures in the aorta, the arteries and veins (of both the head and feet) and the right atrium are about 100, 95, 5 and 1 mmHg, respectively. When standing, the weight of the column of blood in the blood vessels results in an increase in arterial and venous pressure below the level of the heart and a decrease in these pressures above the level of the heart (Fig. 17.4). For each centimetre of blood (1 cmH$_2$O) above or below the level of the heart, pressure changes by 0.74 mmHg. Thus, for a person

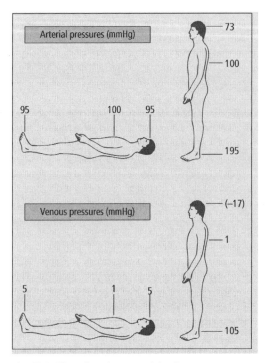

Arterial pressures (mmHg)

73

100

95   100   95

195

Venous pressures (mmHg)

(−17)

1

5   1   5

105

Fig. 17.4 Effect of gravity on arterial and venous pressures.

As blood flows towards the feet, it loses gravitational potential energy and gains potential energy due to pressure. Thus the total fluid energy in the arteries of the feet is the equivalent of 95 mmHg irrespective of a supine or standing posture. Therefore, although the changes in blood pressure on adoption of the standing posture mean that blood flows against a hydrostatic pressure gradient; for instance from the heart (100 mmHg) to the arteries in the feet (195 mmHg), the flow is not against a fluid energy gradient. Similarly, when total fluid energy is considered, it can be seen that it is not difficult for blood to return from the feet to the heart.

Transmural pressure, venous capacity and ultrafiltration

If blood vessels were rigid tubes, no cardiovascular adjustments for the standing posture would be required other than to compensate for decreased blood volume due to increased ultrafiltration across the capillary wall. However, the changes in transmural pressure affect the veins in particular, which tend to empty and collapse above, and progressively fill below, the level of the heart.

The collapse of superficial veins in the neck breaks the column of blood and hence removes the effects of gravity, and the venous pressure approximates to zero. The veins, although collapsed, are not occluded so flow can continue unimpaired through spaces formed where the walls are not in total apposition. As blood accumulates behind the areas of collapse, every time the pressure rises sufficiently above zero some venous flow occurs. Deeper veins are better supported by surrounding tissue and do not collapse as much. Intracranial veins do not collapse at all because the CSF and blood are affected equally by gravity and because the venous sinuses are maintained patent by their structural association with the dura (p. 61). Thus when a person is standing the CBF depends only on the pressure in the carotid arteries; the venous pressures at the exit from the cranium, where the neck veins are collapsed, being zero at all times.

Irrespective of posture, if the mean right atrial pressure equals about 1 mmHg, the height of the uncollapsed column of blood in the external jugu-

1.8 m tall whose head is about 30 cm above the heart in the upright posture, blood pressure at the entrance to the cranial cavity is about 22 mmHg less compared with the pressure in the supine position. Hence the arterial pressure at the entrance to the cranial cavity becomes 73 mmHg and, were it not for the fact that the veins in the neck collapse, the venous pressure at the cranial exit would be ~17 mmHg. Because of venous collapse, the venous pressure is in fact close to zero. In the feet, which are about 130 cm below the heart when standing, there is an increase in pressure of about 100 mmHg and hence the arterial pressure becomes 195 mmHg and the venous pressure becomes 105 mmHg provided that, in the case of the veins, the standing is motionless.

It must be noted that blood flows from a point of high to low total fluid energy. The total fluid energy is the sum of the kinetic energy and the potential energy due to pressure, plus that due to gravity.

lar vein is always about 1.5 cm vertically above the right atrium (which is approximately at the level of the sternal angle). A greater length of uncollapsed vein can obviously be seen the more tilted the subject is towards the supine position. The vertical height of this blood column above the sternal angle is used clinically as a measure of central venous pressure (p. 398), and the pulsations of the a, c and v waves and particularly, the x and y descents (p. 360), can sometimes be distinguished at the top of the column.

Initially, on standing, venous valves prevent backflow from the heart. Veins below the level of the heart are then slowly (30–60 s) distended in proportion to the transmural force by the arterial inflow. This results in an increase of about 500 mL in venous blood volume, most of this being displaced from the thorax. Consequently, were it not for reflex compensations, there would be a reduction in end-diastolic volume which would reduce stroke volume (Starling's law of the heart) and produce systemic hypotension. Furthermore, the increased hydrostatic pressure in the capillaries below the level of the heart would cause considerably more ultrafiltration than usual and over a period of hours this would lead to loss of blood volume and, most noticeably, to **local oedema** in the ankles.

Reflex compensations

The decrease in end-diastolic volume caused by sudden standing is detected by the **atrial stretch receptors** (p. 405) and the decrease in MABP (from both the direct gravitational effect at the level of the carotids and the decrease in $\dot{Q}$) is detected by the **carotid baroreceptors** (p. 403). Therefore, in the space of about 5 s there are reflex increases in sympathetic activity and in adrenaline release, causing:

1 an increase in heart rate and in myocardial contractility tending to restore $\dot{Q}$ towards the supine value;

2 vasoconstriction in the skeletal musculature, skin, kidneys and gut, reducing blood flow to these organs, increasing TPR and decreasing capillary pressure; and

3 venoconstriction in all veins, but in particular in those of the skin and gut, which displaces some blood back to the thorax.

All of these responses contribute to **short-term regulation** and **restoration of MABP**.

Over a longer period of time, **long-term regulation**, the atrial stretch receptors will trigger an increase in antidiuretic hormone secretion. The reduced blood flow to the kidneys enhances the release of renin, which increases circulating concentrations of angiotensin II and aldosterone. These responses, which are similar to those occurring after a mild haemorrhage, augment vasoconstriction and decrease urinary Na^+ excretion, which helps **restore blood volume** towards normal.

One of the most important mechanisms counteracting the long-term effects of standing is the **skeletal muscle venous pump**. The rhythmic contraction of leg muscles reduces venous capacity and assists venous and lymphatic returns (p. 398). Intermittent closure of the venous valves also interrupts the vertical column of blood between the heart and limb and thus reduces the effective hydrostatic pressure. By these means the venous pressure in the feet can be lowered from about 105 mmHg to as little as 30 mmHg. The normal muscular contractions associated with moving around in the standing posture are sufficient to achieve this and hence there is less of an increase in venous capacity and no local oedema. Prolonged standing, venous obstruction or pregnancy can overstretch the veins and lead to incompetent venous valves. The consequent ineffectiveness of the skeletal muscle venous pump results in the excessive distension of, in particular, superficial veins which fill with sluggishly moving blood—the condition known as **varicose veins**.

Restoration of the MABP may be inadequate during motionless standing or when suddenly standing (particularly in hypotensive patients or in patients with an impaired sympathetic system or in subjects in a hot environment where venodilation in the skin predominates). If the MABP declines to a level (about 50 mmHg) below which myogenic autoregulation of cerebral blood flow cannot occur, the person becomes **dizzy**, has impaired vision and may even faint. **Fainting** has the advantage of returning the person to the supine position!

Haemorrhage

Loss of 10% of the blood volume (about that given by a blood donor) is easily compensated for and results after a few minutes in little change in MABP. Loss of up to 30% over a relatively brief period (e.g. 30 min) will cause a fall in MABP to about 70 mmHg and signs of **mild shock**. The cardiovascular reflexes initiated by such a fall will eventually compensate completely for the loss of blood volume. However, the rapid loss of a greater volume of blood will result in **severe shock**, which may become irreversible if not treated by blood transfusion or by raising the blood volume by administration of a fluid with similar colloid osmotic pressure to plasma. The signs of shock are described in the next section. Prompt restoration of the lost blood prevents the adverse consequences of intense reflex vasoconstriction in the renal, splanchnic, muscle and skin vascular beds. Thus the drastic reduction in organ perfusion, which deprives the tissue of sufficient O_2 and can lead to permanent damage, in particular to the kidneys (**tubular necrosis**), is avoided.

Following a haemorrhage the decrease in blood volume reduces end-diastolic volume and hence stroke volume, $\dot{Q}$ and MABP. Detection of these reductions by atrial stretch receptors and arterial baroreceptors will result in an immediate increase in sympathetic activity and adrenaline secretion and a slightly slower increase in the secretion of angiotensin II, antidiuretic hormone and aldosterone. The consequent responses (p. 573) are the same as those that follow a change from the supine to the erect posture (p. 418) but are of greater magnitude. These responses may serve to restore $\dot{Q}$ and MABP towards normal. Further restoration can occur only by making good the deficit in blood volume. Approximately 15 min after a blood volume loss of about 25%, at least 500 mL of plasma volume will have been provided by the transfer of interstitial fluid into the capillaries, as a consequence of reduced capillary pressure resulting from the hypotension itself, and from vasoconstriction. In the

next few hours, further restoration of circulation blood volume and replenishment of interstitial fluid occurs because of the increased water and Na^+ retention by the kidneys (urine production is minimal), and because of, when possible, the quenching of thirst. In contrast, replacement of the plasma proteins by hepatic synthesis requires 3–6 days and the formation of new erythrocytes takes a period of about 4 weeks.

The progress of these adjustments to haemorrhage can be examined using the cardiac and vascular function curves (Fig. 17.5), which were described on p. 400. In Fig. 17.5, position A is the normal pre-haemorrhage operating point, $\dot{Q}$ being about 6 L min^{-1} and mean right atrial pressure about 1 mmHg. Immediately after the rapid loss of ~25% of the blood volume, the cardiac function curve is normal but, due to the reduction in blood volume, the vascular function curve is shifted substantially downwards and thus the operating point moves to position B. Position B depicts the resultant low right atrial pressure, reduced end-diastolic volume, small stroke volume and fall in $\dot{Q}$ that will produce hypotension. After about 5 s, baroreceptor and atrial stretch receptor reflexes cause a sympathetic increase in myocardial contractility and vasoconstriction, which moves the cardiac function curve upwards and steepens it. At the same time reflex venoconstriction shifts the vascular function curve upwards a little. Thus position C is reached. After about 15 min, restoration of some of the lost volume (by capillary reabsorption of interstitial fluid) will move the systemic vascular function curve upwards a little further and the improved MABP will result in less sympathetic drive to myocardial contractility and less vasoconstriction and hence a flatter ventricular function curve. Thus position D will be reached. After a few more hours, the cardiovascular system will have returned to the original position of A.

Hypotension, fainting and shock

Hypotension

Arterial systolic pressures below 100 mmHg are taken to indicate **hypotension**. Such pressures are

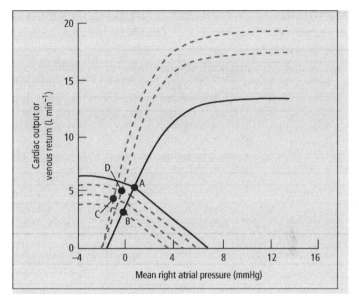

Fig. 17.5 Cardiac and vascular function curves in response to haemorrhage. Operating point: A, prehaemorrhage; B, immediately after a rapid haemorrhage; C, after reflex increase in myocardial contractility, vasoconstriction and venoconstriction; D, after restoration of some of the blood loss.

associated usually with decreases in $\dot{Q}$ but sometimes with decreases in TPR and occasionally in both. Hypotension may be the result of:

1 haemorrhage;

2 cardiovascular disorders such as aortic or mitral stenosis or cardiac failure;

3 loss of tone in resistance and capacitance vessels;

4 allergic or toxic reactions causing vasodilation;

5 visceral or deep pain;

6 standing;

7 coughing or straining (e.g. in defaecation), if the intrathoracic pressure is raised sufficiently to impair venous return;

8 a $\dot{Q}$ during exercise that is insufficient to compensate for the vasodilation in the skeletal musculature; and

9 endocrine disorders, for example Addison's disease (p. 265).

Fainting

The commonest manifestation of acute hypotension is **fainting** (**syncope**), which is the sudden loss of consciousness due to cerebral ischaemia. For this to occur, the MABP must decrease to a level below the range of autoregulation (i.e. below approximately 50 mmHg) such that CBF decreases

and the O_2 delivery to the brain is impaired. It is usually of short duration since the resulting supine position helps elevate the MABP. Fainting that results from sudden bradycardia and diffuse vasodilation is referred to as **vasovagal syncope**. If this is precipitated by strong emotion, the term **psychogenic syncope** is sometimes used. If the cerebral ischaemia is prolonged, this may lead to necrosis of cerebral tissue (**cerebral infarction**). A thrombosis or a rupture in a major cerebral artery (i.e. a **stroke**) leads to local areas of brain **ischaemia** (reduced blood supply) and often to local areas of prolonged or permanent brain damage.

Shock

Hypotension becomes critical only when inadequate blood flow disrupts organ function. This is referred to as **shock**. The signs of shock are pallor, coldness of the skin and sweating, collapse of superficial veins, hyperventilation, tachycardia, reduced urine formation, thirst, decreased body temperature, decreased metabolism and metabolic acidosis. If shock is untreated or sufficiently severe, it is likely to become irreversible with severe hypotension, unconsciousness, central nervous system damage, hypoventilation and further reductions in $\dot{Q}$, which will lead eventually to respiratory and cardiac failure and to death. Inadequate $\dot{Q}$ can arise either from sudden failure of the heart to pump, as in coronary occlusion, or from a severe reduction in blood volume due to dehydration, haemorrhage or plasma loss resulting from burns.

Hypertension

Repeated measurements of arterial diastolic pressure above 90 mmHg in the resting supine subject are taken clinically to indicate the condition of **hypertension**. It is associated with increases in $\dot{Q}$, TPR or blood volume. Clinically, hypertension is classified as primary or essential (95% of cases) and secondary or symptomatic.

The causes of **primary hypertension** are not clear but may include:

1 hereditary factors;
2 a large Na+ intake in the diet; and
3 psychological factors.

Secondary hypertension can be the result of:

1 renal disease causing renal vasoconstriction, reduced renal blood flow, the release of renin and a consequent increase in blood volume;
2 endocrine disorders leading to increased adrenaline secretion or to increased aldosterone or glucocorticoid secretion resulting in Na+ retention; and
3 toxaemia in pregnancy.

In hypertensive patients, the baroreceptor reflex modulates MABP around an elevated set-point. Hypertension can lead to further renal damage, more severe hypertension, ischaemic heart disease, congestive heart failure and strokes.

Myocardial ischaemia

Reduction or cessation of blood flow (**ischaemia**) to the heart can be caused by atherosclerosis or thrombosis of the coronary vessels, by a low aortic diastolic pressure as in cardiac failure or haemorrhage, by a rise in atrial and ventricular diastolic pressures as in cardiac failure or by a high left ventricular systolic pressure as in aortic valve stenosis. The resultant hypoxia of the myocardium affects mainly the left ventricle and, if severe, it leads to myocardial **infarction**, i.e. death (**necrosis**) of cardiac muscle. Treatment of myocardial ischaemia attempts to increase coronary flow (with vasodilating drugs), decrease myocardial O_2 consumption (by reducing preload and afterload with veno- and vasodilating drugs) and decrease heart rate and myocardial contractility (with β-adrenoceptor antagonists).

Cardiac failure

Substantial cardiac (ventricular) failure most commonly results from **myocardial ischaemia**, but may also result from heart valve disease or hypertension. However, a mild reduction in coronary perfusion may cause only **angina pectoris**, which is the term applied to the pain arising from myocardial hypoxia, which is commonly triggered by exercise.

The sequence of events in an instantaneous cardiac failure can be examined using cardiac and vascular function curves (Fig. 17.6). Position A is the normal operating point where $\dot{Q}$ is about 6 L min^{-1} and mean right atrial pressure is about 1 mmHg. When the heart fails, myocardial contractility is insufficient to eject an adequate stroke volume and both $\dot{Q}$ and MABP fall. As the heart becomes engorged with blood, end-diastolic volume and atrial pressures are raised. The cardiac function curve therefore becomes very flat but initially there is no change in the vascular function curve. The new operating point now occurs at position B with a low $\dot{Q}$ and high right atrial pressure.

Reflex mechanisms now come into play to try and minimize the decrease in $\dot{Q}$ and attempt to maintain CBF. Arterial baroreceptors detect the hypotension and their reflexes dominate the opposing reflexes triggered by the atrial stretch receptors detecting the increased end-diastolic volume. The reflex increase in sympathetic activity and adrenaline causes tachycardia, some improvement in myocardial contractility, which together steepen a little the cardiac function curve. Reflex venoconstriction causes a displacement upwards in the vascular function curve. Thus position C is reached within about 1 min.

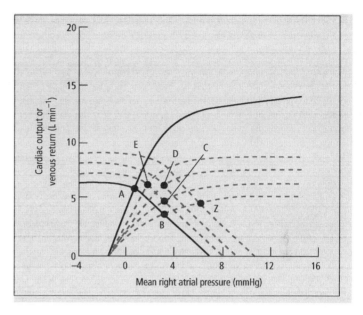

Fig. 17.6 Cardiac and vascular function curves in response to cardiac failure. Operating point: A, pre-failure; B, onset of sudden cardiac failure; C, after short-term reflex adjustments; D, after long-term adjustments; Z, position if short- and long-term mechanisms fail; E, after clinical treatment.

There now follows a sequence of longer-term adjustments over a week or so. The diminished blood flow and vasoconstriction have reduced renal perfusion and hence glomerular filtration. As a consequence there is Na^+ and water retention. Furthermore, the increased sympathetic activity and reduced renal blood flow promote the secretion of renin, which increases circulating angiotension II and aldosterone and thus Na^+ retention is further enhanced. Meanwhile the baroreceptors have promoted antidiuretic hormone production, reinforcing the water retention. Fluid retention in the blood elevates capillary pressures, disturbing the Starling equilibrium and increasing interstitial fluid volume. When fluid retention reaches 3–4 L, generalized oedema results and, if the left atrial pressure has also become raised, there may be pulmonary oedema too. Impaired lung gas exchange will result in cyanosis and hyperventilation, often with dyspnoea (breathlessness). The raised blood volume displaces the vascular function curve upwards even further. During this period of a week or so, some myocardial repair may have occurred, together with some hypertrophy of the undamaged myocardium in response to the prolonged increase in afterload caused by vasoconstriction. Thus an improved cardiac function curve

may eventuate and the new operating point is now at D for this **stable state of chronic compensation** where $\dot{Q}$ is nearly back to normal. However, the heart remains congested, fluid retention is obvious and the ability to exercise is severely limited. Furthermore the hypertrophied myocardium and dilated ventricles worsen the condition because they make greater demands on myocardial O_2 delivery.

Note that when the initial cardiac failure is very severe, even position C cannot be reached because the failing ventricle cannot either respond to the increased sympathetic drive or cope with the increase in afterload from the vasoconstriction. The cardiac function curve either does not improve or gets even flatter. Renal function deteriorates further and fluid retention gets worse, moving the vascular function curve further upwards. Thus position Z rather than C eventuates. To prevent death from **congestive heart failure**, clinical intervention is required.

Administration of digoxin or other cardiac glycosides may be able to increase myocardial contractility and therefore steepen the cardiac function curve. They appear to act by inhibiting the sarcolemmal Na^+–K^+–ATPase so that the Na^+ gradient across the membrane falls, decreasing

Na$^+$–Ca^{2+} counter-transport (Fig. 15.20). Thus Ca^{2+} expulsion from the cell slows down and intracellular Ca^{2+} accumulates, making more Ca^{2+} available for the contractile process. Administration of vasodilating drugs will reduce the afterload and therefore also help steepen the cardiac function curve. Administration of diuretics reduces fluid retention and venodilating drugs increase venous capacity; these changes will move the vascular function curve downwards. After successful clinical treatment the operating point will shift to position E and eventually back to the normal position A.

Chapter 18

Respiration

18.1 Introduction

In biochemical terms, **cellular respiration** is the oxidation of organic substances by the passage of electrons through the coenzyme chain to molecular O_2. In the process O_2 acts as an electron acceptor and is converted to water. During oxidation, CO_2 is produced and energy is stored in the high energy bonds of adenosine triphosphate. Physiologists use the term respiration in a broader sense to include:

1 diffusion of O_2 and CO_2 between capillaries and cells;

2 carriage of these gases in the blood; and

3 gas exchange between blood and the external environment, which involves not only diffusion across the lung capillaries but also the bulk movement of gases in and out of the lung.

Diffusion of O_2 and CO_2 between the cells and systemic capillaries and between pulmonary capillaries and the gas of the alveoli occurs over short interstitial distances and through thin capillary walls. The quantity of gas transferred (**gas exchange**) is usually expressed as the rate of O_2 **consumption** and CO_2 **production** by the body as a whole.

For gases to be exchanged with the environment, they have to be moved into (inspiration) and out of (expiration) the alveoli of the lungs by **bulk flow**, commonly termed breathing. This results from pressure gradients generated by the

action of respiratory muscles and is aided in expiration by elastic recoil of the lungs and contraction of abdominal muscles. Bulk movement of gases, and the volumes and pressures involved, are the topic of **lung mechanics**. The volume of gas moved per minute is called the pulmonary **ventilation**. That part of each inspiration, which reaches the **alveoli** is available for gas exchange by diffusion; the remainder occupies the conducting airways (**dead space**) across which no gas exchange occurs.

Gas transport around the body depends on the flow of blood in the cardiovascular system. For adequate and efficient gas exchange, not only must the alveoli be ventilated but there must be sufficient blood flow to perfuse the alveolar capillaries. The ratio of ventilation to **blood perfusion** must be reasonably uniform throughout the lung. Gas exchange at most tissues depends on a blood flow proportional to the metabolic need—much of this is provided by alterations in arteriolar tone in response to local metabolites (metabolic regulation, p. 388).

Haemoglobin in the red blood cells plays a central role in the chemical combination of O_2 and CO_2 with blood. Carriage of CO_2 in the blood also leads to the formation of H^+ and HCO_3^- ions and thus affects **acid–base balance**.

In a normal healthy person at sea level, ventilation and the partial pressures of O_2 and CO_2 in arterial blood remain, at rest, remarkably constant.

If metabolic demands change, e.g. in exercise, or if the conditions under which O_2 is supplied alter, e.g. at altitude, then appropriate alterations in ventilation and blood flow occur by **reflex regulation**. The respiratory centres in the brain not only integrate chemoreceptor and mechanoreceptor information but they also generate the rhythmicity of breathing.

Additional functions of the respiratory system

The lungs also have functions other than gas exchange.

1 the pulmonary capillary bed acts as a blood filter preventing particles like small clots, detached cells or air bubbles from reaching the systemic circulation where they may obstruct capillary blood flow within essential organs such as the brain;

2 the airways remove airborne particles by phagocytosis or mucociliary action aided by coughing;

3 ventilation of the airways contributes to heat loss (p. 605) and water loss (p. 571);

4 the pulmonary vessels are an important reservoir for blood (p. 410);

5 the larynx is used for the production of sound (phonation);

6 the pharynx is the conduit for both swallowing and airflow; and

7 the lung tissue has many metabolic functions, such as:

(a) conversion of angiotensin I to angiotensin II;

(b) synthesis and removal of bradykinin and certain prostaglandins;

(c) storage and release of serotonin and histamine;

(d) inactivation of noradrenaline and adrenaline;

(e) synthesis of peptides like substance P and opiates;

(f) secretion of heparin by mast cells; and

(g) secretion of immunoglobulins in the bronchial mucus.

These non-respiratory functions of the respiratory system are not the main focus of this chapter and will only be touched upon briefly in subsequent sections.

Symbols and abbreviations

For use in respiratory physiology there is an agreed set of symbols and abbreviations (Table 18.1).

The anatomy of the respiratory system

On inspiration, air passes through the **upper respiratory tract** (nose, pharynx, larynx) into the trachea (Fig. 18.1); air can also gain entry to the pharynx via the mouth. The conchae of the paired **nasal cavities** create a vast surface area, which is lined by ciliated columnar epithelium containing mucus-secreting cells; there are also coarse hairs or vibrissae at the nostrils and a dense vascular network in the submucosa. In the nasal cavities the air is **filtered** to remove foreign particles, **warmed** to 37°C and **humidified**. Sensory nerve endings of the trigeminal nerve detect irritants in the nasal mucosa and trigger sneezing. In the **pharynx**, sensory endings of the glossopharyngeal nerve detect irritants that cause the aspiration reflex. The pharynx serves as a common passageway for food and liquid entering from the mouth and for gas entering from the nasal cavities. During swallowing, food and fluid are deflected from the entrance to the larynx by a cartilaginous flap called the **epiglottis**.

The **larynx** is a cartilaginous 'box' that contains the **vocal cords** separated by a space between them called the **glottis**, which closes during swallowing. Vibration of these cords as air passes through the glottis produces sound, the amplitude and pitch of which can be altered by the speed of air movement and the size of the glottis, respectively. Changes in glottal aperture also occur in normal breathing. The glottis dilates during inspiration and constricts during expiration; the constriction increases airway resistance and therefore prolongs (brakes) expiration. Laryngeal muscles controlling the glottis are skeletal and are innervated by the recurrent laryngeal nerve. Another vagal branch, the superior laryngeal nerve, contains afferent fibres from mucosal irritant receptors, which initiate the cough reflex.

The **lower respiratory tract** commences with the **trachea** (diameter ~2.5 cm) which divides into

Table 18.1 Glossary of symbols.

Gas exchange*		
General variables	V	Gas volume in general. Pressure, temperature and percentage saturation with water vapour must be stated
	$\dot{V}$	Gas volume per unit of time
	P	Gas pressure in general
	F	Fractional concentration in dry gas phase
	$\dot{Q}$	Volume flow of blood
	C	Content in blood phase
	f	Respiratory frequency—breaths per unit of time
	R	Respiratory exchange ratio in general (volume CO_2/volume O_2)
	D	Diffusing capacity in general (volume per unit of time per unit pressure difference)
Symbols for the gas phase	I	Inspired gas
	E	Expired gas
	A	Alveolar gas
	T	Tidal gas
	D	Dead-space gas
	B	Barometric
Symbols for the blood phase	a	Arterial
	v	Venous
	c	Capillary
Special symbols and abbreviations	$\bar{x}$	Dash above any symbol indicates a mean value
	$\dot{x}$	Dot above any symbol indicates a time derivative
	x'	Apostrophe following a symbol indicates an 'end' value
	STPD	Standard temperature, pressure, dry (0°C, 760 mmHg)
	BTPS	Body temperature, pressure, saturated with water
	ATPS	Ambient temperature, pressure, saturated with water
Examples	$F_A O_2$	Fraction of O_2 in the alveolar air
	$\dot{V}O_2$	Volume of O_2 consumed per minute
	$P_c O_2$	Partial pressure of O_2 in the capillary blood

* From Otis, A.B. (1964) In: Fenn, W.O. & Rahn, H. (eds) *Handbook of Physiology*, Section 3, *Respiration*, vol. 1, pp. 681–98. American Physiological Society, Washington.

the two main **bronchi**, one to each lung (Fig. 18.1). These subdivide repeatedly within the lung until the alveoli are reached, after some 23 'generations' or divisions. The first 16 generations are the **conducting airways**. The walls of the trachea and bronchi down to the 11th generations (diameter ~1 mm) are supported by cartilage, comprising C-shaped rings in the trachea and incomplete plates in the bronchi, have bands of smooth muscle and are lined by a ciliated pseudostratified columnar epithelium. Mucoserous glands in the submucosa and mucus-secreting goblet cells in the epithelium produce a fluid that contributes to humidification and helps trap particles and soluble pollutants.

These are then moved towards the pharynx by the action of the cilia (the so-called mucociliary escalator). The smooth muscle is innervated by parasympathetic fibres from the vagus nerves, which cause bronchoconstriction; the role of sympathetic innervation is unclear.

The 12th to 16th divisions of the airways are called the **bronchioles** (diameter <1 mm), which lack cartilage and therefore are susceptible to collapse when compressed by strong expirations. The lining epithelium is cuboidal and it contains many secretory neuroepithelial bodies and—in place of globlet cells—Clara cells; the functions of both are under investigation. The main components of the

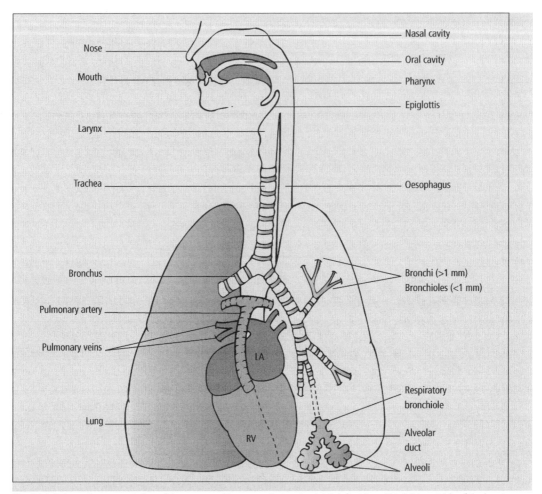

Fig. 18.1 Schematic representation of the upper and lower respiratory tract. LA, left atrium; RV, right ventricle of the heart.

bronchiolar wall are elastic fibres and smooth muscle. Nerve endings of the superior laryngeal nerve sensitive to stretch and irritants are found throughout the lower airways.

The 17th to 19th generations are the **respiratory bronchioles**, which give rise to a few single alveoli and form the **transitional zone**. The 20th to 22nd generations are the **alveolar ducts**, which are ~500 μm in diameter and are completely lined by alveoli (Fig. 18.2). The airways end blindly in clusters of numerous alveoli (the alveolar sacs), which can intercommunicate through the pores of Kohn. The alveolar ducts and alveoli comprise the **respiratory zone** where gas exchange occurs.

There are 300–600 million alveoli in the lungs and, since each **alveolus** at the end of a normal expiration is ~100 μm in diameter, they provide 50–90 m^2 of surface area for gas exchange. The alveoli abut with one another so that the wall (interalveolar septum) of one is shared with another. The alveolar wall is, in effect, a huge dense capillary network and has a number of very thin layers through which gas molecules must diffuse. These layers comprise the fluid lining layer, the alveolar epithelium, the interstitium and the capillary endothelium (total average thickness ~1 μm) and are referred to collectively as the alveolar–capillary membrane or air–blood barrier (Fig. 18.3). The

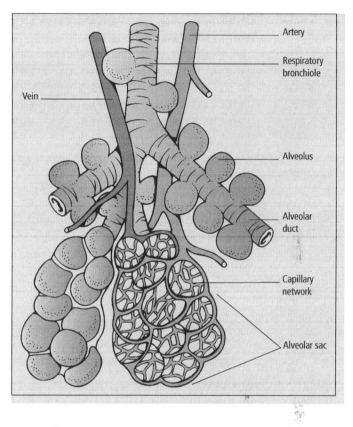

Fig. 18.2 Structure of the terminal airways and alveoli. The capillary networks are shown for only one alveolar sac.

interstitium contains reticular and elastic fibres, which confer on the lungs some elasticity. The alveolar epithelial cells are of two kinds: type I, by far the most numerous, are thin squamous cells; type II are cuboidal in shape and have villi at their apical surface. They store surfactant in lamellar bodies and secrete it into the fluid-lining layer. Alveolar macrophages rove over the surface of the alveoli and provide the last line of defence against foreign particles.

Alveolar capillaries receive blood low in O_2 and high in CO_2 through the pulmonary circulation (p. 410), while capillaries supplying the walls of the larger airways receive oxygenated blood from the aorta through the bronchial part of the systemic circulation (p. 410).

18.2 Lung mechanics

The thorax is a sealed compartment lined on the inside by a smooth moist membrane (the parietal pleura). There is a similar membrane (the pulmonary pleura) on the outer surface of the lungs and the cohesive force of the narrow liquid-filled space between the pleura ensures that the lungs do not collapse away from the chest wall. Air is drawn into the lungs by the action of inspiratory muscles (diaphragm, external intercostals, neck and back muscles) which enlarge the thorax and hence the lungs. At rest the diaphragm is the main inspiratory muscle. Expiration at rest is achieved entirely by elastic recoil of the lungs, which pulls the diaphragm up and the chest inwards. More forceful expirations require contraction of the abdominal and internal intercostal muscles. The volume in the lungs at maximum inspiration is called the total lung capacity (TLC; ~6 L) and its subcomponents are inspiratory reserve volume (IRV), tidal volume (V_T), expiratory reserve volume (ERV) and residual volume (RV). The first three volumes comprise the vital capacity (VC); the last two volumes comprise the functional residual capacity (FRC).

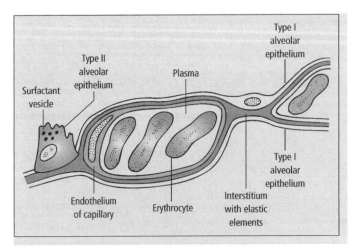

Fig. 18.3 Structure of the shared wall of two alveoli. The very thin fluid lining layer covering the alveolar epithelium is omitted.

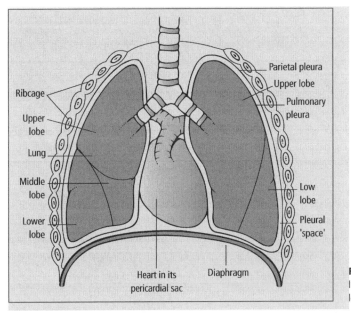

Fig. 18.4 Association between the lungs and the thorax showing the lung lobes.

The thorax and respiratory muscles

The lower part of the trachea and the paired lungs are contained within the **thorax**, which is a closed compartment. It is sealed at the top by connective tissue and muscles, which are attached to the sternum, upper ribs and vertebral column, and is totally separated from the abdomen by the upward dome of a thin sheet of skeletal muscle, the diaphragm (Fig. 18.4). In the midline, membranes associated with the pericardium of the heart, large blood vessels and the oesophagus create separate right and left compartments such that, should one lung collapse, the other can remain inflated. The inner surface of the ribcage and diaphragm is lined by a moist membrane, the **parietal pleura**, which is continuous with the midline membranes. Firmly attached to the outer surface of the lungs is another moist epithelial membrane, the visceral or **pulmonary pleura**. The **pleural space** (also called inter- or intrapleural space) between the parietal and pulmonary pleura is filled with a thin film of liquid which produces strong cohesive forces that prevent the pleura from separating but permit them to slide with ease over each other. If air is allowed to enter the pleural space (**pneumothorax**), the lungs no longer remain attached to the thoracic walls and collapse. Usually the cohesive attachment of the lung to the chest ensures that when the chest enlarges, so too do the lungs, and when the lungs elastically recoil, the chest correspondingly shrinks.

The dimensions of the chest are altered by the contraction of the skeletal muscles of respiration (Fig. 18.5); those not active during quiet breathing are called the accessory muscles. During quiet breathing **inspiration** is achieved mainly by contraction of the **diaphragm**, which is innervated bilaterally by the **phrenic nerves** arising from cervical roots 3–5 of the spinal cord. Contraction of the diaphragm has the double action of depressing the floor of the thorax and raising the ribcage at its point of origin, thus elongating and widening the thorax, respectively, and hence increasing its volume. The **parasternal intercostal muscles** are also activated during quiet inspiration and assist raising the ribcage. As the dome of the diaphragm becomes flattened by the contraction, the abdominal viscera are pushed against a relaxed abdominal wall. Between the ribs, extending diagonally

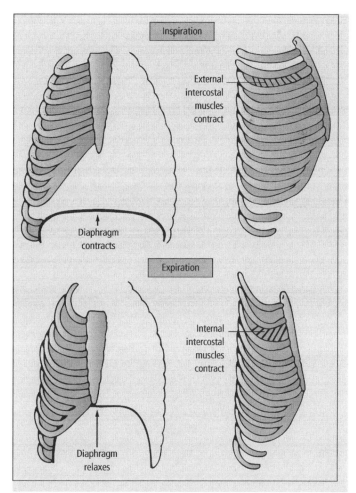

Fig. 18.5 Diaphragm and intercostal muscles.

downwards as they come forwards, are the **external intercostal muscles**, which favour inspiration by elevating the anterior end of each rib, causing an increase in the width of the chest. However contraction of the external intercostal muscles is pronounced only during stimulated breathing or lateral bending of the trunk; their action is primarily to support the chest wall in the intercostal spaces. Larger strenuous inspirations also need the assistance of the **accessory muscles** of inspiration, such as the sternomastoid muscle and scalene muscles of the neck and back, to raise the sternum.

During quiet breathing **expiration** is a passive event. No muscular contraction is involved and the thorax shrinks as a result of **passive elastic recoil** of elements in the lung stretched during the previous inspiration. Forceful expirations require the elastic recoil to be aided by muscle activity from the accessory muscles of expiration. In stimulated breathing the **internal intercostal muscles** extend diagonally upwards as they come forwards and their contraction depresses the ribcage. Contraction of **abdominal muscles** drives the diaphragm upwards into a highly domed shape expelling gas from the lungs—it is the more important expiratory muscle. Expiration commences slowly because some inspiratory diaphragmatic activity continues into the first phase of expiration and it is prolonged by the braking effect that arises from expiratory constriction of the glottis. When the rate of breathing increases, the duration of

expiration shortens markedly because the next inspiratory effort is timed to start earlier; furthermore, there is now expiratory muscle activity and removal of some of the braking.

Lung volumes

The volume of air breathed in and out of the lungs is called the **tidal volume (V_T)**. At rest this volume is about 500 mL in healthy young adults (~70 kg). At the end of a normal inspiration the extra volume that can be inhaled with maximal voluntary inspiratory effort is the **inspiratory reserve volume (IRV)**—about 3 L (Fig. 18.6). At the end of a normal expiration the maximal volume that can be voluntary exhaled is the **expiratory reserve volume (ERV)**—about 1.3–1.5 L. These volumes are readily measured by mouth-breathing in and out of a **spirometer** using breaths that are not rapidly forced. One cannot, however, expel all the gas from the lungs—there remains after maximal exhalation a volume of about 1.2 L called the **residual volume (RV)**. This volume can only leave the lungs if they collapse away from the chest wall, for example in pneumothorax when air emboli break the cohesive film in the pleural space; even then about 200 mL remains trapped—the so-called minimal volume. RV can be measured by the **helium dilution technique** or **body plethysmography**.

Combinations of volumes are referred to as capacities. Thus the volume remaining in the lungs

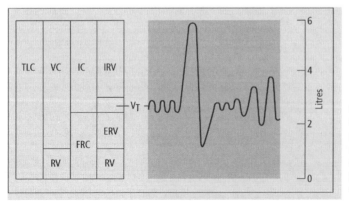

Fig. 18.6 The subdivisions of lung volume. ERV, expiratory reserve volume; FRC, functional residual capacity; IC, inspiratory capacity; RV, residual volume; TLC, total lung capacity; VC, vital capacity; V_T, tidal volume.

at the end of a normal expiration, comprising the ERV and RV, is the **functional residual capacity (FRC)**—about 2.5 L (Fig. 18.6). This is a substantial volume and, apart from the ~150 mL dead space volume in the airways (p. 488), is the volume of gas normally filling the alveoli at the start of the inspiration. The volume of gas that can be shifted in and out of the lungs during maximal inspiration and expiration, about 5 L, comprising the IRV, V_T and ERV, is the **vital capacity (VC)**. The total volume of gas (about 6 L) occupying the lungs at maximal inspiration includes in addition the RV and is the **total lung capacity (TLC)**. Terms such as inspiratory capacity (IRV + V_T) and expiratory capacity (V_T + ERV) are also used.

These volumes and capacities increase with body size and are slightly smaller in females. With ageing there is a reduction in elastic recoil of the lungs and stiffening of the chest wall, which leads to a gradual increase in RV and FRC (particularly the former as ERV decreases), and a fall in VC with little change in TLC. Thus, in a younger person RV tends to be smaller than ERV; in an older person the RV is the larger. When lying down compared with standing, the RV does not change but FRC (and hence ERV) decrease because the outward elastic recoil of the chest is reduced (p. 436) as the weight of the abdominal contents no longer pulls the diaphragm downwards. When FRC is so reduced, more lung volume is available as the IRV. Because there is a greater blood volume in the thorax when lying down (p. 417), TLC and VC may decrease a little.

Lung volumes and capacities can also be affected by lung diseases. For instance, in **restrictive lung diseases** like **pulmonary fibrosis**, the alveoli are so stiff that their expansion is restricted and all volumes and capacities are therefore less than normal. To compensate, the work of breathing is minimized (p. 445) by V_T becoming shallower and the frequency of breathing more rapid—such a pattern also maintains the product of the two, i.e. ventilation, close to normal. In **obstructive lung diseases**, like **asthma** (where the airways are narrowed by bronchoconstriction), **chronic bronchitis** (where plugs of mucus and inflammatory swelling of the bronchial mucosa obstruct the airways) and **em-**physema, vigorous expiration can raise pleural pressure so much that air is trapped in the alveoli, raising the RV and hence the FRC. There is little change in IRV but the ERV and VC are often reduced. In emphysema these volume changes are greater because destruction of alveolar tissue leads to loss of elastic recoil and the loss of radial traction this provides. The latter normally keeps small airways patent (p. 442). To compensate, V_T may be deeper and breathing frequency slower.

Lung-related pressures

Air enters and leaves the lungs by flowing down pressure gradients between the mouth and the alveoli. The required changes in alveolar pressure are created by outwards and inwards movements of the chest, which at the same time cause changes in pleural pressure. When the gas is stationary, the alveolar pressure is the same as at the mouth (atmospheric). Whether air is flowing (a dynamic event) or not (a static event), the pleural pressure is affected by the inward elastic recoil of the lungs and, at volumes below ~4 L, by the outward elastic recoil of the chest. The recoil of lungs and chest in opposite directions creates a negative pressure in the pleural space (–5 cmH$_2$O at FRC). The recoil forces are dependent on the degree of inflation. To examine these correctly, transmural pressures should be considered—the most important being the transpulmonary pressure (alveolar pressure minus pleural pressure).

There are four pressures related to breathing (Fig. 18.7a)—**mouth pressure** (P_{mo}), **body surface pressure** (P_{bs}, which is atmospheric unless in a pressure suit), intrapulmonary or **alveolar pressure** (P_{alv}) and intrapleural or **pleural pressure** (P_{pl}). (Cardiovascular physiologists also refer to pleural pressure as intrathoracic pressure.)

The air that enters and leaves the lungs does so by bulk flow down the pressure gradient between the mouth (or nose) and the alveoli—thus the pressure gradient for airflow is $P_{mo} - P_{alv}$. Airflow is a dynamic condition, and the pressure gradient is affected by airflow rate, airway resistance and frictional resistance of lung tissue (p. 441). Changes in P_{alv} required for airflow are created by outwards

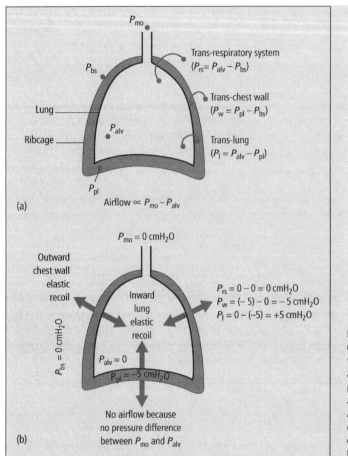

P_{mo}

Trans-respiratory system
($P_{rs} = P_{alv} - P_{bs}$)

P_{bs}

Trans-chest wall
($P_w = P_{pl} - P_{bs}$)

Lung

P_{alv}

Ribcage

Trans-lung
($P_l = P_{alv} - P_{pl}$)

P_{pl}

(a)   Airflow ∝ $P_{mo} - P_{alv}$

$P_{mo} = 0$ cmH$_2$O

Outward
chest wall
elastic
recoil

Inward
lung
elastic
recoil

$P_{rs} = 0 - 0 = 0$ cmH$_2$O
$P_w = (-5) - 0 = -5$ cmH$_2$O
$P_l = 0 - (-5) = +5$ cmH$_2$O

$P_{bs} = 0$ cmH$_2$O

$P_{alv} = 0$

$P_{pl} = -5$ cmH$_2$O

No airflow because
no pressure difference
between P_{mo} and P_{alv}

(b)

Fig. 18.7 (a) Lung-related pressures (on left: P_{alv}, P_{bs}, P_{mo} and P_{pl}) and transmural pressures (on right: P_{rs}, P_w and P_l). Airflow is dependent on the pressure gradient between the mouth and alveoli. (b) Lung-related pressures at functional residual capacity (FRC) due to outward elastic recoil of the chest and inward elastic recoil of the lungs.

and inwards movement of the chest and are seen also as changes in P_{pl}.

When air is not flowing (a static condition), P_{pl} is a consequence only of the elastic recoil forces resulting from the degree of inflation or deflation of the respiratory system. Such elastic recoil creates pressure differences across the alveolar wall and across the chest wall. The relevant **transmural** pressures ($P_{in} - P_{out}$) are:

1 trans-respiratory system pressure (P_{rs}) between alveoli and the body surface, i.e. $P_{alv} - P_{bs}$;

2 trans-chest wall pressure (P_w) between the pleural space and body surface, i.e. $P_{pl} - P_{bs}$; and

3 trans-lung or transpulmonary pressure (P_l) between alveoli and the pleural space, i.e. $P_{alv} - P_{pl}$.

These transmural pressures are rather small, and are measured with water manometers and expressed in cmH$_2$O rather than mmHg (1 cmH$_2$O = 0.76 mmHg).

Pressures at FRC

A **static** condition of no airflow occurs naturally at the end of a normal expiration at rest, i.e. at FRC. As no air is flowing, P_{mo} and P_{alv} are at the same pressure (atmospheric pressure, which on a standard day is 760 mmHg, but is used as a reference of zero pressure). At FRC P_{pl} is negative at about −5 cmH$_2$O (Fig. 18.7b). This **subatmospheric** pressure arises from **elastic recoil** of the lungs and chest wall in opposite directions; the lungs recoil inwards and the chest recoils outwards. The two surfaces do not normally separate as they are held together by the cohesive action of the film of liquid in the pleural space. In this static condition at FRC:

$$P_l = +5\,cmH_2O \text{ (i.e. } P_{alv} - P_{pl} = 0 - (-5)\text{)};$$
$$P_w = -5\,cmH_2O \text{ (i.e. } P_{pl} - P_{bs} = (-5) - 0\text{)}; \text{ and}$$
$$P_{rs} = 0\,cmH_2O \text{ (i.e. } P_{alv} - P_{bs} = 0 - 0\text{)}.$$

This zero pressure for P_{rs} indicates that at FRC the whole respiratory system is at its elastic equilibrium. Note also that at any lung volume, if there is no airflow, $P_w = -P_l$. Furthermore pressures, in contrast to volumes, are independent of body size.

P_{pl} of $-5\,cmH_2O$ is an average value for a person in an upright posture. The weight of the lungs causes them to pull away from the thorax more at the apex (top) than at the base of the lung. Thus, when the trunk is upright, the P_{pl} is $-10\,cmH_2O$ at the apex and $-2.5\,cmH_2O$ at the base of the lung (1 cm of vertical height progressing down the lungs equals a P_{pl} of about $+0.2\,cmH_2O$).

Elastic properties of the respiratory system

The elastic recoil produced by the lungs alone, chest alone and lungs plus chest are estimated from volume and pressure measurements made when respiratory muscles are voluntarily relaxed and the volume prevented from escaping by occlusion of the mouth. The elastic recoil force of lungs plus chest is given by the pressure at the mouth, that for the chest alone by the pleural pressure and that for the lungs alone by the transpulmonary pressure (mouth pressure minus pleural pressure). The ease with which each structure stretches (compliance) is measured as the change in volume/change in pressure. Disease rarely affects chest wall compliance but diseased lungs can become either stiff or floppy. Elastic recoil is expressed as the elastance, which is the reciprocal of compliance (i.e. change in pressure/change in volume). Only a quarter to a third of the lungs' elastic recoil is caused by the elastic fibres of its alveolar walls; most is caused by surface tension at the alveolar tissue–gas interface.

Static pressure–volume relationships

Elastic properties of the lungs and chest wall, individually and when operating together (i.e. the respiratory system as a whole), are examined by determining pressures over the entire range of volumes that the lung can contain (Fig. 18.8).

These pressure and volume measurements must be made at different degrees of deflation and inflation at moments when breathing movements are voluntarily stopped, i.e. no air is flowing in or out (static conditions). At each step a spirometer tube attached to the mouth is occluded and, without closing the glottis, the thoracic muscles are then **relaxed**. Measurements are made of the volume by the spirometer, and P_{pl} either by a catheter placed in the pleural space or, more simply, by one inserted via the nose into the lower third of the oesophagus. As this part of the oesophagus is in the intrathoracic compartment, its pressure reflects that of the pleural space provided that there are no oesophageal contractions. P_{alv} is technically impossible to measure because of the tiny size of the alveoli—under static conditions, however, it equals P_{mo} because no air is flowing. P_{bs} is atmospheric at all times.

P_{mo} is a measure of the **elastic recoil** of the **lungs and thorax in combination**. In this artificial situation where the airways are not open to the atmosphere, P_{mo} and therefore P_{alv} is negative, zero or positive depending on the lung volume as depicted in Fig. 18.8. The respiratory system is at its equilibrium point or resting volume—the FRC—when the P_{mo} it produces is zero. At volumes above this, P_{mo} is positive as the system attempts to collapse and recoil inwards, and at volumes below FRC it is negative as the elastic recoil forces are now directed outwards (Fig. 18.8).

The **elastic recoil force** of the **thorax** alone is estimated from P_{pl} since the P_w equals $P_{pl} - P_{bs}$ and $P_{bs} = 0$. The equilibrium position for the thorax occurs at a volume of about 4 L; at volumes above and below 4 L, P_{pl} is positive (from inward recoil forces) and negative (from outward recoil forces;

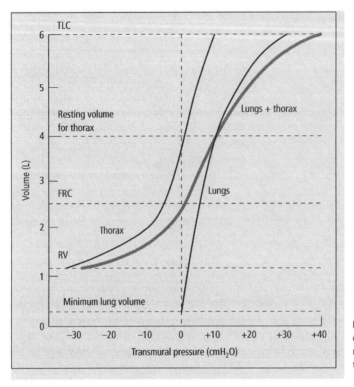

Fig. 18.8 Relaxation pressure volume curves for the thorax, lungs and the respiratory system as a whole (lungs + thorax).

Fig. 18.8), respectively. Since the pleural film binds the chest to the lungs, the chest is at the same volume as the lungs and vice versa. At FRC (2.5 L) this volume is much smaller than the equilibrium volume of the chest and thus the outwards recoil force of the chest creates a subatmospheric pressure of $-5\,cmH_2O$ in the pleural space.

The **elastic recoil force** of the **lungs** alone is represented by P_l, that is $P_{alv} - P_{pl}$ or, in this case, $P_{mo} - P_{pl}$. At all volumes the elastic recoil force of the lungs is inwards so that P_l is always positive. By extrapolation (as in Fig. 18.8) the equilibrium position (zero pressure) for the lungs occurs close to zero volume (the minimal volume of ~200 mL) which can only be achieved if the RV is expelled (as can happen in a pneumothorax). At FRC the lungs' inward recoil force (P_l) is $+5\,cmH_2O$. Since the chest recoil force (P_{pl}) at FRC is equal but opposite ($-5\,cmH_2O$) to the lung recoil force, the respiratory system as a whole is at equilibrium (P_{alv} or $P_{mo} = 0$).

When a person lies down, the chest's outward recoil force, and therefore that of the total respiratory system, is less because gravity is no longer pulling the abdominal contents away from the diaphragm. As a consequence the equilibrium point is at a lower FRC (at a P_{pl} and P_l of about -4 and $+4\,cmH_2O$, respectively).

Compliance and elastance

The ease with which an organ can be stretched is called its **compliance**. It is defined as the change in volume per unit change in pressure ($\Delta V/\Delta P$) and the more compliant an organ, the greater the volume achieved for a particular pressure change. Compliance can be measured for respiratory organs from static pressure–volume curves, usually from the steepest portions, which occur around FRC. At high volumes near TLC the inelastic elements limit the degree of stretch and thus the curves in Fig. 18.8 flatten near TLC and the compliances become very low. The compliance of healthy adult lungs around FRC is about 0.2 L cmH$_2$O^{-1}. The slope of the thorax curve around FRC is similar to that of the lung curve (Fig. 18.8) so that chest compliance is also about 0.2 L cmH$_2$O^{-1}. For the respiratory system as a whole, its slope in Fig. 18.8, and therefore its compliance, is much less (about 0.1 L cmH$_2$O^{-1}). This is because the lungs and thorax are in series with each other and their compliances, like electrical conductances are summed as reciprocals.

Because lung volumes but not lung pressures vary with body size, compliance values, as measured above, will be large in an adult compared with a small child. Measurements can be standardized by expressing them relative to the subject's FRC (i.e. $\Delta V / \Delta P$/FRC)—this is called **specific compliance**. If the FRC is 2.5 L and lung compliance is 0.2 L cmH$_2$O^{-1}, then the specific lung compliance is 0.08 cmH$_2$O^{-1} and in health this value would be similar for mammals of all sizes.

Changes in chest wall compliance are uncommon; however, lung compliance is altered by various **lung diseases**. In diseases associated with increased fibrous tissue in the alveoli (**pulmonary fibrosis**, an example of a restrictive lung disease), the lung becomes stiff—its compliance decreases. The stiffer lung requires a greater transpulmonary and therefore greater pleural pressure to achieve the same inspired volume as a normal lung; thus the inspiratory muscles have to work harder. In diseases where there is destruction of alveolar tissue creating alveoli with large air spaces (as in **emphysema**), only small pressure changes are required to inflate the very compliant lungs. However, an increased compliance is not an advantage because much of expiration is usually produced by passive **elastic recoil**—in these floppy lungs there is little recoil. More expiratory muscle activity is self-defeating as airways collapse in the absence of radial traction (p. 442).

The elastic properties of the lung, as with blood vessels (p. 377), can be described by the **elastic resistance** or **elastance** ($\Delta V / \Delta P$), the reciprocal of the compliance. The elastance of the lungs and chest

separately are both 5 cmH$_2$O L^{-1} and, as the lungs and chest are in series, their elastances, like electrical resistances, are additive and the combined elastance is thus 10 cmH$_2$O L^{-1}.

The elastic resistance of the lung is due to two components. About a quarter to a third results from the **elastin fibres** in the alveolar interstitium; the remainder results from the **surface tension** at the interface between the gas in the alveoli and the liquid surface of the alveolar wall. (The interface is variously called the gas–liquid or air–tissue or alveolar interface.)

The magnitude of these two components can be demonstrated by pressure–volume curves determined in lungs removed from the body which are either gas-filled or liquid-filled (Fig. 18.9). The elastance of the gas-filled lung (5 cmH$_2$O L^{-1}) will be similar to that of the lung adhering to the thorax (provided that it has not been deflated below RV). When all the gas in the alveoli is experimentally replaced with liquid (saline), there is no surface tension because there is no longer a gas–liquid interface. Thus the elastance of the liquid-filled lungs is only 1.25 cmH$_2$O L^{-1}—a measure now only

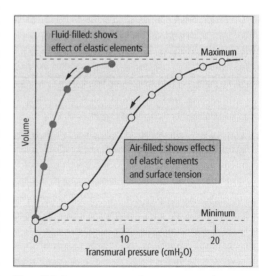

Fig. 18.9 Lung pressure–volume curves when gas-filled and liquid-filled, constructed during deflation of the lung.

of the elastic resistance of the interstitial elastin fibres.

Alveolar surface tension and surfactant

According to the law of Laplace, the alveolar surface tension for a particular alveolar radius must be opposed by an appropriate transmural pressure— the transpulmonary pressure. If the fluid lining the alveoli was purely interstitial fluid, the transmural pressure required for even moderate inflation would be enormous. However, the surface tension is lowered considerably by surfactant secreted by the alveolar type II cells. Furthermore, surfactant lowers surface tension to a greater degree when it is aggregated into a smaller surface area; this permits small alveoli, at the same transmural pressure as nearby larger alveoli, to remain stable and not to empty into the larger ones. Alveolar stability is also achieved by mechanical support from the surrounding alveoli. Surfactant, by reducing the transmural pressure, also prevents the alveolar gas space from filling up with fluid ultrafiltered from the lung capillaries. Breathing is periodically interrupted by the large inflation of a sigh, which serves to replenish some of the surfactant molecules and restore lung compliance to normal.

Surface tension at a gas–liquid interface is inversely proportional to the radius of curvature. The smaller the radius of a spherical alveolus, the greater the transmural pressure ($P_{in} - P_{out}$, i.e. $P_{alv} - P_{pl}$, which is the same as transpulmonary pressure) required to oppose the surface tension. This relationship between surface tension (T), transmural pressure (P_t) and radius (r) is described by the law of Laplace (p. 378) as $P_t = 2T/r$ in which the thickness (u) component has been omitted because the alveolar wall is so thin.

Reduction of surface tension by surfactant

If the liquid lining the alveoli was pure interstitial fluid, the surface tension would be very high, creating a P_{pl} as great as $-30\,cmH_2O$, even at FRC. The alveolar fluid contains a substance called **surfactant**, which has detergent-like properties and substantially lowers the surface tension to

about one-sixth. Surfactant is a mixture of phospholipids (mainly desaturated phosphatidylcholine) secreted by the alveolar type II epithelial cells. Surfactant secretion is stimulated by alveolar expansion and β-adrenergic mechanisms; turnover is very rapid, with a half-life of about 2 h.

The surface tension of interstitial fluid is ~70 dyn cm^{-1} (0.07 N m^{-1}), and with an alveolar radius of ~50 μm at FRC, the transmural pressure without surfactant would be $2 \times 70/0.005 = 28\,000$ dyn cm^{-1} (28 N m^{-1}), which is 28 cmH_2O. As the inside pressure P_{alv} is zero, the outside pressure P_{alv} is therefore $-28\,cmH_2O$. However, because of surfactant, the alveolar surface tension (at FRC) is ~12 dyn cm^{-1} and thus the P_{pl} is actually $-5\,cmH_2O$.

In the human fetus surfactant secretion by the type II alveolar cells is not established until the 30th week; thus premature babies are deficient in lung surfactant (**newborn respiratory distress syndrome**). Without surfactant the premature lungs have such a high surface tension that a lot of inspiratory effort is needed to generate enough negative P_{pl} even to inflate the lungs a little. As soon as inspiratory efforts stop, the high elastance of the lungs causes them to recoil very rapidly to very low volumes. Factors reducing production of surfactant or increasing its rate of destruction may contribute to **adult respiratory distress syndrome**.

Alveolar stability

In any one part of the lung the alveoli are unlikely to be exactly the same size and yet they will all be subjected at any one moment to the same transmural pressure. Imagine one larger and one smaller alveolus in the same alveolar sac or interconnected by an airway. If the surface tension of the two alveoli were the same, then the law of Laplace ($P_t = 2T/r$) would indicate that the small alveolus would require a larger P_t than the large alveolus to keep it open. The smaller alveolus would therefore be unstable and empty into the larger. Because the surface tension in the small alveolus reduces virtually in proportion to the reduction in its radius, its required P_t is the same as

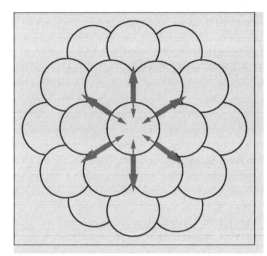

Fig. 18.10 Stability of alveoli produced by mechanical interaction with neighbouring alveoli.

for the larger alveolus and thus the small alveoli do not collapse.

A second and more important factor contributes to alveolar stability. This is the mechanical interaction conferred by the geometry of adjacent alveoli (Fig. 18.10). Any alveolus tending to collapse will be liable to pull away from its neighbours, but at the same time will be held open by its attachment to them. This mechanical interaction is termed **alveolar interdependence**.

Reduction of ultrafiltration by surfactant

Surfactant not only lowers the overall alveolar surface tension and confers alveolar stability, but it also assists in preventing the air spaces of the alveoli from filling up with liquid. As the alveolar walls contain a massive network of capillaries, the forces causing ultrafiltration and reabsorption of liquid across the capillary wall (Starling equilibrium; p. 393) have to be considered. Surfactant, by lowering the pleural pressure, decreases the hydrostatic pressure gradient and therefore reduces the amount of fluid ultrafiltered.

In systemic capillaries the hydrostatic pressures in the plasma and interstitial fluid on average are 24 and −2 mmHg, respectively, and their colloid osmotic pressures are 25 and 0 mmHg, so that ultrafiltration forces (Δ26 mmHg) are slightly in excess of reabsorption forces (Δ25 mmHg). The colloid osmotic pressures, and therefore reabsorption forces, are the same for the pulmonary capillaries; the hydrostatic ultrafiltration forces are, however, different. Pulmonary capillary pressure is low (10 mmHg; p. 410) and interstitial pressure is effectively that of the pleural space (at FRC this is −5 cmH$_2$O or −4 mmHg) so the ultrafiltration force (Δ14 mmHg) is considerably less than the reabsorption force (Δ25 mmHg) and the lungs remain dry. Only when pleural pressures reach −16 mmHg (−21 cmH$_2$O), during, for example, large inflations, will there be net ultrafiltration. The pulmonary circulation has a very extensive lymphatic network to prevent any permanent fluid accumulation. If surfactant was not present, the pleural pressure even at FRC would be −30 cmH$_2$O (−23 mmHg) and the ultrafiltration force (Δ33 mmHg) would be well in excess of reabsorption and the alveolar air spaces would be flooded with liquid.

Sighs and surfactant

A **sigh** is a reflexly generated (p. 483) single deep breath that occurs after a period of quiet breathing. Quiet breathing around FRC does not cause much breath-by-breath alteration in the alveolar surface area and, as a consequence, in the tightly compressed surface film the surfactant molecules are gradually squeezed away from the surface. The progressive lowering of surfactant concentration at the surface layer causes the surface tension to rise gradually so that the lung has more elastic resistance or, expressed another way, becomes less compliant. The purpose of the large inflation, which stretches and unfolds the alveolar surface area, is to spread out the surfactant molecules, allowing newly released molecules to come to the surface. After the sigh, when breathing is back at volumes near FRC, these extra molecules return the alveolar surface tension to its usual ~12 dyn cm^{-1}.

Hysteresis

Most textbooks place undue emphasis on the

phenomenon of a **hysteresis** loop present in the tension–area relationship of a surface film of surfactant (Fig. 18.11a) or in the pressure–volume relationship determined in an air-filled, but not a liquid-filled, isolated lung (Fig. 18.11b). Hysteresis is the term used to describe the fact that a particular area during expansion results in a higher surface tension than during compression; similarly, attaining any particular volume during inflation requires a larger pressure than during deflation. In the case of tension–area measurements, the hysteresis is greater the more it is compressed/expanded to its limits and is thought to be due to the time it takes even in these step-by-step (i.e. static) measurements for surfactant molecules to realign themselves at the changing surface area of the interface. In the case of the static pressure–volume relationship, hysteresis is only seen if the lungs are first deflated to their minimum volume. In other words, a collapsed lung does not significantly inflate until a fairly large transmural pressure, the critical opening pressure (~8 cmH₂O), is reached. The hysteresis is very small for volume changes between RV and TLC and virtually negligible for the normal tidal volume occurring at FRC; this hysteresis is caused by surfactant.

Resistance to airflow

The resistance to airflow in and out of the lungs is due mainly to friction in the airways with a very small contribution from friction within the lung tissue. Airway resistance is determined by the viscosity of air and the radii of the airways (Poiseuille equation). As the airways branch extensively in a parallel manner, the total resistance is very small and an alveolar-to-mouth pressure gradient of 1 cmH₂O is sufficient to cause airflow. The major sites of airway resistance are the upper respiratory tract and the medium-sized bronchi. Airways not supported by cartilage can have their calibre enlarged by the radial traction, which results from an increased lung volume, producing more alveolar elastic recoil. Conversely, they can be compressed to the point of collapse during forced expirations. Contraction of smooth muscle in the airway walls also produces changes in calibre. Bronchoconstriction is caused by parasympathetic activity and by local release of chemicals like histamine; bronchodilation results from activation of smooth muscle β₂-receptors by substances like adrenaline. Mucus secretion into the airway lumen can also increase airway resistance. Airway resistance is

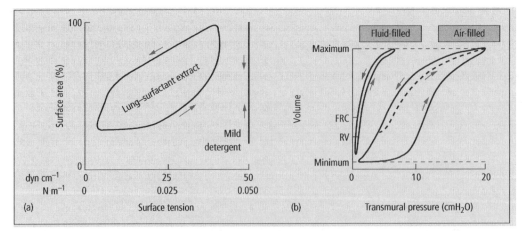

Fig. 18.11 (a) Surface tension–surface area curves for lung fluid extract compared with a mild detergent. (b) Inflation and deflation pressure–volume curves in air-filled and fluid-filled lungs. Note that there is virtually no hysteresis in the fluid-filled lung and little hysteresis if inflation starts at RV or FRC.

assessed by measuring the expiratory forced vital capacity (FVC), the volume so expired in the first second (FEV_1), the forced expiratory flow rate (FEF), the peak flow rate and the width of a dynamic pressure–volume loop.

Airflow into the lungs requires a pressure gradient between the atmosphere (i.e. the nose or mouth; P_{mo}) and the alveoli (P_{alv}). For a particular pressure gradient (ΔP), the magnitude of the airflow (volume/unit of time, $\dot{V}$) depends mainly on the frictional resistance (R) encountered in the airways, as described by the Poiseuille equation where $\dot{V} = \Delta P/R$ and $R = 8\eta l/\pi r^4$ (p. 373). P_{mo} is normally zero and for a 500 mL V_T typical of quiet breathing where airflow rises to about $0.5\,Ls^{-1}$, P_{alv} reaches about $-1\,cmH_2O$ during inspiration, sucking gas into the alveoli, and about $+1\,cmH_2O$ during expiration, pushing gas out of the alveoli. These pressure gradients for airflow are tiny, particularly when compared with those for blood flow, because air has a much lower viscosity (η) than blood and flows through tubes that are much wider. Airflow resistance for quiet breathing is typically about 2 $cmH_2O\,s\,L^{-1}$, i.e. $(\Delta 1\,cmH_2O)/(0.5\,L\,s^{-1})$.

Airway resistance accounts for 80–90% of the resistance to airflow. The other factors that contribute are the inertia to movement of the respiratory system and the frictional (viscous) resistance encountered at the lung–chest wall surface and within the chest and lung tissues as the elements move against each other. All are negligible except for the frictional resistance of lung tissue, which in health causes only 10–20% of the airflow resistance. Lung tissue resistance can increase in such conditions as pulmonary fibrosis. The airway resistance plus the lung tissue resistance are often referred to as the **pulmonary resistance**—both are non-elastic resistances. Inertia becomes appreciable only during rapid respiratory actions like sneezing and coughing.

Distribution of airway resistance

During wakefulness about 40–50% of airway resistance is found in the upper respiratory tract (nasal passages, pharynx and larynx) and this resistance is significantly reduced when one switches from nose to mouth breathing—this commonly occurs during the high airflow of exercise. Most techniques used for measuring breathing impose mouth breathing and therefore do not include the consequences of nasal resistances. Narrowing of the glottis during expiration increases laryngeal resistance and, as mentioned earlier, is part of the expiratory braking mechanism. During sleep the resistance in the upper respiratory tract is increased; in patients with obstructive sleep apnoea this can lead to complete cessation of airflow due to occlusion of the pharynx (p. 489).

Below the larynx most of the resistance resides, not in the bronchioles, but in the trachea and bronchi down to about the seventh generation. Although the highest individual resistance is indeed to be found in the bronchiole with the smallest radius, the branching of the bronchial tree creates an enormous number of parallel tubes, the resistances of which add as reciprocals (p. 374) so that the total resistance is low. Thus, beyond the segmental bronchi, the airway resistance correspondingly falls as the total cross-sectional area of the airways progressively increases with each successive generation of branching towards the alveoli. The medium-sized bronchi (2–4 mm in diameter) around the fourth generation are normally the site of greatest resistance. The resistance of the airways beyond the 15th generation is virtually zero. Those pulmonary disorders, which reduce the calibre of small airways, are difficult to detect by measures of airway resistance as they contribute such a small proportion of the resistance.

Effect of lung volume on airway calibre and resistance

The pressure inside the airways is either zero or, when air is flowing, graded from mouth to alveoli; the pressure outside the airway wall (the pleural pressure) is caused by elastic recoil of the alveoli. Thus, larger lung volumes, by producing more elastic recoil, increase the transmural pressure ($P_{in} - P_{out}$) across the airway wall and, in those airways not stiffened by cartilage, the calibre of their lumen enlarges and so the resistance to airflow falls. (Contraction of airway smooth muscle can help stiffen the airway wall.) In effect, airways are supported and pulled outwards by the elastic recoil of the alveolar tissue surrounding them—an action referred to as **radial traction**. At small lung volumes, airway transmural pressure is low, the radial traction is less and the airways become narrower and hence airflow resistance increases. The greatest changes in resistance in fact occur at low volumes—those between FRC and RV.

In obstructive lung diseases breathing occurs at a higher FRC and, in asthma, where alveolar tissue is normal, this provides more radial traction in an attempt to open up the constricted airways a little. When the elastic recoil is reduced by destruction of alveolar tissue, as in emphysema, the airways are actually narrower not because the disease has affected the airway structure but because some of the radial traction has been lost.

Below FRC the increase in airway resistance can be dramatically exaggerated by collapse of airways not supported by cartilage. To expel air and reach volumes below FRC requires expiratory muscle contraction, which, if done forcefully and rapidly, generates positive pleural pressures (as high as $+100\,cmH_2O$). This positive pressure surrounding the airways is uniform along its length but in the lumen of the airway, pressure will fall from positive values at the alveolar end to zero at the mouth, so that at some point along the airway the positive pressure outside will exceed that inside. Depending on the pressure difference and the extent of cartilaginous support, the airway at this point will be compressed and possibly collapsed. This **dynamic airway compression** or collapse limits the maximum rates of expiratory flow. The lung volume at which airway collapse occurs during forced expirations after a maximum inspiration is called the **closing volume**. In young healthy adults the closing volume occurs just before RV is reached but with ageing it occurs at volumes just above FRC. In emphysema where there is less radial traction, or in obstructive lung disease where airways are already narrow, dynamic airway compression occurs not only at lung volumes above FRC but also with only mild expiratory muscle effort. The wheezing noise during such expirations is due to vibration of the collapsed airways and the turbulent flow.

Effect of bronchial smooth muscle on airway resistance

Smooth muscle in all of the airways (trachea to alveolar duct) is under the control of the autonomic nervous system but since the medium-sized bronchi are the major site of airway resistance, it is control of their smooth muscle tone that physiologically alters airway resistance—hence the term **bronchomotor control**.

Bronchoconstriction is produced in a number of ways.

1 It is caused by increased activity in vagal **parasympathetic** fibres (via their postganglionic cholinergic fibres). The parasympathetic contribution to the resting bronchomotor tone can be abolished by atropine (an antagonist of muscarinic acetylcholine receptors) and as a result there is a 30% reduction in airways resistance. Parasympathetically mediated bronchoconstriction occurs as a reflex effect of stimulating irritant and cough receptors in the airways (p. 483)—the bronchoconstriction both limits the entry of the irritant and increases expiratory airflow velocity to dislodge and expel the irritant. Parasympathetic activity also **increases mucus secretion** into the airways, which in itself decreases the calibre of the airways.

2 Substantial bronchoconstriction and mucus secretion can also be caused directly by **local chemical mediators** such as histamine and leukotrienes released from mast cells in the airways, for example, during allergic **asthma** attacks.

3 The calibre of very small airways close to the alveoli is also dependent on CO_2 **levels**. If parts of the lung become overventilated, there is a decrease in local airway CO_2 that has a direct effect on the smooth muscle, causing local airway constriction and subsequently reduction in the ventilation of nearby alveoli. The significance of this mechanism is explained on p. 463.

Relaxation of bronchial smooth muscle (**bronchodilation**) results from activation of β_2-

adrenoceptors by circulating adrenaline or therapeutically administered sympathomimetics (e.g. isoprenaline and salbutamol). In humans few of these β_2-receptors are activated by transmitter release from sympathetic nerves. In addition bronchodilation can be produced by a **non-adrenergic non-cholinergic** innervation of the bronchial smooth muscle in which vasoactive intestinal polypeptide may be the neurotransmitter. A second type of peptidergic innervation, releasing the neurotransmitter substance P and other neurokinins, is also present—it appears to be involved in the bronchoconstrictions accompanying bronchospasm. Mucus secretion into the airways is mainly under vagal cholinergic control and its volume and composition are modulated by sympathetic (α and β adrenergic) and peptidergic mechanisms, and by inflammatory mediators.

Forced expiratory assessment of airway resistance

As the direct measurement of resistance from $P_{mo} - P_{alv}$ and $\dot{V}$ is difficult, airway resistance is usually assessed indirectly, either from the width of the dynamic pressure–volume loop (p. 445) or from a forced expiration into a spirometer where expiration is preceded by a maximal inspiration (Fig. 18.12). The volume exhaled is the **forced vital capacity** (FVC) and even in health it is a little smaller than VC (measured without forceful breathing) because expiratory forces compress the small airways (p. 442). In obstructive diseases airflow is retarded by narrow airways, causing FVC to be quite a lot smaller than the VC. Loss of radial traction resulting in more small airway compression in emphysema exaggerates this difference further.

Forced expired volume in the first second (**FEV$_1$**) is a more sensitive measure of changes in airway resistance—in health it is about 80% of the FVC. In obstructive disease the **FEV$_1$/FVC ratio** is less than 80% as the decrease in FEV$_1$ is greater than the decrease in FVC. In restrictive diseases, where all lung volumes are smaller (p. 433), both FVC and FEV$_1$ will be smaller but their ratio does not decrease; if anything, it may increase.

As shown in Fig. 18.12, a similar indicator of airway resistance is **forced expiratory flow rate** (**FEF**)—also called the maximal mid-expiratory flow rate. This is simply the slope ($\Delta V/\Delta time$) of a straight line drawn between volumes at 25% and

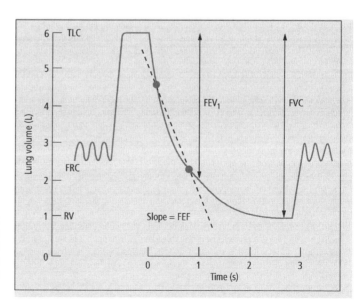

Fig. 18.12 Measurement from a spirometer of the volume expired in the first second (FEV$_1$), the forced vital capacity (FVC) and forced expiratory flow rate (FEF). RV, residual volume; TLC, total lung capacity.

75% of FVC on the expiratory curve. The fastest rate of airflow occurs soon after the beginning of a forced expiration and this is measured by expiring rapidly and forcefully into a peak flow meter. For a 70-kg healthy male, the typical peak expiratory flow rate is ~600 L min^{-1}.

Pressure and volume during the breathing cycle

Pleural pressure during the breathing cycle is the consequence of two forces, one due to elastic recoil, which is proportional to the degree of inflation, and the other due to the negative (inspiration) and positive (expiration) alveolar pressures generated to overcome the resistance to airflow. As air is flowing, the pressure–volume relationship is referred to as dynamic and is seen to be a loop. The width of the loop is an estimate of airflow resistance. The slope of the line drawn between the points of minimum and maximum volume of the breath, when airflow is zero, measures the elastic recoil, i.e. lung compliance. The area enclosed by the loop is a measure of the work of breathing (costing for a normal breath at rest only about 5% of the body's total O_2 consumption). With slow deep breaths most of the extra work is against the elasticity of the alveoli, while with rapid shallow breaths most of the extra work is against the airway resistance. Maximal respiratory muscle forces can be estimated from the mouth pressures generated during maximal inspiratory (Müller's manoeuvre) or expiratory (Valsalva's manoeuvre) effort against an obstructed mouth.

During the **dynamic** event of air moving, P_{pl} is the consequence of two forces. The first is the elastic recoil of the lungs alone, as already described for static conditions in Fig. 18.8. The second is the additional dynamic pressure required to overcome the resistance to airflow; this is the negative P_{alv} of inspiration (-1 cmH$_2$O for a V_T of 500 mL) created by inspiratory muscle contraction, and the positive P_{alv} of expiration ($+1$ cmH$_2$O) from recoil of lung tissue compressing the alveoli. (During deeper or more forceful breathing, expiratory muscle contraction will contribute to the compression of alveoli.) The apportioning of P_{pl} to its compo-

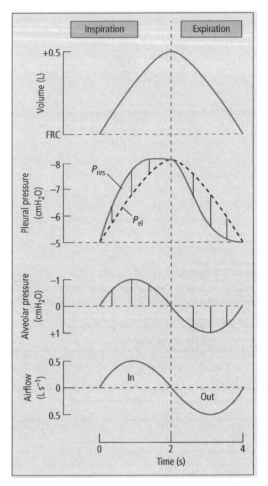

Fig. 18.13 Pressures and volume during the breathing cycle. P_{el}, pressure due to elastic recoil; P_{res}, pressure required to overcome airway resistance and cause airflow.

nents of elastic recoil (P_{el}) and airway resistance (P_{res}) at different moments during inspiration and expiration is portrayed in Fig. 18.13.

When interpreting this diagram, note that:

1 as P_{el} is dependent on lung volume, the time-based shapes of these graphs are identical;

2 there is a brief moment of zero flow whenever airflow reverses direction, i.e. at the transition between inspiration and expiration and vice versa;

3 inward airflow reaches its peak near mid-inspiration and outward airflow peaks near mid-expiration at about 0.5 L s^{-1};

4 given that mouth pressure is zero, P_{alv} is also the measure of P_{res} and its time-based shape is identical to that of the airflow it permits;

5 P_{pl} during dynamic breathing is due to the combined effect of P_{el} and P_{res}; and

6 P_{pl} at the beginning of inspiration (i.e. at FRC) is $-5\,cmH_2O$ and at the end of a 500-mL breath in is $-8\,cmH_2O$ (which in mmHg is -3 and -5, respectively).

In reality the duration of inspiration is shorter than expiration and airflow rates are somewhat greater than depicted, especially in inspiration, and occur earlier in each breathing phase. Airflow also increases whenever the same tidal volume is shifted in a shorter time or with larger tidal volumes (although a large volume taken over a longer time could leave the flow rate unchanged). As faster breathing usually accompanies deeper breaths, airflow rates can reach values in excess of 6 Ls^{-1} with a P_{alv} of $+12\,cmH_2O$ in expiration and $-12\,cmH_2O$ in inspiration. Even for 500-mL breaths, P_{alv} can be greater or smaller than 1 cmH_2O if the airways are bronchoconstricted or bronchodilated, respectively. A maximal forced inspiratory effort can produce a P_{pl} as low as $-80\,cmH_2O$ at peak inspiratory flow rates; for maximal forced expiratory efforts P_{pl} can be as high as $+100\,cmH_2O$.

Dynamic pressure–volume relationship

Figure 18.13 illustrates the time course of the volume and P_{pl} changes during one breath cycle. If for each moment the volume is now plotted against the P_{pl} (Fig. 18.14), the curve for expiration (CFA) does not follow the same path as for inspiration (ABC) and a loop results in which, at any particular volume, P_{pl} in expiration is less negative than in inspiration except at the end of inspiration (C) and end of expiration (A). If that part of the P_{pl} that is due only to P_{el} is plotted against volume, a single straight line results for both inspiration and expiration (AC). The slope of this line ($\Delta V/\Delta P$) is identical to that determined under static conditions for the lung alone (Fig. 18.8) and it is of course the measure of **lung compliance**. As the breathing manoeuvres required for static conditions are often difficult for the subject to achieve, lung compliance is usually measured quickly and simply by drawing a straight line between points A and C determined during dynamic conditions—in fact A and C represent static conditions because airflow at these points has ceased momentarily.

The **inspiratory–expiratory loop** (Fig. 18.14) is often called a hysteresis loop; very little, if any, hysteresis is due to tissue resistance (p. 440) or surfactant, the effect of which is only evident when preceded by deflation to near-zero volume (p. 440). The hysteresis in Fig. 18.14 is due almost entirely to airway resistance and the need to generate negative and positive P_{alv} in inspiration and expiration (Fig. 18.14). Thus, P_{pl} is more negative in inspiration and less negative in expiration than the elastic recoil depicted by line AC. The width of the loop (measured in cmH_2O at its widest point parallel to the pressure axis) indicates the magnitude of **airway resistance**—a true measure ($cmH_2O\,s\,L^{-1}$) requires flow rate to be measured too (p. 441). When airway resistance increases, e.g. during the bronchoconstriction of asthma, the loop is much wider (Fig. 18.14b).

Work of breathing

The area of the dynamic pressure–volume loop can be used to estimate the physical work that must be done by the respiratory muscles to overcome the elastic recoil of the lung and the non-elastic resistance of the airways. (Area is the product of pressure ($g\,cm^{-2}$) $\times$ volume (cm^3) and this has the same final dimensions ($g\,cm^{-1}$) as the strict measure of work, which is force $\times$ distance.) The area ABCDA in Fig. 18.14 represents the inspiratory work required to inhale 500 mL (a tidal volume typical of quiet breathing). This inspiratory work is divisible into two parts—that used to oppose the elastic recoil of the lung (AECDA) and that used to overcome airway resistance, allowing inspiratory airflow (ABCEA). Some of the energy used to stretch the elastic elements is stored as elastic energy whereas the rest, including the energy used to overcome the frictional resistance to airflow, is dissipated and lost as heat. During a normal 500-mL expiration no extra energy is required

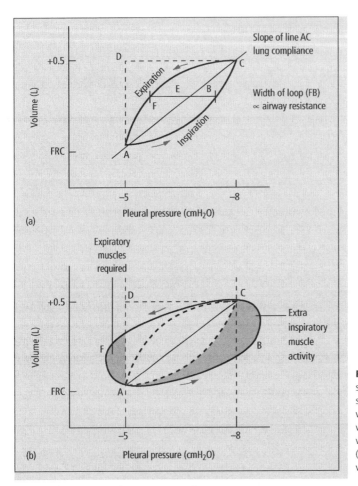

Fig. 18.14 Pressure–volume relationships during dynamic conditions. The slope of AC measures compliance; width of loop (FB) is an estimate of airway resistance; areas of loop indicate work of breathing. (a) Normal lung; (b) during asthma (depicted assuming volume has not increased).

because the elastic energy is released from storage when the lungs are permitted to recoil. This passive elastic recoil finally vanishes as FRC is approached, but on the way was more than sufficient to provide the mechanical work (AECFA) required to overcome the airway resistance encountered by expiratory airflow. (Although not depicted here, expiratory resistance is usually greater than inspiratory due to narrowing of the tracheobronchial tree and glottis.)

Faster breathing rates require higher flow rates and therefore a larger P_{alv}—this will widen both sides of the hysteresis loop and is indicative of the increased work against resistive forces. When just the tidal volume increases, point C in Fig. 18.14a will be at a higher volume and pressure and thus

the work (AECDA) done to overcome the elastic recoil of the lungs will have increased.

When airway resistance increases (e.g. in asthma) lung compliance does not change (Fig. 18.14b), but the wider inspiratory side of the loop indicates the greater inspiratory muscle work now required to overcome the airway resistance, such that the pleural pressure during inspiration at B may even become more negative than at end-inspiration. Similarly, the width of the expiratory side of the loop will be greater and if the pleural pressure at F becomes less than at end-expiration, expiration can no longer be purely passive and the work component to the left of the vertical AD line has to be supplied by expiratory muscle contraction.

Effect of breathing pattern

At a particular level of ventilation the work of breathing depends on the pattern of ventilation — the same ventilation can be achieved by either slow deep breaths or rapid shallow breaths. With slow deep breaths most of the work is against the elasticity of the alveoli (static) while with rapid shallow breaths most of the work is against the resistance to airflow through the airways (dynamic; Fig. 18.15). Large tidal volumes increase the elastic work of breathing to a greater extent than high breathing frequencies increase the resistive work of breathing. Breathing is regulated to a pattern that is the most economical, i.e. produces minimum total work, explaining why at rest breathing frequency is usually about 12–15 breaths per minute. Resistive work for a particular breath pattern increases in obstructive airway diseases so patients breathe more slowly to minimize the extra work of breathing. Elastic work increases in lung diseases that cause stiffer lungs, and therefore to minimize the work patients take smaller breaths more frequently.

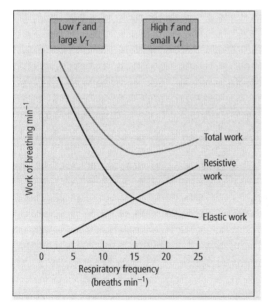

Fig. 18.15 Relationship of work of breathing to breathing frequency (*f*) at a constant level of ventilation. Work is done against elastic resistance and airflow resistance. V_T, tidal volume.

Metabolic cost of breathing

In a healthy person at rest respiratory muscles consume about 5% of the body's total O_2 consumption; this rises to about 30% in maximal voluntary hyperventilation. In lung or chest disease the metabolic cost can be this high even at rest, imposing a severe limitation on the amount of exercise such patients can perform.

Maximal respiratory muscle forces

The full strength of respiratory muscle contraction can be estimated by the maximum alveolar pressures generated during inspiratory and expiratory efforts against a closed glottis or an obstructed mouth. Respiratory muscle weakness can be detected by such measurements. Inspiratory effort (Müller's manoeuvre) at RV gives the greatest negative value (about –120 cmH$_2$O); expiratory effort (Valsalva's manoeuvre, as in straining during defecation) at TLC gives the greatest positive value (about +200 cmH$_2$O). These pressures are those in the alveoli but are measured at the mouth. As the lung's transmural pressure at RV and FRC would be its usual 2 cmH$_2$O and 30 cmH$_2$O, respectively (Fig. 18.8), because this is dependent only on elastic recoil, the pleural pressure in maximum inspiratory and expiratory effort would be –122 cmH$_2$O and +170 cmH$_2$O. The large positive pleural pressures generated in the Valsalva's manoeuvre, while aiding defecation, will compress intrathoracic veins, impeding venous return (p. 399), and may lead to fainting.

18.3 Ventilation, gas exchange, alveolar gases and diffusion

The volume per minute that ventilates the lung is the product of the volume of each tidal breath and their frequency. Of the 500 mL tidal volume breathed in at rest, about two-thirds reaches the alveoli (alveolar volume) and is available for gas exchange; the remaining third is not available because it fills the conducting airways (anatomical dead space) or does not come into contact with alveolar capillaries (alveolar dead space). The latter is very small. The two dead spaces comprise the physiological dead space which is estimated using the Bohr equation. The gases exchanged in the lungs and tissues are O_2 and CO_2 and the ratio of CO_2 production to O_2 consumption is the respiratory exchange ratio (or, at steady state, the respiratory quotient or RQ). The ventilatory requirement and O_2 extraction coefficient indicate how much of the ventilated air is actually utilized. Volumes are usually measured under ATPS (ambient temperature, pressure, saturated with water) conditions, but should be stated in units of BTPS (body temperature, pressure, saturated with water) for ventilation and STPD (standard temperature, pressure, dry (O°C, 760 mmHg)) for gas exchange (see Table 18.1).

Ventilation and its components

In a healthy ~70-kg person at rest, the duration of each breath (total breath time, T_T) is about 4–5 s, of which about one-third is spent inspiring (inspiratory time, T_I) and two-thirds expiring (expiratory time, T_E). The **frequency** of breathing (*f*) ranges from 12 to 15 breaths min^{-1} and the volume of each breath (V_T) from 500 to 600 mL. The product of the two, $f \times V_T$, is the **ventilation** ($\dot{V}_E$) of about 6–7 L min^{-1}. (Note that the dot above the V symbol indicates the volume is expressed per unit of time and the subscripts identify the particular component of the gas phase; see Table 18.1). $\dot{V}_E$ is also referred to as the pulmonary ventilation. The subscript indicates that $\dot{V}_E$ is typically calculated from measurement of an expired (V_E) not an inspired (V_I) tidal volume. Strictly speaking, V_T is the average of V_I and V_E; the latter is slightly smaller because less CO_2 is produced by the body in exchange for the O_2 consumed.

At the end of a 500-mL inspiration, about a third of the breath (~150 mL) fills the conducting airways and is called the **dead space** (V_D)—'dead' because it cannot be used for gas exchange. Approximately 350 mL of the tidal volume has reached the alveoli (the **alveolar volume**, V_A) to mix with the rest of the gas in the alveoli and be available for gas exchange with the blood. As the

volume in the alveoli at the end of expiration is about 2.5 L (the FRC), the V_A adds only 12% more to the volume and thus serves as a source of alveolar gas replenishment rather than replacement. The inspired alveolar volume mixes by diffusion with the gas in the FRC (p. 440). At rest with a V_A of 350 mL and a breathing frequency of 12 min^{-1}, the amount of gas ventilating the alveoli per minute, the **alveolar ventilation** ($\dot{V}_A$), is 4.2 L min^{-1} (*f* × V_A). Similarly, the gas in the airways that is not available for gas exchange is 1.8 L min^{-1} (*f* × V_D)—the **dead-space ventilation** ($\dot{V}_D$).

All these volumes are dependent on gender, age, physical training and body mass—for instance, the larger the person the greater the volume, while in a smaller person the breathing frequency is higher. In severe exercise the values for a 70-kg person can become as great as $f \sim 50\,min^{-1}$, $V_T \sim 3.0\,L$ and $\dot{V}_E \sim 150\,L\,min^{-1}$. As *f* becomes greater, the duration of each breath (T_T) becomes shorter and the times spent inspiring (T_I) and expiring (T_E) become about equal. Note that the maximum V_T of exercise is much smaller than the vital capacity of 5.0 L, which can only be sustained for a few breaths. Although during exercise there is a small increase in V_D (to no more than ~350 mL) due to mainly passive and some active bronchodilation, most of the increased V_T ventilates the alveoli (at least four-fifths in severe exercise compared with two-thirds at rest).

Different breathing patterns have a marked effect on the alveolar ventilation. For instance, deep slow breathing (e.g. $V_T = 1\,L$, $f = 6\,min^{-1}$) still gives a resting $\dot{V}_E$ of 6 L min^{-1} but it is comprised of a $\dot{V}_D$ of 0.9 L min^{-1} (150 mL × 6 min^{-1}) and $\dot{V}_A$ of 5.1 L min^{-1} (850 mL × 6 min^{-1}). Compared with normal breathing, this provides proportionately more ventilation of the alveoli and less wastage per minute in the dead space; however, the work of breathing with such a pattern is costly (p. 445). On the other hand shallow panting (e.g. $V_T = 250\,mL$, $f = 24\,min^{-1}$, $\dot{V}_E = 6\,L\,min^{-1}$) not only has a high energetic cost but it is also very wasteful as it has a $\dot{V}_D$ of 3.6 L min^{-1} (150 mL × 24 min^{-1}) and a $\dot{V}_A$ of only 2.4 L min^{-1} (100 mL × 24 min^{-1}).

Anatomical, alveolar and physiological dead space

V_D comprises not only the volume of the conducting airways (the **anatomical dead space**) but also that part of the alveolar volume (**alveolar dead space**) occupying alveoli that are inadequately perfused with blood and therefore not fully participating in gas exchange. In health the alveolar dead space is less than 5 mL but in various lung diseases it can be larger due to inequalities between alveolar ventilation and blood flow (p. 465). **Physiological dead space** equals anatomical dead space plus alveolar dead space.

The dead space, as well as alveolar volume and the alveolar and dead space ventilations, can be estimated using the **Bohr equation**. The principle behind this equation is that in an expirate the total amount of a gas exhaled equals the amount of that gas coming from both the dead space and the alveoli. The amount of a gas in each compartment = volume (V) of that compartment × fractional composition (F) of the gas concerned; so for CO_2:

$$V_E \times F_E co_2 = V_D \times F_I co_2 + V_A \times F_A co_2$$

This equation can be written either for the volumes (V) of these compartments or for their ventilations (volume/min, $\dot{V}$). Since $F_I co_2$ is virtually zero, the equation simplifies to:

$$V_E \times F_E co_2 = V_A \times F_A co_2 \qquad (18.1)$$

V_E is measured as the volume of a single expirate (or a number of them collected over a known time in a bag), $F_E co_2$ is a gas sample taken from the bag which is a mixture of alveolar and dead-space gases (hence the term mixed-expired) and $F_A co_2$ is a gas sample representing the average alveolar gas value which is obtained about two-thirds of the way through expiration (see Fig. 18.16) or more easily but less accurately at the very end of an expiration (hence the term end-expired or end-tidal). The unknown V_A is calculated and V_D determined knowing:

$$V_E = V_D + V_A \qquad (18.2)$$

When equation (18.2) is substituted into equation (18.1) and rearranged knowing $V_E = V_T$, the equation becomes:

$$V_D = \frac{F_A co_2 - F_E co_2}{F_A co_2} \cdot V_T$$

This is the final format in which the Bohr equation is usually given, but for the beginner it is harder to understand.

Gas exchange

At rest an adult consumes about 250–300 mL min^{-1} of O_2 (the **O_2 consumption**, $\dot{V}o_2$) and produces in exchange about 200–250 mL min^{-1} of CO_2 (the **CO_2 production**, $\dot{V}co_2$). The ratio of CO_2 produced to O_2 consumed, $\dot{V}co_2/\dot{V}o_2$, is called the **respiratory exchange ratio** (R). In steady-state conditions, it is common to use the term **RQ**, which depends entirely on the chemical nature of the combusted food. If the substrates are solely carbohydrates the RQ is 1.0, while for a fuel of protein the RQ is 0.81 and for fat 0.7. Since our tissues oxidize a mixture of these three substrates, the RQ is on average 0.82. The R value is not the same as the RQ value during the transition from one steady state to another—for instance, at the beginning of hyperventilation the excreted CO_2 is greater than that produced metabolically because initially extra CO_2, derived from the large stores in tissue and blood (p. 475), is blown off. Thus, although the RQ may still be 0.82, the R value may have risen to as much as 1.4. An R value lower than 0.82 occurs under conditions where CO_2 stores are being replenished.

Gas consumption or production can be calculated from the difference in the amount of the gas that enters and leaves the lungs per minute. Therefore $\dot{V}_I$ and its gas fraction (e.g. $F_I o_2$) and $\dot{V}_E$ and its gas fraction (e.g. $F_E o_2$) have to be measured. Thus:

$$\dot{V}o_2 = \dot{V} \times F_I o_2 - \dot{V}_E \times F_E o_2$$

and, as $\dot{V}_I$ is virtually the same as $\dot{V}_E$,

$$\dot{V}o_2 = \dot{V}_E (F_I o_2 - F_E o_2)$$

Similarly,

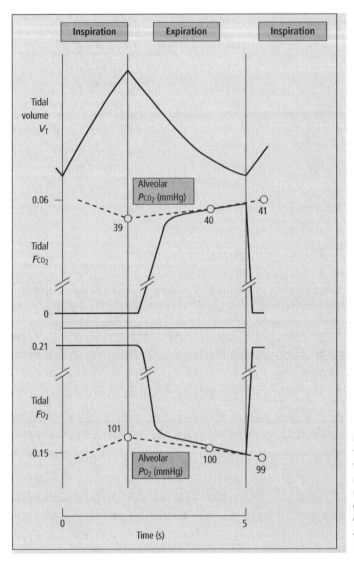

Fig. 18.16 Tidal volume (V_T) and fractions of CO_2 and O_2 measured at the mouth (Fco_2 and Fo_2) during inspiration and expiration. Dashed lines represent the changes in alveolar gas composition (expressed in mmHg) during the breathing cycle. Time axis is for a breathing frequency of $12 \, min^{-1}$.

$$\dot{V}co_2 = \dot{V}_E \times F_Eco_2 - \dot{V} \times F_Ico_2$$

and, as F_Ico_2 is close to zero,

$$\dot{V}co_2 = \dot{V}_E \times F_Eco_2$$

$\dot{V}_E$ is slightly smaller than $\dot{V}_I$ whenever less CO_2 is produced than O_2 consumed (i.e. the R value is <1.0). The exact difference can be calculated using inspired and expired N_2 fractions, since N_2 is not consumed or produced.

The ratio of ventilation to O_2 consumption ($\dot{V}_E/\dot{V}o_2$) is called the **ventilatory requirement**

and at rest is ~25 ($7.5/0.3 \, L \, min^{-1}$). It shows what a large quantity of air enters the lungs relative to the amount of O_2 consumed. A better expression is the **O_2 extraction coefficient**, which takes into account how much of the incoming air is actually O_2. This coefficient is the amount of O_2 used/amount of O_2 inspired, expressed as a percentage:

$$\dot{V}o_2 / (\dot{V}_I \times F_Io_2) \times 100$$

At rest the O_2 extraction coefficient is 15–20%, showing how little of the O_2 entering is actually used—there is in effect a large reserve available should the next few breaths be impeded. Neither of these ratios takes into account the O_2 reserves held in the 2.5 L of the FRC. In severe exercise $\dot{V}_{O_2}$ may be as great as 2–3 L min^{-1} depending on the person's ability to perform physical work—the more work the person is capable of, the greater the $\dot{V}_{O_2}$. Highly trained athletes may have a maximum $\dot{V}_{O_2}$ as high as 5–6 L min^{-1}. In severe exercise the stimuli to ventilation (p. 621) are such that breathing is far in excess of the $\dot{V}_{O_2}$ ensuring high enough alveolar P_{O_2} in a diffusion-limited situation (p. 459); thus the ventilatory requirement may be as high as 50 and the O_2 extraction coefficient as low as 10%. Furthermore, as the excessive breathing blows off CO_2 from its body stores, R values are greater than 1.0 in the initial stages of severe exercise.

The gas laws and ATPS, BTPS and STPD conditions

As a gas expands when heated and shrinks when compressed, the numerical value ascribed to its volume (V) or the volume/unit of time ($\dot{V}$) is dependent on the prevailing temperature (T) and pressure (P). Allowance must also be made for the volume occupied by water vapour. The partial pressure of water vapour (P_{H_2O}) depends entirely on the degree of saturation and the prevailing temperature.

In the lungs, gases are at body temperature (273 + 37 K), body pressure (which is at the same pressure as the ambient barometric pressure) and fully saturated with water vapour ($P_{H_2O} = 47$ mmHg) at that temperature (these are **BTPS** conditions). However, expired volumes are usually collected at ambient temperature, which as a rule is lower than body temperature, so the volume shrinks and some of the water vapour condenses. In this situation the gas is at ambient temperature, ambient pressure and saturated with water vapour at that temperature (i.e. **ATPS**). Since it is the volume the gas occupied when it was in the lungs that is important, the volume at ATPS must be converted to its volume at BTPS. Similarly, the volumes of CO_2 produced and O_2 consumed are usually calcu-

lated from volumes collected at ATPS but in this case they are reported as they would be under standard conditions of physical chemistry—these are standard temperature (0°C), standard pressure (760 mmHg) and completely dry ($P_{H_2O} = 0$ mmHg) (i.e. **STPD**)—as it is the amount of gas that is relevant.

Partial pressures of inspired, expired and alveolar gas

In the gas phase the partial pressure of a gas is proportional to its fractional share of the total volume of a dry gas mixture (Dalton's law). Expired gas is a mixture of that from both the dead space (which has the same composition as the inspired air) and the alveoli. The partial pressures of alveolar O_2 and CO_2 fluctuate very slightly during the breathing cycle as they are influenced by the tidal effect of inspired gas and the continuous effect of diffusional gas exchange between the blood and the alveoli. The mean alveolar P_{O_2} and P_{CO_2} are usually 100 and 40 mmHg, respectively, but can be raised or lowered by three fundamental determinants—the inspired gas composition, the magnitude of metabolism and the magnitude of alveolar ventilation—as described in the so-called alveolar gas equations.

Each gas in a dry mixture exerts a **partial pressure** (P_{gas}), which is proportional to its fractional share (F_{gas}) of the total volume. This is **Dalton's law** and when applied to respiratory gases P_{H_2O} must be subtracted from the total pressure (the barometric pressure, P_B, in mmHg):

$$P_{gas} = F_{gas}(P_B = P_{H_2O})$$

Although the air breathed has a variable humidity, once it has been inspired beyond the nasal passages it virtually becomes fully saturated with water vapour at a value (P_{H_2O} 47 mmHg) dictated by the body's temperature (37°C). Thus:

$$P_{gas} = F_{gas}(P_B - 47)\text{mmHg}$$

The fractional composition and partial pressures for inspired (P_I), mixed-expired (P_E) and mean alveolar gases (P_A) are given in Table 18.2 for O_2, CO_2 and N_2, when P_B is 760 mmHg (standard P_B at sea level). Note that the composition of the mixed-expired gas, at least for normal breathing (p. 448), is a mixture of one-third dead-space gas (equivalent in gas composition to inspired gas) and two-thirds alveolar gas. Inspired gases at sea level when fully saturated with water are P_1O_2 150 mmHg and P_1CO_2 virtually zero (0.2 mmHg). Typical values for alveolar gases under normal healthy conditions are **P_AO_2 100 mmHg and P_ACO_2 40 mmHg.**

As shown in Fig. 18.16, the composition of the **alveolar gas** fluctuates very slightly during the breathing cycle. Alveolar gas is influenced by the tidal effect of inspired gas from the airways and the continuous effect of diffusional gas exchange with the blood perfusing the alveoli. The alveolar gas fluctuation at rest is small because these two effects are dampened by the size of the total alveolar gas volume (the 2.5 L of FRC). At the beginning of inspiration the gas that first enters the alveoli is inspired from the dead space which contains alveolar gas left there from the preceding expiration—thus the P_{CO_2} in the alveoli continues to rise and P_{O_2} to fall. Only when the dead space is cleared does inspired fresh air enter the alveoli, diluting the alveolar gas to a small degree—thus, the P_{CO_2} now falls and P_{O_2} rises. Throughout expiration, gas flows out of the alveoli and the alveolar gas is modified only by alveolar blood perfusion, which continually supplies CO_2 to, and removes O_2 from, the gas phase. The rise in P_{CO_2} and fall in P_{O_2} during expiration are often referred to as the **alveolar slope** (or less correctly, the alveolar plateau if the rise and fall are slight). The alveolar P_{CO_2} and P_{O_2} approach the mean value about two-thirds through expiration (Fig. 18.16) but if the alveolar slope is slight, the end-expired values can be used instead and this will only slightly overestimate P_ACO_2 and slightly underestimate P_AO_2.

Determinants of alveolar O_2 and CO_2 and the alveolar gas equations

There are three fundamental determinants of alveolar gas composition—the inspired gas composition and the magnitudes of alveolar ventilation and metabolism. Note also that the effect of metabolism on alveolar gases depends on both an adequate blood perfusion of the alveoli and the matching of this perfusion to the alveolar ventilation; p. 465.

Alveolar P_{O_2}

P_AO_2 will decrease whenever there is a fall in the P_{O_2} inspired into the alveoli from the atmosphere. As $P_1O_2 = (P_B - P_{H_2O}) \times F_1O_2$, a fall in P_1O_2 can occur either at altitude where, although F_1O_2 is still 0.21, the P_B is less than 760 mmHg, or when the fractional composition of the atmosphere falls below the usual 0.21, as in poorly ventilated environments. P_AO_2 will also decrease if less than the usual volume of inspired gas ventilates the alveoli (i.e. if there is an impairment of $\dot{V}_A$), and if more O_2 than usual is extracted from the alveolar gas into the blood stream (i.e. if the body's $\dot{V}O_2$ increases). The relationship between these determinants is expressed in the **alveolar gas equation for O_2**:

Table 18.2 Fractional composition (*F*) and partial pressures (*P*, in mmHg) of inspired (*F*$_1$ or *P*$_1$), mixed-expired (*F*$_E$ or *P*$_E$) and mean alveolar gas (*F*$_A$ or *P*$_A$) for O_2, CO_2 and N_2 when P_B is 760 mmHg and all these compartments are fully saturated with water vapour at 37°C. Note that fractions for gases are given for a 'dry' gas mixture.

	F_1	F_E	F_A	P_1	P_E	P_A
O_2	0.2093	0.163	0.140	149	116	100
CO_2	0.0003	0.037	0.056	0.2	26	40
N_2	0.7904	0.800	0.804	563	571	573
H_2O	—	—	—	47	47	47

$$P_A o_2 = P_I o_2 - \frac{\dot{V} o_2 \times 863}{\dot{V}_A}$$

where 863 is a conversion factor which, first, accounts for the $\dot{V} o_2$ being in STPD units and $\dot{V}_A$ in BTPS units (both are in $L min^{-1}$) and second, permits the fractional expression ($\dot{V} o_2 / \dot{V}_A$) to be converted into partial pressures so that it can be subtracted from $P_I o_2$. A graphical expression of the O_2 alveolar gas equation is shown in Fig. 18.17. Each curve portrays the relationship between $P_A o_2$ and one of its determinants, $\dot{V}_A$, for different values of $P_I o_2$ or $\dot{V} o_2$. As $P_A o_2$ is the dependent variable, it is depicted on the vertical axis. The relationship between $P_A o_2$ and $\dot{V}_A$ is hyperbolic such that for resting conditions (middle curves), where $P_I o_2$ is 150 mmHg ($F_I o_2 = 0.21$) and $\dot{V} o_2$ is 300 mL min^{-1} STPD, a normal alveolar ventilation ($\dot{V}_A$) of 5 L min^{-1} BTPS produces the normal alveolar $P o_2$ of 100 mmHg (point A). When hypoventilation occurs, $P_A o_2$ decreases; when hyperventilation occurs, $P_A o_2$ increases and approaches, but can never reach, the inspired $P o_2$ value of 150 mmHg as there is continuous O_2 consumption.

A raised hyperbolic curve results from either a decrease in $\dot{V} o_2$ (depressed metabolism) or an increase in $P_I o_2$—the magnitude of the change determines the degree of upwards shift (Fig. 18.17). Thus, for instance, if $P_I o_2$ were to increase, the $P_A o_2$ will be elevated (point B) without any need for an increase in $\dot{V}_A$. Similarly, a downward-shifted hyperbolic curve shows the lower $P_A o_2$ values for each particular level of $\dot{V}_A$ when either $\dot{V} o_2$ increases (e.g. during exercise) or $P_I o_2$ decreases (e.g. the hypoxia of altitude). Clearly, in these two situations, to prevent $P_A o_2$ from falling to point Y or C (Fig. 18.17), an increase in $\dot{V}_A$ is required. In the case of exercise the increase in $\dot{V}_A$ exactly matches the increase in $\dot{V} o_2$ and $P_A o_2$ remains constant (point Z), whereas at altitude the fall in $P_A o_2$ can only be minimized (point D). In intense exercise the increase in breathing may be such that $P_A o_2$ is greater than 100 mmHg.

Alveolar Pco_2

$P_A co_2$ is also determined by the inspired gas composition and the magnitudes of alveolar ventilation and metabolism. In this case $P_A co_2$ will increase if there is CO_2 in the inspired gas (i.e. $P_I co_2$ increases), if ventilation is depressed (i.e. $\dot{V}_a$ decreases) or if more CO_2 than usual is produced by metabolism and carried to the alveoli (i.e. $\dot{V} co_2$ increases). Converse changes will decrease $P_A co_2$ and the most obvious example is that caused by voluntary hyperventilation. The **alveolar gas equation for CO_2** is derived in a similar fashion to that for O_2 and is:

$$P_A co_2 = P_I co_2 + \frac{\dot{V} co_2 \times 863}{\dot{V}_A} \text{ or } P_A co_2 = \frac{\dot{V} co_2 \times 863}{\dot{V}_A}$$

as $P_I co_2$ is frequently omitted because it is normally near zero (0.214 mmHg). (Note that the truncated form of this equation is independent of ambient pressure and is used clinically to measure $\dot{V}_A$, often with $P_a co_2$ substituted for $P_A co_2$.)

The graphical relationship between $P_A co_2$ and $\dot{V}_A$ for normal conditions of a $P_I co_2$ of 0 mmHg and a resting $\dot{V} co_2$ of 250 mL min^{-1} STPD is shown in Fig. 18.18 such that a typical $\dot{V}_A$ of 5 L min^{-1} BTPS produces the normal $P_A co_2$ of 40 mmHg (point A). Hypoventilation elevates $P_A co_2$ while hyperventilation decreases $P_A co_2$, though this never falls to the inspired $P co_2$ value of 0 mmHg because of the metabolic production of CO_2. Upward-shifted hyperbolic curves (Fig. 18.18) result in situations where $\dot{V} co_2$ increases (an in exercise) or $P_I co_2$ increases (hypercapnia); downward-shifted curves (not illustrated) occur for decreases in $\dot{V} co_2$. Clearly, to prevent $P_A co_2$ from rising to point Y or C (Fig. 18.18) when $\dot{V} co_2$ or $P_I co_2$ increases, an increase in $\dot{V}_A$ is required. In the case of exercise the increase in $\dot{V}_A$ matches the increase in $\dot{V} co_2$ and $P_A co_2$ remains constant (point Z), whereas during hypercapnia the rise in $P_A co_2$ can only be minimized (point D). Clinically (for inspired $P co_2$ conditions of 0 mmHg) the adequacy of $\dot{V}_A$ for tissue metabolism is judged by how much the $P_A co_2$, or more usually $P_a co_2$, deviates from 40 mmHg.

The alveolar gas equation

The equations for alveolar O_2 and CO_2 when combined give:

$$P_AO_2 = P_IO_2 - \frac{P_ACO_2}{R} + F$$

where R is the respiratory gas exchange ratio ($\dot{V}CO_2/\dot{V}O_2$) and F is a small correction factor (1–

3 mmHg, which can be ignored except for exact calculations) derived from the N_2 correction and required when R is less than 1. Furthermore, P_aCO_2 frequently replaces P_ACO_2 in the above equation, particularly for clinical use, because there is rarely a

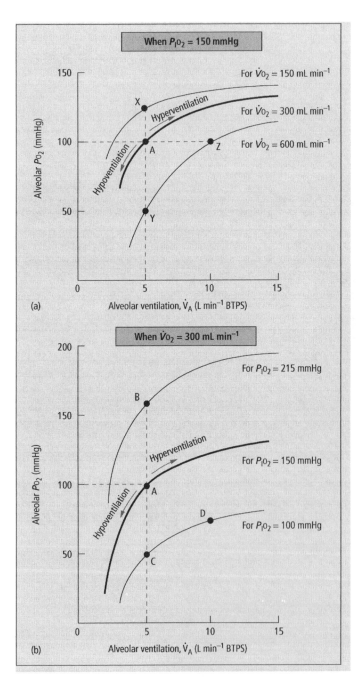

(a)

(b)

Fig. 18.17 P_AO_2 resulting from different alveolar ventilations (a) when P_IO_2 remains at the normal inspired level of 150 mmHg during three levels of $\dot{V}O_2$ and (b) when $\dot{V}O_2$ remains at the normal level of 300 mL min^{-1} STPD (standard temperature, pressure, dry) during three conditions of P_IO_2. In each case the middle curve has been calculated for normal metabolic and inspired O_2 conditions ($\dot{V}O_2 = 300$ mL min^{-1} STPD and $P_IO_2 = 150$ mmHg) with point A indicating that a normal $\dot{V}_A$ of 5 L min^{-1} BTPS (body temperature, pressure, saturated with water) produces a P_AO_2 of 100 mmHg; hypoventilation lowers and hyperventilation increases P_AO_2. The upper curve represents either decreased metabolism (a) or increased P_IO_2 (b) and the new P_AO_2 that results (points X and B) if there is no alteration in $\dot{V}_A$. The lower curve represents the situation in exercise (a) or at altitude (b), with points Y and C indicating the consequences if there is no reflex alteration in $\dot{V}_A$ compared with the actual reflex increase in $\dot{V}_A$ that occurs in exercise (point Z) or at altitude (point D).

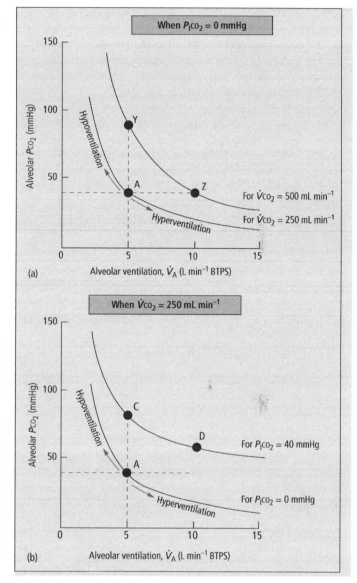

Fig. 18.18 $P_A co_2$ resulting from different alveolar ventilations for normal metabolic and inspired CO_2 conditions ($\dot{V} co_2 = 250$ mL min^{-1} STPD and $P_I co_2 = 0$ mmHg) where point A indicates that a normal $\dot{V}_A$ of 5 L min^{-1} BTPS produces a $P_A co_2$ of 40 mmHg and hypoventilation increases and hyperventilation lowers $P_A co_2$. The upper curve represents either increased metabolism (a) or increased $P_I co_2$ (b) and the new $P_A co_2$ which would result (points Y and C) if there was no alteration in $\dot{V}_A$ compared with the actual $P_A co_2$ achieved due to the reflex increase in $\dot{V}_A$ that occurs in exercise (point Z) or during hypercapnia (point D).

difference between the two (p. 458). The advantage of this combined alveolar gas equation (often called *the* alveolar gas equation) is that $P_a co_2$ is relatively easy to measure from an arterial blood sample, $P_I o_2$ is known (150 mmHg at sea level), the R value is assumed to be 0.8–0.85 and thus $P_A o_2$ can be calculated. $P_a o_2$ is always less than $P_A o_2$ and the magnitude of the $P_{A-a} o_2$ gradient can be an important clinical measure (p. 466).

Partial pressures of gases in solution in the blood

In the lungs O_2 and CO_2 in the capillaries equilibrate with the alveolar gases so that the blood leaving the lungs, which becomes the arterial blood of the body, has a $P o_2$ of 100 mmHg and $P co_2$ of 40 mmHg. Venous blood leaves the various tissues at different partial pressures and finally enters the lungs as mixed venous blood with a P_{O_2} of 40 mmHg and P_{CO_2} of 46 mmHg. Gas movement across the capillary walls of the lungs and tissues occurs by diffusion down a partial-pressure gradient and is dependent on the molecular weight and solubility of the gas, on the surface area available and on the distance travelled (Fick's law of diffusion). Usually most of the diffusion has occurred by the time the blood has traversed a third of the length of the capillary. Diseases that thicken the alveolar–capillary membrane or reduce the alveolar surface area cause a reduction in the pulmonary diffusing capacity for O_2. Successful gas transfer and maintenance of the partial pressure gradients rely not only on alveolar ventilation but also on blood flow through the lungs and tissues. The relationship between the amount of O_2 transferred, the cardiac output and the arteriovenous difference in O_2 content is expressed in the Fick principle. Increased cardiac output and greater O_2 extraction from the blood, causing a decrease in O_2 content of venous blood, allow for increased O_2 consumption.

When a liquid is exposed to a gas phase for long enough to reach equilibrium the partial pressures of the gases in the liquid and gas phase are identical. Note, however, that the content of the gas (millilitre of gas per litre of medium) may be very different between the two phases depending on the solubility of the gas in the liquid; p. 467. Given the large surface area and thinness of the air-to-blood barrier (p. 428), sufficient contact time occurs in the alveoli to permit the capillary blood leaving the alveoli to come to the same partial pressures as the alveolar gas. Thus, for rest-

ing normal conditions, $P_{A}O_2$ and end-pulmonary capillary blood P_{O_2} ($P_{c}O_2$) are both 100 mmHg and $P_{A}CO_2$ and $P_{c}CO_2$ are both 40 mmHg (Table 18.3 and Fig. 18.19). The end-pulmonary capillary blood leaves the lungs in the pulmonary veins to become the arterial blood for the rest of the body. Partial pressures in arterial blood are: $P_{a}CO_2$ 40 mmHg and $P_{a}O_2$ ~95 mmHg (Table 18.3 and Fig. 18.19).

The P_{O_2} in arterial blood is less than end-pulmonary capillary blood for the following reasons. The 1–2% of the cardiac output that comes through the bronchial and coronary circulations (p. 411) bypasses the alveoli and drains, respectively, into the pulmonary veins and directly into the left heart itself, and this modifies slightly the arterial blood composition (such venous admixture is referred to as a shunt; p. 461). Because of differences in the respective shapes of CO_2 and O_2 blood dissociation curves (p. 475), this venous admixture has a negligible effect on $P_{a}CO_2$ but lowers by a few mmHg the $P_{a}O_2$. A further lowering of $P_{a}O_2$ occurs as a consequence of alveolar ventilation and alveolar perfusion not being in the same proportion throughout the lungs (p. 465).

The blood that enters the alveolar capillaries via the pulmonary arteries is a mixture of all the venous blood coming from all the organs, each metabolizing at different rates (p. 410). This mixed venous ($\bar{v}$) blood for a resting person typically has a $P_{\bar{v}}CO_2$ of 46 mmHg and a $P_{\bar{v}}CO_2$ of 40 mmHg (Table 18.3 and Fig. 18.19). As sufficient time is allowed for equilibrium to occur as blood transits through the tissues capillaries, the interstitial fluid (ISF) bathing the 'typical' cell is said as an approxima-

Table 18.3 Partial pressure of gases in the alveoli and blood. Note that water cannot exist in a vapour form in a liquid (blood) phase.

	Partial pressure (mmHg)			
	O_2	CO_2	N_2	H_2O
Alveolar gas (P_A)	100	40	573	47
End-pulmonary capillary blood (P_c')	100	40	573	—
Systemic arterial blood (P_a)	95	40	573	—
Mixed venous blood ($P_{\bar{v}}$)	40	46	573	—

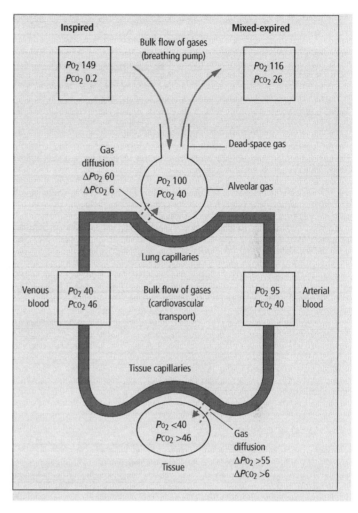

Inspired

P_{O_2} 149
P_{CO_2} 0.2

Bulk flow of gases
(breathing pump)

Mixed-expired

P_{O_2} 116
P_{CO_2} 26

Dead-space gas

Gas
diffusion
ΔP_{O_2} 60
ΔP_{CO_2} 6

P_{O_2} 100
P_{CO_2} 40

Alveolar gas

Lung capillaries

Venous
blood

P_{O_2} 40
P_{CO_2} 46

Bulk flow of gases
(cardiovascular
transport)

P_{O_2} 95
P_{CO_2} 40

Arterial
blood

Tissue capillaries

$P_{O_2} <40$
$P_{CO_2} >46$

Gas
diffusion
$\Delta P_{O_2} >55$
$\Delta P_{CO_2} >6$

Tissue

Fig. 18.19 P_{O_2} and P_{CO_2} (mmHg) in various parts of the respiratory and cardiovascular system. Bulk flow of gases occurs between atmosphere and lungs (breathing pump) and around the body in the blood stream (cardiovascular transport). Gases move across capillary walls by diffusion.

tion to be at a P_{CO_2} of 46 mmHg and P_{O_2} of 40 mmHg.

Diffusion

Gases move by diffusion down gradients of partial pressure (not concentration) between alveolar gas and pulmonary capillary blood and between systemic capillary blood and ISF. In Fig. 18.19 at both sites of diffusion the initial P_{O_2} and P_{CO_2} gradients are $\Delta 60$ and $\Delta 6$ mmHg, respectively. As **Fick's law of diffusion** states, the amount of gas diffusing in unit time through the resistance of a barrier is inversely proportional to the thickness of the barrier and directly proportional to the surface area of the

barrier, the diffusion constant (D) for that gas through that barrier, and the partial pressure gradient of the gas across the barrier.

As stated by Graham's law, the diffusion constant is directly proportional to the solubility of the gas, which is dependent on temperature, and inversely proportional to the square root of its molecular mass (M_r). For biological membranes at 37°C the diffusion constant for CO_2 is 23 times greater than for O_2 because, despite its larger M_r (44 vs. 32), CO_2 is very much more soluble than O_2 in plasma (0.65 vs. 0.031 mL L^{-1} mmHg^{-1}). Thus, given that the volume per unit time of CO_2 produced and O_2 consumed is similar, CO_2 diffusion occurs down much smaller partial-pressure gradients. Furthermore, because of its high diffusion constant, CO_2 diffusion is rarely impeded.

In the lungs, because of difficulties of their individual measurement, the surface area of the alveoli, the diffusion constant for O_2 and the thickness of the air–blood barrier (which is not only the alveolar–capillary membrane but also the distance within the capillary to the centre of the red blood cells) are all lumped together and called the **pulmonary diffusing capacity** for O_2 (D_LO_2). Thus:

$$D_LO_2 = \frac{area \times Do_2}{thickness} \quad and\ so \quad \dot{V}o_2 = D_LO_2 \times \Delta Po_2$$

This equation is *not* used to measure $\dot{V}O_2$ but is in fact rearranged to permit measurement of D_LO_2:

$$D_LO_2 = \frac{\dot{V}o_2}{\Delta Po_2} \quad or \quad D_LO_2 = \frac{\dot{V}o_2}{P_AO_2 - P_{\bar{c}}O_2}$$

where $P_{\bar{c}}O_2$ is the mean pulmonary capillary Po_2 averaged over the entire length of the capillary (Fig. 18.20). Again there is a problem of measurement—$P_{\bar{c}}O_2$ can only be deduced from a prior knowledge of all the other variables in the equation.

The problem is solved by measuring instead the pulmonary diffusing capacity for CO. This is because $P_{\bar{c}}co$ can be taken as zero on account of the very high affinity between CO and haemoglobin, such that little CO is actually in solution in the plasma (p. 472)—thus $D_Lco = \dot{V}co/P_aco$. Measurements are made after a subject inspires a gas mixture containing a small amount of CO (about 0.1%) for a few breaths. Then P_aco is measured from the first end-expiratory sample and $\dot{V}co$ by the rate at which CO disappears from the alveoli into the blood over a 10-s breath-hold (estimated by measuring CO in the alveoli at the beginning and end of the breath-hold). D_Lco so measured at rest is about 25 mL min^{-1} mmHg^{-1}. Because of the M_r and solubility differences between CO and O_2, D_LO_2 is 1.23 × D_Lco, i.e. ~30 mL min^{-1} mmHg^{-1}. Similarly, the pulmonary diffusing capacity for CO_2 (D_LCO_2) is 23 times greater than D_LO_2.

Figure 18.20 depicts the calculated Po_2 profile of blood along the length of the pulmonary capilliary

from when it enters the capillary as mixed venous blood ($P_{\bar{v}}O_2$ 40 mmHg) to when it finally leaves 0.75 s later as end-capillary blood (P_cO_2) at a composition identical to alveolar (P_AO_2 100 mmHg). The initial Po_2 gradient is Δ60 mmHg (100–40) and as O_2 rapidly diffuses into the blood elevating the capillary Po_2, the gradient gets smaller and smaller as the blood moves along the capillary. When breathing air, most of the diffusion in a healthy lung is complete about one-third of the way along the lung capillary. By equalizing the shaded areas below and above a particular Po_2 (Fig. 18.20), the mean pulmonary capillary Po_2 ($P_{\bar{c}}O_2$) can be estimated—normally ~90 mmHg. With reference to the equation $\dot{V}o_2 = D_LO_2 \times (P_AO_2 - P_{\bar{c}}O_2)$, one can see that at rest the appropriate values are: $\dot{V}o_2$ ~300 mL min^{-1}, D_LO_2 ~30 mL min^{-1} mmHg^{-1}, P_AO_2 100 mmHg and $P_{\bar{c}}O_2$ 90 mmHg, indicating that the average partial-pressure gradient for diffusion is 10 mmHg.

In exercise D_LO_2 increases by up to two- to three-fold because the larger tidal volumes, by inflating the alveoli more, increase the alveolar surface area and because more pulmonary capillaries are perfused. There is, however, no alteration in the thickness of the air–blood barrier. In heavy exercise P_AO_2 can be elevated to 110–120 mmHg because of high ventilation (p. 453), the $P_{\bar{v}}O_2$ of blood entering the alveoli can be as low as 20 mmHg and, because transit time through the pulmonary capillary can shorten to 0.25 s (p. 410), the mean $P_{\bar{c}}O_2$ can be some 30–40 mmHg lower than at rest. These will all increase the initial and average ΔPo_2 gradients for diffusion. In heavy exercise transit time may be too short to permit end-pulmonary P_cO_2 to equilibrate with P_AO_2 and as a consequence P_aO_2 may fall to ~90 mmHg (p. 420). This is detected as a widening of the alveolar–arterial Po_2 difference (p. 466).

Lung diseases, which either thicken the air–blood barrier (e.g. pulmonary oedema and pulmonary fibrosis, the latter caused for example by sarcoidosis or asbestosis) or reduce the alveolar surface area (e.g. alveolar collapse as in atelectasis or loss of alveolar septa as in emphysema), can reduce D_LO_2 considerably such that, even after a normal resting transit time of 0.75 s, end-pulmonary

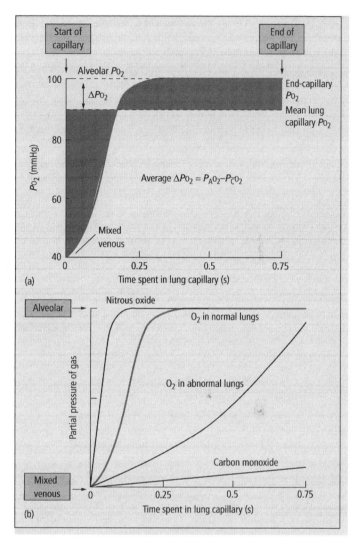

Fig. 18.20 (a) Pulmonary capillary P_{O_2} as a function of time spent in the capillary of a normal lung. (Blood P_{O_2} changes slowly at the beginning of the capillary because at these low levels of P_{O_2} most of the O_2 diffusing into the blood combines with haemoglobin and causes very little increase in P_{O_2}.) (b) Time course of changes in capillary partial pressure for different gases in the normal lung (N_2O, O_2 and CO) and abnormal lung (O_2).

Figure labels: Start of capillary; End of capillary; Alveolar P_{O_2}; ΔP_{O_2}; End-capillary P_{O_2}; Mean lung capillary P_{O_2}; Average $\Delta P_{O_2} = P_A O_2 - P_{\bar{C}} O_2$; Mixed venous; P_{O_2} (mmHg); Time spent in lung capillary (s); (a)

(b) Alveolar; Nitrous oxide; O_2 in normal lungs; O_2 in abnormal lungs; Carbon monoxide; Mixed venous; Partial pressure of gas; Time spent in lung capillary (s)

$P_{\bar{c}}O_2$ may not reach the $P_A O_2$ level (Fig. 18.20). Hence $P_a O_2$ may be well below the normal 100 mmHg so that the alveolar–arterial P_{O_2} difference widens. This is exacerbated even more during exercise or in conditions when the initial mixed venous to alveolar P_{O_2} gradient is already low (e.g. at altitude).

Transfer of gases across the alveolar–capillary membrane may be diffusion-limited or perfusion-limited. If the end-capillary is less than the alveolar partial pressure for the gas in question, its transfer is **diffusion-limited** (e.g. CO in all instances, O_2 in very strenuous exercise, O_2 at rest

with a moderately severe abnormality of the alveolar–capillary membrane, and CO_2 with exceptionally severe alveolar–capillary abnormality). If the blood equilibrates with the alveolar gas early in its passage through the capillary (e.g. O_2, CO_2 and the anaesthetic gas, N_2O), the transfer of that gas is **perfusion-limited** and gas transfer would increase if pulmonary capillary flow increased.

Fick's law of diffusion also applies to diffusion between cells and tissue capillaries. Although it is not easy to quantify, and varies from organ to organ, the concept of a tissue-diffusing capacity akin to that for the lung is important. As expected from Fick's law, such a tissue-diffusing capacity is proportional to the diffusion constant of the gas concerned and the surface area of the organ's capillaries and inversely proportional to the distance from the capillary to the cell's mitochondria. When O_2 and CO_2 metabolism by the tissue increases, the capillary surface area increases and, in contrast to the situation in the lung, the diffusion distance decreases. This is a consequence of metabolic regulation (p. 388)—ensuring that more capillaries in the tissue are perfused and therefore 'open', which both increases the surface area for gas exchange and permits any one cell to be closer than it was to an open capillary. In contrast to the lung, capillary transit time through active tissues does not alter much (p. 392).

Fick principle

Another equation concerned with gas transfer states, in the case of O_2, that:

$$\dot{V}_{O_2} = \dot{Q}(C_aO_2 - C_{\bar{v}}O_2)$$

where $\dot{V}_{O_2}$ is the O_2 consumption (mL min^{-1}). $\dot{Q}$ is the cardiac output (L min^{-1}) and C_aO_2 and $C_{\bar{v}}O_2$ are, respectively, the arterial and mixed-venous content of O_2 (mL of O_2 L^{-1} blood). For CO_2 the equation is:

$$\dot{V}_{CO_2} = \dot{Q}(C_{\bar{v}}CO_2 - C_aCO_2)$$

These equations illustrate the **Fick principle**. It is often used to measure not gas transfer but $\dot{Q}$ and blood flow to individual organs (e.g. p. 553), and as a technique it is called the Fick method. (The equation is also referred to as the Fick equation and must not be confused with that for Fick's law of diffusion.)

The Fick equation illustrates how dependent gas transfer is on the rate of blood flow through the lungs and tissues. At rest typical values are $\dot{V}_{O_2}$ 300 mL min^{-1}, $\dot{Q}$ 6 L min^{-1}, C_aO_2 195 mL L^{-1} and $C_{\bar{v}}O_2$ 145 mL L^{-1}. Were $\dot{Q}$ to fall due to various cardiovascular disorders (p. 472), $\dot{V}_{O_2}$ can only be maintained by extracting a greater amount of O_2 from the circulating blood—thus $C_{\bar{v}}O_2$ falls. C_aO_2 is

dependent on alveolar P_{O_2} and the haemoglobin concentration (p. 467) and in these particular cardiovascular disorders neither of these will change. The arteriovenous O_2 difference ($C_aO_2 - C_{\bar{v}}O_2$) therefore widens, but only because $C_{\bar{v}}O_2$ falls. Some organs extract more O_2 out of the circulating blood than others, so the content of O_2 in their venous blood, and hence their arteriovenous O_2 difference, differ.

During exercise C_aO_2 remains virtually unchanged and the increase in O_2 delivery to the exercising muscles is achieved by an increase in $\dot{Q}$ and this, coupled with a greater extraction of O_2 from the blood (i.e. $C_{\bar{v}}O_2$ decreases), permits the increased consumption of O_2. Typical values for strenuous exercise are $\dot{V}_{O_2}$ 3000 mL min^{-1}, $\dot{Q}$ 20 L min^{-1}, C_aO_2 195 mL L^{-1} and $C_{\bar{v}}O_2$ 45 mL L^{-1}, with obvious widening of the arteriovenous O_2 difference.

The similarity of the Fick equation, $\dot{V}_{O_2} = \dot{Q}(C_aO_2 - C_{\bar{v}}O_2)$, to the ventilatory equation used on p. 450 to measure O_2 consumption, $\dot{V}_{O_2} = \dot{V}_E(F_IO_2 - F_EO_2)$, is obvious—the first is based on blood variables and the second on ventilatory variables. The version using alveolar ventilation, $\dot{V}_{O_2} = \dot{V}_A(F_IO_2 - F_AO_2)$, is more relevant here as gas transfer in the lungs is ultimately dependent on both $\dot{Q}$ and $\dot{V}_A$. It was stated on p. 450 that R is the ratio of $\dot{V}_{CO_2}/\dot{V}_{O_2}$. From the $\dot{V}_{O_2}$ equations just summarized and the equivalent ones for $\dot{V}_{CO_2}$, it is apparent that R can also be calculated from:

1 $(F_ECO_2 - F_ICO_2)/(F_IO_2 - F_EO_2)$;
2 $(F_ACO_2 - F_ICO_2)/(F_IO_2 - F_AO_2)$; and
3 $(C_{\bar{v}}CO_2 - C_aCO_2)/(C_aO_2 - C_{\bar{v}}O_2)$.

18.4 Shunts, regional ventilation and perfusion, and the V$_A$/Q ratio

P_aO_2 (~95 mmHg) is always less than P_AO_2 or P_cO_2 (100 mmHg). This alveolar–arterial P_{O_2} difference arises because of first, venous admixture from the coronary and bronchial circulations (normal anatomical shunts) which bypass the alveolar capillaries, and second, the consequences of an uneven base-to-apex distribution of the ratio of alveolar ventilation to blood perfusion ($\dot{V}_A/\dot{Q}$ ratio) which is due to gravity. The base of the lung receives 2.5 times more $\dot{V}_A$ and six times more $\dot{Q}$ than the lung apex when in the upright posture. Small spontaneous alterations in $\dot{V}_A/\dot{Q}$ are mitigated by local mechanisms, restoring either of the two components towards normal. For instance, too low a $\dot{V}_A$ would produce locally high CO_2 and low O_2, causing the nearby bronchioles to dilate and the pulmonary arterioles to constrict, the former improving local ventilation and the latter reducing local blood flow to match the ventilation. The alveolar–arterial Po_2 difference becomes wider in various lung diseases where there are intra-pulmonary shunts, abnormal anatomical shunts, inequality of the $\dot{V}_A/\dot{Q}$ ratio or impairment of pulmonary diffusion.

Shunts

Any venous blood that is added to blood in the systemic arteries (**venous admixture**) without going through ventilated areas of the lungs is referred to as a right-to-left (R–L) **shunt**. In the normal lung there are two main **anatomical** sources of such a shunt—some coronary venous blood drains via Thebesian veins into the left ventricle and some of the bronchial circulation returns via the pulmonary veins. Because of differences in the respective shapes of CO_2 and O_2 blood dissociation curves (p. 476), venous admixture from shunts has a negligible effect on P_aCO_2 but lowers P_aO_2 by a few mmHg relative to P_AO_2, thus creating an alveolar–arterial Po_2 difference (p. 475).

Normally only 1–2% of the cardiac output bypasses the alveoli. This can be viewed as wasted perfusion, analogous to the concept of wasted (dead-space) ventilation (p. 448). For wasted ventilation the basis of the Bohr equation (written usually for CO_2) states:

$$\dot{V}_E \times F_ECO_2 \quad = \dot{V}_D \times F_ICO_2 \quad + \dot{V}_A \times F_ACO_2$$

total ventilation = wasted ventilation + useful ventilation

For wasted or shunted perfusion the statement (written usually for O_2) is:

$$\dot{Q}_t \times C_aO_2 \quad = \dot{Q}_s \times C_{\bar{v}}O_2 \quad + \dot{Q}_c \times C_aO_2$$

total perfusion = wasted perfusion + useful perfusion

Note that these equations can be condensed to $\dot{V}_E = \dot{V}_D + \dot{V}_A$ and $\dot{Q}_t = \dot{Q}_s + \dot{Q}_c$ but the same cannot be done for the fraction (F) or content (C) because they cannot be added without knowing the volume (or flow rate) of each. Furthermore, the O_2 must be expressed in units of content not partial pressure in the shunt statement because the shape of the O_2 haemoglobin dissociation curve (O_2 content vs. Po_2) is not linear but sigmoidal (p. 470).

Shunted blood flow ($\dot{Q}_s$), containing the unmodified mixed-venous content of O_2 ($C_{\bar{v}}O_2$), is added to the pulmonary capillary blood flow ($\dot{Q}_c$) which, as it has passed through ventilated alveoli, has a normal oxygenated pulmonary end-capillary content (C_cO_2), to give the total pulmonary blood flow ($\dot{Q}t$, i.e. cardiac output). The mixed blood comprises the final arterial content of O_2 (C_aO_2), which is less than C_cO_2 by an amount dependent on the venous admixture. Flow is usually given in units of litres of blood per minute and content in millilitres of O_2 per litre of blood. A rearrangement of the equation given to illustrate the shunt statement produces the form known as the **shunt equation**:

$$\frac{\dot{Q}_s}{\dot{Q}_t} = \frac{C_cO_2 - C_aO_2}{C_cO_2 - C_{\bar{v}}O_2}$$

in which $\dot{Q}_s$ can be calculated after measurement of each of the other variables. $\dot{Q}_t$ is first measured using the Fick principle (p. 460). C_cO_2 is difficult to sample and is estimated from the O_2 content vs. Po_2 relationship of the O_2 haemoglobin dissociation curve and the assumption that its Po_2 is the same as alveolar Po_2. The C_aO_2 is measured from an arterial gas sample and $C_{\bar{v}}O_2$ from a venous blood sample, which for accuracy should be from the pulmonary artery as this contains a true sample of the body's mixed-venous gases. As the shunted blood from the bronchial circulation may not have a composition identical to mixed-venous, the shunt equation has some limitations.

Pathological R–L shunts can occur on an anatomical basis in cardiovascular diseases (e.g. patent ductus arteriosus at birth, and atrial or ventricular septal defects—the so-called 'hole-in-the-heart') and on a functional basis from intra-pulmonary shunts in pulmonary diseases (e.g.

blockage of bronchi or bronchioles with mucus, and bronchiolar or alveolar collapse in which the alveoli that are not ventilated but are still perfused constitute a shunt). A shunt-like effect can also occur if the alveolar ventilation to some of the alveoli is just reduced rather than abolished (see alveolar ventilation/perfusion ratio; p. 465)—when this occurs it contributes a hidden augmentation of the $\dot{Q}_s$ calculated by the shunt equation. A true shunt can be distinguished from the effect of a poor ventilation/perfusion ratio by breathing 100% O_2—the shunted blood will not come into contact with the high alveolar O_2 and so nothing will change (thus the final C_aO_2 will *not* improve), whereas the C_aO_2 in poorly ventilated alveoli will gain some benefit from exposure to high alveolar O_2 (thus the final C_aO_2 will increase).

The term **physiological shunt** was coined to refer to the presence of all types of shunts in health and disease and to be a term similar in concept to that of the physiological dead space (p. 449). However, some use it to refer only to those anatomical shunts normally present in health, as all other types of shunts are pathological.

Regional variations in ventilation

In the upright posture when breathing normally at FRC, the base (bottom) of the lungs receives ~2.5 times more ventilation per unit of lung volume than the apex (top) of the lungs (see Fig. 18.21). This can be measured by a bank of radioactive counters placed along the chest of a subject who is breathing tracer amounts of radioactive xenon gas. When in the supine position, the base and apex are in fact ventilated equally but it is the dorsal region of the lungs that now receives a higher ventilation relative to the ventral regions. The effects of gravity are the cause of these regional variations in ventilation—the lowermost regions are called the gravity-dependent regions and receive the better ventilation.

Gravity results in the weight of the lungs tending to pull them away from the chest very slightly at the base and very strongly at the apex. This causes P_{pl} at FRC to be $-2.5 \, \text{cmH}_2\text{O}$ at the base and $-10 \, \text{cm} \, \text{H}_2\text{O}$ at the apex of an upright lung (p. 434). The

consequences of this are that the basal regions with the lower transmural pressure ($P_{alv} - P_{pl}$) will begin inspiration at FRC containing less gas than the apical regions (Fig. 18.21). However, because basal regions are on the steep part of the compliance curve, they will inflate more easily during inspiration and thus, for the same inspiration-to-expiration P_{pl} of $\Delta 3 \, \text{cmH}_2\text{O}$ as in the apical regions, the Δ volume and resulting ventilation achieved will be greater (Fig. 18.21).

Effect of lung disease

When the lungs become stiffer because of age or lung diseases, the base of the lungs may be operating on the lower flat part of the compliance curve (Fig. 18.21), in which case ventilation of the basal may become less than that of the apical regions. Furthermore, as P_{pl} at the base may even become positive, small airways may be intermittently or totally closed due to compression (p. 441), thus pro-

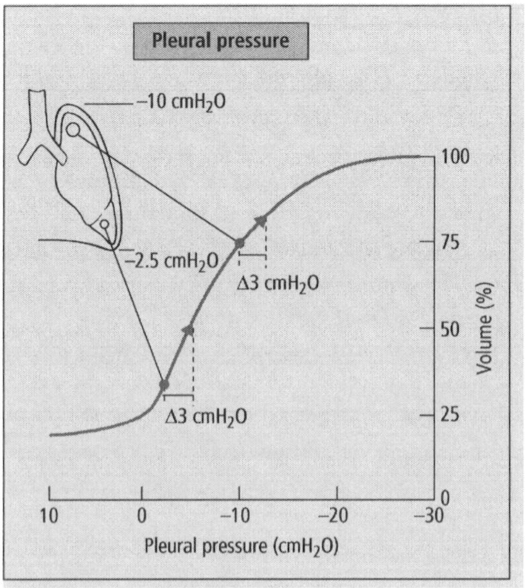

Fig. 18.21 Effect of the upright posture on P_{pl} at the apex and base of the lung at functional residual capacity (FRC). Alveoli (depicted as an open circle in the lung) are more inflated at the apex than at the base and are therefore further up the compliance curve. Blue arrow heads indicate volume increment during each inspiration at the apex compared with the base.

ducing intermittent basal ventilation or trapping gas in the alveoli. These effects can occur in healthy young people but only when deliberately breathing at low lung volumes below FRC.

Throughout the lungs uneven ventilation can occur if, due to disease, some areas have less compliant alveoli or the airways supplying some alveoli but not others have an increased resistance due to bronchoconstriction, inflammation, blockage or compression.

Regional variations in pulmonary blood flow

The regional distribution of pulmonary blood flow can also be measured by a bank of radioactive counters on the chest of a subject, this time after the subject has received an intravenous injection of radioactive xenon dissolved in saline. In the upright posture the base receives approximately six times more blood flow per unit of lung volume than the apex of the lungs (see Fig. 18.22). As with regional variations in ventilation, this base-to-apex gradation disappears on lying down and if supine, the blood flow is now greater in the gravity-dependent dorsal region.

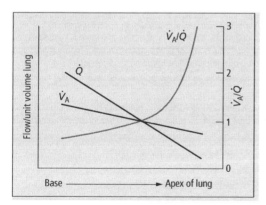

Fig. 18.22 Effect of gravity in the upright posture on pressure at the arterial (a) and venous (v) ends of pulmonary capillaries (cap.). Distension of vessels increases blood flow at the base of the lung; collapse of vessels reduces blood flow at the apex of the lung (the −4 cmH₂O in parentheses indicates the pressure that would occur if the vessels were rigid).

Gravity does not affect the extravascular pressure in the region of the alveoli (i.e. the alveolar pressure, which is ~0 cmH$_2$O) but it does affect the hydrostatic pressure inside blood vessels (p. 418). In the lung at the level of the tricuspid valve, the pressure in the pulmonary artery is 25 mmHg systolic/8 mmHg diastolic (p. 410) falling, though still with a marked pulse (see Fig. 16.6), to ~12 mmHg at the arterial end and to ~8 mmHg at the venous end of the pulmonary capillaries. These pressures at the arterial and venous ends of the capillary convert to ~16 and ~11 cmH$_2$O.

In the upright posture the base of the lung in an adult will be some 10 cm below and the apex some 15 cm above the tricuspid valve and so the blood pressures increase by 10 cmH$_2$O at the base and fall by 15 cmH$_2$O at the apex of the lung (Fig. 18.23). As pulmonary vessels have very thin walls, such changes in intravascular pressure relative to extravascular pressure (i.e. the transmural pressure, $P_{in} - P_{out}$) cause distension of vessels at the base and compression at the apex. Thus, for example, at the arterial end of the capillary the 16 cmH$_2$O becomes at the base 26 cmH$_2$O, the vessels distend and perfusion increases, while at the apex the pressure is only 1 cmH$_2$O and the vessels tend to collapse (Fig. 18.23). However, given the systolic/diastolic pulse, this pressure at the apex will become positive in systole and more negative in diastole and thus at the apex flow will actually be intermittent. Should pulmonary arterial pressure fall (e.g. after a haemorrhage), apical flow may cease entirely. Alveoli that are ventilated but not perfused constitute the alveolar dead space (p. 448). In exercise the elevation in pulmonary arterial blood pressure ensures that apical regions are perfused continuously.

Just below the apex arterial pressure will always exceed alveolar pressure but the gravitational effects on venous pressure are such (Fig. 18.23) that alveolar pressure is greater than venous pressure. Not only will there be some compression of the veins near the capillary, but also the pressure gradient causing blood flow is actually the difference between arterial and alveolar pressure. Only in the middle and lower regions of the lungs will venous exceed alveolar pressure, thus permitting the arte-

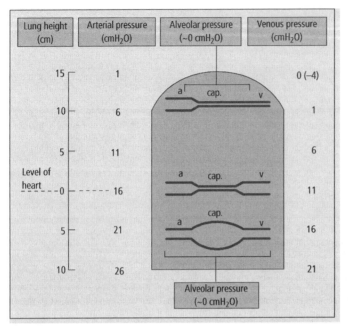

Lung height (cm)	Arterial pressure (cmH$_2$O)	Alveolar pressure (~0 cmH$_2$O)	Venous pressure (cmH$_2$O)

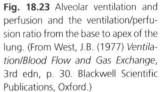

Fig. 18.23 Alveolar ventilation and perfusion and the ventilation/perfusion ratio from the base to apex of the lung. (From West, J.B. (1977) *Ventilation/Blood Flow and Gas Exchange*, 3rd edn, p. 30. Blackwell Scientific Publications, Oxford.)

rial-to-venous pressure gradient to determine blood flow.

Effect of lung disease

Uneven perfusion of some alveoli with respect to others can occur because of local blockage by emboli and thrombi, local compression (e.g. by oedema or tumours), local damage to blood vessels by disease and local collapse or overexpansion of alveoli. Because pulmonary blood pressure is relatively low, uneven perfusion is easily precipitated by pulmonary hypotension.

Effect of breathing on lung perfusion

The extravascular pressure in the vicinity of the pulmonary capillaries is the alveolar pressure, which fluctuates around 0cmH$_2$O, becoming −1 cmH$_2$O in inspiration and +1cmH$_2$O in expiration (p. 441) — greater airflow will cause greater fluctuations. Thus perfusion also depends on the phase and magnitude of the breathing cycle being augmented during inspiration by vessel dilation. On the other hand, deep inspirations actually compress, not dilate, the alveolar vessels because the

walls of the alveoli become so stretched that the vessels within them are compressed. During a normal expiration perfusion may cease at the apex because alveolar pressure may exceed arterial pressure. Furthermore, clinical treatment with positive-pressure ventilation can cause alveolar pressure to exceed arterial pressure throughout the breathing cycle, resulting in cessation of perfusion, particularly at the apex of the lung or, if recumbent, in the gravity non-dependent regions.

Pulmonary vascular resistance

In the pulmonary circuit a distinction between arteries and arterioles is not usually made and arteries, capillaries and veins each contribute one-third of the total pulmonary resistance (p. 410). For pulmonary arteries and veins away from the alveolar region, the extravascular pressure is not the alveolar but the pleural pressure. During inspiration towards TLC the increasingly negative pleural pressure and radial traction (p. 442) from surrounding lung tissue dilates arteries and veins, lowering their resistance and hence increasing pulmonary blood flow. This effect is, however, small and the overall pulmonary vascular resistance at large lung vol-

umes is in fact raised markedly by compression of capillaries within stretched alveolar walls. During expiration from FRC towards RV the effect on capillaries is small but loss of radial traction and positive pleural pressures, particularly with a forced expiration, compress pulmonary arteries and veins, increasing their resistance considerably. Thus pulmonary vascular resistance is least near FRC.

Ventilation/perfusion ratios

Adequate exchange of O_2 and CO_2 between alveoli and blood, and the maintenance of partial-pressure gradients down which these gases diffuse, require that $\dot{V}_A$ and $\dot{Q}$ be reasonably well matched in each of the alveolar units throughout the lung.

The ratio $\dot{V}_A/\dot{Q}$ is in fact a fourth determinant of alveolar gas partial pressures for a particular alveolar unit. It cannot be included in the format of the alveolar gas equations (p. 452) because these relate to the lung as a whole. The amount of O_2 (or CO_2) in an alveolus obviously depends on how much is added to the alveolus per minute, which is determined by local $\dot{V}_A$, and how much is removed (or added) per minute by the blood, which is determined by local $\dot{Q}$.

In adults at rest, typically $\dot{V}_A$ is $5\,L\,min^{-1}$ and $\dot{Q}$ is $6\,L\,min^{-1}$, giving for the lung as a whole an overall $\dot{V}_A/\dot{Q}$ ratio of 0.83 (although in different individuals, as $\dot{V}_A$ and $\dot{Q}$ can range between 4 and $6\,L\,min^{-1}$, the $\dot{V}_A/\dot{Q}$ ranges from 0.8 to 1.2). These ratios of $\dot{V}_A/\dot{Q}$ produce on average an alveolar Po_2 of 100 mmHg and Pco_2 of 40 mmHg. If, however, a group of alveoli is unventilated (i.e. the $\dot{V}_A/\dot{Q}$ becomes zero), the gases in these alveoli will soon become the same as the blood entering them—that is, the mixed-venous values of Po_2 40 mmHg and Pco_2 46 mmHg. On the other hand, if these alveoli receive normal ventilation but are unperfused (i.e. the $\dot{V}_A/\dot{Q}$ becomes infinite) their gases soon become identical to inspired gases at a Po_2 of 150 mmHg and Pco_2 of 0 mmHg. These are of course extreme examples used to illustrate the fact that alveolar–capillary units with a low $\dot{V}_A/\dot{Q}$ ratio have a low alveolar Po_2 and high Pco_2 and those with a high $\dot{V}_A/\dot{Q}$ ratio have a high alveolar

Po_2 and a low Pco_2. Not surprisingly, even in the normal lung, all $300–600 \times 10^6$ alveolar units are not ventilated and perfused absolutely equally. Mismatching of $\dot{V}_A/\dot{Q}$ occurs in diseases where there is uneven ventilation (p. 461) or uneven perfusion.

Local control of $\dot{V}_A/\dot{Q}$ matching

Two mechanisms work together to minimize mismatching of $\dot{V}_A/\dot{Q}$ in small groups of alveolar–capillary units. One affects the bronchioles to alter the local distribution of ventilation, the other affects the small pulmonary vessels to alter the local distribution of blood flow. If a group of alveoli are underventilated or overperfused (i.e. the $\dot{V}_A/\dot{Q}$ ratio has decreased) their alveolar Po_2 will be low and Pco_2 high. Bronchiolar smooth muscle is not particularly sensitive to Po_2 but in response to high airway Pco_2 it will relax. The resulting bronchodilation reduces the local airway resistance and hence increases airflow to the alveoli those bronchioles supply. Thus local ventilation increases and the $\dot{V}_A/\dot{Q}$ ratio returns towards normal. Smooth muscle of small pulmonary arterioles is not particularly sensitive to Pco_2 but in response to low Po_2 it contracts. The resulting vasoconstriction increases vascular resistance, reducing the blood flow to the pulmonary capillaries and thus returning the local $\dot{V}_A/\dot{Q}$ ratio towards normal. Conversely, in a group of alveoli that are overventilated or underperfused (i.e. $\dot{V}_A/\dot{Q}$ has increased), the alveolar Po_2 will be high and the Pco_2 low, and the $\dot{V}_A/\dot{Q}$ ratio will be adjusted back towards normal by local bronchoconstriction and vasodilation.

Such a vasoconstricting response to low Po_2 is unique to pulmonary arterioles—in all systemic arterioles the response is one of vasodilation. Pulmonary vessels respond more to the airway than blood Po_2 and the effect of low O_2 may be mediated by release of some vasoconstrictor substance rather than by a direct effect on the smooth muscle. The vasoconstricting response to low O_2 is, however, a disadvantage in the generalized hypoxia of high altitude or chronic obstructive lung disease because all pulmonary arterioles throughout the lung constrict.

Variation in $\dot{V}_A/\dot{Q}$ due to gravity

A normal cause of variation in $\dot{V}_A/\dot{Q}$ is based on regional variations in $\dot{V}_A$ and in $\dot{Q}$ (Fig. 18.23) that are induced by gravity and particularly evident in the upright posture. Both $\dot{V}_A$ and $\dot{Q}$ decrease from base to apex of the lungs but, as the reduction in $\dot{Q}$ (six-fold) is greater than the reduction in $\dot{V}_A$ (2.5-fold), their ratio *increases* from base to apex. Thus, the base of the lung, although well ventilated and perfused, has a $\dot{V}_A/\dot{Q}$ ratio falling to about 0.6, and therefore contains alveoli with a slightly lower P_AO_2 and higher P_ACO_2 than areas with a $\dot{V}_A/\dot{Q}$ ratio of 1.0. In contrast, at the apex of the lung there are very large increases in the $\dot{V}_A/\dot{Q}$ ratio rising to more than 3.0 over a short distance and the apex therefore contains alveoli with a very much higher P_AO_2 and lower P_ACO_2. The shape of the $\dot{V}_A/\dot{Q}$ line clearly shows that the variation in the ratio is in fact quite small in most of the lung, i.e. in the lower 75% of the lungs. In exercise the apex of the lung becomes better perfused so there is far less gravity-induced variation in the $\dot{V}_A/\dot{Q}$ ratios. The poor perfusion of the apical regions causes them to contribute little to overall gas exchanges. Furthermore the high $\dot{V}_A/\dot{Q}$ ratio of the apical regions means that the relative overventilation flushes out more CO_2 from the blood—in contrast, no extra O_2 is absorbed because, as the Po_2 is already high, the blood is already virtually fully saturated. Thus the $\dot{V}CO_2/\dot{V}O_2$, i.e. *R*, is high in the apical units and, conversely, low in the basal units.

As stated above, Po_2 is low (and Pco_2 high) in the alveolar gas and end-capillary blood of basal compared with apical regions. As total ventilation of basal is greater than apical regions, the alveolar gas from the basal region will make a greater contribution to the final expired alveolar gas mix. Similarly, the contribution from basal regions will dominate the final blood gas composition but to a much greater extent because the basal-to-apical gradation in blood flow is far greater. Thus the mixed blood leaving the lungs (the eventual arterial Po_2 for the rest of the body) will have a lower arterial Po_2 than the final alveolar Po_2. Moreover, when mixing within the blood phase is considered, one must sum the O_2 in units of content, not partial pressure, because of the non-linear shape of the oxyhaemoglobin dissociation curve (p. 470). Thus blood from the apical areas with a high $\dot{V}_A/\dot{Q}$ ratio, although having a high Po_2, will not have a higher O_2 content and therefore cannot compensate adequately for the low O_2 content of blood from the basal regions. As a consequence, the lowering of arterial Po_2 is exaggerated.

Assessment of $\dot{V}_A/\dot{Q}$ inequality

As the measurement of $\dot{V}_A/\dot{Q}$ inequality is difficult, its presence is indirectly assessed from the magnitude of the alveolar–arterial Po_2 difference. Often an 'ideal' alveolar Po_2 is calculated using the alveolar gas equation (p. 453) which assumes no $\dot{V}_A/\dot{Q}$ inequality. The presence of low $\dot{V}_A/\dot{Q}$ units is assessed with the shunt equation (p. 460) while pretending that there are no anatomical shunts and assuming that all the lowered P_aO_2 is due to blood passing through unventilated alveoli. The presence of high $\dot{V}_A/\dot{Q}$ units is assessed by calculating the physiological dead space, using arterial and mixed-expired Pco_2 in the Bohr equation (p. 449), and assuming that the alveolar dead space component of physiological dead space (p. 449) is entirely caused by ventilation of unperfused alveoli.

Alveolar–arterial Po_2 and Pco_2 differences

In healthy upright lungs P_aO_2 is usually 5–10 mmHg lower than P_AO_2. Half of this alveolar–arterial Po_2 difference is caused by the gravity-induced variations in $\dot{V}_A/\dot{Q}$; the rest is a consequence of anatomical shunts and any alveolar units receiving no ventilation. The alveolar–arterial Po_2 difference increases in heavy exercise and in diseases, which produce excessive $\dot{V}_A/\dot{Q}$ inequality, increased shunting or impaired diffusion across the alveolar–capillary membrane. The low P_aO_2 resulting from $\dot{V}_A/\dot{Q}$ abnormalities or impaired diffusion can be improved by high O_2 breathing, but not that due to shunts.

The effects of $\dot{V}_A/\dot{Q}$ and shunts also cause arterial Pco_2 to be greater than alveolar Pco_2 but the difference is less than 1 mmHg because the CO_2 blood dissociation curve (content vs. P_{CO_2}) in the physiological range is not only linear but also very steep (p. 475). Thus large changes in CO_2 content occur for only very small changes in P_{CO_2}. An arterial–alveolar P_{CO_2} difference may be just detectable if $\dot{V}_A/\dot{Q}$ mismatching is severe or the alveolar–capillary membrane is grossly thickened.

18.5 Blood gas transport

O₂ carriage

Nearly all of the O_2 in the blood is carried in the red blood cells bound to the haem part of haemoglobin; a very small amount (~1%) is carried in physical solution. The amount of O_2 per litre of blood thus depends on the haemoglobin concentration and its degree of saturation. This in turn depends on P_{O_2}. Typically in arterial blood with a P_{O_2} of 95 mmHg, the haemoglobin saturation is 97% and, if the haemoglobin concentration is $150 \, g \, L^{-1}$, the O_2 content is $195 \, mL \, L^{-1}$; in venous blood P_{O_2} is 40 mmHg, haemoglobin saturation 70% and O_2 content $140 \, mL \, L^{-1}$. Each haemoglobin molecule binds four O_2 molecules to different degrees, giving rise to the sigmoidal shape of the oxyhaemoglobin dissociation curve in which O_2 content, or percentage of haemoglobin saturation, is plotted against blood P_{O_2}. An increase in blood temperature and in the amount of CO_2, H^+ or 2,3-bisphosphoglycerate (2,3-BPG) bound to the globin part of haemoglobin decreases the affinity of haemoglobin for O_2 and thus shifts the curve to the right; opposing changes shift the curve to the left. Shifts are described as an increase (right shift) or decrease (left shift) in the P_{50} (i.e. the P_{O_2} at which 50% saturation of the haemoglobin molecule occurs). Shifts in either direction caused by changes in CO_2 and H^+ are called the Bohr effect.

The amount of O_2 physically dissolved in the blood depends on its solubility and is proportional to its partial pressure (Henry's law: gas content = solubility × partial pressure). At 37°C the solubility of O_2 in blood is $0.03 \, mL \, L^{-1}$ for every mmHg increase in partial pressure. Thus arterial blood at a P_{O_2} of 100 mmHg will contain in physical solution 3 mL of O_2 per litre of blood. If this was the only

means of gas carriage, the body's resting O_2 consumption of 300 mL of O_2 per minute would require an impossibly high $\dot{Q}$ of at least $100 \, L \, min^{-1}$ with no O_2 left behind in the venous blood. Fortunately, the combination of O_2 with haemoglobin in the red blood cells results in about $200 \, mL \, L^{-1}$ being carried in arterial blood; only about 1.5% of the total is therefore in physical solution.

The **haemoglobin concentration** in the blood is typically taken as $150 \, g \, L^{-1}$ (but see Chapter 13, Table 13.3 for normal range) and each gram of haemoglobin when fully saturated with O_2 has combined with 1.34 mL of O_2. The term **O_2 capacity** of the blood is used to indicate how much O_2 per litre of blood is attached to the haemoglobin when fully saturated with O_2—it therefore depends on the individual's haemoglobin (Hb) concentration:

$$O_2 \text{ capacity} = 1.34 \times Hb \text{ concentration}$$
$$(mL \, O_2 \, L^{-1} \text{ blood}) = (mL \, O_2 \, g^{-1} \, Hb)$$
$$\times (g \, Hb \, L^{-1} \text{ blood})$$

When the haemoglobin concentration is $150 \, g \, L^{-1}$ the O_2 capacity is $201 \, mL \, O_2 \, L^{-1}$, whereas in an anaemic person with a haemoglobin of, say, $100 \, g \, L^{-1}$, the O_2 capacity is much reduced, at $134 \, mL \, O_2 \, L^{-1}$. The blood, even arterial, is rarely fully saturated with O_2 as this requires a high P_{O_2} of nearly 300 mmHg. The expression **O_2 saturation of Hb** (%) describes whether the sites on the haemoglobin molecules which carry O_2 are fully or partially occupied:

$$O_2 \text{ saturation of Hb (\%)}$$
$$= \frac{O_2 \text{ bound to Hb} (mL \, O_2 \, L^{-1})}{O_2 \text{ capacity} (mL \, O_2 \, L^{-1})} \times 100$$

Note that the amount of O_2 bound to the haemoglobin equals the total O_2 content of the blood sample minus the amount of O_2 in physical solution. Stated another way:

Total O_2 content $= 1.34 \times Hb$ concentration
$$\times \% \text{ saturation} + (P_{O_2} \times 0.03)$$

Thus, for a healthy person with a typical arterial blood P_{O_2} of 95 mmHg, which causes 97% saturation, the O_2 bound to haemoglobin is $195 \, mL \, L^{-1}$ (assuming a haemoglobin concentration of

$150\,g\,L^{-1}$), that in solution is $2.9\,mL\,L^{-1}$ and the total is $197.9\,mL\,L^{-1}$. For venous blood with a Po_2 of $40\,mmHg$ causing 70% saturation of haemoglobin, the O_2 bound to haemoglobin is 140.7, that in solution is 1.2 and the total is $141.9\,mL\,L^{-1}$.

Haemoglobin

The haemoglobin molecule is a globular protein (M_r 64 500) composed of four subunits. Each subunit comprises a haem group contained within a crevice in a polypeptide chain. **Haem** consists of a **protoporphyrin ring** surrounding an iron atom in the ferrous state (Fig. 18.24). The iron is bonded to four nitrogens of the protoporphyrin ring; iron can form two more additional bonds—one with O_2, and the other to the proximal histidine of a polypeptide chain. There are two α and two β polypeptide chains in each haemoglobin molecule in an adult (p. 299); the four chains together are referred to as the **globin**. Globin cannot combine with O_2 but it can bind to CO_2 and H^+ ions and, in the case of β chains, to the molecule **2,3-BPG**, for-

merly known as 2,3-diphosphoglycerate, which is a metabolite of red blood cells (p. 299).

Because there are four subunits, each molecule of haemoglobin can combine through its haem groups with up to four molecules of O_2. When no O_2 is bound the so-called deoxyhaemoglobin molecules give the blood a dark blue–purple colour. As O_2 binds to the haemoglobin converting it to oxyhaemoglobin, the blood colour changes to a red when finally well oxygenated. The term **oxygenation** is used because the Hb–O_2 association is reversible; it is not an oxidation—this would consume O_2 permanently and therefore O_2 could not be released later to the tissues. The oxygenation process can be written in four stages as:

1 $Hb + O_2 = HbO_2$
2 $HbO_2 + O_2 = Hb(O_2)_2$
3 $Hb(O_2)_2 + O_2 = Hb(O_2)_3$
4 $Hb(O_2)_3 + O_2 = Hb(O_2)_4$

Deoxygenated haemoglobin exists in a 'tense' state compared with **oxygenated** haemoglobin which exists in a 'relaxed' state (Fig. 18.25). In the tense deoxy state strong ionic bonds (salt-bridges) form between the four polypeptide chains, making them immobile and keeping them apart, particularly the β chains which also have salt-bridge connections to the 2,3-BPG wedged between them. The consequence of this is that the ferrous ions do not lie in the plane of the protoporhyrin rings and these therefore adopt a bent shape. As O_2 attaches to the haem groups, the ferrous ions move into and straighten up the plane of the protoporphyrin rings. Furthermore, the ionic bonds between the polypeptide chains become broken, allowing the haemoglobin molecule to extrude the 2,3-BPG and change its configuration into its relaxed state. The attachment of one O_2 molecule facilitates the uptake of the subsequent ones. This **cooperative effect** on the **affinity of O_2 for haemoglobin** is referred to as the **haem–haem interaction** and gives rise to the sigmoidal shape of the oxyhaemoglobin dissociation curve.

Changes in the O_2 **affinity** of haemoglobin are also brought about by altered levels of Pco_2, pH and 2,3-BPG. These directly affect the globin and through salt-bridges make the haemoglobin molecule more tense or more relaxed and thus change

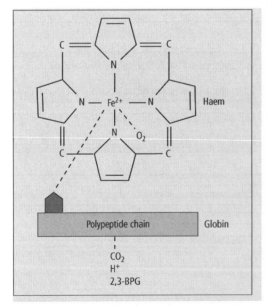

Fig. 18.24 Structure of one of the subunits of the haemoglobin molecule (note that the polypeptide chain is actually coiled and much longer than shown). 2,3-BPG, 2,3-bisphosphoglycerate; Fe^{2+}, ferrous iron.

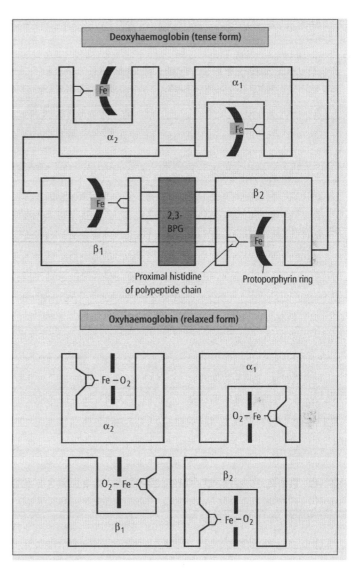

Fig. 18.25 The four subunits of haemoglobin in their deoxygenated (tense) and oxygenated (relaxed) forms. The ferrous iron and the proto-porphyrin ring lie in a crevice created by the foldings of the α and β polypeptide chains. Thin lines indicate salt-bridges. 2,3-BPG, 2,3-bisphos-phoglycerate; Fe, ferrous iron.

the affinity of the haem for O_2. As the initial site of action is at a spatially distinct site, the change in O_2 affinity is due to an **allosteric interaction**.

CO_2 decreases the affinity of haem for O_2 because it binds to terminal amino groups on all four polypeptide chains to produce carbamates ($R-NH_2 + CO_2 = R-NHCOOH$), which form salt-bridges stabilizing the tense form. Similarly, H^+ ions bind to the polypeptide chains, specifically to the amino groups ($R-NH_2 + H^+ = RNH_3^+$), carboxyl groups ($R-NHCOO^- + H^+ = R-NHCOOH$) and, most im-

portantly, to the nitrogen of the imidazole groups ($N + H^+ = NH^+$) of the histidine residues, and thereby promote the tense form. An increased concentration of 2,3-BPG stabilizes the tense form by providing extra cross-links between the β chains.

Thus hypercapnia (increased CO_2) and acidosis (increased H^+) decrease the haemoglobin affinity for O_2. An increased concentration of 2,3-BPG also decreases the haemoglobin affinity for O_2. As the production of 2,3-BPG by the red blood cells increases during chronic (long-term) hypoxia and chronic alkalosis, this counteracts the increased O_2 affinity associated with acute alkalosis.

Sickle-cell anaemia and a deficiency in the enzyme pyruvate kinase of red cells cause increased production of 2,3-BPG, while hexokinase enzyme deficiency results in decreased production. Blood becomes low in 2,3-BPG in chronic acidosis or when stored in blood banks for as little as 1 week (p. 314). This results in haemoglobin with a high O_2 affinity so that, when the blood is transfused, the haemoglobin will not offload its O_2 readily to the tissues.

Oxyhaemoglobin dissociation curve

The amount of O_2 bound to haemoglobin is determined by Po_2 and the relationship between the two is the **oxyhaemoglobin dissociation curve** (Fig. 18.26)—the term association curve is equally appropriate but rarely used. Such a curve is constructed by equilibrating (at the same temperature, pH and Pco_2) a series of blood samples each with a gas mixture containing a different Po_2. The vertical axis is expressed as either the per cent saturation or O_2 content (mLL^{-1}). The values for O_2 content portrayed in Fig. 18.26 are for a person with a haemoglobin concentration of $150\,g\,L^{-1}$ and do *not* include the O_2 content in physical solution.

The oxyhaemoglobin dissociation curve (Fig. 18.26) has a characteristic **sigmoidal shape**, which is due to sequential binding of the four O_2 molecules, one to each of the four haem groups where each combination facilitates the next (the haem–haem interaction). The last binding proceeds very rapidly, which helps to counteract the tendency of the whole process to slow down as the haemoglobin molecule becomes saturated. The **flat upper portion** of the curve occurs around Po_2

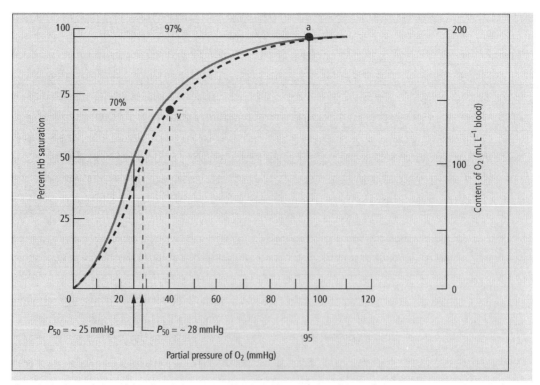

Fig. 18.26 The oxyhaemoglobin dissociation curve. Blue sigmoid curve for conditions of $Pco_2 = 40\,mmHg$ and pH = 7.4. Dashed sigmoid curve for conditions of $Pco_2 = 46\,mmHg$ and pH = 7.37. a, arterial value; v̄, mixed-venous value. Hb, haemoglobin.

values usually encountered in the alveoli (~100 mmHg) where O_2 is associating with the haemoglobin. The advantage of this flatness is that it permits the blood to attain a good saturation with O_2 even if the alveolar Po_2 were to fall to 60 mmHg (the haemoglobin would then be ~90% saturated). This offers some degree of safety for onloading O_2 when at altitude or in diseases producing low P_AO_2 or P_aO_2. Conversely, increases in Po_2 above the normal 100 mmHg by voluntary hyperventilation or by breathing high O_2 will make very little difference to the O_2 content of the blood.

The **steep middle portion** occurs around Po_2 values encountered in the tissues (~40 mmHg) where O_2 is dissociating from the haemoglobin. The advantage of this steepness is that if the tissues were to increase their metabolism, larger quantities of O_2 can be offloaded to the tissues for only a very small decrease in blood Po_2. Thus, during activity decreases in venous Po_2 are relatively small and the blood-to-tissue Po_2 gradient required for diffusion can be maintained with little reduction.

Figure 18.26 also compares the O_2–Hb curve for samples of blood maintained at a pH of 7.4 and Pco_2 of 40 mmHg (normal arterial conditions) with a second curve for blood maintained at pH 7.37 and Pco_2 46 mmHg (resting venous conditions). Clearly, venous conditions have shifted the curve to the right and, for any given Po_2, less O_2 is bound to the haemoglobin or, stated another way, the affinity of haemoglobin for O_2 has decreased and thus more O_2 has been released. A change in O_2 affinity is usually described by the P_{50}, the Po_2 at **which the haemoglobin is 50% saturated**. The P_{50} for arterial conditions is 25 mmHg; it increases to ~28 mmHg in venous blood. In other words, when blood has a decreased O_2 affinity, the P_{50} is increased because the curve itself is shifted to the right. The normal resting arterial values are Po_2 95 mmHg, haemoglobin saturation 97%, haemoglobin O_2 content 195 mL L^{-1}, while the venous values are Po_2 40 mmHg, haemoglobin saturation 70%, haemoglobin O_2 content 141 mL L^{-1}.

Bohr effect

The shift of the O_2–Hb dissociation curve to the right under conditions of increased Pco_2 and decreased pH (as in venous blood) shows how increased H$^+$ ions and CO_2 decrease the O_2 affinity of the haem group by an allosteric interaction with the globin, which promotes the tense form of the haemoglobin molecule. Conversely, when H$^+$ ions and Pco_2 in the blood decrease, the O_2–Hb curve shifts to the left and the P_{50} is decreased (Fig. 18.27) because the relaxed form of the haemoglobin molecule has an increased O_2 affinity. These right and left shifts due to H$^+$ ions and CO_2 are called the **Bohr effect**. An increase in blood temperature and in the 2,3-BPG produced by the red blood cells also shifts the O_2–Hb curve to the right; decreases in temperature and 2,3-BPG cause the curve to shift to the left (Fig. 18.27). The 2,3-BPG has a known allosteric effect and temperature acts through altering the effective acidity.

Situations altering O_2 affinity

Different situations cause the curve, usually to advantage, to shift to the right or left. As blood enters the **lung** and CO_2 diffuses out of the blood into the alveoli, the reduction in blood Pco_2 and H$^+$ ions shifts the curve to the left (Fig. 18.26). Thus the affinity of haemoglobin for O_2 in the upper part of the curve increases at the site where O_2 is available for onloading. As blood enters the **tissue** capillaries and picks up CO_2, the right shift specifically of the steep part of the curve decreases the affinity of haemoglobin for O_2 at the site where O_2 needs to be released to the tissues.

If the tissues become metabolically more active (e.g. muscles in **exercise**), CO_2 production will increase, more acid will form and more heat will be generated—all factors promoting further shifting of the O_2–Hb curve to the right, which automatically releases more O_2 from the haemoglobin to the tissues that need it in greater supply (Fig. 18.28a). Note that the difference in arteriovenous (a–v) O_2 content is increased in exercise (p. 619). In intensely exercising skeletal muscles, lactic acid production will also raise the concentration of H$^+$ ions in the blood perfusing them—favouring even more offloading of O_2 for any given Po_2. In prolonged severe exercise there is also an increased production of 2,3-BPG—again a factor promoting offloading of O_2 to the muscle. Acidosis would be

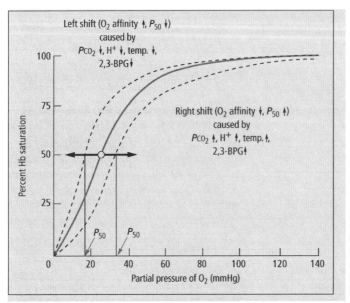

Fig. 18.27 Right and left shifts in the oxyhaemoglobin dissociation curve; blue line for P_{CO_2} 40 mmHg, pH 7.40 and blood temperature 37°C. 2,3-BPG, 2,3-bisphosphoglycerate; Hb, haemoglobin.

expected to decrease production of 2,3-BPG (p. 468) but in this situation the excessively hypoxic state of venous conditions has a stronger effect and increases production. In **circulatory failure**, if O_2 consumption is to be satisfied given the poor cardiac output, the a–vO_2 difference must increase (Fick principle)—the arterial O_2 is unchanged but the venous O_2 falls (Fig. 18.28a). Hypercapnia and acidosis shift the O_2–Hb curve to the right.

At high **altitude** or in diseases causing **chronic hypoxia** a shift of the curve to the right occurs due to increased production of 2,3-BPG (Fig. 18.28b). This ensures that, despite the low P_aO_2 and lower haemoglobin saturation, the usual amount of O_2 will be released to the tissues from the blood for only a small fall in tissue and hence venous P_{O_2}. This effect of 2,3-BPG more than compensates for the effect of hypocapnia, which would act to shift the curve to the left; the hypocapnia is the result of the stimulated breathing caused by the hypoxia of altitude. At altitude the a–vO_2 difference may, in accord with the Fick principle, actually decrease a little (not shown) because the cardiac output may increase.

In **anaemia** the haemoglobin concentration is low and therefore so is the O_2 content (Fig. 18.28c).

The shape of the saturation curve, however, is very similar to normal, unless the anaemia is severe, in which case the curve is shifted to the right due to the increased synthesis of 2,3-BPG caused by chronic hypoxia (Fig. 18.28d). The increase in 2,3-BPG results in more O_2 being released from the haemoglobin to the tissues for a particular P_{O_2}, thus compensating to some extent for the lower O_2 content. The a–vO_2 difference in mild anaemia will not change from normal but in severe anaemia there is a limit to how low the venous P_{O_2} can fall without impairing diffusion gradients between blood and tissues. Thus the a–vO_2 difference becomes smaller (not shown) and, if O_2 metabolism is not to fall, the cardiac output must increase.

Fetal haemoglobin has few β chains; instead there are γ chains (p. 299), which bind 2,3-BPG weakly thus creating fewer salt-bridges. The consequence is a relaxed state for the haemoglobin molecule and therefore, in effect, fetal haemoglobin has a curve which is shifted to the left, indicative of high O_2 affinity (Fig. 18.28e). This left shift more than compensates for the effect of fetal blood acidity, which by itself would cause a right shift. The left shift facilitates the uptake of O_2 by the fetus from the placenta, where not only is the P_{O_2} rather

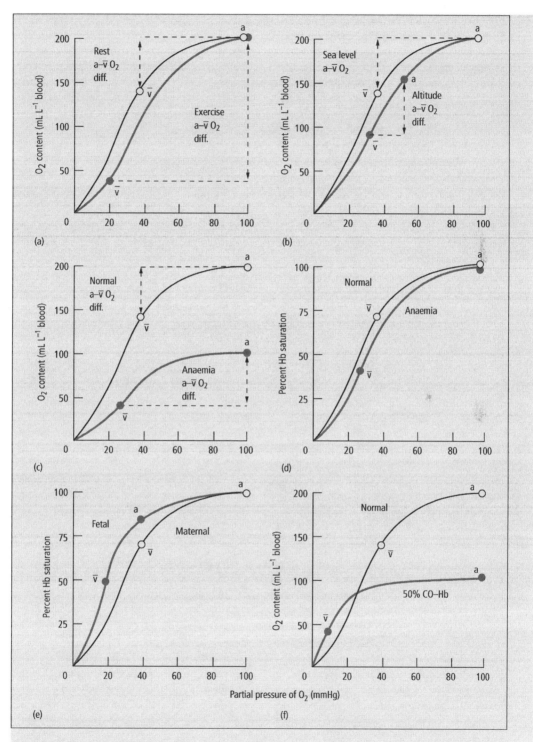

Fig. 18.28 The oxyhaemoglobin dissociation curve in the normal situation compared with (a) intense exercise or circulatory failure, (b) long-term altitude (chronic hypoxia), (c) O_2 content in anaemia, (d) per cent haemoglobin saturation in anaemia, (e) fetal blood and (f) CO poisoning. The O_2 content is given for normal blood, assuming a haemoglobin concentration of $150\,g\,L^{-1}$. Arterial (a) and mixed-venous (v̄) values are shown. Hb, haemoglobin.

low, but also the diffusion distances are greater than in the lung. O_2 transfer to the fetus is also enhanced by the higher haemoglobin concentration of fetal blood.

Carbon monoxide is poisonous because it combines with haem about 250 times more avidly than O_2. For instance, this gas at an environmental concentration of only 0.1%, if breathed for about 100 min, will come to occupy 50% of the haem sites. Given the now reduced O_2 capacity, the O_2 dissociation curve will be displaced below normal (Fig. 18.28f). It also shifts to the left because when CO combines with haem it forms **carboxyhaemoglobin** (CO–Hb), which pulls on the histidine of the polypeptide chains more strongly than oxyhaemoglobin, thus weakening the salt-bridges more and promoting a more relaxed form of haemoglobin. The left shift of the O_2–Hb curve makes the situation even worse, as what little O_2 was bound in the alveoli to the haemoglobin is not released very easily to the tissues. Carboxyhaemoglobin gives a distinctive cherry-red colour to the blood. The treatment for CO poisoning is a blood transfusion, or administration of 100% O_2 or, even better, hyperbaric O_2 (p. 492), which over a number of hours will very slowly displace the CO.

Cyanosis

Cyanosis is a blue–purple colour, most obvious in the skin, nail beds and mucosal membranes, caused by a low O_2 saturation of haemoglobin in the arteriolar blood and is indicative of blood with a low O_2 content. Its presence is detectable when there is at least $50 g L^{-1}$ of deoxyhaemoglobin, but reliable recognition depends on skin pigmentation, suitable illumination and adequate capillary perfusion. At a normal haemoglobin concentration of $150 g L^{-1}$, cyanosis is evident at 66% saturation when the O_2 content is ~130 mL $O_2 L^{-1}$. However, in polycythaemia, in which the haemoglobin concentration is elevated to, say, $250 g L^{-1}$, cyanosis can occur at 80% saturation and would not be indicative of an abnormally low O_2 content. In contrast, in anaemia, where the O_2 content is always low, there may be insufficient deoxyhaemoglobin to allow cyanosis to be seen

(e.g. if haemoglobin concentration was $100 g L^{-1}$, the O_2 content is already low at $134 mL L^{-1}$ and would have to fall to $67 mL L^{-1}$ to be seen as cyanotic). **Central cyanosis** (blue mouth and tongue) is due to poor gas exchange in diseased lungs or to R–L shunts. In **peripheral cyanosis** (blue limbs but pink mucosa) the lungs are healthy but there is poor circulation.

Myoglobin

Myoglobin is not found in the blood, but in skeletal and cardiac muscle cells where it is a respiratory pigment, which aids O_2 delivery. In contrast to haemoglobin, myoglobin only has one haem group and one globin chain and thus has a hyperbolic O_2 dissociation curve (Fig. 18.29), which is independent of pH or P_{CO_2}. Furthermore, its P_{50} is 5 mmHg and it is about 90% saturated at a P_{O_2} of 20 mmHg. O_2 is only extracted from the myoglobin store at the sudden start of exercise (p. 617) at a time when blood perfusion has not yet increased sufficiently to supply the required O_2. The myoglobin store of O_2 is replenished at the end of exercise, when the P_{O_2} of the muscle cells rises above 10 mmHg.

CO$_2$ carriage

The CO_2–blood dissociation curve (CO_2 content plotted against P_{CO_2}) is curvilinear and does not show saturation. Typically, at rest, arterial blood has a P_{CO_2} of 40 mmHg with a CO_2 content of $490 mL L^{-1}$; while venous blood has a P_{CO_2} of 46 mmHg and a CO_2 content of $535 mL L^{-1}$. The CO_2 affinity of blood is decreased by oxygenation of the haem groups as this makes the globin less able to combine with CO_2 and H^+. Conversely, deoxygenated blood has a higher CO_2 affinity. These changes in CO_2 affinity caused by O_2 binding are called collectively the Haldane effect and result in downwards and upwards shifts in the CO_2–blood dissociation curve. CO_2 produced by the tissues is carried not only by the globin part of the haemoglobin molecule (as a carbamino compound, ~30%) but also in physical solution (~10%) and as bicarbonate (~60%). Due to the presence of car-

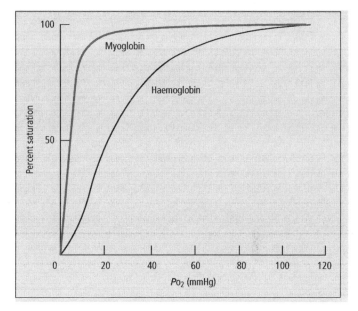

Fig. 18.29 Oxygen dissociation curve for myoglobin compared with haemoglobin.

bonic anhydrase, most of the HCO_3^- (and H^+) is formed in the red cells but the HCO_3^- then diffuses out into the plasma in exchange for chloride. The H^+ ions are buffered by globin. An osmotic imbalance occurs so that water enters the red cells by osmosis, causing them to swell. The pH of the plasma is dependent on the ratio of HCO_3^- to Pco_2 (the Henderson–Hasselbalch equation), so that the pH of arterial and venous blood are 7.40 and 7.37, respectively. The Pco_2 is rapidly controlled by ventilation, whereas HCO_3^- is slowly altered by the kidneys.

CO₂–blood dissociation curve

The shape of the **CO₂–blood dissociation curve** (Fig. 18.30a) differs from that of the O_2–Hb curve — it is not sigmoidal but curvilinear. It rises very steeply in the initial part, is virtually linear over the Pco_2 values normally encountered in the blood and never reaches saturation. Thus CO_2 content cannot be expressed in terms of per cent saturation. The blood also contains about 2.5 times more CO_2 than O_2. Venous blood at a Pco_2 of 46 mmHg has a CO_2 content of 535 mL L^{-1} and arterial blood at a Pco_2 of 40 mmHg has a CO_2 content of 490 mL L^{-1}.

Blood contains only a small part (~2.5 L calculated from ~500 mL of CO_2 per litre of blood × ~5 L of blood) of the total amount of CO_2 in the body. CO_2 stores amount to over 100 L, much of which is dissolved in fat or stored in bone. O_2 stores are minute, amounting to no more than 1.5 L, and are held in the blood, alveoli and myoglobin.

Haldane effect

For each O_2–Hb curve the Pco_2 and pH had to be defined (Fig. 18.26); similarly, for each CO_2–blood curve, the Po_2 must be held constant in the samples being equilibrated with CO_2 (Fig. 18.30b). Under arterial conditions (where Po_2 is 95 mmHg) the CO_2–blood dissociation curve is shifted down compared with venous conditions (where Po_2 is 40 mmHg). If high O_2 is breathed so that 100% O_2 saturation of haemoglobin is achieved, the CO_2–blood curve will shift just a little further down. Conversely, if Po_2 is lower than 40 mmHg (e.g. venous conditions in exercise or at altitude) the CO_2–blood curve will shift even further upwards. A downward shift in the CO_2–blood curve means that for a given Pco_2 the blood can hold less CO_2 content — that is, the **CO₂ affinity** of the blood has decreased. Conversely, an upward shift in the curve for a given Pco_2 indicates that the

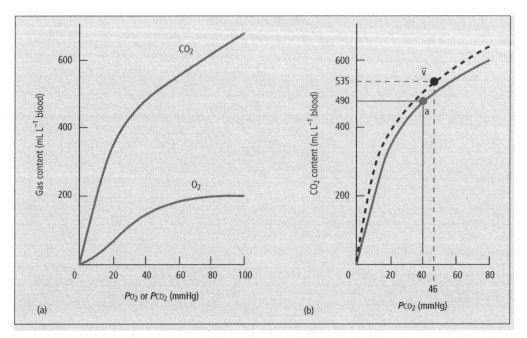

Fig. 18.30 (a) Comparison of O_2– and CO_2–blood dissociation curves. (b) The CO_2–blood dissociation curve, where a is the arterial and v̄ the mixed-venous value. The blue curve is for a P_{O_2} condition of 100 mmHg when haemoglobin is nearly 100% oxygenated; the dashed curve is for a P_{O_2} condition of 40 mmHg when haemoglobin is ~70% oxygenated.

blood has a higher CO_2 affinity and can hold more CO_2 content. (As blood does not saturate with CO_2, an equivalent of the P_{50} of the O_2–Hb curve cannnot be used.)

The effect of changes in O_2 on CO_2 carriage is called the **Haldane effect** (whereas the effect of CO_2/H^+ on O_2 carriage is the Bohr effect). As with the Bohr effect, the Haldane effect is due to allosteric interactions (p. 471) within the haemoglobin molecule.

When the haem group is fully oxygenated, promoting the relaxed form of the haemoglobin molecule which has no salt-bridges, the imidazole groups in the globin chains are more dissociated (i.e. a stronger acid) and thus a weaker buffer. Globin is therefore less able to combine with H^+ ions and to form carbamino compounds (see below) with CO_2. The deoxygenated haemoglobin molecule, by contrast, is a weaker acid and thus a stronger buffer and can form more carbamino compound.

Forms in which CO_2 are carried

CO_2 is carried in the blood in three forms: in **physical solution**, as carbamino compounds and as bicarbonate (Table 18.4). CO_2 is very much more soluble than O_2—its solubility coefficient is 0.65 mL of CO_2 per litre of blood per mmHg of P_{CO_2}. At an arterial P_{CO_2} of 40 mmHg and a venous P_{CO_2} of 46 mmHg, 26 and 30 mL of CO_2 per litre of blood, respectively, are therefore carried dissolved in physical solution. This is about 5–6% of the total CO_2 content (cf. only 1% of O_2 content is carried in solution).

Some 5–10% of the total CO_2 is carried in the form of **carbamino compounds** which are formed when CO_2 combines with the terminal amine groups of plasma proteins and, in particular, of the globin chain of the haemoglobin molecule. The reaction is R–NH_2 + CO_2 = R–NHCOOH.

The remaining 85–90% of the total CO_2 is carried as **bicarbonate**. CO_2 is hydrated by water into carbonic acid which is a weak acid and thus it partially dissociates into H^+ ions and bicarbonate, i.e. $H_2O + CO_2 \leftrightarrow H_2CO_3 \leftrightarrow H^+ + HCO_3^-$. The hydration step is slow in the plasma but is accelerated (to as short as ~0.1 s) in the red blood cells by the enzyme **carbonic anhydrase**. Although most of the bicarbonate is formed in the red blood cells, only about a quarter of it remains there; the rest ends up in the plasma.

Table 18.4 shows not only the proportions in which the three forms of CO_2 are carried in arterial and venous blood but also, and more importantly, the proportions in which the CO_2 produced by the tissues is carried. As the newly produced CO_2 converts arterial into venous blood, 8% goes into physical solution, 30% forms carbamino compounds and 62% converts to bicarbonate. In other words, the carbamino form increases its contribution to the total. Figure 18.31 identifies how much of each is formed in the plasma compared with red blood cells.

Chloride shift

As bicarbonate is formed primarily in the red blood cell rather than in the plasma, the bicarbonate will diffuse out of the cell down its concentration gradient into the plasma (hence more bicarbonate is carried in the plasma—the proportional amount determined by the volume of plasma relative to red blood cells). To preserve electroneutrality, the anion chloride moves from the plasma into the red blood cell (Fig. 18.31). This HCO_3^-/Cl^- exchange is known as the **chloride shift** or Hamburger phenomenon.

Fate of H^+ ions

H^+ ions are produced not only as carbonic acid dissociates into bicarbonate, but also by the dissociation of the carbamino compounds (weak acids)

attached to the globin chains and plasma proteins (Fig. 18.31). The differential production of H^+ ions in the red cells compared with plasma also creates a potential concentration gradient for diffusion. However, not only is the red-cell membrane impermeable to H^+, but also a greater problem exists in the high acidity levels developing in both the plasma and red cell; the problem is solved by buffering. Plasma proteins buffer H^+ ions produced in the plasma where the buffering reaction is $R–NH_2 + H^+ = R–NH_3^+$. The H^+ ions produced in the red cell are buffered mainly by the imidazole groups (p. 468) of the haemoglobin polypeptide chains, and this addition of H^+ (and CO_2) to the globin chain promotes the release of O_2 from the haem (Fig. 18.31). As the haem becomes deoxygenated it becomes a weaker acid and therefore a better buffer, so the concomitant loss of O_2 aids the buffering (and the formation of carbamino compounds). The degree of buffering is so good that the pH of venous blood (7.37) is only a little more acid than arterial blood (pH 7.40).

Osmotic balance

Each haemoglobin molecule can buffer many H^+ ions. This leaves many HCO_3^- (or Cl^-) ions as free ions constituting a pool of osmotically active particles and causing H_2O to move from the plasma into the cell (Fig. 18.31). As a consequence of **osmosis** the red cell swells; the increase in cellular volume can be detected as about a 3% greater haematocrit in venous compared with arterial blood.

Acid–base balance

Even though plasma proteins and haemoglobin act as blood buffers for H^+, the third buffer of the blood is the carbonic acid–bicarbonate system:

Table 18.4 Proportions in which CO_2 is transported in the blood.

	% Arterial (a)	% Venous (v̄)	% (v̄ − a)*
Physically dissolved	5.5	5.8	8.0
Carbamino compound	4.9	7.2	30.0
HCO_2^-	89.6	87.0	62.0

* Percentage of newly produced CO_2 in each form.

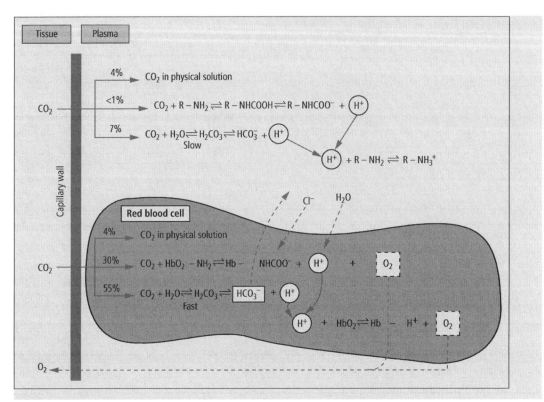

Fig. 18.31 The forms and proportions in which CO_2 is carried in the plasma and red blood cells. Also shown are the chloride shift, buffering, O_2 exchange and osmosis. Hb, haemoglobin.

$H_2O + CO_2 \leftrightarrow H_2CO_3 \leftrightarrow H^+ + HCO_3^-$. This may seem surprising, as it is a producer of H^+ ions in the first place. However, because it is a weak acid with a pK′ of 6.1, it is a good physiological buffer. When there is an increase in H^+ the mass reaction is pushed to the left, effectively buffering the H^+ by producing CO_2. This CO_2 is then excreted very rapidly by the lungs through H^+-stimulated breathing (p. 484). If CO_2 in the body increases as a result of CO_2 in the atmosphere or impaired breathing, the mass reaction is pushed to the right and the H^+ so produced is buffered by increased plasma HCO_3^- under the regulation of the kidney, albeit slowly (Table 21.2).

When the law of mass action is solved for H^+ and put into pH notation, the equation derived is called the **Henderson–Hasselbalch equation**. When applied to the carbonic acid–bicarbonate system this equation is written as:

$$pH = pK' + \log \frac{[HCO_3^-]}{0.03 \times Pco_2}$$

where pK′ is 6.1, $[HCO_3^-]$ is in mmol L^{-1}, 0.03 is the solubility of CO_2 expressed in mmol L^{-1} mmHg^{-1} and Pco_2 is in mmHg. The denominator (0.03 × Pco_2) is in this form as a substitute for $[H_2CO_3]$, which is difficult to measure. At a Pco_2 of 40 mmHg, the pH is 7.40 as the $[HCO_3^-]$ is usually 24 mmol L^{-1}; for venous conditions Pco_2 is 46 mmHg, pH 7.37 and $[HCO_3^-]$ 25.7 mmol L^{-1}. The equation makes it clear that pH depends on the ratio of $[HCO_3^-]$ to Pco_2 (the 'buffer pair'); the former is controlled slowly by the kidneys and the latter rapidly by the lungs. A primary change in one of the buffer pair is compensated for by a secondary change in the other in the appropriate direction (Table 21.2). If the primary change is an alteration in CO_2, it is called **respiratory acidosis** or **alkalosis**; if it is an alteration in $[HCO_3^-]$ it is **metabolic acidosis** or **alkalosis**. Whole-body buffering also involves buffers in the interstitial and intracellular fluids. Further details on acid–base balance are the domain of fluid and electrolyte balance (Chapter 21).

18.6 Regulation of respiration

Breathing occurs rhythmically. The rhythmicity is generated within the respiratory centres which are found in specific areas of the medulla oblongata (dorsal respiratory group (DRG), ventral respiratory group (VRG) and pre Bötzinger complex) and pons (pontine respiratory group, PRG). The depth and frequency of the resting rhythm are determined by feedback to the respiratory centres from mechanoreceptors in the lungs and chest wall. Some stimuli, e.g. temperature, pain, and emotion, affect breathing via higher brain centres (hypothalamus and limbic system), which then influence the respiratory centre. Breathing is also under appreciable voluntary control from the cerebral cortex (e.g. in breath-holding, taking large breaths or speaking) and this pathway bypasses the respiratory centres. Superimposed on the normal pattern of breathing are protective reflexes of short duration, which are initiated, for example, by irritants as in coughing or sneezing. The principal control of ventilation is from chemoreceptors located peripherally (carotid and aortic bodies) and centrally (intracranial chemoreceptors). The peripheral chemoreceptors monitor arterial P_{O_2}, P_{CO_2} and pH, while the central chemoreceptors monitor brain P_{CO_2} and pH; together they regulate breathing to provide arterial P_{O_2}, P_{CO_2} and acid–base homeostasis. Breathing is more sensitive to stimulation by high CO_2 (hypercapnia) than low O_2 (hypoxia) so ventilation is matched to metabolism through the CO_2 produced rather than the O_2 consumed.

Respiratory centres

Historical background

In the early 1920s, Lumsden performed brainstem transections and concluded that respiratory control was provided by centres that he called the pneumotaxic centre (in the upper pons), the apneustic centre (in the lower pons), and the inspiratory and expiratory centres (in the medulla oblongata). The pontine centres were postulated because a transection between upper and lower pons, effectively removing the pneumotaxic centre, produces slow deep breathing. If done in conjunction with a bilateral vagotomy, to remove vagal sensory input from the lungs, inspirations become prolonged, separated by only brief expirations (a pattern referred to as apneustic breathing). This led to the conclusion that the pneumotaxic centre normally promoted expiration and the apneustic centre normally promoted inspiration; the two together finely tuned the normal breathing pattern.

Postulation of the medullary inspiratory and expiratory centres arose because, after a transection between the pons and medulla, breathing was dominated by prolonged expiratory spasms and irregular short inspiratory gasps (hence the terms gasping centre and inspiratory centre were used interchangeably). However, more refined techniques for pons ablation have since demonstrated that the medulla by itself will produce a relatively normal pattern of rhythmic inspiration/expiration. This pattern becomes slower and deeper when the incoming vagal sensory information is blocked. As breathing is abolished only by a transection between the medulla and spinal cord, the rhythmic drive to the respiratory muscles must be generated within the medulla.

Current concepts

No specific group of neurones has ever been found in the so-called apneustic centre; consequently this concept, and any theories of respiratory control involving it, have been abandoned. The pneumotaxic centre is now referred to as the **pontine respiratory group (PRG)** and it is now known to comprise expiratory neurones in the **nucleus parabrachialis medialis** and inspiratory neurones in the **nucleus parabrachialis lateralis** and the laterally sited **Kölliker–Fuse nucleus** (Fig. 18.32a). Modern evidence indicates that rather than

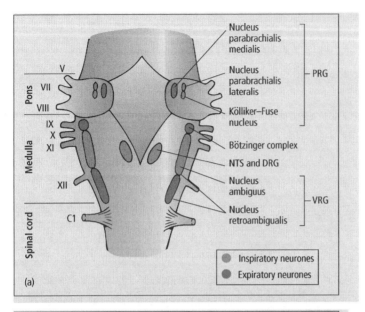

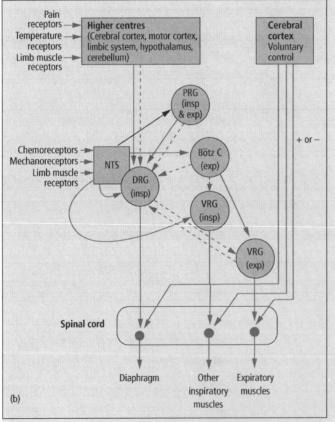

Fig. 18.32 (a) Location in the brain of neuronal groups constituting the respiratory centres. (b) Schematic representation of the well-established interconnections between neuronal groups, including sensory receptor inputs (solid blue lines, excitatory; dashed blue lines, inhibitory). Bötz C, Bötzinger complex; exp, expiration; insp, inspiration; NTS, nucleus of the tractus solitarius; PRG, pontine respiratory group; VRG, ventral respiratory group.

inspiratory and expiratory centres, the medulla is composed of three bilateral aggregations of respiratory neurones known as the DRG, the VRG and the Bötzinger complex. They receive sensory information and, after integration, adjust appropriately the efferent activity to the respiratory muscles. The pontine nuclei somehow modulate DRG and possibly VRG activity.

The **dorsal respiratory group (DRG)** is part of the **nucleus of the tractus solitarius** from which it receives afferent information from respiratory-related mechanoreceptors and chemoreceptors. It is composed mainly of inspiratory neurones. These are upper motor (premotor) neurones projecting ipsilaterally down the spinal cord to the lower motor neurones of mainly the phrenic nerves, which supply the diaphragm. The DRG inspiratory neurones also have inhibitory actions on the expiratory neurones in the **ventral respiratory group (VRG)** (Fig. 18.32b).

The **VRG** is located rostrally in the nucleus ambiguus and caudally in the nucleus retroambigualis. The **nucleus ambiguus** contains not only premotor inspiratory neurones but also motor neurones to the laryngeal muscles and parasympathetic neurones to the bronchioles and heart. The rostral part of the **nucleus retroambigualis** contains more inspiratory premotor neurones and, like those of the nucleus ambiguus, they mainly supply the external intercostals and accessory muscles rather than the diaphragm. These inspiratory VRG neurones receive sensory input and behave like those in the DRG. In the caudal part of the **nucleus retroambigualis** are mainly found the expiratory premotor neurones supplying the internal intercostal and abdominal muscles. During resting breathing, in which expiration is passive, the activity in these VRG expiratory neurones is insufficient to discharge their lower motor neurones. The VRG expiratory neurones appear to have inhibitory effects on inspiratory neurones late in the inspiratory phase, contributing to the termination of inspiration, the so-called inspiratory cut-off switch.

The **Bötzinger complex** is just rostral to the nucleus ambiguus and is composed entirely of expiratory neurones. It receives sensory input relayed through the nucleus of the tractus solitarius and has an inhibitory effect on the inspiratory neurones of the DRG and VRG and an excitatory effect on the expiratory neurones of the VRG. The **pre-Bötzinger complex** (rostral to the Bötzinger complex) is thought to form the kernel of the respiratory rhythm generator. During resting breathing the neurones in this complex display cyclical firing, which persists even when the neuronal complex is isolated. The precise mechanism by which the pre-Bötzinger complex generates respiratory rhythm is not clear. It may be that some neurones have pacemaker properties and spontaneously discharge in a phasic manner, inhibiting when they do so the expiratory neurones. An alternative hypothesis is that there is a neural network of local re-excitation with inspiratory and expiratory neuronal pools, causing reciprocal inhibition between the phasic firing of the two pools.

Higher brain centres

There is evidence that the **hypothalamus** provides a continual background excitatory drive to the DRG. Furthermore, the hypothalamic **temperature-regulating centres** receive inputs from cutaneous and deep-core thermoreceptors (p. 607) such that both hot and cold cutaneous stimuli increase breathing, as do a fever and mild hypothermia. Activation of the **defence reaction centre** (p. 409) in the hypothalamus also stimulates breathing.

Evidence also suggests that the **cerebral cortex** influences breathing by providing a continual inhibitory drive to both the hypothalamus and the DRG. The cerebral cortex and **limbic system** integrate emotional and painful stimuli and, via the hypothalamus, have both excitatory and inhibitory effects on the respiratory centres, which produce a wide variety of respiratory expressions of emotion and pain.

During exercise the **cerebral motor cortex** activates—with a feed-forward command—the DRG to increase breathing in proportion to the degree of exercise (p. 621). Limb muscle receptors (p. 621) appear to cause some of the ventilatory increase occurring in exercise (p. 621), and some of their input is integrated by **cerebellar nuclei** (p. 408).

All **voluntary** control of respiration—as in taking large breaths, performing forced expirations, hyperventilating deliberately, speaking or breath-holding—stems from the cerebral cortex, but it bypasses the respiratory centres and travels in the pyramidal system directly to the lower motor neurones (Fig. 18.32b). In these circumstances the cortex can, for a short time, override respiratory reflexes but eventually the reflex control takes precedence.

Mechanoreceptors and the pattern of breathing

Input in the vagal nerves from stretch and irritant receptors of the lung acts on the so-called inspiratory cut-off switch and helps determine the V_T and f that produce a particular level of ventilation. f is dependent on the time spent in the T_I and T_E phases of breathing. If these lung receptor inputs are removed by a vagotomy (and the pontine nuclei are intact), breathing is slow and deep—this is the basic pattern generated by the respiratory centres. With vagal input the normal breathing pattern is achieved—one that is relatively fast and shallow.

Lung-stretch receptors are in the smooth muscle of the trachea and lower airways and are stimulated in proportion to the degree of lung inflation by the accompanying increase in transmural pressure. Their nervous discharge shows little adaptation to a sustained inflation but, during normal breathing, increases and decreases in phase with inspiration and expiration. This phasic afferent information inhibits directly, and via the PRG, the inspiratory neurones of the DRG while the inspiration is in progress. The outcome of this vagal input is a shorter T_I and smaller V_T; the vagal input also lengthens the duration of the next T_E by inhibiting the occurrence of the next inspiration.

Lung-irritant receptors are also stimulated during inspiration but they affect only the duration of the next T_E by shortening it via an excitatory input to the DRG, which promotes an earlier occurrence of the next inspiration. As the lung-irritant effect on T_E dominates that from the lung-stretch recep-

tors, the two receptor types together produce the normal breathing pattern of a shallow V_T and short T_I and T_E.

The vagal effect on breathing is more pronounced in the newborn and anaesthetized state; furthermore, the potency of the lung-stretch receptor reflex is also species-dependent. In conscious adult humans this reflex appears to be weak in the resting V_T range but at the higher V_T of exercise or of breathing driven by hypoxia or hypercapnia, the effects of the lung-stretch receptor reflex become more apparent. Thus, although the breathing pattern at rest is altered little by heart–lung transplantation, f in these patients does not increase as much during stimulated breathing.

The breathing pattern, particularly in humans, is also determined by **proprioceptors** (joint receptors, Golgi tendon organs and muscle spindles) that are present in the chest wall and diaphragm (the latter has mainly tendon organs) and provide information about thoracic inflation. Proprioceptors also provide feedback, which enables the strength of the contraction to be varied so that a certain V_T can be achieved if the airway resistance changes. The proprioceptor reflex is integrated within the spinal cord. Since one becomes aware of changes in chest compliance and airways resistance, it is assumed that the stretch afferents relay to the sensory cortex as well as to the respiratory centres. The distressful sensation of breathlessness is called **dyspnoea** but which receptors provoke this sensation is not known; chest-wall afferents have been implicated, but all respiratory mechanoreceptors as well as higher brain centres are likely to contribute.

Mechanoreceptors and protective reflexes

Mechanoreceptors having reflex effects on respiration are found in the upper airways (nose, epipharynx, larynx and trachea). In the lower airways (bronchi to alveolar ducts) there are lung-stretch, lung-irritant and bronchial C receptors and, in the alveoli, pulmonary C (or juxtacapillary) receptors. All of these mechanoreceptors provide protective reflexes affecting both ventilation and bronchomotor tone. As the cardiovascular system has a large role to play in gas transport, most of these respiratory mechanoreceptors also cause cardiovascular reflexes (p. 406). Similarly, some of the mechanoreceptors located in the cardiovascular system also elicit respiratory reflexes — baroreceptors or ventricular vagal afferents depress, while ventricular sympathetic afferents augment breathing.

Nerve endings of the trigeminal (Vth) nerves in the **nasal mucosa** are excited by chemical and mechanical irritants and reflexly cause a **sneeze** and broncholaryngeal constriction. A sneeze is a number of superimposed inspirations followed by a strong and rapid expiration and then a short pause in the expiratory position. Stimulation by liquids produces only a long pause in breathing, i.e. an apnoea, which is well developed in diving mammals.

Glossopharyngeal nerve endings in the epithelium of the **epipharynx** are excited by mechanical irritants such as a blockage and this results in the **aspiration reflex** and bronchodilation. The aspiration reflex is a powerful inspiration, which attempts to pull the blockage into the pharynx. A **negative pressure pharyngeal reflex**, which activates the genioglossus muscle (tongue), has also been demonstrated in response to excessive negative intraluminal pressure. Excessive pressures, up to −20 to 30 cmH$_2$O can be generated by breathing against an occluded airway, such as may occur during sleep in patients with obstructive sleep apnoea (p. 489). Activation of the negative pressure reflex triggers the re-opening of the upper airway; impairment of this is implicated in this condition.

Vagal nerve endings in the epithelium of the **larynx** and **trachea** are excited by mechanical and chemical irritants and reflexly cause a **cough** and broncholaryngeal constriction. A cough is a large slow inspiration followed, initially against a closed glottis, by rapid and powerful expirations. As in the sneeze, the broncholaryngeal constriction increases expiratory airflow velocity, helping to expel the irritants. Mild stimulation of these receptors causes slow, deep breathing.

As described earlier, **lung-stretch receptors** are involved in determining the pattern of breathing and are slowly adapting vagal nerve endings in the smooth muscle of the trachea and lower airways. Experimentally, if these receptors are stimulated by a sustained inflation (followed by occlusion of the airways), there is a reflex cessation of diaphragmatic activity and the duration of the pause is proportional to the degree of inflation. Conversely, a sustained deflation with an occluded airway promotes strong and frequent inspiratory efforts. These responses are called the **Hering–Breuer reflex**, and in real life can be viewed as protective, preventing too much inflation or too much deflation. Stimulation of these receptors also causes bronchodilation.

Lung-irritant receptors are vagal nerve endings in the epithelia of the trachea and lower airways that are stimulated by mechanical or chemical irritants such as mucus, noxious gases or tobacco smoke. The protective reflex initiated is an increase in f and V_T, together with broncholaryngeal constriction. Histamine released in **asthma** probably stimulates the lung-irritant receptors. These receptors can also be stimulated by large deflations and inflations, but the response rapidly adapts (hence their alternative name of rapidly adapting lung-stretch receptors). In this reflex the response is a short-lived, intense inspiration. Thus the lung-irritant receptors permit, and may even trigger, the augmented breaths or **sighs** that punctuate normal breathing. These sighs serve to re-inflate and reset the compliance of alveoli that have gradually collapsed with time during quiet breathing (p. 438). The role of the lung-irritant receptors in determining the pattern of breathing has already been considered.

Bronchial C and **pulmonary C** receptors are vagal nerve endings of unmyelinated (C) fibres lying respectively in the bronchial interstitium or next to capillaries in the alveolar interstitium. Pulmonary C receptors, because of their position, are also called **juxtacapillary** or **J receptors**. Bronchial and pulmonary C receptors are usually silent and therefore do not play a role in the regulation of normal breathing. Both are stimulated by mechanical distortion or increases in ISF pressure. Large inflations stimulate the bronchial C receptors, though with rapid adaptation, while lung congestion or oedema stimulates the pulmonary C receptors. Both receptor types are also stimulated by substances such as histamine, bradykinin and prostaglandins, that are released in lung disease. The reflex initiated is broncholaryngeal constriction, apnoea followed by rapid shallow breathing and, if the stimulus is severe, the so-called J reflex which is an inhibition of spinal motor neurones, thus relaxing skeletal muscles. A general depression of somatic (and cardiovascular; p. 406) activity is a most appropriate response to serious lung damage.

Respiratory chemoreceptors

As some of the mechanoreceptors can also respond to certain chemical stimuli, the term chemoreceptors is usually reserved for those receptors monitoring, directly or indirectly, blood gases. Chemoreceptors maintain homeostasis of arterial Po2, Pco2 and pH and assist in ensuring that V.E is appropriate to the level of metabolism. They are stimulated by a rise in Paco2 (hypercapnia), a rise in arterial [H+] (acidosis) and a fall in Pao2 (hypoxia), and reflexly cause an increase in V.E (and of course in V.A). As described previously, V.A is one of the determinants of the alveolar and hence blood gas composition (p. 452), so that the reflex increase in V.A lowers Paco2 and elevates Pao2, thus restoring alveolar and arterial gases back towards normal (Pco2 40 mmHg and Po2 100 mmHg). Since V.E is more sensitive to increases in Paco2 than to decreases in Pao2 (Fig. 18.33), the controlling link between V.E and metabolism is the CO2 produced rather than the O2 consumed. The precision of control is such that in healthy individuals Paco2 and PAco2 remain remarkably constant (± 2 mmHg) over a wide range of metabolic rates.

Ventilatory chemosensitivity

The sensitivity of breathing to hypercapnia and hypoxia can be experimentally determined by altering the composition of the inspired gas (the $F_I co_2$ or $F_I o_2$). When, for example, the $F_I co_2$ is

raised, $P_A co_2$ and hence $P_a co_2$ increase (p. 453). Some minutes later the final (i.e. steady-state) increase in $P_a co_2$ is less than the initial increase because the reflex stimulation of $\dot{V}_E$ lowers the $P_a co_2$. However, in the face of altered inspired gases, the $\dot{V}_E$ increase can never restore $P_a co_2$ (or $P_a o_2$) to normal (see Figs 18.17 and 18.18).

In **hypercapnia** (respiratory acidosis) the steady-state responses show that the $\dot{V}_E$ is linearly related to $P_a co_2$ (Fig. 18.33a, solid blue line). Note also that at lower $P_a co_2$ values $\dot{V}_E$ becomes less sensitive to $P_a co_2$ and at higher $P_a co_2$ values $\dot{V}_E$ sensitivity is reduced due to CO2 narcosis of the respiratory and other neural centres in the brain. During such hypercapnia tests, the $P_a o_2$ will progressively increase from the normal ~100 to up to ~120 mmHg because of hyperventilation. If the inspired O2 is deliberately decreased experimentally to maintain the $P_a o_2$ constant at, say, 50 mmHg during the hypercapnia tests, the $\dot{V}_E$ –$P_a co_2$ curve not only shifts upwards but also steepens its slope (Fig. 18.33a, dashed line). This steepening indicates increased $\dot{V}_E$ sensitivity and is referred to as a multiplicative or potentiating interaction between hypoxia and hypercapnia; apparently it is well developed only in humans. Although not illustrated here, $\dot{V}_E$ is also linearly related to arterial pH—as pH decreases (acidosis), $\dot{V}_E$ increases.

In hypoxia $\dot{V}_E$ is inversely related to $P_a o_2$ with a curve that steepens progressively as the hypoxia becomes more severe (Fig. 18.33b). At $P_a o_2$ values below 30 mmHg, the low O2 severely depresses brain activity, which decreases $\dot{V}_E$. Hypoxia occurs naturally and progressively as one ascends to high altitude; lowering the $F_I o_2$ can simulate this. As the reflex increase in $\dot{V}_E$ will also progressively lower $P_a co_2$ and arterial [H+] which, in their turn, will depress $\dot{V}_E$, the $\dot{V}_E$ at a particular $P_a o_2$ at simulated altitude is less (Fig. 18.33b, dotted line) than when the $P_a co_2$ is held constant at its normal ~40 mmHg by adding a little CO2 to the inspired gas during the hypoxia tests (solid blue line). The potentiating interaction between hypoxia and hypercapnia can also be seen as a steeper curve (Fig. 18.33b, dashed line) when the $P_a co_2$ is held elevated and constant at, say, 45 mmHg whilst the sensitivity to $P_a o_2$ is tested.

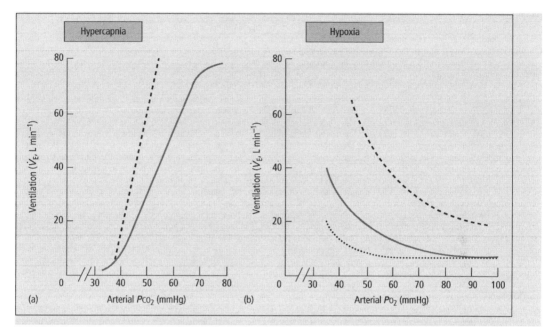

Fig. 18.33 (a) Ventilatory sensitivity to hypercapnia while O_2 is experimentally maintained constant (solid blue line for normoxia, $P_{a}O_2 = 100\,mmHg$; dashed line for hypoxia, $P_{a}O_2 = 50\,mmHg$). (b) Ventilatory sensitivity to hypoxia at simulated altitudes where $P_{a}CO_2$ falls progressively because of the $\dot{V}_E$ response (dotted line) and at sea level while CO_2 is experimentally maintained constant (solid blue line for normocapnia, $P_{a}CO_2 = 40\,mmHg$; dashed line for hypercapnia, $P_{a}CO_2 = 45\,mmHg$).

Peripheral chemoreceptors

The arterial or **peripheral chemoreceptors** are located in the **carotid** and **aortic bodies** and are stimulated by arterial hypoxia, hypercapnia and acidity. After removal of the peripheral chemoreceptors, all the $\dot{V}_E$ response to acute hypoxia, approximately 20% of the response to hypercapnia and nearly all the response to acute metabolic acidosis are lost. Peripheral chemoreceptors also cause bronchoconstriction, elicit cardiovascular reflexes (p. 406) and increase secretion of antidiuretic hormone and adrenaline.

The **carotid bodies** are small nodules found bilaterally at the bifurcation of the internal and external carotid arteries (Fig. 18.34). The dense capillary network of each carotid body is supplied by a branch from the external carotid artery and the venous blood drains into the internal jugular vein. The blood flow of $20\,mL\,g^{-1}\,min^{-1}$ is so great that the O_2 consumption of the carotid body causes only a tiny a–vO_2 difference. Thus, their capil-

lary gas tensions are very close to arterial values and any change reaches equilibrium in the carotid body within seconds. The carotid bodies are said therefore to monitor arterial P_{O_2}, P_{CO_2} and pH. Increased plasma [K$^+$] is now known to also be an excitatory stimulus (p. 622).

The capillaries of the carotid body are surrounded by **glomus cells**, supportive **sustentacular cells** and sensory nerve endings of a branch of the IXth cranial nerve (**glossopharyngeal nerve**). Despite much research, it is still not known precisely how the carotid body senses its stimuli. Although some evidence suggests that the nerve endings themselves are chemosensitive, the glomus cells, which are metabolically very active and rich in a variety of neurotransmitters (e.g. dopamine, acetylcholine, substance P), are considered most likely to be the chemosensitive element.

The **aortic bodies** are scattered over the aortic arch and the main arteries of that area (Fig. 18.34) and are innervated by the Xth cranial nerve (**vagus nerve**). They are anatomically similar to the

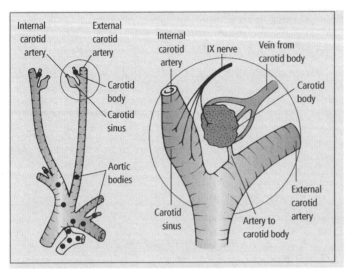

Fig. 18.34 Location of aortic and carotid bodies on the aortic arch and near the carotid arteries, respectively. Enlargement shows the vasculature and innervation of the carotid body.

carotid bodies but less vascular and hence respond more sluggishly. Furthermore they are not as sensitive as the carotid bodies to hypoxia, hypercapnia and acidity. Their reflex effect on respiration is weak; their role is predominantly for cardiovascular reflexes (p. 406). As the aortic bodies have a lower blood flow, their capillary gas tensions and nerve activity are, in contrast to the carotid bodies, affected by anaemia, CO poisoning and hypotension. Thus in these conditions the aortic bodies may have important reflex effects on $\dot{V}_E$.

Central chemoreceptors

The intracranial or **central chemoreceptors** are located at a depth of about 500 μm in discrete areas near the **ventrolateral surface** of the **medulla oblongata** (Fig. 18.35). Evidence also exists for deeper, more widespread locations. Within any of these areas, no precise structure has yet been identified anatomically but it is presumed that nerve endings here monitor the brain ISF. The central chemoreceptors are stimulated by arterial hypercapnia, cause cardiovascular reflexes (p. 406), and are responsible for about 80% of the $\dot{V}_E$ response to hypercapnia. They are, however, insensitive to hypoxia.

Central chemoreceptors are only slightly stimulated by acute increases in arterial acidity. This is because of the presence of a blood–brain barrier (p. 59), which greatly restricts movements of ions (but not of O_2 and CO_2) and the extent to which arterial H^+ can influence the brain ISF. Since H^+ and HCO_3^- ions do not readily cross this barrier, most of the arterial $[H^+]$ changes in acute metabolic acidosis and alkalosis are not reflected in the brain ISF. During chronic metabolic acidosis or alkalosis, there is a slow leak of HCO_3^- down its concentration gradient between blood and ISF (see below), but equilibrium is never reached.

During acute hypercapnia (**acute respiratory acidosis**) the increase in blood P_{CO_2} immediately increases P_{CO_2} in the brain ISF. However, since the relative blood flow to the brain is about 40 times less than that to the carotid bodies, it takes 5–10 min to reach the final steady state (or even longer, considering the vast stores of CO_2 (p. 475) in fatty tissue and bone which are poorly perfused and contribute to the final CO_2 equilibrium). This ISF CO_2 is then hydrated to H_2CO_3, which dissociates into HCO_3^- and H^+. It is now believed that not just ISF H^+ but also ISF P_{CO_2} are the stimuli to the central chemoreceptors. The formation of H_2CO_3 may be accelerated by carbonic anhydrase, which has been found in capillary endothelia and large neurones within the ventrolateral location of the central chemoreceptors.

The pH and P_{CO_2} of brain ISF are influenced

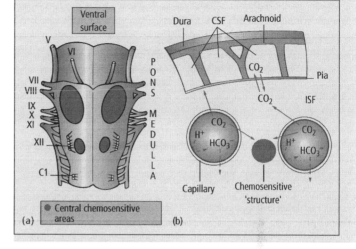

Fig. 18.35 (a) Location of the central chemosensitive areas on the ventral surface of the medulla oblongata. (b) The position of the chemosensitive structure in relation to the capillaries and the cerebrospinal fluid (CSF). ISF, interstitial fluid.

mainly by the composition of arterial blood but also to some degree by the rate of cerebral blood flow, the metabolism of the brain cells and by the slowly flowing cerebrospinal fluid on the surface of the medulla (Fig. 18.35). Since the location of the central chemoreceptors was first identified by applying acidic cerebrospinal fluid to the brain surface, it has been implied that the receptors monitor cerebrospinal fluid pH. However, cerebrospinal fluid is physiologically some distance from the chemosensitive structures and its pH is dependent on ISF pH, blood $P\text{CO}_2$ and on nearby vascularity. Thus, the cerebrospinal fluid pH changes slowly and may be somewhat different to that of the ISF pH at the site of the receptor.

During **chronic respiratory acidosis**, brain ISF pH is restored towards normal. This reduces the stimulus to the central chemoreceptors so that the chronic $\dot{V}_E$ response is less than the acute one. Such homoeostasis of brain pH is essential for the viability of the neurones of the brain. Brain ISF pH is restored by a gradual increase in ISF [HCO_3^-], resulting from three mechanisms.

Rapid and slow changes in central chemoreceptor activity also occur during metabolic acidosis and hypoxia. Although acidosis and hypoxia stimulate the carotid bodies, the increased $\dot{V}_E$ produces arterial hypocapnia which rapidly decreases brain ISF H+ and $P\text{CO}_2$ and thus decreases stimulation of the central chemoreceptors. Thus, the initial $\dot{V}_E$ re-

sponse to the acidosis and hypoxia is quickly dampened to give the acute steady-state response. However, very gradually HCO_3^- will move from the ISF to the brain cells and, to a small extent, to the plasma. In hypoxia there is also an increase in lactic acid formation in the glial cells. All this will restore brain ISF pH towards normal and reduce the depression of the central chemoreceptors. Thus, the response to chronic metabolic acidosis and chronic hypoxia will become augmented compared with the acute response. This is the basis of the gradual increase in $\dot{V}_E$ that typifies acclimatization to altitude (p. 490).

18.7 Pathophysiology: Respiration in disease and under extreme conditions

Hypoxia can be the result of respiratory diseases; sleep apnoea is one such example. Hypoxia and hypercapnia result from cessation of breathing (apnoea) caused either by sleep-related reduction in output from the central respiratory controller—central sleep apnoea—or by a sleep-related collapse of the pharyngeal airway—obstructive sleep apnoea. Hypoxia also occurs in healthy individuals at high altitude where the decreased P_B lowers the inspired $P\text{O}_2$. Physiological adjustments occur in response to short-term (acute) hypoxia and develop further during acclimatization to long-term (chronic) hypoxia. At high altitude the initial adjustment may be accompanied by acute mountain sickness and, even after acclimatization, chronic mountain sickness may suddenly appear. Diving is a condition where breathing must occur while submerged at increased P_B (hyperbarism). Breathhold, snorkel and scuba diving create different problems—the first is limited by O_2 stores, the second requires breathing against an increased pressure on the chest, and the third can lead to nitrogen narcosis at depth and, on ascent, to decompression sickness. Breathing pure O_2, either at normal atmospheric pressure or under hyperbaric conditions for the medical treatment of hypoxia, is associated with the dangers of O_2 toxicity, alveoli collapse (atelectasis) and impaired blood CO_2 carriage.

Types of hypoxia

Hypoxia is a term used to denote a P_AO_2 that is below the normal range of 90–100 mmHg. Blood and tissue, when low in Po_2, can also be referred to as hypoxic, although there is a specific term, **hypoxaemia**, for a P_aO_2 below the normal range of 80–90 mmHg. The ultimate consequence of any respiratory disease is a **deficiency of O_2 in the tissues**—this is also referred to as hypoxia, which can lead to confusion, as it may not necessarily be accompanied by a low P_aO_2. The classification of hypoxia into four main types helps clarify this:

1 hypoxic hypoxia, in which P_aO_2 is abnormally low (i.e. hypoxaemia);

2 anaemic hypoxia, in which P_aO_2 is normal but the haemoglobin concentration and therefore the O_2 content are reduced, and thus to compensate venous Po_2 is low (Fig. 18.28c)—CO poisoning and methaemoglobin formation (p. 474) are also categorized as anaemic hypoxia;

3 stagnant or **ischaemic hypoxia**, in which blood flow to a tissue is so low (e.g. in circulatory failure) that delivery of O_2, carried in otherwise normal blood, is inadequate and thus venous blood is less oxygenated than usual (Fig. 18.28a); and

4 histotoxic hypoxia, in which P_aO_2 and perfusion are normal but due to a toxic agent (e.g. cyanide poisoning) the cells cannot utilize the O_2 properly and venous Po_2 is therefore more oxygenated than usual.

Hypoxic hypoxia (hypoxaemia)

This will occur if there is a decrease in P_AO_2 caused, as shown by the alveolar gas equation for O_2 (p. 452), either by a **low inspired Po_2** (e.g. at high altitude) or by **hypoventilation**. Hypoventilation results from:

1 drugs like barbiturates or morphine, which depress the respiratory centres;

2 damage to the respiratory centres (as in stroke) or to respiratory muscles or their nerves;

3 interference with neuromuscular transmission, as in myasthenia gravis;

4 injury to, or a stiff, chest wall;

5 stiff lungs;

6 obstructed airways; and

7 an imposed dead space from, for example, snorkel-breathing.

Hypoventilation during central and obstructive sleep apnoea

During sleep (p. 215) the respiratory system is greatly compromised; even in healthy people sleep is associated with significant hypoventilation and a sustained respiratory acidosis, as a result of increased pharyngeal resistance (up to four times). In addition, many of the reflexes that protect airway patency or augment respiration to maintain ventilation in the face of increased resistance to airflow are reduced or lost in sleep (p. 441). These effects can predispose to sleep related-breathing disorders of **central sleep apnoea** (CSA) and **obstructive sleep apnoea** (OSA).

Central sleep apnoea—hypo and hyperventilation

CSA is the cessation of breathing during sleep due to an absence of neural output from the respiratory control centres (Fig. 18.36). It can occur in patients with damage to the respiratory

Fig. 18.36 (a) Central sleep apnoea showing cessation of airflow due to absence of efferent respiratory drive. (b) Obstructive sleep apnoea showing cessation of airflow despite continuous respiratory drive, indicating an occluded pharyngeal airway—ribcage and abdominal movements are equal and opposite—paradoxical breathing. (From Vazir *et al.* (2005) *Br J Cardiol*, **12**, 219–23.)

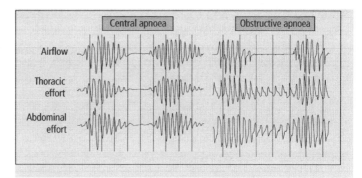

control centre as a result of stroke (e.g. lateral medullary syndrome), it may be congenital (as in congenital hypoventilation syndrome) or—most commonly—it can occur in patients with congestive heart failure (CHF). In patients with CHF $P_a\text{CO}_2$ is reduced at sleep onset as a result of hyperventilation. Therefore the $P_a\text{CO}_2$ is below the sleep-related **hypocapnic apnoeic threshold** (i.e. the loss of conscious inputs to breathing unmasks a highly sensitive hypocapnic-dependent apnoeic threshold). If $P_a\text{CO}_2$ is below this threshold at sleep onset, respiration will be reduced or stop. The hypocapnic apnoeic threshold is typically 2–4 mmHg below sleeping eupnic values. During wakefulness, equivalent levels of $P_a\text{CO}_2$ can maintain respiration, reflecting the importance of conscious inputs to respiratory control. CHF patients with CSA are hypocapnic, due to chronic hyperventilation. The hyperventilation may initially be precipitated by vagally-mediated stimulation of pulmonary irritant receptors, associated with pulmonary congestion. CHF patients with CSA have pulmonary artery occlusion pressure (the pulmonary artery wedge pressure, an indication of pulmonary congestion) and a lower $P_a\text{CO}_2$.

CSA results in repeated apnoeas that produce transient hypoxaemia and arousals from sleep. The termination of each hypoxic event is associated with a surge in sympathetic nervous system activation. Elevated sympathetic nervous system activation and raised catecholamine levels may induce atrial and ventricular arrhythmias resulting in increased mortality in CHF patients with CSA.

Obstructive sleep apnoea—hypo and hyperventilation

OSA is a common disorder occurring in 1–4% of middle-aged men, rising to over 20% in the elderly; the prevalence of OSA in females increases postmenopause (Fig. 18.36). There is a direct link between OSA and the development of systemic hypertension. During wakefulness pharyngeal lumen patency is maintained by activation of pharyngeal muscles; however, during sleep these muscles become hypotonic. In patients with OSA, the negative intralumenal pressure produced by the respiratory pump muscles during inspiration, together with a lack of compensation by the pharyngeal dilator muscles, results in airway collapse. OSA patients are also more likely to have an anatomically smaller pharyngeal airway during sleep, and/or an increase in extralumenal pressure (pharyngeal adipose tissue). The partial or complete pharyngeal airway occlusion occurs at sleep-onset, and this leads to hypoxia with hypercapnia; the occlusion is terminated on arousal from sleep. This cycle can occur hundreds of times a night, leading to repetitive hypoxia, hypercapnia and autonomic activation. Daytime symptoms include excessive sleepiness, nocturnal choking, morning headaches and lethargy. The most notable cardiovascular changes are an acute increase in heart rate, systemic blood pressure and peripheral vasoconstriction that occur at the termination of an apnoeic episode.

Chronic and acute and respiratory failure

Respiratory failure is defined by hypoxia, P_aO_2 < 60 mmHg; **type I respiratory failure** is hypoxia with normocapnia (normal P_aCO_2); **type II respiratory failure** is hypoxia and hypercapnia, P_aCO_2 > 50 mmHg. A further distinction is made between acute and chronic respiratory failure: the former develops in minutes to hours, and the latter over days. Type I respiratory failure occurs as a result of a failure of the O_2 exchange mechanism (e.g. pulmonary oedema, p. 411); type II respiratory failure occurs in disorders in which alveolar ventilation is limited relative to the rate of CO_2 production (e.g. restrictive and obstructive lung disease). Treatment depends on the underlying pathophysiology (e.g. non-invasive ventilation in restrictive and obstructive lung disease).

The low inspired Po_2 of high altitude

As given by Dalton's law ($Po_2 = Fo_2 \times P_B$), a reduction in the inspired Po_2 can result from either a fall in F_IO_2 or a decrease in P_B. Hypoxia has long been studied in healthy individuals acutely and chronically exposed to the low Po_2 of high altitude. As one ascends a mountain, P_B and thus the inspired Po_2, and therefore P_AO_2, fall (Table 18.5). Because hypoxia stimulates breathing, Po_2 in the table has been calculated using incremental increases in alveolar ventilation typical of that shown earlier in Fig. 18.33.

Acute hypoxia

A number of responses to hypoxia occur acutely.

1 Respiratory function: there is hyperventilation (Fig. 18. 33) and consequential lowering of P_aCO_2 (hypocapnia or respiratory alkalosis). The exact magnitude is hard to predict because of the interaction of a number of factors. For example, hypoxia directly depresses the respiratory centres but stimulates ventilation via the peripheral chemoreceptors. However, the hyperventilation blows off CO_2 at a rate greater than it is being produced metabolically. Thus, the person becomes hypocapnic and arterial pH rises. These in turn, through peripheral and central chemoreceptors, inhibit ventilation. The net effect at moderate altitude is commonly an approximate doubling of ventilation at rest, but individual responses vary considerably.

2 Cardiovascular function: there is tachycardia and an increase in cardiac output, while arterial blood pressure usually remains about normal or is even decreased. Once more, in any individual, the effect is hard to predict quantitatively because of interactive processes (see Chapter 14).

3 Cerebral function: this is very sensitive to the severity and speed of onset of hypoxia. Severe and sudden hypoxia will result in rapid loss of consciousness. Moderate hypoxia of relatively gradual onset may cause only such changes as lack of judgement and psychomotor disturbance.

Table 18.5 Effect of barometric pressure (P_B) on the partial pressure of inspired (P_IO_2) and alveolar O_2 (P_AO_2).

Height above sea level		P_B (mmHg)	P_IO_2* (mmHg)	P_AO_2 (mmHg)
Feet	Metres			
0	0	760	149	100
8500	2591	550	103	68
14000	4267	450	84	48
21000	6401	350	63	36
28000	8534	250	42	30

* In moist tracheal air.

4 Blood: the degree of deoxygenation is detectable as cyanosis (p. 474). Venous Po_2 is low and the a–vO_2 difference (Fig. 18.28b) depends on the extent of any increase in $\dot{Q}$. Furthermore acutely, but not chronically, the hypocapnia causes a left shift in the oxyhaemoglobin curve, making it difficult to offload what little O_2 there is in the blood.

After 8–24 h newcomers to high altitude frequently develop symptoms of **acute mountain sickness** which last 4–8 days. The symptoms are dizziness, headache, vomiting, nausea, breathlessness (dyspnoea; p. 482), irritability, insomnia, fatigue, loss of appetite and heart palpitations. The cause is not known but it appears to be associated with cerebral oedema.

Chronic hypoxia

Over subsequent weeks and months most people acclimatize to living at high altitude, although the ability to perform strenuous exercise may be limited. However, no human communities live permanently above 5500 m (18 000 feet) because further acclimatization becomes impossible; instead there is a slow deterioration in all aspects of performance. **Acclimatization** is the process whereby the body tries to compensate and improve the O_2 delivery to the tissues. These same processes may occur in patients who have been hypoxic for a long time due to respiratory disease. The various compensating mechanisms of acclimatization are listed below (permanent residents born and bred at high altitude have some extra attributes which are not included here).

1 Respiratory function: the hyperventilation continues and in fact increases because of restoration of brain ISF pH (p. 486). Pulmonary diffusing capacity can increase up to threefold as a result of more open pulmonary capillaries, increased pulmonary capillary blood volume and greater alveolar surface area. Cyanosis therefore may be absent at rest but will become apparent during exercise.

2 Kidney function: the kidneys excrete bicarbonate with eventual correction of the respiratory alkalosis; this takes 2–3 weeks.

3 Cardiovascular function: $\dot{Q}$ and heart rate tend to come back to sea-level values. However, hypox-

ic vasoconstriction of small pulmonary arteries (p. 466) leads to pulmonary hypertension and right ventricular hypertrophy—these responses have no apparent physiological advantage. The vasoconstriction also precipitates muscularization of pulmonary arterioles, which are normally devoid of smooth muscle.

4 Tissue function: there is an increase in the capillarity of many tissues and in the concentration of cytochrome oxidase; the former improves O_2 transfer and the latter permits the mitochondria to utilize the O_2 more effectively. The myoglobin content of skeletal muscle also increases, which raises the reserve store of O_2; myoglobin may also facilitate intracellular diffusion.

5 Blood: there is an increase in 2,3-BPG production, which shifts the oxyhaemoglobin curve to the right (Fig. 18.28b) to enable O_2 to be offloaded to the tissues more easily. Furthermore, hypoxia increases erythropoietin secretion (p. 294), leading to an increased red-cell count (polycythaemia). Depending on the altitude elevation, the haemoglobin concentration may increase to as much as $200\,g\,L^{-1}$ and thus, despite the low P_{aO_2} and percentage of haemoglobin saturation, the arterial O_2 content at altitude will not fall as much. There is a disadvantage to this—the increased blood viscosity increases quite considerably the work of the heart.

Some individuals, apparently successfully acclimatized, gradually or even suddenly fail in their compensating responses. Their ventilation falls, producing dyspnoea and cyanosis. Haematocrit and pulmonary arterial pressure increase further, leading to right heart failure. In sudden failure, pulmonary oedema is the most dominant feature. These are all the symptoms of **chronic mountain sickness**. The only course of action is to remove the person to a lower altitude.

Increased ambient pressure and diving

During submersion in water, the pressure increases by 1 atm (1 atm = 760 mmHg) for every 10 m (33 feet) of descent. The increased pressure (**hyperbarism**) itself is unlikely to have any effect on the solid tissues or liquids of the body. It is the gas-filled cavities of the body that are affected—the air-filled nasal sinuses, the middle ear, the gastrointestinal tract and the lungs. Gas will be compressed during the descent and will expand during the ascent. It is important for the cavities to communicate with the outside pressure (by opening the nose and mouth/glottis and, in the case of the middle ear, the eustachian tube), particularly during a rapid ascent. Submersion also poses the problems of hypothermia, distortion of information reaching the special sense organs, i.e. disturbance of vision and hearing, and the need to breathe under water. A dive may be:

1 short enough to be accomplished on such air as can be inhaled at the surface—single-breath diving;

2 carried out at a shallow depth such that connection with the atmosphere can be maintained through a tube—snorkel diving; or

3 long enough to demand a continual supply of air, in which case the air must be supplied at whatever the increased ambient pressure—conventional and scuba diving.

Single-breath diving is basically, **breath-holding** with the additional complicating factor of submersion. Suppose one takes a deep breath and goes down to 10 m (+1 atm). The P_{O_2} and P_{CO_2} will approximately double—not quite, because both gases will pass along their gradients into the blood. After a brief period (20–30 s), the combined effect, through stimulation of respiratory receptors, of rising P_{CO_2} (the most potent stimulus), falling P_{O_2} and, as lung O_2 stores are used up, decreasing lung volume is sufficient to force the diver to the surface. The danger lies in the temptation to hyperventilate before submerging in an attempt to prolong the dive. The initial hypocapnia resulting from the prior hyperventilation may permit a longer stay at depth but by then the P_{O_2} has reached a rather low level. On ascent, as the ambient pressure drops, the P_{O_2} is very rapidly lowered further, to levels at which unconsciousness is likely to occur. Standard advice before such a dive is that four maximum breaths are allowable.

The problem in **snorkel diving** is essentially one of lung mechanics because the person is breathing to and from the surface pressure, which is 1 atm.

Alveolar pressure is therefore, on average, ~1 mmHg (p. 441) either side of atmospheric pressure. This must be counteracted by the action of the inspiratory muscles if the chest is not to collapse. The maximum subatmospheric P_{pl} that can be generated is of the order of 100 mmHg (p. 447), equivalent to a submerged pressure of ~1.2 m. If one considers that maximum respiratory muscular effort can only occur for short periods, and if one also takes into account the increased dead space of the snorkel tube, it is clear that a snorkel diver is confined to a snorkel length of about 0.4 m.

Conventional and scuba diving is being submerged within a closed chamber while breathing its compressed gases. **Scuba** (self-contained underwater breathing apparatus) **diving** involves breathing gases through a regulated valve system from a pressurized tank carried by the diver. In either case the pressure of the gas breathed and the pressure on the outside of the chest are equal but the problem is that of breathing N_2 (and O_2) at pressures greater than 1 atm. N_2 breathed at a pressure greater than ~4 atm (~30 m below the surface) is at such a dissolved concentration in the tissues that it results in **nitrogen narcosis**—a condition also known as 'rapture of the deep'. The mechanism causing this narcosis is not known but the symptoms are euphoria, loss of memory, clumsiness and impaired intellectual function resembling alcohol intoxication. When diving at depths of more than 30 m there are dangers, not at depth but as the diver ascends. The N_2, though inert, dissolves in the body fluids (especially the fatty tissues) in proportion to its partial pressure. If the ascent is too quick, the ambient pressure decreases too rapidly and the N_2 comes out of solution and forms tiny bubbles in the tissues and blood. Such bubbles can form emboli in the cerebral, myocardial or pulmonary circulations or in the tissue of the brain itself and in the joints. The symptoms of **decompression sickness** are paralysis, myocardial damage, coughing and dyspnoea which divers call 'the chokes', and severe pain in the joints ('the bends'). Treatment is by recompression in a pressure chamber, followed some time later by a gradual decompression. The problem of N_2 narcosis can be avoided by breathing a mixture of **helium** and O_2, because helium is only half as soluble as N_2 so that less is dissolved in the tissues. Helium has two other advantages: it has a low density, which decreases gas-flow resistance and therefore the work of breathing, and it is a much smaller molecule and can therefore diffuse more rapidly through the tissues, which makes it less likely to come out of solution and form bubbles. Even helium is a narcotic at very great depths, producing tremors, drowsiness and decreased manual dexterity.

Breathing pure O_2

Pure O_2 should not be breathed during diving or for prolonged medical treatment because it produces **oxygen toxicity**. At only 1 atm, 100% O_2 for even 12 h produces tracheobronchial irritation, and after a few days leads to thickening of the alveolar–capillary membrane. Neonates are even more susceptible because the lung damage is more extreme (bronchopulmonary dysplasia) and the developing vascular tissue of the retina becomes opaque (retrolental fibroplasia). Pure O_2 at pressures greater than 3 atm even for short periods affects the central nervous system and causes convulsions. Thus, when diving to great depths the fraction of O_2 in the mix delivered from the tanks is decreased to prevent the occurrence of high P_{O_2} in the blood and tissues.

Breathing pure O_2 at 1 atm can also cause alveolar collapse (**atelectasis**) of those alveoli beyond an obstructed airway. This is because O_2 is much more soluble than N_2, so it is absorbed out of the alveolus into the blood very much more quickly than N_2. The usual presence of 80% N_2 in the alveolus, by delaying alveolar gas absorption, acts as a 'splint' supporting the alveolus.

When breathing pure O_2 at 3 atm, the resting O_2 consumption can be satisfied entirely by the O_2 in physical solution. However, the carriage of CO_2 now has to take place without the assistance of desaturation of haemoglobin (the Haldane effect), so the usual amount of CO_2 loaded into the blood from the tissues (45 mL of CO_2 per litre of blood) raises the venous P_{CO_2} to ~56 instead of 46 mmHg (Fig. 18.30b).

Hyperbaric O_2, provided it is at pressures of less than 3 atm for less than 5 h, is of value for correcting CO poisoning as the high P_{O_2} helps displace CO from the haemoglobin molecule and raises the amount of O_2 dissolved in the blood.

Chapter 19

Digestive System

19.1 Structure and organization

The role of this system is to digest food and absorb nutrients and water. To achieve this, ingested material is subject to an orderly and controlled process of modification as it passes from mouth to anus. During this passage, fluids containing enzymes that break down complex molecules are secreted into the lumen of the gut. The secretory processes are regulated and coordinated by the enteric nervous system and intestinal hormones. Products of this digestion are absorbed across the epithelial cells, principally in the small intestine. The activity of the smooth muscle responsible for gastric and intestinal motility is also regulated and coordinated by the enteric nervous system and by intestinal hormones.

All the water, nutrient, vitamins, minerals and electrolytes required for growth and maintenance are absorbed from the digestive tract and transported to other tissues by the blood stream. However, only a small portion of the ingested solid material—small lipid- and water-soluble molecules—may be absorbed unchanged. The complex macromolecules that form the bulk of the diet must first be reduced to simpler, metabolizable forms by **digestion**, which is accomplished in the lumen of the digestive tract.

The **digestive tract** is a tube extending from the mouth to the anus and includes the pharynx, oesophagus, stomach, small intestine and large intestine (Fig. 19.1). Food entering the tract is mixed and propelled along mainly as a result of smooth muscle activity. As ingested material progresses through the tract, complex molecular structures are broken down by hydrolytic enzymes acting in either acidic or neutral environments. The digestive fluids are secreted from glandular tissue that forms part of the gut wall or from glands that lie outside the intestinal tract and whose ducts enter the digestive tract (the salivary glands, pancreas and liver).

The **digestive process** starts in the mouth where the food may be ground and mixed with saliva. Here the addition of a salivary amylase to the food begins the breakdown of starches. After passage through the pharynx and oesophagus, this material enters the stomach where it is acted on by acid-dependent gastric proteases. However, digestion in the stomach is limited and one of the main functions of the stomach is to store partially digested material (chyme) for slow release into the small intestine. The final phases of digestion occur in the small intestine and colon. In the small intestine the chyme is broken down by the actions of pancreatic enzymes (e.g. protease, lipase and amylase) and enzymes released from desquamated epithelial cells. Most of the products of digestion are absorbed by the small intestine and the residue passes into the large intestine (colon). In the colon there is little digestion but the actions of the normal bacterial flora on dietary fibre (e.g. cellulose)

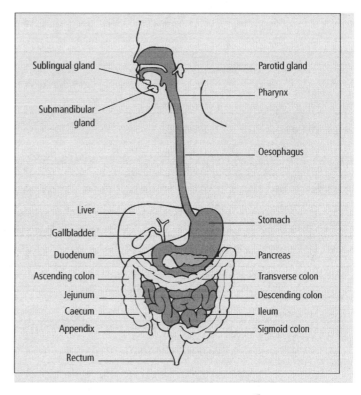

Fig. 19.1 Anatomy of the human digestive tract.

Labels (clockwise): Sublingual gland, Parotid gland, Pharynx, Submandibular gland, Oesophagus, Liver, Stomach, Gallbladder, Duodenum, Pancreas, Ascending colon, Transverse colon, Jejunum, Descending colon, Caecum, Ileum, Appendix, Sigmoid colon, Rectum.

result in formation of gases (e.g. methane and H_2) and in the synthesis of short-chain fatty acids and vitamins (e.g. butyrate, vitamin K), which may be absorbed. In addition, the colon has some capacity to absorb water and to absorb and secrete ions. The solid waste products and undigested material are expelled as faeces.

Structure of the digestive tract

From the mouth to the anus, the digestive canal is lined by a mucous membrane (**mucosa**). In the mouth, oesophagus and anus, where there can be considerable abrasion, the epithelial layer is of a stratified squamous variety some 10–15 cells thick. In regions devoted to absorption and secretion, a single-layered columnar epithelium is found (Fig. 19.2). Absorption is enhanced in these regions by folding and by the formation of both villi— finger-like projections of the mucosa—and microvilli, which form a **brush border** on the luminal surface of the epithelial cells.

Striated or smooth muscle surrounds the mucosa of the digestive tract. The striated muscle is found in the upper regions of the tract (the mouth, pharynx and upper oesophagus) and at the anus. In between, the tract is surrounded by an external layer of smooth muscle, the **muscularis externa**, composed of an outer layer with its fibres oriented in a longitudinal direction and an inner layer containing fibres with a circular orientation (Fig. 19.2). This part of the tract also contains a thinner, smooth-muscle layer, the **muscularis mucosae**, at the base of the mucous membrane and extending into the villi in the small intestine (Fig. 19.2a). The thicker outer coat is involved in the propulsion and mixing of food, while the muscularis mucosae may control the folding and shape of the mucosa.

The **blood vessels**, **lymphatics** and **neurones** to the intestinal tract travel in the mesenteries. The blood vessels entering the tract branch to supply the external muscle layer, the submucosa and the mucosa. The final vascular supply within these

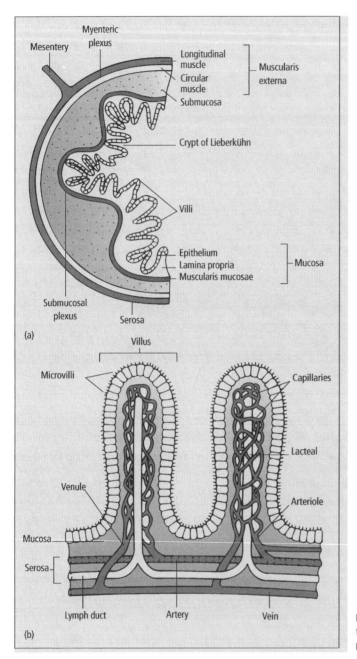

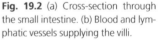

Fig. 19.2 (a) Cross-section through the small intestine. (b) Blood and lymphatic vessels supplying the villi.

regions may vary from a simple rectilinear network in the muscle layers to a basket-like arrangement in the villi of the small intestine (Fig. 19.2b).

Intrinsic nerves in the tract between the lower oesophagus and the rectum comprise the **enteric nervous system**, in which the number (10^8) of neurones approaches that found in the spinal cord. These neurones are grouped in the **myenteric (Auerbach's) plexus**, which lies between the outer longitudinal and circular muscle layer, and in the submucosal (Meissner's) plexus, which lies between the circular muscles and the muscularis mucosae (Fig. 19.2a). These intrinsic networks are composed of excitatory and inhibitory motor neurones projecting to the smooth muscle fibres, excitatory neurones serving secretory cells and hormone-releasing cells, and interneurones. The input of these plexuses comes from the autonomic nervous system and from intrinsic chemoreceptors and mechanoreceptors, which may have their sensory terminals in the epithelial sheet (Fig. 19.3).

Regulation of the digestive system

In general, the motor and secretory activity of the gastrointestinal tract is regulated and coordinated by nerves and hormones. The hormones and many of the neurotransmitters and neuromodulators involved are peptides, and in some cases the same peptide can serve as both hormone and neurotransmitter. The general term **regulatory peptide** is sometimes used to describe such peptides that act as either neurotranmitters/modulators, hormones or in a local paracrine manner.

   Nervous control can be subdivided into intrinsic and extrinsic components. **Intrinsic nervous control** involves local reflexes confined to the wall of the gut itself and effective over short distances (centimetres). Such intrinsic reflexes include the peristaltic reflex (p. 504). Receptors responsive to a variety of stimuli (e.g. stretch, pH, osmolarity,

products of digestion) activate **intrinsic primary afferent neurones (IPAN)** whose cell bodies are located in the intramural plexuses. The IPAN synapse within the plexuses (either directly or via interneurones) with efferent neurones supplying nearby smooth muscle, secretory cells or hormone-producing cells. Individual enteric neurones contain a range of substances that may act as neurotransmitters or neuromodulators; these include acetylcholine (ACh), nitric oxide (NO, synthesized by nitric oxide synthase, NOS), γ-aminobutyric acid (GABA), 5-hydroxytryptamine (5-HT, serotonin) and a variety of peptides (Table 19.1). The different combinations of substances, which are related to the function and location of individual enteric neurones, has been called 'chemical coding'. Usually one substance acts as the primary transmitter, with one or more subsidiary transmitter or modulator. Some useful generalizations may be made in relation to this multiplicity of neurotransmitters: neurones of the myenteric plexus project predominantly to the circular muscle layer; neurones of the submucosal plexus project into the mucosa and submucosa. Neurones containing vasoactive intestinal polypeptide (VIP) and NOS are generally inhibitory; neurones containing tachykinins (e.g. substance P, SP; neurokinin A, NKA) are generally cholinergic and excitatory. There is increasing evidence that most of the neurally-induced relaxation of smooth muscle in the digestive tract (e.g. sphincter relaxation, gastric

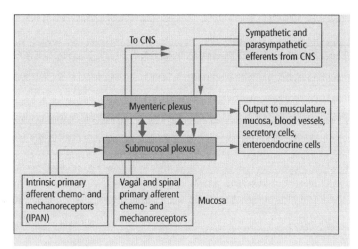

Fig. 19.3 Intrinsic and extrinsic nerves of the gastrointestinal tract.

Table 19.1 Gut peptides. CCK, cholecystokinin; CGRP, calcitonin gene-related peptide; GIP, glucose-dependent insulinotropic peptide; GRP, gastrin-releasing peptide; NKA, neurokinin A: PACAP, pituitary adenylate cyclase-activating peptide; PHI, peptide histidine isoleucine; SP, substance P; VIP, vasoactive intestinal polypeptide. (PHI is a co-product of the VIP precursor; it is co-secreted with, and has virtually identical biological functions to VIP.)

	Neurotransmitter/modulator	Endocrine	Paracrine
CCK	+	+	+
CGRP	+		
Enteroglucagons		+	
Galanin	+		
Gastrin		+	
Ghrelin		+	
GIP		+	
GRP	+		
Opioids	+		
Motilin		+	
Neuropeptide Y	+		
Neurotensin	+	+	
PACAP	+		
Pancreatic polypeptide		+	
Peptide YY		+	
Secretin		+	
Somatostatin	+	+	+
Tachykinins (SP, NKA).	+		
VIP/PHI	+		

Table 19.2 Major enteric neurone types in small intestine and their main neurotransmitters. Primary transmitter in bold. ACh, acetylcholine; NO, nitric oxide; TK, tachykinin; VIP, vasoactive intestinal polypeptide.

Enteric neurone type	Main transmitters	Functions
Excitatory motor neurone	**ACh**, TK	contraction of intestinal smooth muscle
Inhibitory motor neurone	**NO**, VIP	relaxation of intestinal smooth muscle
Interneurone	**ACh**	neurone-neurone relay within plexus
Cholinergic secretomotor/vasodilator	**ACh**	intestinal secretion, vasodilation
Non-cholinergic secretomotor/vasodilator	**VIP**	intestinal secretion, vasodilation
Intrinsic primary afferent (IPAN)	**TK**, ACh	stretch/chemoreceptors

receptive relaxation and peristaltic relaxation) is caused by neural release of NO, possibly in association with VIP. Table 19.2 summarizes some of the recognized roles of enteric neurotransmitters. Some (rare) gut tumours can produce regulatory peptides that may then be released into the blood and have hormone-like actions. For example, some pancreatic islet cell tumours produce VIP, which stimulates water and electrolyte secretion by the pancreas and small intestine and can produce excessive watery diarrhoea (p. 538).

Extrinsic nervous control involves the central nervous system and allows regulation and coordination of gastrointestinal activity over greater distances. Afferent fibres run in association with the autonomic nerves supplying the gut. They carry information from chemoreceptors and mechanoreceptors located in the gut wall; the transmitted information may be either unconscious or perceived. Painful or uncomfortable sensations are generally mediated by spinal afferent fibres, with cell bodies in the dorsal root ganglia, while sensations such as fullness or satiety are mediated by vagal afferent fibres, with cell bodies in the nodose ganglia. The efferent outflow, conveyed by **sympathetic** or **parasympathetic** nerves from the central nervous system, changes neuronal activity within the intramural plexuses or acts directly on effector cells in secretory organs (salivary glands, liver, pancreas). Examples of such extrinsic reflexes include the **gastrocolic reflex** (see p. 506) as well as more complex coordinated behaviour (e.g. chewing and swallowing).

In addition to nervous control, there is **hormonal regulation** of motility and secretion. A variety of peptides secreted by enteroendocrine cells within the epithelial cell layer, function as hormones (Table 19.1 and p. 521). Some of these enteroendocrine cells (open type) are exposed directly to the luminal contents, and are therefore presumed to be influenced by them; others (closed type) lie deeper in the epithelial cell layer and would seem to be controlled by nerves or by other hormones. Released hormones (e.g. gastrin, secretin, cholecystokinin (CCK)) enter capillaries to be transported through the circulation to exert **endocrine** effects on more distant parts of the alimentary system or on other organs. In addition, they may diffuse into the wall of the gut and act locally to alter gut activity (**paracrine effect**).

As well as these physiological peptides, bacteria in the gut lumen, cells involved in the immune system (e.g. phagocytes, mast cells, lymphocytes) and mesenchymal cells in the gut wall (e.g. endothelium, fibroblasts, smooth muscle) release chemicals that can modulate motility and secretion (p. 532).

Whereas the effects of nerves can be rapidly initiated or terminated and sharply localized, the effects of hormones are slower in onset and offset and tend to be more diffuse. Exclusive neural control in the digestive system is found in the upper part of the tract (mouth, oesophagus) and at its termination (anus), where rapid but short-lasting responses are required. Both nerves and hormones play important roles in the control and regulation of gastric activity. In the intestine, motility is more dependent on neural mechanisms; however, hormonal control is more important in regulating liver and pancreatic secretions.

19.2 Motility of the digestive tract

Both longitudinal movement and mixing of the luminal contents are essential if efficient digestion and absorption are to be maintained. In the mouth and upper oesophagus, where the movement of food is rapid, motility is controlled directly by the central nervous system. Where the movement is concerned mainly with mixing and slow propulsion (during digestion and absorption), the motility is regulated by a combination of mechanisms inherent in the muscle (**myogenic mechanisms**), by **neural mechanisms** and, to a lesser extent, by **hormones**.

The general properties of skeletal and smooth muscle that are responsible for motility have been discussed in Chapter 5. The motility of the lower tract is largely under the influence of the myenteric plexus, which in turn is influenced by the extrinsic nerves (parasympathetic and sympathetic) and the submucosal plexus (Fig. 19.3). Most **parasympathetic fibres** are **excitatory** and the **sympathetic fibres** are **inhibitory**. The sympathetic inhibition may be direct or by presynaptic inhibition at excitatory synapses. In addition, inhibition of smooth muscle is mediated by non-cholinergic, non-adrenergic (NANC) fibres that release NO and VIP.

Mouth and oesophagus

Chewing (mastication)

When food enters the mouth, chewing movements (mastication) reduce the size of the particles and mix them with saliva; both of these actions contribute to the taste, odour and swallowing of food. The mechanical effects are accomplished by the cutting action of the incisor teeth and the crushing movements of the molar teeth.

Although the chewing movements are under voluntary control, much chewing occurs involuntarily. Chewing involves the coordinated action of the mandible, tongue, cheeks and palate. The lower jaw is usually held closed as a result of reflex (muscle spindle) activity but a conscious decision or the presence of food in the mouth may momentarily inhibit this reflex and initiate jaw opening. The alternate activation and inhibition of nerves supplying the muscles controlling opening and closing, results in chewing. The appropriate rhythm, force and degree of occlusion are provided reflexly, and as the reflex is unilateral the chewing force is exerted largely on the side containing the bolus of food.

Swallowing (deglutition)

Swallowing results in the movement of food from the mouth to the oesophagus (Fig. 19.4), movement down the oesophagus and movement from the oesophagus to the stomach. Initially, the tongue forces a bolus of food to the rear of the mouth. The stimulation of receptors in the posterior wall and soft palate then results in activation of the **swallowing reflex**. This activity is coordinated within a **swallowing centre** in the medulla oblongata and the reflex, once initiated, cannot be stopped. It involves the elevation of the **soft palate** to close the nasopharynx, the raising of the **larynx** to close its entrance, the approximation of the vocal cords to close the **glottis**, the inhibition of breathing, and the relaxation of the **upper oesphageal sphincter**. As the bolus enters the

pharynx, the epiglottis is tilted back and this assists in the closure of the lower respiratory tract. Collectively these processes seal off the nasal passages and the lower respiratory tract. Lesions in the region of the swallowing centre, for example in stroke, which interfere with this coordinated activity, may be fatal. Once the tongue has passed the food into the pharynx, the pharyngeal skeletal muscles contract and propel the bolus of food into the oesophagus. The pressure generated, which can be up to 100 mmHg above atmospheric, normally provides the major force propelling the food into the oesophagus.

Oesophagus

In the oesophagus, a **peristaltic wave** (a ring of contraction preceded by a region of relaxation) propels viscous material towards the stomach. Fluid material travelling under the influence of the pressure generated by swallowing and by gravity may arrive at the stomach before the contractile wave. The peristaltic wave travels at approximately $5 \, \text{cm s}^{-1}$ and takes about 8 s to travel the length of the oesophagus. The pressures generated by peristalsis in the oesophagus range from 30 to 120 mmHg. The **primary peristaltic wave**, which is initiated by the medullary swallowing centre, normally clears the oesophagus of food, but if particles remain in the oesophagus **secondary peristaltic waves** may begin. These waves arise as a result of distension or

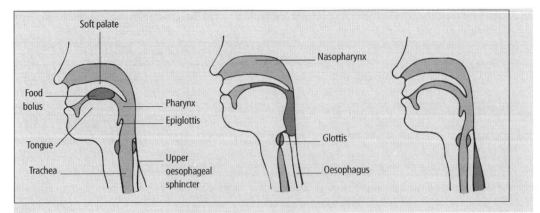

Fig. 19.4 Movement of a bolus of food from the mouth to the oesophagus.

irritation of the oesophagus and involve the swallowing centre. The secondary waves, which arise without any awareness, commence at the upper oesophageal sphincter and progress to the stomach. The movement of the food bolus from the oesophagus to the stomach is accomplished after relaxation of the **lower oesophageal sphincter (LOS)**. This sphincter comprises the terminal 4 cm of the oesophagus, is anatomically not much different from adjacent areas, and is normally closed. Pressure recordings from this region show that the sphincter relaxes some 1–2 s after swallowing is initiated, remains relaxed for 8–9 s and then contracts. The relaxation is mediated by the inhibitory neurotransmitters NO and VIP. Between swallowing movements, the tone of this sphincter is maintained by slight contraction of the smooth muscle layer, primarily by intrinsic (myogenic) activity of the muscle. The resting pressure of the closed sphincter (10–15 mmHg) prevents reflux of the stomach contents, which would otherwise occur, because the pressure in the stomach (5–10 mmHg) is higher than that in the thoracic oesophagus (–5 mmHg, p. 433).

Stomach

The stomach receives, stores, breaks down and partially digests food prior to its gradual release into the small intestine. The stomach has three outer smooth-muscle layers (the longitudinal, circular and oblique layers). Functionally, for both motility and secretion, the stomach can be divided into two regions (Fig. 19.5). The proximal stomach, comprised of fundus and body (corpus), is highly distensible, with a relatively thin layer of smooth muscle that has a basal tone, is lined by a secreting mucosa (p. 510), and acts as a reservoir for food. The distal stomach (antrum) is much less distensible, has basal smooth-muscle electrical activity, and displays phasic peristaltic contractions that serve to grind up food into smaller particles before they pass through the pyloric canal.

Gastric motility

As food enters the stomach, the proximal region relaxes to accommodate the meal with little or no increase in intragastric pressure. The relaxation is a consequence of both **receptive relaxation**, a vago-vagal reflex initiated by the passage of food along the oesophagus, and **adaptive relaxation** induced by the presence of food in the proximal region. Both processes involve the activation of postganglionic NANC myenteric inhibitory neurones, with NO and VIP as the most likely transmitters. In the fed state, continuous peristaltic waves at the rate of about three per minute, sweep from the

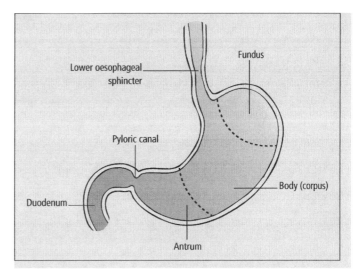

Fig. 19.5 Functional divisions of the stomach.

Lower oesophageal sphincter

Fundus

Pyloric canal

Body (corpus)

Duodenum

Antrum

proximal stomach towards the pyloric sphincter (Fig. 19.6). During these contractions, the pressure in the distal region may rise to 30 mmHg or more. The **pyloric sphincter**, which is normally relaxed, closes rapidly during each contraction so that only

small quantities of fluid containing small particles of food (**chyme**) enter the small intestine through the pyloric sphincter. Most of the content in the antrum is squirted back into the body of the stomach (Fig. 19.6). This produces a shearing effect that fragments larger food particles and is termed **retropulsion**.

Control of gastric motility

The contractile activity of the stomach is regulated by **myogenic**, **neural** and **hormonal** mechanisms. The frequency of the contractions and their coordination depend on the spread of **slow waves** of depolarization (30–60 mV) throughout the smooth muscle layers (Fig. 19.7). This rhythmic depolarization (**basic electrical rhythm**) originates from specialized cells within the muscle layers, **the interstitial cells of Cajal (ICC)**. An area along the greater curvature of the proximal stomach generates electrical potentials at the greatest frequency (about three per minute) and thus acts as the dominant pacemaker, which drives the more distal areas at this rhythm. Slow waves can be initiated in neighbouring regions of smooth muscle by passive current spread through gap junctions. Thus the slow waves are conducted around and along the stomach wall. The slow waves of the stomach are larger than those in the small intestine and may have superimposed on them a number of small spike-like potentials (Fig. 19.7) that initiate con-

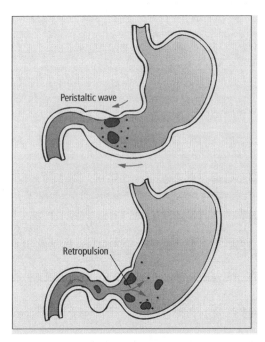

Fig. 19.6 Movement of an antral peristaltic wave towards the pylorus, forcing a small quantity of chyme into the duodenum and the remainder back into the distal stomach (retropulsion).

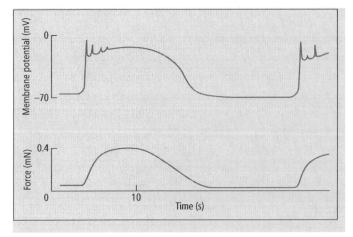

Fig. 19.7 Rhythmic depolarization of the membrane potential (slow waves) of gastric smooth muscle may initiate small spikes and contractions. (In the small intestine the slow waves are usually smaller and the action potentials larger than those illustrated here. See Fig. 5.19.)

tractions. Also, the slow wave itself may reach a potential at which contraction is initiated; the amplitude of the contraction is then dependent on the degree by, and the time for which this threshold is exceeded. Thus, during normal digestion, it is the slow waves that determine the frequency and conduction velocity of the peristaltic contractions. The ionic basis of the slow waves in the smooth muscle has been attributed to permeability changes associated with an influx of Ca^{2+} followed by an efflux of K^+.

The force of gastric contractions is regulated primarily by neural mechanisms. Vagal stimulation of cholinergic motor nerves depolarizes the smooth-muscle cells. Subsequent slow waves thus lower the membrane potential further and for a longer time. The resulting potentials in the smooth-muscle cells then induce a more powerful contraction. In contrast to this, NANC inhibitory nerve fibres cause hyperpolarization, and thus inhibit gastric motility. Although a number of hormones such as gastrin and secretin can be demonstrated experimentally to affect gastric motility, the extent to which they are important at their circulating physiological concentrations is questionable.

Gastric emptying

The rate at which the stomach empties is determined by the contents of the organ and by its motility. Liquids are emptied faster than solids, with the rate of emptying being approximately exponential. Solids empty more slowly since they must first be reduced to a small particle size. Carbohydrate-rich meals empty most rapidly, protein-rich meals empty more slowly and fatty meals slowest of all. The slow emptying of fatty (and protein) meals is explained by the release of CCK from the upper intestinal epithelium in response to the appearance there of fat or protein. CCK acts (in an endocrine or paracrine manner) at CCK1 receptors on the terminals of vagal afferent fibres in the upper gut that form the afferent arm of a vagovagal reflex. The efferent arm acts to cause gastric relaxation (in the manner described for receptive relaxation above) and thereby slows emptying. Meals of high osmolarity or low pH also tend to delay gas-

tric emptying; this has been attributed to the activation of duodenal osmoreceptors and chemoreceptors. By regulating gastric motility, gastric emptying is controlled very precisely so that the load presented to the duodenum at any one time is optimally matched to the digestive and absorptive capacities of the small intestine.

Vomiting

Vomiting results in the rapid expulsion of the stomach contents through the mouth. It is preceded by a large retrograde contraction, initiated and coordinated by central, peripheral and enteric nervous systems that forces intestinal contents into the stomach. It involves:

1 forceful inspiratory movements when the glottis and nasopharynx are closed;

2 relaxation of the lower oesophageal sphincter; and

3 contraction of the abdominal and thoracic muscles.

When the descent of the diaphragm coincides with contraction of the abdominal muscles, the elevation of abdominal pressure forces the gastric contents out through the mouth. Integration of the vomiting sequence occurs in a **vomiting centre** in the medulla oblongata that is anatomically and functionally associated with the centres governing respiration. It is influenced by the adjacent **chemoreceptor trigger zone** in the area postrema, which may be stimulated by a variety of drugs (e.g. morphine and its derivatives) that induce vomiting, as well as being involved in the vomiting associated with radiation and with motion sickness.

Small intestine

Following a meal, most of the digestion and absorption of food takes place in the duodenum and jejunum. Thus the motility of this section serves to mix the chyme from the stomach with the digestive juices secreted by the pancreas and liver and also to expose the luminal contents to the intestinal wall across which absorption occurs. In addition, the intestinal contents are propelled toward the large intestine, a process that normally takes some 4–6 h.

Motility of the small intestine

Following a meal, the above functions are accomplished by three main motility patterns — **segmentation**, **pendular contractions** and **peristalsis**.

Segmentation is the alternate contraction and relaxation of complete segments of the small intestine and reflects the activity of the circular muscle (Fig. 19.8). As the chyme from one contracting segment is forced into adjacent relaxed areas, this motility pattern thoroughly mixes the luminal contents. The contracting segments may be short or long; the latter are more effective in displacing the contents into adjoining regions. The frequency of the segmental contractions decreases down the length of the human small intestine from about 12 to nine contractions per minute. Although the contractile band does not progress, this pattern has some propulsive action because of the decreased frequency of segmentation from duodenum to ileum.

Pendular movements involve contraction of longitudinal muscle. This moves the wall of the intestine over the contents of the lumen and so serves to mix and propel the chyme through the small intestine.

Short **peristaltic contractions** travelling 10–15 cm are an important propulsive force in the small intestine. The peristaltic reflex entails local co-ordination of excitatory and inhibitory motor neurones, which act in combination to propel a bolus of material along the gut by contracting the circular muscle above the bolus, and relaxing the muscle below it (Fig. 19.9). This reflex can be elicited by luminal distension, or by chemical or mechanical stimulation of the mucosa, mediated by release of 5-HT from enterochromaffin (EC) cells (Fig. 19.9).

Control of small intestinal motility

The motility of the small intestine depends primarily on **myogenic** and **neural** mechanisms. As in the stomach, the rhythmic contractile activity of the small intestine results from regular slow waves of depolarization of the smooth muscle cells (Fig. 5.19). Contraction in a segment of the small intestine is coordinated by the spread of slow-wave activity from cell to cell with consequent initiation of action potentials. In each portion, the ICC act as a

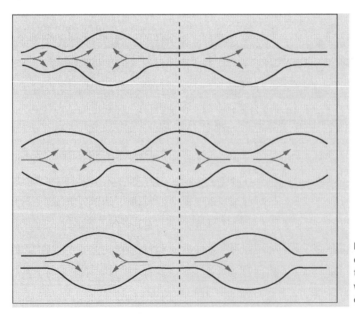

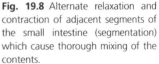

Fig. 19.8 Alternate relaxation and contraction of adjacent segments of the small intestine (segmentation) which cause thorough mixing of the contents.

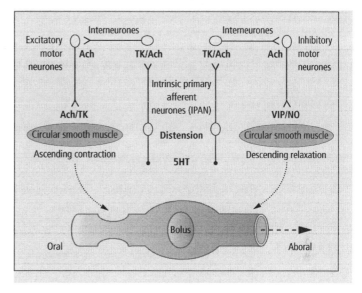

Fig. 19.9. Local coordination of excitatory and inhibitory motor neurones to propel a bolus of food along the small intestine (peristalsis) by ascending contraction and descending relaxation of the circular smooth muscle.

pacemaker to drive the electrical activity. The small intestine exhibits a decrease in the frequency of contractions along its length. This decrease is the result of successive portions of the intestine, from the duodenum to the ileum, having a lower intrinsic frequency of slow-wave generation. This is propagated to adjacent smooth-muscle cells. However, as the activity spreads, more distal portions are unable to follow this high frequency and a new pacemaker region operating at a slower rate then takes over.

Both the intrinsic and extrinsic nerves play a role in regulating intestinal motility. Stimulation of the postganglionic, cholinergic, enteric nerves increases the amplitude of contractions, while stimulation of the sympathetic or NANC inhibitory nerves inhibits contractions. Since the motility of the small intestine continues in the absence of extrinsic nerve supply, it seems likely that the neural regulation of motility is mainly intrinsic. This argument is supported by the observation that isolated segments of the small intestine increase their contractile activity in response to distension, or chemical stimulation of the mucosa.

The extrinsic nerves, however, also play a role and their importance is indicated by the presence of the following reflexes.

1 The **intestinointestinal inhibitory reflex** in which distension of one intestinal segment causes complete intestinal inhibition.
2 The **anointestinal inhibitory reflex** in which distension of the anus causes intestinal inhibition.
3 The **gastrointestinal reflex** in which food entering the stomach causes excitation of intestinal motility.

The role of hormones in the control of intestinal motility is less clear.

For chyme to enter the large intestine, it must pass through the **ileocaecal sphincter** which in humans is approximately 4 cm long. At rest this sphincter is closed by a pressure of some 20 mmHg. During normal movements, this pressure is reduced in association with peristaltic contractions in the terminal ileum and the chyme moves into the large intestine.

Large intestine and rectum

The large intestine stores undigested remnants prior to defecation, plays a role in salt and water balance and contains bacteria (largely anaerobic). The bacteria break down cellulose and other complex carbohydrates, forming short-chain fatty acids (e.g. butyrate), ammonia and gases (methane and hydrogen). They also synthesize, and are an important source of, vitamin K. The progression of chyme through the large intestine is relatively slow (12–18 h).

Colonic motility

The motility of the colon is in some ways similar to that found in the small intestine. The colon is inactive for a large proportion of the time but when contractions occur they may be either of a **segmental** or **peristaltic** nature. The segmental contractions have a slower frequency (three to four per minute) than in the small intestine and the deep but restricted infoldings of the wall form distinct pouches called **haustra**. This movement slowly mixes the luminal contents and improves absorption of salt and water.

Propulsive activity, **mass movements**, occurs infrequently (two to three times each day) and results in the development of relatively high pressures (80–100 mmHg) that drive part of the colonic contents towards the rectum. These contractions may travel 30 cm or more.

Defecation

The rectum is normally empty, but its distension by the mass movement of faecal material from the colon induces relaxation of the smooth muscle of the **internal anal sphincter** and the urge to defecate. In paraplegics this and the contraction of the rectum will lead to automatic defecation, but normally contraction of the **external anal sphincter**, which contains skeletal muscle, allows retention of the rectal contents. When conditions permit, voluntary relaxation of the external sphincter allows defecation to proceed. The expulsion of the faecal mass may be assisted by raising the intra-abdominal pressure as a result of forced expiratory movements against a closed glottis.

Control of colonic and rectal motility

The motility of the colon is largely dependent on **myogenic** and **neural** mechanisms. Slow waves are propagated through the muscle layers but their activity has less directional coordination than that in the stomach and small intestine. Indeed, reverse slow-wave activity and contractions can be recorded in the distal colon and serve to keep the rectum empty between periods of mass peristalsis. The intrinsic nervous plexus plays an important role in the coordination and conduction of contractions as distension can induce coordinated local peristalsis. Loss of the plexus (as in Hirschsprung's and in Chagas' disease) results in marked constriction of the affected segment with pronounced colonic distension proximal to the segment. The motility of the colon is also influenced by the extrinsic nerve supply as illustrated by the **gastrocolic** and **duodenocolic** reflexes, which stimulate motility after material has entered the stomach or duodenum, respectively. Mass movements may follow such reflex activity and result in the urge to defecate.

Defecation is normally a voluntary act involving higher centres of the brain and also the medulla and spinal cord. Rectal distension causes the rectal muscle to contract and the internal anal sphincter to relax. These actions involve intrinsic and extrinsic cholinergic pathways and, in the case of relaxation, also NANC inhibitory fibres. Afferent impulses from the rectum pass to the sacral cord and higher centres. Depending on the situation, the higher centres will either augment or inhibit the sacral centre. If defecation proceeds, the parasympathetic discharge along the pelvic nerves to the colon and rectum is augmented and the somatic motor activity in the pudendal nerve to the external anal sphincter ceases. This defecation reflex is facilitated by the tactile stimulation, which accompanies passage of the faeces through the anus.

Motility during the interdigestive period

During **fasting** quite different patterns of motility are observed. Under these conditions there is a coordinated pattern of alternating quiescence and activity that involves the stomach and small intestine, referred to as the **migrating motor complex (MMC)**. This develops 4–5 h after a meal and recurs at about 100 min intervals until food is again consumed. A period of smooth-muscle inactivity (phase I) is followed by a period of irregular contractions (phase II) leading to a short period (5–10 min) of intense activity (phase III) with regular and forceful contractions. In the stomach these periods involve an increase in muscle tone in the proximal stomach with superimposed phasic contractions, and phasic contractions at the rate of about three per minute in the distal stomach that can generate pressures exceeding 100 mmHg. In the human, these periods of activity precede, but are coordinated with, the activity patterns found in the small intestine that are initiated in the duodenum and slowly spread to the ileocaecal junction. These coordinated bursts of smooth-muscle activity serve to empty the residual contents of the stomach, including basal gastric secretions, and refluxed duodenal contents, including biliary and pancreatic secretions, as well as indigestible solids into the small intestine and to sweep the contents of the small intestine towards the colon. The MMC may also help prevent bacterial overgrowth in the small intestine. The coordination of the MMC may in part be regulated by the hormone motilin. In humans, with meals eaten at regular intervals during the day, the motility pattern associated with food intake occurs throughout the day and the interdigestive activity just described usually develops only at night.

19.3 Secretions of the digestive system

There are five major secretory tissues in the digestive system—the **salivary glands, stomach, pancreas, hepatic–biliary system** and **intestine** (Fig. 19.10). The first four of these have been studied extensively but rather less is known about the secretions of the intestine. Representative values for the compositions of the various secretions are given in Table 19.3.

Salivary secretions

In the human, three pairs of salivary glands are found—the **parotid, submandibular** (also called the submaxillary) and **sublingual**. There are also numerous small mucus-secreting glands throughout the mouth and pharynx.

In the salivary glands, acini that contain secretory cells drain into ducts that coalesce and finally open into the oral cavity (Fig. 19.11).

About 1.5 L of saliva is secreted daily, of which one-quarter comes from the submandibular glands and two-thirds from the parotids. Secretion occurs at a continuous basal rate of $0.3 \, mL \, min^{-1}$ but, when stimulated by acidic foods, such as lemon juice, it can reach a maximum flow of $4–5 \, mL \, min^{-1}$.

Table 19.3 Volumes and representative values for osmolarity, pH and ionic concentrations of plasma and gastrointestinal secretions.

	Volume (L day^{-1})	Osmolarity (mosmol L^{-1})	pH	Na$^+$ (mM)	K$^+$ (mM)	Cl$^-$ (mM)	HCO$_3^-$ (mM)
Plasma	(3.0 total)	300	7.4	150	5	110	24
Saliva	1.5	100	7.5	40	15	25	30
Gastric juice	3.0	200	1.0	50	10	100	0
Pancreatic juice	1.5	300	7.8	140	10	70	80
Bile	0.5	300	7.5	140	5	80	20

1 Volumes given are average values in humans for 24-h samples of secretion.

2 Values depend upon flow rates and therefore can vary quite widely.

3 In gastric juice HCO$_3^-$ secreted by the surface cells reacts with H$^+$ and is converted to CO$_2$ and H$_2$O. Since H$^+$ and HCO$_3^-$ are thereby removed from the solution, the measured osmolarity is less than the osmolarity of the original secretions.

4 In the jejunum, pH rises from proximal to distal regions.

5 There is also an isosmotic secretion of NaCl from crypt cells in the small intestine. Normally, this may be up to 2 L per 24 h.

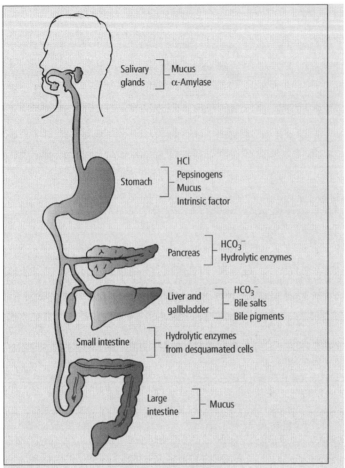

Salivary glands — Mucus
α-Amylase

Stomach — HCl
Pepsinogens
Mucus
Intrinsic factor

Pancreas — HCO$_3^-$
Hydrolytic enzymes

Liver and gallbladder — HCO$_3^-$
Bile salts
Bile pigments

Small intestine — Hydrolytic enzymes from desquamated cells

Large intestine — Mucus

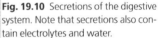

Fig. 19.10 Secretions of the digestive system. Note that secretions also contain electrolytes and water.

Saliva contains a **mucous** secretion, mainly from the sublingual and submandibular glands, and a **serous** secretion of water and ions, mainly from the parotid and submandibular glands. It also contains the enzymes, α amylase (ptyalin), secreted by the parotid glands and involved in initiating carbohydrate digestion, and a lipase (**lingual lipase**) secreted by glands within the mucosa of the tongue and which contributes to fat digestion. Other substances found in the saliva are lysozyme, immunoglobulin A (IgA) and blood group antigens.

Functions of saliva

The water, salts and protein secreted by the salivary glands serve several functions. Water and mucin form a **lubricant** that moistens foods, helps swallowing and aids in speech. In addition, the water facilitates **taste** (see Chapter 7) by partially dissolving ingested material. Saliva helps in the maintenance of oral epithelium and teeth by preventing epithelial dehydration and inhibiting the proliferation of bacteria. The bactericidal effect of the enzyme lysozyme may contribute to the latter effect. Dental caries are also inhibited by salivary HCO$_3^-$, which neutralizes residual acid (ingested or produced by oral bacteria). The digestion of carbohydrates is initiated in the mouth by the secretion of salivary α amylase. But the rapid passage of food through the mouth and oesophagus means that little digestion of carbohydrate occurs before

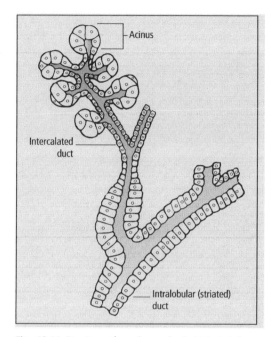

Fig. 19.11 Structure of a salivary gland. (Adapted from Leeson, C.R. (1967) In: Code, C.F. (ed.) *Handbook of Physiology*, Section 6, *Alimentary Canal*, vol. 2, pp. 463–95. Williams & Wilkins, Baltimore.)

it reaches the stomach. The effectiveness of the amylase depends on its dispersion through the food bolus and the rapidity of its inactivation by gastric acid.

Formation of saliva

The serous secretion entering the mouth is hypo-osmotic when compared with plasma and has less Na^+ and Cl^- but more K^+ than plasma (Table 19.3). In the acini, Cl^- secretion (Fig. 1.15) results in the formation of an isosmotic, relatively protein-free secretion with an ionic composition similar to that of plasma, although HCO_3^- (40 mM) is a little higher. As this primary secretion passes through the ducts, Na^+ is actively reabsorbed, accompanied by Cl^-, and small quantities of K^+ are secreted. Since the duct epithelium has a low hydraulic conductivity, the reabsorbed ions are not accompanied by water and so a hypo-osmotic secretion is produced. The actual composition of the serous secre-

tion varies with the flow rate; the higher the rate, the closer the ionic composition is to that of the primary secretion (Fig. 19.12). Note that Na^+–K^+ exchange in the ducts is stimulated by aldosterone, a hormone involved in electrolyte balance. Nitrate is actively taken up from the circulation by the salivary glands and re-secreted so that nitrate concentrations in saliva are considerably higher than those in plasma. A proportion of the salivary nitrate is reduced to nitrite by the action of bacteria in the oral cavity and thus enters the gastric lumen in swallowed saliva. In the acidic environment of the stomach, the nitrite may provide the substrate for generation of nitric oxide and potentially carcinogenic N-nitrosocompounds.

Control of salivary secretion

Increases in salivary flow may result from stimulation of receptors in the mouth, pharynx and oesophagus. Food in the mouth stimulates taste receptors and irritates the oral mucosa, while chewing activates a variety of mechanoreceptors, such as pressure receptors adjacent to teeth and the muscle spindles of masticatory muscles.

Such increases in salivation are reflex actions controlled solely by nervous activity. Afferent sensory fibres carry information to **salivatory centres** in the pons and medulla of the brain, while efferent autonomic fibres supply the glands. The salivatory centres also receive impulses from higher centres of the brain and so the sight, smell and thought of food may also cause salivation, whereas sleep, fatigue, dehydration and fear can inhibit salivation.

In contrast to their actions in other viscera, the parasympathetic and sympathetic fibres have a similar, but not identical, effect in salivation. **Parasympathetic** stimulation, which is of major importance in humans, causes a prolonged copious secretion accompanied by vasodilation. ACh released by parasympathetic fibres induces the secretion of electrolytes and water through a Ca^{2+}-dependent process initiated through the polyphosphoinositide system. The vasodilation is due to release of VIP, a co-transmitter with ACh in a proportion of postganglionic parasympathetic nerves;

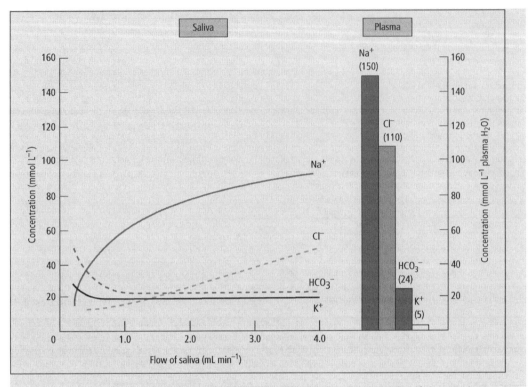

Fig. 19.12 Composition of saliva at different rates of flow. For comparison, the ionic composition of plasma is shown on the right. (Modified from Thayson, J.H., Thorn, N.A. & Schwartz, I.L. (1954) *Am J Physiol*, **178**, 155–9.)

NO may also contribute to the vasodilation. **Sympathetic** stimulation produces a small quantity of thick mucous saliva, which is accompanied by vasoconstriction.

Gastric secretions

Tubular glands in the mucosa of the proximal region (the oxyntic mucosa) secrete the gastric juice containing pepsinogens, acid and mucus. The glands secrete into numerous gastric pits (100 per mm^2), which open into the stomach lumen. Stem cells, which lie in the neck region of the glands, continuously replenish all cell types of the gastric epithelium. The neck region also contains mucus-secreting **mucous neck cells**. **Chief cells** secreting **pepsinogens** tend to lie deep within the gland and **parietal cells** secreting **acid** lie closer to the gland opening. Scattered throughout the gland are small numbers of **enteroendocrine cells**, the most important of which are histamine-secreting, **enterochromaffin-like (ECL) cells** and somastostatin-secreting **D-cells**. The superficial region of the glands and the rest of the gastric epithelium are composed of **surface mucous cells** that secrete a bicarbonate-rich alkaline mucus (Fig. 19.13). The glands in the antrum are essentially free of parietal cells, but have numerous mucus-secreting cells and some pepsinogen-secreting cells, and also contain the G-cells that synthesize and release gastrin into the interstitial fluid.

In total, 2–3 L of an isosmotic gastric juice is secreted each day. At rest, the stomach secretes an HCO$_3^-$-rich isosmotic fluid at a rate of 15–20 mL h^{-1}. But with the appropriate stimuli the stomach secretes acidic gastric juice at rates that may exceed 150 mL h^{-1}. Stimulated gastric secretions contain acid, pepsinogens, mucus, and intrinsic factor.

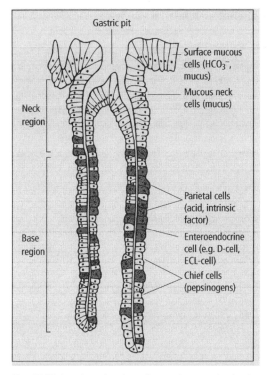

Fig. 19.13 Location of major cell types in a gastric gland. D-cells secrete somatostatin, ECL cells secrete histamine. (Adapted from Ito, S. & Winchester, R.J. (1963) *J Cell Biol*, **16**, 541–77.)

The **pepsins** have maximum proteolytic activities between pH 2 and 3 and are formed from precursor pepsinogens by the action of acid or by the autocatalytic action of pepsins. They initiate the breakdown of proteins by cleaving peptide bonds adjacent to aromatic amino acids, which results in the production of polypeptides of widely differing sizes. Note that since peptic digestion is incomplete, significant quantities of protein leave the stomach to be digested in the small intestine. A **gastric lipase** is also secreted and contributes to fat digestion.

One non-digestive but essential component of gastric juice is **intrinsic factor**. This heat-labile glycoprotein (M_r 60 000) is necessary for absorption of cobalamin (vitamin B_{12}) in the ileum. Intrinsic factor is secreted by the parietal cells in humans and its concentration rises concomitantly with the acid concentration. The amount of intrinsic factor secreted in 24 h is sufficient to bind 50–200 µg of cobalamin, 10–50 times the amount needed for the daily supply of the vitamin. The secretion of intrinsic factor is markedly depressed in gastric atrophy (where parietal cells are absent or reduced in number), and body stores of cobalamin are reduced resulting, if untreated, in **pernicious anaemia** (p. 537).

Functions of gastric secretions

Gastric **hydrochloric acid** is produced by the parietal cells as an isosmotic secretion (150 mM HCl, pH 0.8), which mixes with fluid within the stomach so that the final acid concentration of the gastric contents is somewhat lower. An acid environment is necessary for the activation and optimum activity of the gastric proteolytic enzymes, the pepsinogens, and it denatures ingested proteins, breaking up connective tissue and cells. The acid also plays a protective role, destroying bacteria and other potential pathogens.

The secreted **mucus** forms a viscid gel on the surface of the epithelial cells that creates an unstirred layer of HCO_3^- ions (secreted by these cells) and thus protects them from exposure to the acid and pepsin in the lumen of the stomach (see p. 535).

Formation of gastric secretions

Mucus, ions and water make up the bulk of the gastric juice secreted by the proximal and distal regions. The composition of the gastric secretions is not constant but varies with the flow rate (Fig. 19.14). The basal secretion produced by the surface mucous cells is plasma-like in composition but is modified extensively as gastric secretion increases through secretion of acid by the parietal cells of the proximal region. Table 19.3 gives representative values for the average composition of gastric juice over a 24-h period.

HCl is secreted by parietal cells in an energy-dependent process and the key element is the **H^+,K^+–ATPase**, or **proton pump**. At rest parietal cells contain numerous membranous structures, the tubulovesicles, which are rich in H^+,K^+–ATPase. The tubulovesicles lie adjacent to a system of

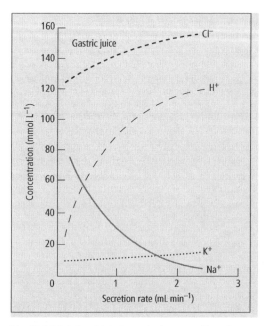

Fig. 19.14 Relationship between ionic composition of gastric juice and its rate of secretion. (After Nordgren, B. (1963) *Acta Physiol Scand*, Suppl. 202, 1–83.)

canals or canaliculi, which run throughout the cytoplasmic space and open into the lumen of the gastric glands (Fig. 19.15). When parietal cells are stimulated to secrete acid the tubulovesicles fuse with the canaliculi (Fig. 19.15), and at the same time there is an increase in canalicular membrane permeability to K^+ and Cl^-. The movement of K^+ into the lumen allows intracellular H^+ to be exchanged (one for one) with K^+, through cycles of phosphorylation and dephosphorylation of the H^+,K^+–ATPase. There is therefore a net secretion of HCl (Fig. 19.16). The water accompanying the HCl is driven out of the cell by the efflux of ions. The composition of the acidic fluid secreted by the parietal cell is therefore largely isosmotic HCl with a little KCl. For each mole of H^+ secreted, an equivalent amount of base (OH^-) is produced. In the parietal cell carbonic anhydrase catalyses the reaction that combines OH^- with CO_2 to give HCO_3^-. The HCO_3^- then passes out of the cell into the blood via a Cl^-/HCO_3^- exchanger; the exchange thereby providing a source of Cl^- to accompany the secretion of H^+. During the increased gastric acid secretion that follows a meal, sufficient HCO_3^- may be produced to

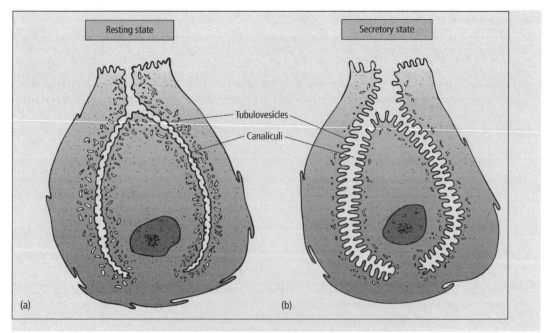

Fig. 19.15 Appearances of parietal cells in (a) the resting state and (b) after a secretory stimulus.

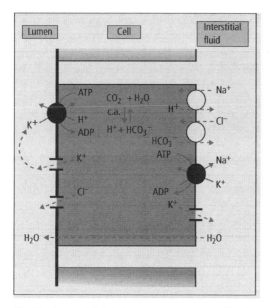

Fig. 19.16 A model of the isosmotic secretion of HCl by the parietal cells. c.a., carbonic anhydrase.

raise the pH of both blood and urine; this is termed the **postprandial alkaline tide.**

Specific inhibitors of the H^+,K^+–ATPase — **proton pump inhibitors (PPI)** are used therapeutically to completely inhibit gastric acid secretion, e.g. for peptic ulcers or gastro-oesophageal reflux disease.

Figure 19.16 illustrates a model for the formation and secretion of gastric acid. The high concentration gradient for H^+ between the lumen of the stomach and the plasma ($10^6:1$) appears to be maintained not only by H^+ transport, but also by the general impermeability of the apical membranes and tight junctions of the mucosa.

Pepsinogens are synthesized in the chief cells, stored in granules and secreted by exocytosis as inactive precursors. Secretion in an inactive form helps prevent autodigestion of the chief cells. **Intrinsic factor** is synthesized and secreted by the parietal cells.

Control of gastric secretion

During the phases of gastric secretion described below, stimulation of acid secretion is generally accompanied by an increase in secretion of enzymes, and in motility and hence gastric emptying (p. 503).

Histamine, secreted from the ECL cells in response to gastrin, is the primary modulator of acid secretion (Fig. 19.17). Histamine acts in a paracrine fashion at H_2 receptors on parietal cells, stimulating adenylyl cyclase via the G protein, $G_{s\alpha}$, and activating the H^+,K^+–ATPase by elevating cyclic adenosine monophosphate (cAMP). Blockade of H_2 receptors by specific inhibitors such as ranitidine or famotidine is used clinically to prevent gastric acid secretion. CCK2 (gastrin) and muscarinic M_3 receptors are present on parietal cells, and binding of gastrin or ACh causes a rise of intracellular calcium. Gastrin or ACh alone are relatively weak direct stimulants of parietal cell acid secretion, but they may act to enhance the effects of histamine. Acid secretion from the parietal cell is inhibited by somatostatin acting at somatostatin type 2 receptors either directly on parietal cells, or indirectly on ECL cells to inhibit histamine secretion.

The physiological stimulus for acid secretion is food. Traditionally, food-stimulated gastric secretion is described in three phases: cephalic, gastric and intestinal, which refer to the sites of origin of the stimuli for secretion. Although these three phases occur consecutively, there is considerable overlap between them.

Cephalic phase

The cephalic phase initiates acid secretion through central mechanisms. The initiating events may be either psychological or physical. Thus the thought, sight or smell of food, chewing actions or the presence of food in the mouth or pharynx, stimulate the dorsal motor nucleus of the vagus to increase parasympathetic output to the stomach. Efferent parasympathetic fibres in the vagus nerve excite postganglionic fibres in the myenteric and submucosal plexuses of the stomach, which in turn release ACh in the vicinity of the parietal cells of the proximal region. Other efferent parasympathetic vagal fibres stimulate postganglionic enteric neurones in the antral region of the stomach to release gastrin-releasing peptide (GRP) which stimulates

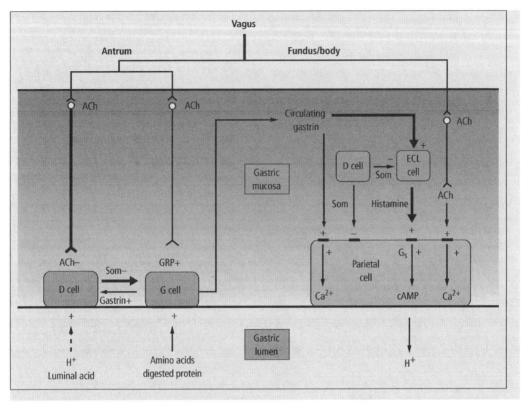

Fig. 19.17 Schematic diagram of the control of gastric acid secretion. D cell, somatostatin-secreting cell; Som, somatostatin; G cell, gastrin-secreting cell. ACh, acetylcholine; cAMP, cyclic adenosine monophosphate; ECL, enterochromaffin-like; GRP, gastrin-releasing peptide; G_s, adenylyl cyclase-stimulating G protein.

G-cells of the distal stomach mucosa to release gastrin; this travels via the blood supply to act on ECL cells in the proximal region. GRP may also stimulate acid secretion by gastrin-independent mechanisms. The cephalic phase accounts for about 30% of the gastric secretory response to a meal.

Gastric phase

The entry of food into the stomach initiates the gastric phase of secretion, by both distension of the stomach and the chemical nature of the food. Distension of the stomach stimulates nerves of the enteric nervous system, which in turn stimulate acid secretion via both a local intrinsic reflex and an extrinsic vagovagal reflex. The efferent vagal pathway is the same as that activated during the cephalic phase. A number of chemical constituents of food stimulate acid secretion, the most

important being products of protein digestion, particularly aromatic amino acids. They act directly on the open type G-cells in the antrum that are exposed to the luminal contents (Fig. 19.17) to stimulate release of gastrin into the blood. The gastric phase accounts for about 60% of the response to a meal.

Control of acidity

In addition to the stimulation of acid secretion, there is also a negative feedback, by which low luminal gastric pH (below about three) inhibits the release of gastrin from G-cells in the distal region. This is due mainly to a local paracrine effect of somatostatin released from neighbouring open type D-cells in response to luminal acid (Fig. 19.17). Although gastrin stimulation is only one of the pathways involved in control of acid secretion, it is the most significant. Thus feedback inhibition limits acid secretion both during feeding and between meals; the latter function may be important as the interdigestive secretions, though small, are acidic and unbuffered by ingested material.

Intestinal phase

Hormones may be involved in the continuation of acid secretion, albeit at a reduced rate, in response to the entry of chyme into the small intestine. However, this is of relatively minor significance and probably contributes no more than 10% of the total gastric secretion following a meal. Of more overall importance is the fact that chyme entering the intestine normally decreases gastric secretion and motility. This negative feedback thus matches the delivery of chyme to the handling capacity of the upper small intestine and is of great physiological importance. A decreased pH, fat and hyperosmolarity in the duodenum causes the suppression of gastric activity and also inhibits gastric emptying. The decrease in gastric emptying is primarily mediated by CCK. The inhibition of gastric secretion is largely hormonal, and the active principle is usually referred to as **enterogastrone**. It is likely that a number of hormones contribute to the enterogastrone effect; candidates include CCK, glucose-dependent insulinotropic polypeptide (GIP) and the glucagon-like peptides.

Pancreatic exocrine secretions

The pancreas consists of two portions—exocrine and endocrine, of which only the exocrine will be considered here. The digestive secretions of the pancreas are initially formed in acini that are similar to those in salivary glands. A system of ducts from the acini unites with the bile duct to form a common duct, which enters the upper duodenum. The entrance of this common duct into the duodenum is controlled by the **sphincter of Oddi**.

The pancreas secretes about 1.5 L of fluid each day. At rest (low flow rates) the secretion is plasmalike; with higher flow rates, an **alkaline fluid** rich in HCO_3^- is secreted. Representative values for its volume and composition are shown in Table 19.3. With the appropriate stimulus the pancreas will

also secrete **hydrolytic enzymes** that act on all the major groups of nutrients.

Functions of pancreatic secretions

The HCO_3^--rich secretion of the pancreas and also, to a lesser extent, of the liver contributes to the neutralization of the acid chyme, which enters the duodenum from the stomach. Thus a favourable pH is established for the pancreatic enzymes, which have optimal activities in the 6.7–9.0 pH range. A pH profile of the gastrointestinal tract is shown in Fig. 19.18.

The pancreatic enzymes or their precursors are secreted along with the aqueous secretion and include:

1 protease precursors—trypsinogen, chymotrypsinogen and procarboxypeptidases—which are secreted by the pancreas and activated in the small intestine. The activation is initiated by the conversion of trypsinogen to trypsin by the intestinal enzyme **enteropepdidase** (enterokinase), found on the apical plasma membrane of the intestinal epithelial cells. The trypsin in turn activates trypsinogen autocatalytically and also activates the other precursors;

2 an active α amylase, which is similar in action to the salivary α amylase and splits α1,4-glycosidic bonds and hydrolyses starch to mainly maltose;

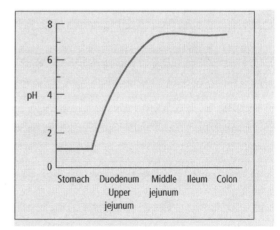

Fig. 19.18 A pH profile of the gastrointestinal tract.

3 lipases and colipase, which act on triglycerides and phospholipids;

4 a number of other enzymes, e.g. **ribonuclease**, **elastase** and **collagenase**, which act on specific macromolecules.

The major pancreatic enzymes, their substrates, actions and products are listed in Table 19.4.

Formation of pancreatic secretions

Two groups of cells contribute to the secretion — the acinar cells and the duct cells. Acinar cells respond to CCK and ACh with an increase in intracellular Ca^{2+}, mediated via the polyphosphoinositide system (Fig. 2.8); this stimulates an exocytotic secretion of enzyme precursors and enzymes and the production of an isosmotic NaCl secretion. In the human, this involves the Cl^- secretory process illustrated in Fig. 1.15.

The enzymes of the pancreatic secretions are all synthesized in the same cells and released in parallel. However, the ratio is not necessarily constant and examination of the pancreatic secretions of individuals on widely differing diets (e.g. high-protein or carbohydrate) shows that these secretions can change to suit the diet.

The duct cells lining the intra- and interlobular ducts produce an isosmotic HCO_3^--rich secretion. This is stimulated by secretin via a cAMP-mediated mechanism, and the HCO_3^- concentration may reach 150 mM. The precise ionic basis for the production of such high concentrations of secreted bicarbonate is not yet fully elucidated, but one simplified model of possible pathways is illustrated in Fig. 19.19.

Since the pancreatic fluid is a mixture of an isosmotic Cl^- secretion from acinar cells and an isosmotic HCO_3^--rich secretion from duct cells, the Cl^- and HCO_3^- composition of the secretion which emerges from the pancreas is not fixed, but varies from about 40 mM HCO_3^- and 110 mM Cl^- at basal flow rates (~0.2 mL min^{-1}) to 120 mM HCO_3^- and 30 mM Cl^- at high flow rates (~2 mL min^{-1}).

Control of pancreatic secretions

Between meals pancreatic secretion occurs at very

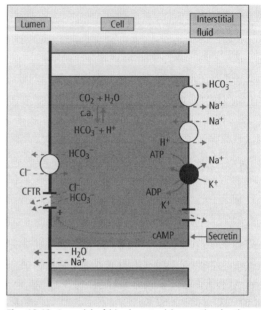

Fig. 19.19 A model of bicarbonate-rich secretion by the duct cells of the exocrine pancreas. c.a., carbonic anhydrase; CFTR, cystic fibrosis transmembrane conductance regulator.

low rates, except during the interdigestive motor cycle (p. 506), when brief increases in pancreatic enzyme and HCO_3^- secretion occur. Although as with gastric secretion, cephalic and gastric phases of pancreatic secretion can be recognized, the major control is exerted during the intestinal phase when nerves and, more importantly, intestinal hormones regulate pancreatic secretion. The entry of chyme into the duodenum is generally followed by the secretion of an HCO_3^- and enzyme-rich fluid from the pancreas. The hormones responsible for this secretion are secretin and CCK. **Secretin** (and a small quantity of CCK) is released from the mucosa of the duodenum and upper jejunum in response to acid chyme. It acts on the duct cells and stimulates secretion of HCO_3^--rich fluid. The release of **CCK** is stimulated by the **products of digestion** (particularly fat and protein) in the upper small intestine. It stimulates the release of an enzyme-rich secretion from acinar cells. In addition, several peptides may inhibit secretion, including somatostatin, pancreatic polypeptide and glucagon (which inhibits duct secretion).

Table 19.4 Pancreatic enzymes: their substrates and products.

Precursor	Enzyme	Substrate	Action	Products
Trypsinogen	Trypsin	Protein and polypeptides	Endopeptidase that cleaves peptide bonds on the C-terminal side of arginine or lysine	Peptides
Chymotrypsinogen	Chymotrypsin	Protein and polypeptides	Endopeptidase that cleaves peptide bonds on the C-terminal side of tyrosine and phenylalanine	Peptides
Procarboxypeptidase A	Carboxypeptidase A	Protein and polypeptides	Exopeptidase that hydrolyses peptide bonds adjacent to most C-terminal amino acids	Amino acids
Procarboxypeptidase B	Carboxypeptidase B	Protein and polypeptides	Hydrolyses mainly bonds adjacent to C-terminal arginine or lysine	Amino acids
Proelastase	Elastase	Elastin and protein	Hydrolyses peptide bonds adjacent to neutral amino acids	Peptides
	Lipase	Triglycerides	Cleaves fatty acids From positions 1 and 3 of triglycerides	Free fatty acids and 2-monoglycerides
Procolipase	Colipase	Triglycerides	Exposes the active site of lipase to substrate	
	Phospholipase A	Lecithin or cephalin	Cleaves off a fatty acid	Free fatty acid and lysolecithin or lysocephalin
	Cholesterol ester hydrolase	Cholesterol and fatty acids	Cleaves off cholesterol	Cholesterol and free fatty acids
	Deoxyribonuclease	DNA	Hydrolyses DNA	Nucleotides
	Ribonucleases	RNA	Hydrolyses RNA	Nucleotides
	α Amylase	Polysaccharides	Hydrolyses α1, 4-glycosidic bonds	Maltose and glucose

Finally, the mix of enzymes secreted is affected by diet. For example, pancreatic amylase and chymotrypsin levels increase when the diet is rich in carbohydrates and proteins, respectively.

Biliary secretions

Bile is formed as a primary secretion of the **hepatic cells** (hepatocytes) into the **biliary canaliculi**, and is modified by the addition of secretions from the duct system through which it passes. The ducts finally coalesce to form the common hepatic duct. The cystic duct from the gallbladder joins the common hepatic duct to form the common bile duct. This merges with the pancreatic duct as the two enter the wall of the duodenum; their opening into the duodenum is controlled by the **sphincter of Oddi**.

About 0.5 L of bile enters the duodenum each day. It is produced continuously but between meals the contraction of the sphincter of Oddi causes it to accumulate in the **gallbladder**. Following a meal, bile is ejected by contraction of the gallbladder and enters the duodenum after relaxation of the sphincter of Oddi. The bile contains two components, which are important in digestion, namely, **bile salts** and HCO_3^-.

Functions of biliary secretions

As discussed on p. 528, the **bile salts** are important in the **digestion** and **absorption of fats** and in the absorption of **fat-soluble vitamins** because of their emulsifying action, particularly in the presence of lecithin and monoglycerides. The HCO_3^- secreted by both the hepatocytes and the duct cells aids in the **neutralization** of acid chyme, which enters the duodenum from the stomach.

The biliary system provides an **excretory route** for bile pigments, cholesterol, steroids, heavy metals and a variety of drugs.

Formation of biliary secretions

Bile formation is primarily the result of active secretion of organic and inorganic anions. Quantitatively the most important organic anions are the bile acids, and bile flow increases linearly with the amount of bile acids secreted. The secretion of HCO_3^-, glutathione, bilirubin and other organic anions, also contributes to the volume of bile secreted. Bile acids (cholic and chenodeoxycholic acids in humans) are synthesized in the liver from cholesterol and are conjugated with the amino acids taurine or glycine to form bile salts. Conjugation, by lowering the pK of the bile acids from about seven to much more acidic values, results in much of the bile acid being in the ionized (bile salt) form, which is both more water-soluble and less lipid-soluble. This has two advantages—the solubility of the bile acids at the low pH of the upper small intestine is enhanced, and passive absorption from the upper small intestine is limited so that the bile salts remain within the intestinal lumen.

Of particular importance in the regulation of bile production is the recycling of bile salts. These are reabsorbed to a limited extent throughout the small intestine by passive diffusion. More importantly, in the terminal ileum they are reabsorbed by the apical sodium-dependent bile transporter, **ASBT**, an example of secondary active transport. Delaying a significant fraction of absorption until the terminal ileum ensures that substantial amounts of bile salts remain throughout the small intestine to promote fat absorption.

Reabsorbed bile salts are carried to the liver in the portal circulation. More than 90% of the bile salts secreted into the small intestine are reabsorbed and returned to the liver in the portal circulation, mostly bound to plasma proteins. This recirculation of bile salts is economic in that the total pool (~3.5 g) is recycled as much as six to eight times in a 24-h period (equivalent to a bile secretion of about 30 g per day); this is referred to as the **enterohepatic circulation**.

The hepatocytes reaccumulate the bile salts from the portal blood by Na^+-dependent co-transport and Na^+-independent transport mechanisms in their basolateral membranes. Conjugated bile salts are preferentially absorbed by the Na^+-dependent mechanism, while unconjugated bile salts are carried mainly by the Na^+-independent transporter. Both reabsorbed and newly synthesized bile salts

are then secreted across the canalicular membrane of the hepatocytes by adenosine triphosphate (ATP)-dependent primary transporters. HCO_3^- is also secreted by the hepatocytes. The tight junctions, which hold adjacent hepatocytes together and form the only barrier between the plasma and the canaliculi, are relatively leaky. Therefore, the secretion of bile salts and HCO_3^- is accompanied by the movement of water and low M_r solutes from the blood to the canaliculi, and this primary secretion is isosmotic. The duct cells also secrete an HCO_3^--rich solution by a mechanism which may be similar to that in the pancreatic duct cells.

The gallbladder

Between meals the gallbladder (volume 20–50 mL) stores and concentrates bile. Following a meal the gallbladder contracts and ejects bile, which enters the duodenum after relaxation of the sphincter of Oddi. Contraction of the gallbladder and relaxation of the sphincter of Oddi are stimulated by the hormonal action of **CCK** released after a meal.

The bile salts are concentrated in the gallbladder by the active reabsorption of Na^+. In the human, Cl^- and HCO_3^- may follow passively. Water also follows passively driven by the osmotic gradient. The bile salts may be concentrated about three-fold depending on the time between meals. This results in the formation of micelles, which are cylindrical aggregates of bile salts that contain phospholipids and cholesterol, as well as holding an appreciable number of inorganic ions. Because each micelle contains many molecules, the osmolarity of gallbladder bile is not substantially greater than that of plasma, despite the removal of the water and the concentration of the bile salts.

Bile pigments, phospholipids, principally lecithins, and cholesterol are also concentrated in the gallbladder bile.

Control of biliary secretion

Biliary secretion is controlled by bile salts delivered to the liver by the portal circulation, circulating hormones and, to a small extent, by autonomic nerves. The most potent stimulators of bile salt secretion are the bile salts themselves, which are reabsorbed in the terminal ileum and returned to the liver in the portal circulation. The greater the quantity of bile salts recycled, the smaller the production of new bile salts by the hepatocytes. Normally, 0.2 to 0.6 g of bile salts is synthesized each day—10–20% of the total pool. This replaces bile salts lost in the faeces. The liver can synthesize as much as 5 g bile salts each day, but cannot match the daily recirculated secretion of about 30 g.

Hormonal control of biliary secretion is exerted largely by **secretin**, released as a result of acid chyme in the duodenum, which increases the production of the HCO_3^--rich secretion from the duct cells (as in the pancreas). Nervous control plays only a minor role in regulating biliary secretion.

Bile pigments and jaundice

The breakdown of red cells in macrophages results in the degradation of the haem groups of haemoglobin with the formation of **biliverdin**. During this reaction, a molecule of CO is released. Biliverdin is reduced to **bilirubin**, which enters the blood, becomes attached to albumin and is carried to the liver. This is termed **unconjugated bilirubin**. Here, it is removed from the plasma by an anion transport system that extracts almost 100% of the load. Microsomal enzymes in the hepatocyte make bilirubin water-soluble by conjugating it with glucuronic acid, and bilirubin is secreted into the bile mainly as the diglucuronide. In the intestine, little of this **conjugated bilirubin** is absorbed. However, bacteria in the large intestine convert some of the bilirubin into a number of products. One of these, **stercobilinogen**, is excreted in the faeces as **stercobilin**. Another, **urobilinogen**, is readily absorbed from the gut, passes back to the liver and is taken up and released back into the bile. A small amount of the absorbed urobilinogen enters the systemic circulation and is excreted in the urine as urobilin.

Jaundice, a yellow coloration of skin, sclera and mucous membranes, is detectable when plasma levels of bilirubin are elevated above some $35\,\mu M$. This can result from increased bilirubin formation (e.g. in haemolytic anaemia), decreased uptake by hepatocytes, disordered cellular conjugation, impaired secretion into the canaliculi or obstruction to biliary drainage. Increased production or failure of hepatocyte uptake results in increased unconjugated bilirubin, which, being bound to albumin, is not excreted in the urine. In contrast, in duct obstruction, the level of conjugated bilirubin is increased as is urinary bilirubin.

Intestinal secretions

The epithelial lining of the small intestine consists of villi and crypts (Fig. 19.20), whereas the large intestine is devoid of villi. Whilst the crypts have generally been considered as sites of secretion of an isosmotic NaCl solution, and the villi and surface cells of the large intestine sites of absorption, this is almost certainly an oversimplification. There is increasing evidence that crypt and villus enterocytes may exhibit both secretion and absorption. The primary secretory process involves the secretion of Cl^-. The cells accumulate Cl^- from the interstitial fluid across the basolateral membrane via the $Na^+–K^+–2Cl^-$ co-transporter. Secretion occurs when apical membrane Cl^- channels (primarily the cystic fibrosis transmembrane conductance regulator, **CFTR**) are activated and Cl^- passes down its electrochemical gradient from the cells to the lumen. The leaky paracellular pathway allows Na^+ and H_2O to follow readily (Fig. 1.15). Under basal conditions ~2 L per 24 h is secreted by the small intestine. This secretion is stimulated by cholinergic nerves, which increase cytosolic Ca^{2+}, and by a variety of peptides, one of which—VIP—acting through increased cell cAMP, may be the most relevant physiologically. A variety of bacterial toxins (e.g. cholera toxin) can activate this secretory process by stimulating the G protein and increasing cAMP (Fig. 2.7), causing diarrhoea (p. 538).

In some regions the secretion of an alkaline fluid or a K^+-rich fluid may also occur. In the duodenum, **Brunner's glands**, as well as mucus-secreting cells which are found throughout the intestinal tract, produce a highly viscid secretion that lies on the surface of the duodenal epithelial cells and contains alkaline (HCO_3^--rich) fluid secreted by these

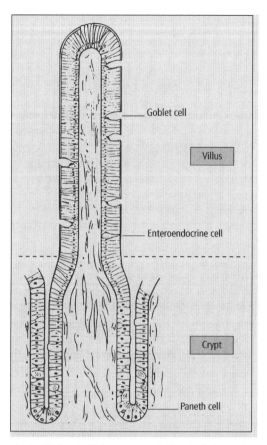

Fig. 19.20 A typical jejunal crypt and villus. At the base, the Paneth cells are thought to have some immunological role in protecting against infection from ingested organisms. The villous cells are constantly being renewed by cells derived from rapidly dividing cells (stem cells) near the base of the crypt. These migrate to the tip of the villus and are shed, a process that in the human takes about 2–3 days. A few cells along the villus become specialized to secrete hormones (enteroendocrine cells) and there are also some mucus-secreting goblet cells.

cells. This may protect the duodenum from the acid chyme entering from the stomach. The rate of secretion is increased by parasympathetic activity and by secretin.

In the ileum and proximal colon, mucus and an alkaline solution rich in HCO_3^- are produced. This involves an HCO_3^-/Cl^- exchange so that the luminal contents are higher in HCO_3^- than plasma but lower in Cl^-. In the colon some of the HCO_3^- may be neutralized by organic acids (generated by bacterial action) in the lumen. The contents of the colon are also rich in K⁺. This is a consequence of both the diffusion of K⁺ into the lumen down the electrical gradient established by Na⁺ absorption and also secondary active secretion of K⁺ (see Fig. 19.24). This involves the accumulation of K⁺ in the cells from the interstitial fluid via the Na⁺–K⁺–2Cl⁻ co-transporter and the Na⁺,K⁺–ATPase. The K⁺ then passes down its electrochemical gradient from the cells to the lumen via K⁺ channels. The absorption of Na⁺ and secretion of K⁺ is enhanced by aldosterone.

Aspects of the control of intestinal secretion are discussed with absorption on p. 531.

Fluid collected from the small intestine, in the absence of gastric, pancreatic and biliary secretions, contains a variety of enzymes. Many of these, e.g. aminopeptidases, amylases and phosphatases, are important in the digestive process and are found in the brush-border region. They are not, however, intestinal secretions but are released from desquamated intestinal cells.

19.4 Gastrointestinal hormones

The gastrointestinal hormones are **peptides** produced by enteroendocrine cells in the gastrointestinal mucosa and are involved in the control of gastrointestinal secretion and to a lesser extent, motility. The enteroendocrine cells have sometimes been referred to as APUD cells (amine precursor uptake and decarboxylation), and were previously thought to be of neuroectodermal origin. It is now clear that like other endocrine cells, enteroendocrine cells are derived from endoderm. Enteroendocrine cells are of either open-type, which have apical processes that contact the lumen of the gut, or closed-type which do not.

Of the many peptides identified in the gastrointestinal mucosa (Table 19.1), a number are recognized to be hormonal regulators of gastrointestinal function under physiological conditions. Thus they are released into the blood in response to a physiological stimulus (e.g. feeding) and produce effects at a different region of the gut, independent of any nervous connections. The open type endocrine cells of the gastrointestinal mucosa are ex-

posed on their luminal surfaces to the contents of the gastrointestinal tract and constituents of the chyme can cause the release of their hormones into the blood stream. In addition, both intrinsic and extrinsic nervous reflexes can cause release of some of these hormones, which not only act through the blood stream but also may diffuse locally and have **paracrine** actions. Peptide hormones are removed from the circulation during passage across most capillary beds to which they are presented, but may also be preferentially removed by organs such as liver and kidney. Several of the peptide hormones are secreted in forms of different chain length; in general the longer forms have a longer half-life in the circulation.

The gastrointestinal hormones can be classified on the basis of their chemical structure into a number of groups or families:

1 Gastrin and CCK, which share five identical amino acids at their biologically active carboxyl end (Fig. 19.21). CCK-like bioactivity is defined by the presence of a sulphated tyrosyl residue at position 7 from the carboxyl end of the peptide; gastrin has a tyrosyl residue at position 6 from the carboxyl end, which may or may not be sulphated (Fig. 19.21). Peptides of the gastrin/CCK family act at two receptors: the CCK1 (or CCK-A) receptor, which has high affinity for CCK and low affinity for gastrin, and the CCK2 (or gastrin/CCK-B) receptor, which has high affinity for both peptides.

2 Secretin, GIP and enteroglucagons, which have sequences of amino acids in common. (The neurotransmitters VIP, peptide histidine isoleucine (PHI)

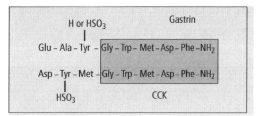

Fig. 19.21 Amino acid sequences at the carboxyl terminal of gastrin and cholecystokinin (CCK). The common pentapeptide amide is boxed. Gastrin-like or CCK-like bioactivities are defined by the position of a sulphated tyrosyl residue.

and pituitary adenylate cyclase-activating peptide (PACAP) are also closely related structurally to this group.)

3 Peptide YY (PYY) and pancreatic polypeptide (PP) share significant sequence homology (as does neuropeptide Y, NPY).

4 Other peptides, e.g. somatostatin, ghrelin, motilin.

The main actions of the individual gastrointestinal hormones on digestive function are outlined below and summarized in Table 19.5. It should also be noted that some of the gastrointestinal hor-

mones may have an important trophic effect on their target glands, e.g. gastrin stimulates the growth of the gastric mucosa and CCK stimulates the growth of acinar cells in the pancreas.

Gastrin

The main circulating forms of gastrin are a 17-amino-acid amidated peptide (G17) and an amino-terminally extended form, G34, which are equally active at the CCK2 receptor. Both G17 and G34 may have their tyrosyl residue sulphated

Table 19.5 Properties and functions of the major gastrointestinal hormones. ACh, acetylcholine; CCK, cholecystokinin; GIP, glucose-dependent insulinotropic peptide; GLP, glucagon-like peptide.

	Released by		**Physiological effects**
Gastrin	**G**-cells in stomach and upper small intestine in response to products of digestion, extrinsic nerve stimulation, antral distension	↑	Secretion of HCl, pepsinogen and intrinsic factor Trophic effect on gastric acid-secreting mucosa
CCK	**I**-cells in upper small intestine in response to products of digestion (fat and protein)	↑ ↓	Secretion of enzyme-rich fluid from pancreatic acinar cells Contraction of gallbladder and relaxation of sphincter of Oddi Gastric emptying Trophic effect on pancreatic acinar cells
Secretin	**S**-cells in upper small intestine in response to ↓ upper intestine pH, fatty acids in upper intestine	↑	Secretion of HCO_3^--rich fluid from pancreatic and hepatic duct cells
GIP	**K**-cells in upper small intestine in response to fat, amino acids and glucose		Releases insulin from pancreatic β-cells
Proglucagon-derived peptides (enteroglucagons and GLP)	**L**-cells in distal ileum and colon in response to glucose and fat in the lumen in these regions		Enhanced intestinal glucose uptake Trophic effect on intestinal crypt cells
Somatostatin	**D**-cells in distal stomach in response to acid **D**-cells in proximal stomach in response to CCK and ACh **D**-cells in intestine and pancreatic islets in response to glucose, fats and bile salts in the intestinal lumen	↓ ↓ ↓ ↓	Gastrin release Gastric acid, histamine and pepsin secretion Inhibits trophic effects of gastrin Pancreatic enzyme secretion Insulin and glucagon release

(Fig. 19.21), but this modification is of little functional consequence for acid secretion.

The properties of gastrin are determined by the carboxyl terminal tetrapeptide amide sequence (trp–met–asp–phe–NH$_2$). Pentagastrin, a synthetic product containing this peptide sequence, has all the properties of gastrin but is less potent. It is used clinically to assess an inability to secrete hydrochloric acid (HCl; **achlorhydria**), and as a provocative test for some tumours, such as medullary thyroid carcinoma.

The gastrins are produced by G-cells in the mucosa lining the antral region of the stomach (Fig. 19.17) and, in humans, the duodenum. The primary stimulus for gastrin secretion is the presence of food in the antrum, notably aromatic amino acids (e.g. phe, tyr) and peptides, as well as calcium and unknown components of coffee, beer and wine (but not caffeine or ethanol). Gastrin is also released by nervous activity in extrinsic pathways during the cephalic phase of gastric secretion, an effect mediated via the vagus nerve and GRP may be one of the neurotransmitters involved. Finally, local nervous reflexes may also stimulate gastrin release, in response to the presence of food in the stomach.

Release of gastrin is inhibited physiologically by somatostatin secreted from neighbouring antral D-cells in response to increasing gastric acidity (Fig. 19.17). In rare cases, gastrin may be produced by tumours (gastrinomas) in the gastrointestinal tract (typically in the pancreas) and this can result in severe peptic ulceration (Zollinger–Ellison syndrome).

Gastrin is carried in the blood stream and **stimulates gastric secretion** of HCl, pepsinogen and intrinsic factor. It also has a trophic effect, stimulating the growth of the acid secreting gastric mucosa, particularly ECL cells. The physiological functions of gastrin are mediated through the CCK2 receptor.

Cholecystokinin

The main physiological forms of CCK are peptides of 58, 39, 33 and 8 amino acid residues; all possess a sulphated tyrosine residue at position seven from the carboxyl terminus and activate the CCK1 receptor. Because circulating concentrations of CCK are much lower than those of gastrin, CCK is not an important physiological activator of CCK2 receptors that mediate acid secretion in the stomach. CCK is produced by I-cells in the mucosa lining the duodenum and jejunum. It is released into the blood in response to the **products of digestion**—especially fatty acids containing 12 or more carbons, peptides and amino acids—in the duodenum and jejunum. The release of CCK in response to food may be partly mediated by CCK-releasing factors secreted into the intestinal lumen.

CCK travels in the blood stream and stimulates enzyme-rich secretion from the acinar cells of the pancreas via the phosphoinositide system and raised intracellular Ca^{2+}. It also potentiates the effects of secretin on HCO$_3^-$ secretion by duct cells. It has a direct effect to contract the gallbladder, and relaxes the sphincter of Oddi by releasing the inhibitory neurotransmitters VIP and NO. It also stimulates the growth of acinar cells in the pancreas. CCK inhibits gastric emptying through stimulation of vagal afferent fibres (p. 503) and also inhibits food intake.

Secretin

Secretin was the first hormone to be discovered (Bayliss and Starling, 1902). Secretin contains 27 amino acids; of these, 14 occupy the same relative position as in glucagon. The full molecule is required for activity. Secretin is produced by S-cells in the mucosa lining the duodenum and jejunum, and its major stimulus for release into the blood is increased acidity in the duodenum and jejunum. It is also released by fatty acids. It is blood-borne and stimulates the duct cells in the pancreas and liver, and Brunner's glands, via cAMP, to produce increased volumes of HCO$_3^-$-rich secretions. This effect is potentiated by CCK and by the neurotransmitter ACh, both of which act through the polyphosphoinositide system and Ca^{2+}. In some species, secretin inhibits acid secretion, but this is unlikely to be physiologically important in humans.

Glucose-dependent insulinotropic peptide

GIP, a 42-amino-acid polypeptide, is produced by K-cells in the mucosa lining the duodenum and upper jejunum. GIP is secreted in response to fat, amino acids and glucose in the upper intestine, and its main physiological function is stimulation of insulin secretion from β-cells of the pancreas; it is therefore an **incretin**. There is also evidence to suggest a role for GIP in regulating triglyceride synthesis in adipocytes. GIP was originally called gastric inhibitory polypeptide, but inhibition of gastric acid secretion is no longer considered to be a physiological function of this hormone.

Enteroglucagons

The glucagon gene is expressed in L-cells of the distal ileum and colon, but the glucagon precursor (proglucagon) is not processed to glucagon. Instead a number of peptides are generated from it that contain, or are related to glucagon. The glucagon-containing peptides (glicentin, oxyntomodulin) are generally referred to as **enteroglucagons**; their physiological functions remain uncertain. The glucagon-like peptide GLP-1 stimulates pancreatic β-cell function and inhibits food intake. GLP-2 enhances glucose uptake by intestinal enterocytes. The various proglucagon-derived peptides are released in response to the presence of glucose and fats in the ileal lumen. Since most of these substances have normally been absorbed before the ileum is reached, blood concentrations of these hormones are not normally high.

Somatostatin

Somatostatin, first identified as a hypothalamic inhibitor of the release of growth hormone from the anterior pituitary (p. 247), is produced by two types of D-cell, in several regions of the gastrointestinal epithelium and in response to various stimuli. Its effects are generally inhibitory. Peptides of 14 or 28 amino acids are secreted that act at a family of at least five receptors (SSTR1-5). In the antral mucosa of the stomach, specialized open type D-cells se-

crete somatostatin in response to low luminal pH; the peptide acts in a local paracrine manner to inhibit gastrin secretion from adjacent G-cells (Fig. 19.17). In the body of the stomach, closed type D-cells secrete somatostatin in response to CCK and ACh; the peptide acts locally to inhibit histamine secretion from ECL cells, HCl secretion from parietal cells (Fig. 19.17), and pepsinogen secretion from chief cells. Somatostatin released from D-cells in the pancreas and in the intestinal mucosa in response to glucose, fats and bile salts, inhibits pancreatic and biliary secretion, blood flow, and the release of a range of hormones (especially insulin and glucagon from the pancreas).

Other gastrointestinal hormones

Motilin is a 22-amino-acid polypeptide produced by M-cells of the duodenal mucosa. Its release into the blood is correlated with increases in gastrointestinal motor activity. Its physiological function remains uncertain, but it may have a role in coordination of the interdigestive, migrating motor complex (MMC).

Ghrelin is a 28-amino-acid peptide, related to motilin, and found principally in X-cells in the body of the stomach. It is the endogenous ligand for the growth hormone secretagogue receptor. Ghrelin concentrations are highest in the interdigestive period and it is a powerful stimulus of appetite. A range of other biological properties related to digestive function have been described, but its physiological role remains to be established.

PYY is a 36-amino acid peptide found in L-cells in the lower ileum and colon. The principal stimulus for its secretion is fat in the lumen of the ileum; it has inhibitory actions on gastrointestinal motility and gastric and pancreatic secretions. PYY may contribute to the so-called 'ileal brake' mechanism whereby the appearance of fat in the distal gut inhibits transit through the proximal intestine thus prolonging the time available for digestion and absorption.

PP is a 36-amino-acid peptide produced by F-cells found mainly in the pancreatic islets, but also scattered throughout the exocrine tissue. Its release into the blood is stimulated by protein meals and although it inhibits pancreatic enzyme and bicarbonate secretion, its physiological status remains uncertain.

Neurotensin is a 13-amino-acid polypeptide produced by N-cells found in the mucosa lining the ileum. Its release into the blood is stimulated by the presence of fat, but its physiological status is uncertain.

As well as the hormones, other chemicals play a role in regulating and coordinating gastrointestinal function. For example, the **prostaglandins** are synthesized, released and degraded in the gastrointestinal tract and when ingested or injected can influence motility and secretion, and **histamine** has important effects on gastric acid secretion and in linking the immune system and the enteric nervous system (p. 534). Although 5-HT is recognized to be an enteric neurotransmitter, about 90% of the body's store of this amine is found in EC cells scattered throughout the gut epithelium from distal stomach to colon. Secretion of 5-HT occurs during mechanical or chemical stimulation of the epithelium and may lead to changes in motility e.g. peristalsis and secretion. Disorders of 5-HT signalling have been implicated in conditions of intestinal motility dysfunction such as inflammatory bowel syndrome (IBS) and ulcerative colitis. 5-HT is also involved in mediating sensations of nausea and vomiting (emesis), particularly in response to cytotoxic anticancer drugs. 5-HT released from EC cells in response to these agents stimulates the terminals of vagal afferent fibres, which in turn activate the vomiting centre in the brainstem. The action of 5-HT on vagal afferent fibres appears to be mediated by the 5-HT_3 class of receptor, and antagonists of this receptor (e.g. ondansetron) can be effective against chemotherapy-induced emesis.

19.5 Absorption

Absorption may be defined as the net passage of a substance from the lumen of the gut across the epithelium to the interstitial fluid. Two important factors influencing absorption are the available surface area and the flux of molecules across the epithelium (amount per minute per unit area), i.e.

$$\text{Amount absorbed/min} = \text{area} \times \text{flux}$$

In the gut, the surface area available for absorption is greatly expanded by loops or coils of the gut, by mucosal infoldings (Fig. 19.2a) that increase the surface area of the loops, by villi (Fig. 19.2b), and by microvilli which form the brush borders of the luminal surface of the cells. In an adult, the total surface area available for absorption in the gut is approximately $400\,\text{m}^2$, which is equivalent to 200 times the external surface area of the body!

The flux of molecules across the epithelium depends on their ability to penetrate the epithelial membranes and also on the driving force for their transport, i.e. their electrochemical potential gradient. The ability of a substance to cross the epithelium depends on its lipid solubility, its size, and on the presence of specific carrier molecules in the membrane (p. 6). Carrier-mediated transport may be downhill, i.e. facilitated diffusion, or uphill, i.e. primary active transport, or secondary active transport (co-transport or counter-transport), as discussed in Fig. 1.6. Furthermore, the leakier the paracellular pathway between the epithelial cells, the more readily organic solutes of small relative molecular mass, ions and water, can cross the epithelium.

The concentration of many substances in the lumen is determined by their rate of digestion. Absorption also depends on the time in contact with the absorptive surfaces, so control of motility is essential to allow normal absorption to take place. The concentration of the products of digestion in the interstitial fluid depends on their rate of removal by the blood, which in turn depends on the blood flow. The blood vessels in the villi are arranged in loops (Fig. 19.2b) so that the distance for diffusion in the interstitial fluid from the basolateral epithelial cell membrane to the capillaries is minimized. The volume of blood flowing to the gastrointestinal tract represents 20–30% of the cardiac output at rest. The rate of capillary blood flow is a thousand times greater than that of the lymphatic flow. Thus substances such as glucose, amino acids, ions and water, which readily enter the capillaries, are removed from them and pass through the portal circulation to the liver. Only those substances, chylomicrons (small lipid aggregations; p. 529), which do not readily cross the capillary basement membrane are transported predominantly by the lymphatic circulation. Such substances enter the venous blood via the thoracic duct and are thus not exclusively transported directly to the liver after absorption.

Absorption in the mouth

Normally, little of the constituents of a meal are absorbed in the mouth. However, some lipid-soluble drugs can be administered by placing them either under the tongue or next to the cheek.

Absorption in the stomach

In the stomach, the H^+ concentration is up to one million times greater than that in the plasma, while the Na^+ concentration can be as low as one-tenth of that in the plasma. This implies the existence of a gastric mucosal barrier in which both the apical plasma membrane of the epithelial cells and the tight junctions between these cells are very impermeable to ions. It is not surprising therefore, that little absorption normally occurs in the stomach. However, lipid-soluble substances, e.g. alcohol (ethanol) and organic acids such as acetyl-

salicylic acid (aspirin) in their non-ionized form, are absorbed to some extent across the stomach wall, although never as fast as from the small intestine.

Absorption in the intestine

The products of digestion are absorbed predominantly in the small intestine (Fig. 19.22). Absorption of salts and water also occurs in the small intestine and, to a more limited extent, in the large intestine. Table 19.6 gives typical volumes per day and ion concentrations found at the end of the different segments of the intestine.

Carbohydrates

A large portion of ingested carbohydrates are polysaccharides (starch and glycogen) and disaccharides (sucrose and lactose) which are mainly hydrolysed to monosaccharides before absorption occurs. This involves an initial luminal digestion to short-chain polysaccharides, disaccharides and monosaccharides by the salivary and pancreatic amylases. The polysaccharides and disaccharides are then hydrolysed to monosaccharides by digestive enzymes bound to the brush border of the epithelial cells. Monosaccharides

Table 19.6 Volumes per day and representative values for ionic concentrations of intestinal fluids at the end of each segment.

	Volume (L day^{-1})	Na$^+$ (mM)	K$^+$ (mM)	Cl$^-$ (mM)	HCO$_3^-$ (mM)
At the end of the					
duodenum	9.0	60	15	60	15
jejunum	3.0	140	6	100	30
ileum	1.0	140	8	60	70
colon	0.1	40	90	15	30

1 Volume leaving the duodenum includes ingested water. Therefore fluid is somewhat hypo-osmotic at this stage.
2 Fluid has become isosmotic by the end of the jejunum.
3 In the ileum Cl$^-$ is reabsorbed in exchange for HCO$_3^-$.
4 In the colon, K$^+$ is secreted in exchange for Na$^+$, and HCO$_3^-$ is secreted in exchange for Cl$^-$. However, the buffering of H$^+$ from short-chain organic acids produced by bacterial action consumes some of this HCO$_3^-$ so that the HCO$_3^-$ concentration is lower than in the ileum. These organic anions now balance some of the charges on Na$^+$ and K$^+$ previously balanced by Cl$^-$ and HCO$_3^-$. By the end of the colon, the fluid may actually be hyperosmotic as a consequence of the production of organic solutes by bacterial action.

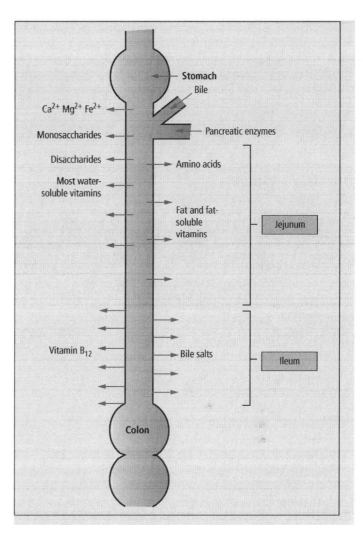

Fig. 19.22 Absorption in the small intestine. (After Booth, C.C. (1968) In: Code, C.F. (ed.) *Handbook of Physiology*, Section 6, *Alimentary Canal*, vol. 2, pp. 1513–27. Williams & Wilkins, Baltimore.)

(principally glucose, galactose and fructose) are largely absorbed in the duodenum and upper jejunum. The absorption of glucose and galactose involves the **sodium glucose-linked transporter, SGLT1** (Fig. 19.23). The activity of this Na^+-dependent co-transporter is greatly influenced by Na^+ in the lumen. The diffusion of Na^+ down its electrochemical gradient provides the driving force for glucose entry into the cell which may be against its concentration gradient. This is an example of secondary active transport, with energy expended by the Na^+/K^+ pump to maintain a low intracellular sodium concentration. Fructose absorption is not dependent on Na^+ and occurs through facilitated

diffusion by the carrier, glucose transporter type 5 (**GLUT5**). The absorbed monosaccharides seem not to be metabolized by the cells but leave across the basolateral membrane by the Na^+-independent carrier **GLUT2**, and then enter the capillaries.

Proteins

Before absorption takes place, the proteins are broken down to peptides or amino acids. About 50% of the digested protein comes from ingested food, 25% from proteins in the gut secretions and 25% from desquamated epithelial cells. Gastric and pancreatic enzymes hydrolyse protein to

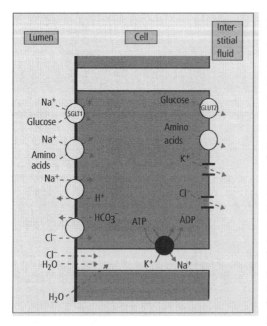

Fig. 19.23 A model of transport mechanisms and of isosmotic fluid absorption in small intestinal villous epithelial cells. SGLT1, sodium glucose-linked transporter type 1; GLUT2, glucose transporter type 2.

short-chain peptides which are further hydrolysed at the brush border to free amino acids or to di- or tripeptides, all of which can enter the intestinal epithelial cells. Absorption normally occurs in the duodenum and upper jejunum and involves at least seven transport systems with somewhat overlapping specificities for the different classes of amino acids (neutral, basic, etc.). The majority of the transporters are Na$^+$-dependent so that amino-acid absorption, like glucose absorption, is increased by luminal Na$^+$ (Fig. 19.23). Some Na$^+$-independent transport of amino acids also occurs. Di- and tripeptides are absorbed rapidly from the lumen by a H$^+$-dependent co-transporter, **peptide transporter type 1 (PEPT1)**, and are hydrolysed to amino acids within the epithelial cells by cytosolic peptidases. Amino acids leave the cell at the basolateral membrane via a separate group of transporters, to enter the hepatic portal blood. In neonates, antibodies and other proteins contained in colostrum may be absorbed in their intact form by pinocytosis.

Lipids

The dietary lipids, up to 150 g per day, are primarily triglycerides, phospholipids, cholesterol and plant sterols. The absorption of lipid is normally an efficient process, and faeces contain less than 5 g of fat per day. Since lipids are not water-soluble, digestion and absorption of these compounds are more complicated than for carbohydrates and proteins. There are a number of stages.

1 Emulsification, digestion and micelle formation. Large lipid droplets must be converted to small lipid droplets (0.5–1 μm in diameter) and these stabilized to prevent coalescence. This process of **emulsification** requires a shearing force provided by gastric and intestinal motility and the presence of stabilizers, of which the physiologically most important are **bile salts**. In the stomach fat digestion is initiated by **lingual lipase** and **gastric lipase**. These liberate short-chain, medium-chain and unsaturated fatty acids. At the normal acidic gastric pH they have little effect on long-chain fatty acids.

In the duodenum, emulsification is enhanced by the combination of bile salts and lecithin so that droplets of about 0.5–1 μm are formed. This gives an enormous surface area. A protein, procolipase, secreted by the pancreas, is converted to its active form, **colipase**, by trypsin in the lumen. Colipase binds to **pancreatic lipase** and also to bile acid and allows the pancreatic lipase to act at the oil–water interface of the emulsion to convert triglycerides to free fatty acids and 2-monoglycerides. These, together with bile salts, lecithin, cholesterol and fat-soluble vitamins, form **micelles**. Micelles are small aggregations (4–6 nm in diameter) of about 20 fat molecules whose hydrocarbon chains interdigitate within a non-aqueous fluid interior and whose polar groups form a negatively charged spherical shell surrounded by cations in aqueous solution. Other major enzymes involved in lipid digestion are listed in Table 19.4.

2 Passage from lumen to cell. The micelles diffuse to the luminal cellular membrane and monoglycerides leave the micelles and diffuse passively across the luminal membrane while free fatty acids are absorbed both by passive diffusion and a sat-

urable uptake mechanism involving a member of the fatty acid transport protein family (FATP 4). The micelles themselves do not cross the membrane. The bile salts are absorbed only slowly from the duodenum and jejunum and so remain active in the upper intestinal lumen of the intestine. Over 90% of the secreted bile salts are eventually absorbed in the terminal ileum by the ASBT.

Note that glycerol and short- and medium-chain length fatty acids (<12 carbons) are sufficiently water-soluble that they can diffuse directly to the luminal cellular membrane and do not require micelles to transport them.

3 Cellular metabolism and synthesis of chylomicrons. Once the long-chain fatty acids have entered the cytosol of the epithelial cells they bind to a fatty acid-binding protein (FABP) and are transported to the smooth endoplasmic reticulum. Here, fatty acids are re-esterified to triglycerides. Then chylomicrons are assembled in the region of the golgi apparatus of the cells. **Chylomicrons** are complexes, about 100 nm in diameter, of triglycerides (87%), cholesterol esters (3%) and fat-soluble vitamins, all of which are enveloped in a hydrophobic coat composed of specific apoproteins (1%), phospholipid (9%) and free cholesterol.

4 Passage from cell to interstitium. Release of the chylomicrons from the cell occurs by exocytosis across the basolateral membrane.

5 Removal by the lymphatic system. The chylomicrons enter the lymphatic lacteals in the villi, not the blood capillaries, reflecting the fact that the endothelial cells lining the lacteals, unlike those in the capillary walls, are not held together by tight junctions and thus allow large molecules to penetrate. The chylomicrons pass through the lymphatic system to the systemic circulation via the thoracic duct.

The blood transports the chylomicrons throughout the body. Capillaries in adipose tissue and muscle contain binding sites for the chylomicrons. Apoprotein CII within the chylomicron activates the enzyme lipoprotein lipase and free fatty acids and monoglycerides are released from the chylomicrons and enter the adipose and muscle cells. The chylomicron remnants are then released from the capillary wall and pass on through the circula-tion to enter liver cells. Thus dietary triglycerides are delivered to peripheral tissues, whereas cholesterol is delivered to the liver.

In contrast, short- to medium-chain fatty acids (<12 carbons) are absorbed from the lumen without requiring micelle formation and tend not to be re-esterified within the epithelial cells. They pass into the capillaries where they bind to albumin, and thence into the portal circulation rather than into the lymphatics. They are thus delivered preferentially to the liver.

Na^+

Under normal conditions, up to 1 mol of Na^+ (equivalent to 58 g NaCl) is absorbed per day. Less than 20% of this is derived from the diet, the remainder having been secreted into the gastrointestinal tract. Since total exchangeable body Na^+ is approximately 3 mol, the importance of Na^+ absorption is obvious, as is the rapid depletion of extracellular fluid volume if Na^+ is lost from the gut in severe vomiting or diarrhoea. Approximately 5–10 mmol of Na^+ is excreted in the faeces daily.

About 90% of Na^+ absorption occurs in the small intestine, chiefly in the jejunum; the remaining 10% occurs in the large intestine. In the small intestine, Na^+ absorption involves predominantly secondary active transport of Na^+ from the lumen to the cell, either in exchange for H^+ or co-transported with organic solutes, and primary active transport from the cell to the interstitial fluid (Fig. 19.23). Thus Na^+ absorption in this segment is increased by glucose and amino acids in the lumen.

The coupling of Na^+ and organic solute movements has important therapeutic implications in the management of cholera and other secretory diarrhoeas. In such cases, the increased net Na^+, Cl^- and H_2O secretion can be offset by oral administration of solutions containing both Na^+ and glucose.

Note that in the small intestine, in particular, the paracellular pathway is leaky and therefore considerable passive movements also occur between the gut lumen and the interstitial fluid. These movements contribute to the rapid equilibration of luminal contents with interstitial fluid. Thus luminal fluid in the small intestine, whatever its initial osmolarity, quickly becomes isosmotic with plasma.

Na⁺ absorption from the large intestine, particularly the distal colon and rectum, is dominated by Na⁺ entry from the lumen through selective channels, whose number is increased by aldosterone. This hormone therefore stimulates the colonic uptake of Na⁺. Some Na⁺ absorption in the colon occurs via a Na⁺/H⁺ exchanger.

K⁺

K⁺ is absorbed throughout the intestinal tract. In the small intestine, the mechanisms involved are not well characterized but diffusion through the paracellular pathway may be the primary route. In the colon, the net movement of K⁺ will depend on a number of transport pathways: (a) paracellular diffusion driven by the electrochemical gradient; (b) secondary active secretion which occurs along the length of the large intestine; and (c) primary active absorption in the distal colon and rectum via a H⁺, K⁺–ATPase in the luminal membrane (Fig. 19.24). K⁺ is secreted into the colonic lumen through K⁺ channels in the apical membrane of the enterocytes. The number of these channels is increased by aldosterone in parallel with Na⁺ channels so that this hormone also enhances K⁺ secretion. The consequence of large intestinal K⁺ secretion is that the faeces normally contain more K⁺ than Na⁺ (Table 19.6). Loss of colonic fluids in chronic or severe diarrhoea may lead to hypokalaemia.

Cl⁻ and HCO₃⁻

Cl⁻ is absorbed from the intestine; HCO₃⁻ is secreted. Absorption of Cl⁻ may be passive, with Cl⁻ driven through the paracellular pathway by the transepithelial electrical gradient generated by Na⁺ absorption. Alternatively, it may involve secondary active transport across the luminal membrane (co-transport with Na⁺ or counter-transport with cell HCO₃⁻ which is thereby secreted) followed by exit across the basolateral membrane. The path-

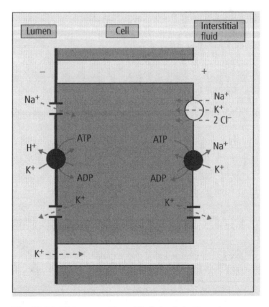

Fig. 19.24 K⁺ transport by epithelial cells in the colon.

ways involved in this HCO₃⁻ loss from the cells remain to be defined but include specific Cl⁻ channels (Fig. 19.23).

In the jejunum, all of these absorptive processes occur. The secondary active transport mechanisms seem to be confined to the villus cells. In contrast, the crypt cells secrete Cl⁻ by the process illustrated in Fig. 1.15. Chloride enters the crypt cells through the basolateral Na⁺/K⁺/2Cl⁻ co-transporter, and leaves via an apical cAMP-dependent chloride channel, cystic fibrosis transmembrane conductance regulator (CFTR).

In the ileum and in the large intestine, the dominant pathway for Cl⁻ absorption appears to be counter-transport across the luminal membrane in exchange for cell HCO₃⁻, which is thereby secreted. The secreted HCO₃⁻ plays a role in the large intestine in buffering H⁺ ions liberated from the short-chain organic acids generated by bacterial action on complex carbohydrates. Thus, although HCO₃⁻ secretion continues in the large intestine, the HCO₃⁻ concentration in the luminal fluid at the end of the colon is actually lower than at the end of the ileum (Table 19.6).

Water

Approximately 8 to 10 L of fluid enters the lumen of the small intestine each day, of which about 2 L is ingested, the remainder being secreted by the salivary glands, stomach, liver, pancreas and intestine itself (Fig. 19.25). The small intestine normally absorbs all but about 1.5 L of this fluid, which then enters the colon. Most of the remaining water is absorbed by the colon, leaving about 0.1 L to be excreted in the faeces.

There is rapid movement of water across the small intestine in response to osmotic gradients. Ions also move freely through the paracellular pathway. Thus the luminal contents rapidly attain the osmolarity of the interstitial fluid. Throughout the intestine, water absorption from an isosmotic luminal solution is secondary to solute absorption and is driven by the resulting osmotic gradient (Fig. 19.23). Coupling between solute and water movements probably occurs within the lateral intercellular spaces.

In addition to the paracellular movement of water, it is now recognized that there is also substantial movement of water across cell membranes, mediated by a family of water transporters known as the aquaporins. Water transport through these channels is bidirectional, and largely driven by osmotic gradients. Around a dozen aquaporins have been identified to date, each with its own characteristic tissue distribution. Within the gastrointestinal (GI) tract, aquaporin 3 is expressed in salivary gland, and aquaporin 10 in upper small intestine. The glucose transporter SGLT1 is also permeable to water and contributes to the osmotically driven transcellular movement.

Movement of this absorbed water from the interstitial fluid to the capillaries is driven by the plasma colloid osmotic pressure. Changes in the capillary hydrostatic or plasma colloid osmotic pressure may influence net water movement between blood and lumen.

In the large intestine, water permeability is lower and osmotic gradients may be generated between the lumen and interstitial fluid. For example, because bacterial action in the large intestine generates osmotically active solutes (e.g. ammonia and short-chain organic acids such as acetic acid),

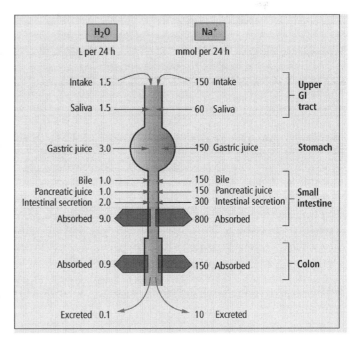

Fig. 19.25 Approximate H_2O and Na^+ movement across the gut over a 24-h period. GI, gastrointestinal.

faeces are normally hyperosmotic to plasma. The normal human colon can apparently absorb as much as 4.5 L of water per day if required.

Regulation of intestinal absorption and secretion

It is important to stress that normally salt and water absorption and secretion are coordinated so that little salt or water loss occurs in the faeces. There is both nervous (Table 19.2) and hormonal control of these processes. However, as well as the physiological mediators, bacteria in the gut lumen, cells involved in the immune system (e.g. phagocytes, mast cells, lymphocytes) and mesenchymal cells in the gut wall (e.g. endothelium, fibroblasts, smooth muscle), release chemicals that can modulate intestinal secretion and absorption. Amongst these are inflammatory mediators such as prostaglandins (e.g. E_2 and I_2), adenosine, histamine and 5-HT. These may act directly on the epithelial cells themselves. In addition, enteric nerve and endocrine cells have receptors for the compounds and the immune cells have receptors for neurotransmitters and hormones. Therefore, there is very close coordination and interaction between these systems in the regulation of intestinal water and electrolyte transport in health and disease. Failure to match absorption to secretion results in secretory diarrhoea (p. 538).

Minerals

Calcium

When dietary Ca^{2+} is plentiful, absorption throughout the intestine by passive paracellular diffusion down a concentration gradient contributes significantly. When dietary Ca^{2+} intake is lower, active absorption is dominant. This occurs largely in the **duodenum** and is regulated by the vitamin D metabolite **1,25-DHCC** (calcitriol). Active absorption involves calcium entry at the enterocyte brush border through voltage-insensitive Ca^{2+} channels, translocation across the cell to the basolateral membrane, and extrusion by a Ca^{2+}–ATPase. The Ca^{2+} transport across the enterocyte is greatly enhanced by **calbindins**, calcium

binding proteins whose synthesis is dependent upon **1,25-dihydroxycholecalciferol** (1,25-DHCC; calcitriol).

Absorption of Ca^{2+} is impaired at an alkaline pH and by the presence in the gut of fat and of other substances such as oxalates and phytates which form insoluble complexes with Ca^{2+}.

Phosphorus

About 1 g of inorganic phosphorus (P_i) is absorbed from the upper small intestine each day, by both passive diffusion and by coupled co-transport with Na^+ across the luminal enterocyte membrane, a process that is stimulated by 1,25-DHCC.

Iron

An average daily diet provides 180–270 μmol of iron. Red meats and sea foods are rich in iron, which is mainly in the ferric state (Fe^{3+}) and in organic form, e.g. as haem and as ferric–protein complexes. Iron is released from the food by acid and proteolytic enzymes in the stomach and small intestine. Reduction to the ferrous state (Fe^{2+}), which is necessary for efficient absorption, is favoured by low pH and reducing agents, such as ascorbic acid and protein sulphydryl groups.

Absorption of iron is regulated to maintain iron balance since there is no physiological mechanism for its excretion. Maximal absorption of iron occurs in the duodenum and upper jejunum and only very small amounts are taken up by the stomach and ileum. Non-haem iron is absorbed via the divalent metal transporter type 1 (DMT1) in the apical membrane. Reduction of insoluble ferric iron to ferrous iron is achieved by a ferrireductase at the enterocyte brush border prior to absorption. Absorption of non-haem iron is limited by dietary substances which form insoluble complexes with iron, e.g. phosphate, phytate and the tannin of tea. Haem iron readily enters the enterocytes by a separate pathway, but the mechanism is not yet clarified. Cytosolic haem oxygenase then releases bound Fe^{2+} which enters the same cytosolic pool as non-haem iron.

Absorption varies directly with the rate of erythropoiesis and inversely with the amount of iron in the body stores, so that 20–30% of dietary iron may be absorbed in iron deficiency but less than 5% when the stores are full.

Once absorbed by the enterocyte, depending upon the body's need, iron is either transferred across the basolateral membrane into the blood via the transporter ferroportin, or sequestered in the enterocyte. Iron transferred to the blood is complexed to transferrin in the interstitial space and it is carried in this form in the blood. Iron not complexed in this way is removed from the portal circulation by the hepatocytes.

Iron not released to the blood after entry into the intestinal mucosal cell is sequestered as ferritin and is ultimately lost from the body when the mucosal cell is shed from the tip of the villus. This is the main route of iron excretion. How intestinal mucosal cells regulate the amount of iron absorbed is not understood.

Vitamins

The pathway followed by vitamins during absorption from the gastrointestinal tract is to a large extent dependent on their lipid and water solubilities. The **fat-soluble** vitamins (A, D, E and K) and their precursors are incorporated into micelles from which they diffuse into the epithelial cells. Like the dietary lipids, the absorption of these vitamins is dependent on the presence of adequate bile salts.

The absorption of many **water-soluble** vitamins is facilitated by the presence of specific metabolically dependent carriers. In some cases (e.g. thiamine, B1 and ascorbic acid, C), these have a Na^+ dependence similar to that for the uptake of sugars and amino acids. The epithelial cells may modify the substance before releasing it to the plasma. For example, **folic acid** (pteroylglutamic acid) is a vitamin (B9) present in foods mainly as a polyglutamate. Folates are absorbed mainly from the duodenum and upper jejunum. Enzymes at the enterocyte brush border first hydrolyze the polyglutamate derivatives to the monoglutamate form, which enters the cells via a sodium-dependent carrier. In the cells reduction and methylation to methyltetrahydrofolate occurs and

this leaves the cells and enters the portal blood. The small intestine has a large absorptive capacity for folate.

The absorption of **cobalamin** (vitamin B_{12}) is further specialized. This vitamin is released in the stomach from complexes with food proteins by acid and proteolytic enzymes. Within the gastric lumen, cobalamin binds to glycoproteins secreted into saliva and gastric juice (known as **R proteins** or haptocorrins). In the duodenum pancreatic enzymes digest the R proteins and cobalamin then combines on a mole-to-mole basis with a glycoprotein, **intrinsic factor**, produced by the gastric parietal cells. This complex resists enzymatic digestion and reaches the terminal ileum where it attaches to specific receptors for intrinsic factor on the brush border of the epithelial cells. (Note that these receptors do not recognize R proteins.) Mucosal uptake of the complex by endocytosis is facilitated by luminal Ca^{2+} and an alkaline or neutral pH. Uptake is followed by degradation of intrinsic factor within the cells and release of the vitamin to the portal blood. Absorption of cobalamin is limited by the number of receptors available in the ileum and a normal diet supplies rather more of the vitamin than can be absorbed. In the portal blood, cobalamin is bound to a transport protein, **transcobalamin II**, which readily releases the vitamin to the bone marrow and other tissues. However, most cobalamin in the blood is tightly bound to another protein, **transcobalamin I**, which gives up little of the vitamin to the tissues, and may represent a longer term storage mechanism.

Gases

Gases in the gut either come from air that has been swallowed or are generated in the gut itself. At any time about 100 mL of gas is present in the intestines, ~60% of which is N_2, mainly from swallowed air. Of the remainder, hydrogen and methane are generated in the colon by bacterial action. CO_2 is formed when secreted HCO_3^- neutralizes gastric acid or organic acids formed by bacterial action in the colon. Odour-generating gases (e.g. H_2S) account for less than 1% of the total gas.

Gases are absorbed from the intestine, diffusing down their gradient of partial pressure to the blood and are then exhaled. Some of the gases generated in the large intestine are expelled through the anus, the total volume per day ranging between about 0.4 and 2.0 L.

19.6 Defence mechanisms in the digestive tract

Large quantities of a variety of micro-organisms, many potentially pathogenic, are ingested with food each day. Several mechanisms provide protection from these:

1 Mucus throughout the tract traps organisms.

2 Gastric acid may destroy organisms. For example, the bacterium causing cholera (*Vibrio cholerae*) is extremely sensitive to acid.

3 Enzymes may digest organisms.

4 Products released by organisms (e.g. enterotoxins) may **stimulate intestinal secretion** and **inhibit fluid absorption** (p. 538). As a consequence there will be increased luminal fluid, and an increased flow rate through the intestine that will wash organisms from the gut. This may result in frank secretory diarrhoea.

5 Antibodies are secreted into the lumen. Of these, **IgA** provides an important defence mechanism, particularly against viruses. IgA is secreted by plasma cells found throughout the tract in the lamina propria, in the form of a dimer linked by a polypeptide, the J chain. The IgA dimer binds to a receptor, the **polyIg receptor** on the basolateral membrane of the epithelial cells and the complex is endocytosed. The IgA is secreted across the epithelial luminal membrane, still attached to part of the receptor, known as the **secretory component**, which protects the IgA dimer from proteolytic cleavage. **Aggregates of lymphoid tissue** (e.g. tonsils, Peyer's patches, and appendix) are also found (p. 306). Immune cell responses can be initiated through signalling of a family of around a dozen membrane-spanning **toll-like receptors**, which recognize conserved structural motifs of pathogens, the so-called pathogen-associated molecular patterns, or PAMP. Individual receptors recognize distinct structural components of pathogens, such as lipoproteins, lipopolysaccharides and nucleic acids.

It is important to stress the intimate relationships in the gut between the immune system and neural pathways. Immunoglobulin bound to mast cell receptors recognizes sensitizing antigens and results in the release of a variety of chemicals from the mast cells including histamine, 5-HT, prostaglandins, leukotrienes and cytokines. Of these, 5-HT and histamine appear to play pivotal roles in stimulating enteric neurones and thereby initiating the increased secretion and motility that may result in watery diarrhoea. As more is learnt about the interplay between the immune system and the enteric and systemic nervous systems, it should become possible to understand on a rational basis the complex interrelationships between psychological and physical factors in a variety of gut diseases.

19.7 Pathophysiology

Oesophagus

If the acid contents of the stomach enter the oesophagus, the sensation of heartburn may be experienced. Occasional symptoms are not uncommon, but chronic heartburn may be indicative of **gastro-oesophageal reflux disease (GORD)**, due to incompetency of the LOS. Gastro-oesophageal reflux may be alleviated by neutralizing or inhibiting gastric acid secretion using antacids, histamine H2 antagonists (e.g. ranitidine) or PPI (e.g. lansoperazole). Alternatively, surgery (usually fundoplication) may be used to strengthen the LOS. Chronic GORD may lead to the pre-cancerous condition of **Barrett's oesophagus** (or Barrett's metaplasia), in which the normal squamous cells of the lower oesophagus are replaced by abnormal columnar epithelium referred to as specialized intestinal metaplasia. Patients with Barrett's oesophagus have an increased risk of developing oesophageal adenocarcinoma.

In the rare condition of achalasia, lower oesophageal motility is disordered as a consequence of destruction of neurones, the LOS fails to relax and passage of food from the oesophagus to the stomach is disrupted. Patients usually present with difficulty in swallowing (dysphagia).

Stomach and upper duodenum

The epithelium of the stomach is normally protected from the potentially damaging effects of secreted HCl and digestive enzymes, by a number of mechanisms. These include tight junctions between the epithelial cells and the presence of a viscid secreted mucus layer, which contains bicarbonate secreted by the epithelial cells in an unstirred layer and thus helps prevent low pH close to the epithelial cell membrane. In addition, maintenance of an adequate mucosal blood flow enhances protection.

When the gastric mucosal barrier is disrupted, the entry of H^+ into the interstitial fluid acidifies the fluid, which damages the epithelial cells and the underlying capillaries, resulting in local haemorrhage. Such **peptic ulceration** of the stomach or duodenum is a relatively common condition, originally attributed to a variety of causes such as hypersecretion of acid, spicy foodstuffs, lifestyle, or stress. It is now recognized that about 90% of duodenal ulcers and 80% of gastric ulcers are caused by infection with the gastric pathogen *Helicobacter pylori (H. pylori)*. This spiral, flagellated bacterium is adapted to survive the harsh environment of the stomach, where it colonizes the gastric mucus and attaches to epithelial cells. Treatment with potent inhibitors of acid secretion (e.g. PPI) may allow ulcers to heal, but they are likely to recur on withdrawal of medication. In contrast, concomitant antibiotic therapy to eradicate infection with *H. pylori* can affect a permanent cure. Infection in gastric corpus with *H. pylori* also causes chronic gastritis (inflammation) and carries an increased risk of gastric cancer.

Peptic ulceration can also be caused by nonsteroidal anti-inflammatory drugs (**NSAIDS**, e.g. aspirin, ibuprofen), which have a topical irritant effect, and in addition inhibit cyclooxygenase (COX) enzymes and thereby reduce local prostaglandin synthesis and decrease gastric bicarbonate secretion.

A number of other agents can disrupt the gastric mucosal barrier. These include bile salts, short-chain fatty acids, ethanol and possibly corticosteroids.

Intestine

Coeliac disease (gluten-induced enteropathy) is an autoimmune disease that affects the villi of the absorptive intestinal epithelium leading to malabsorption (see below). Glutens are a family of proteins found in grains; those from wheat, barley and rye in particular are rich in short peptide sequences that are able to stimulate T-cell production of antibodies. In affected individuals the immune response leads to damage of the intestinal villi, which become flattened, thereby dramatically reducing the epithelial surface area available for absorption. The epithelial damage can usually be reversed, with consequent alleviation of the symptoms, by adopting a gluten-free diet. Hereditary factors play an important but not exclusive role in the development of coeliac disease.

Inflammatory bowel disease (IBD) generally refers to two chronic disorders—**Crohn's Disease** (CD), which may affect any region of the gastrointestinal tract and **ulcerative colitis** (UC), which is largely restricted to the colon. In UC the inflammatory response is confined to the mucosa and submucosa, leading to ulceration; in CD the entire bowel wall is usually involved and narrowing of the bowel (stricture) may occur. Frequent symptoms of IBD are weight loss, diarrhoea and rectal bleeding, and in the case of CD, abdominal pain. Approaches to alleviate the symptoms include the use of immunosuppressive, corticosteroid, antibiotic and anti-inflammatory drugs. Surgical removal of the colon is a definitive treatment for UC, but CD may recur after removal of affected regions of bowel. The aetiology of IBD is not fully understood but there is a strong genetic linkage involving multiple gene loci. At least five significant linkages have been confirmed so far, including the IBD1 locus on chromosome 16 and IBD2 on chromosome 12q. Genes within these loci that have been implicated in IBD include *NOD2* (nucleotide-binding oligomerization domain 2).

The symptoms of UC are sometimes confused with those of **irritable bowel syndrome** (IBS), which include abdominal discomfort and altered bowel habits. There may be alternating bouts of diarrhoea and constipation, although commonly one condition predominates. However, in IBS there is no evidence of organic disease (e.g. inflammation) and it is therefore referred to as a functional disorder. The causes of IBS are unknown and treatment is usually directed at changes in diet and lifestyle.

Lactose intolerance is a common condition that occurs when the body is unable to digest significant amounts of lactose, the main sugar in milk. It is caused by a deficiency of the enzyme lactase, which converts lactose to the absorbable monosaccharides glucose and galactose, at the brush border of intestinal enterocytes. Lactase production begins to decline in early childhood, and in many adults, lactase deficiency may develop progressively over time, but there are significant differences in the susceptibility to this condition of certain ethnic groups. Lactase insufficiency may also result from intestinal injury or disease, or rarely a congenital absence. On reaching the large intestine, undigested lactose is fermented by colonic bacteria, generating osmotically active products (e.g. short chain fatty acids) in the colonic lumen and gases including hydrogen and methane. Frequent symptoms of lactose intolerance are nausea, abdominal pain and diarrhoea; these can be minimized by regulating the lactose content of the diet.

Hirschsprung's disease (aganglionic megacolon) is a congenital condition in which neurones fail to form in a segment of colon during fetal development. The aganglionic segment fails to relax and thus prevents the passage of stool, with consequent hypertrophy and dilation of the bowel above the constriction. In severe cases, symptoms (e.g. constipation, abdominal swelling, vomiting) may develop within a few days of birth, but in other cases may be delayed until childhood or even adulthood. The definitive treatment is surgery to remove the affected section of bowel.

Pancreas

Several mechanisms normally protect the pancreas from digestion by the proteolytic enzymes that it secretes. These include the relative impermeability of the secretory granule membrane, secretion of the enzymes as inactive precursors, and co-storage of the precursors with a trypsin inhibitor. These mechanisms can however fail in the inflammatory condition of **pancreatitis**. Acute pancreatitis can be triggered by obstruction of the pancreatic duct (e.g. by gallstones or duct spasm) or by toxic agents, usually alcohol. The consequences are inhibition of pancreatic secretion, activation of digestive enzymes from their precursors, and the production of pro-inflammatory mediators. Chronic pancreatitis results in slow destruction of the pancreas over many years. Up to 80% of cases are due to alcohol abuse, but the mechanisms involved remain uncertain. Malabsorption caused by lack of digestive enzymes can be ameliorated by oral enzyme supplements; in some cases induction of diabetes due to destruction of the insulin-secreting β-cells of the endocrine pancreas, necessitates insulin replacement therapy.

Liver

Amongst the many important physiological functions of the liver are production of blood proteins, clotting factors, bile, cholesterol and a range of enzymes, regulation of carbohydrate metabolism and storage, and detoxification of drugs including alcohol. Not surprisingly therefore, diseases of the liver can have widespread effects on bodily functions. A range of diseases affect the liver, but perhaps the most common and amongst the potentially most serious are **hepatitis** and **cirrhosis**.

Hepatitis, or inflammation of the liver, may be caused by alcohol abuse, some medications, immune responses, or viral infections. The effects of hepatitis range from the extremes of relatively mild influenza-like symptoms and fatigue, to signs of liver failure, including jaundice (p. 519), ascites, and encephalopathy. Classes of viral infection include hepatitis A, B, C, D and E. Viral hepatitis is extremely contagious, and acute infection can develop into chronic illness, notably with hepatitis B and C. In some individuals, chronic infection with hepatitis B and C may eventually lead to cirrhosis or primary liver cancer. In contrast, many people infected with hepatitis B remain apparently asymptomatic but are carriers of the virus. Current treatment of hepatitis (e.g. combination therapy with interferon and antiviral agents) can be effective in many cases, but prevention of infection remains an extremely important issue. Vaccines are available, notably for hepatitis A and B, and are recommended for groups with high exposure to the disease, such as health care workers.

Cirrhosis is the end stage disease of many forms of chronic liver injury. It represents the progressive destruction of normal liver architecture and its replacement with fibrous or scar tissue. The liver has a remarkable capacity for regeneration, and the earlier stages of damage, **fibrosis,** may be reversed if the insult is removed; cirrhosis is considered essentially irreversible. Because the liver can function in the face of substantial loss of normal tissue, cirrhosis is usually well established before symptoms develop. In addition to the serious consequences of losing normal liver function, the scar tissue obstructs blood flow and raises pressure in the portal circulation. The elevated pressure or **portal hypertension**, leads to fluid build up and swelling of the abdominal cavity (ascites), and engorgement of varicose-like veins or varices (particularly in oesophageal and gastric vasculature), which may rupture with consequent haemorrhage. The most common causes of cirrhosis are chronic excessive alcohol consumption and infection with hepatitis B and C. Less common causes are congenital disorders, autoimmune disease, exposure to environmental toxins and adverse drug reactions.

Gallbladder

Gallstones (cholelithiasis) often develop in the gallbladder. Over 80% of gallstones are cholesterol stones, the remainder being bile pigment stones. Factors that contribute to the formation of choles-

terol stones are excessive concentrations of cholesterol in bile, insufficient bile salt or lecithin, and stasis of the gallbladder. Gallstones are often asymptomatic but blockage of the gallbladder (or other) ducts causes intense pain and can precipitate jaundice (p. 519) and fever. The most common treatment for gallstones is removal of the gallbladder (cholecystectomy).

Malabsorption and diarrhoea

A variety of diseases are associated with an increased need to defecate. Although increased frequency of defecation is often referred to as diarrhoea, it is necessary to distinguish between increased frequency associated with increased bulk of faeces (**malabsorption syndrome**) and increased frequency associated with increased fluid excretion (**watery diarrhoea**).

Malabsorption syndromes

These are usually chronic disorders that arise as a consequence of impaired digestion or absorption of food. The cause may be lack of digestive enzymes (e.g. chronic pancreatitis); lack of bile salts (e.g. obstruction of the common bile duct) which will affect fat digestion and absorption particularly; a loss of absorptive area (e.g. massive bowel resection; diseases involving the epithelium of the small intestine such as gluten-induced enteropathy); or failure of adequate removal from the interstitial fluid of absorbed substances (e.g. obstruction or disruption of the lymphatic drainage; chronic congestive heart failure). The presence of abnormally high amounts of fat in the faeces is termed **steatorrhoea**. As well as the increased mass of faeces, weight loss and symptoms and signs related to nutritional deficiencies of minerals and vitamins will develop as the underlying disease progresses. In Crohn's disease, damage to the small bowel may compromise absorption of cobalamin (vitamin B_{12}) from the terminal ileum leading to anaemia and neurological symptoms. Another more common cause of cobalamin deficiency is **pernicious anaemia** whereby autoantibodies are formed against parietal cells, which therefore fail to secrete the intrinsic factor required for cobalamin absorption. A further consequence of damage to parietal cells is achlorhydria and the loss of acid feedback inhibition of gastrin secretion. The chronic hypergastrinaemia that develops leads to **ECL cell hyperplasia** (since gastrin is a growth factor for ECL cells); in rare cases the hyperplasia may eventually progress to ECL cell tumours, which are usually benign.

Diarrhoea

Increased frequency of defecation associated with fluid faeces is usually acute and can have a number of causes.

1 Stimulation of gut secretion results in **secretory diarrhoea**. Most commonly this is due to viral or bacterial infections, and in the latter case is caused by endotoxins produced by the bacteria. The secretory diarrhoea of cholera is caused by cholera toxin from *Vibrio cholerae*, and travellers' diarrhoea is commonly due to a heat-labile endotoxin from *Escherichia coli*. In both cases, a fragment (A1) of the endotoxin subunit-A enters intestinal enterocytes and constitutively activates the G protein, G_s. This raises cellular cAMP and activates chloride secretion through an apical channel (CFTR); the accompanying water secretion produces the diarrhoea.

In rare cases, gut secretions may be abnormally stimulated due to a peptide secreting tumour such as a gastrinoma (elevated gastric secretions) or a VIPoma (elevated pancreatic, biliary and intestinal secretions).

2 The presence of **non-reabsorbable solutes** in the gut lumen results in **osmotic diarrhoea**. Causes include the ingestion of laxatives such as magnesium sulphate and impaired absorption of digested carbohydrates (e.g. lactose intolerance).

3 Diarrhoea is usually one feature (amongst others) of IBD such as Crohn's disease or UC. This is due to mucosal injury with increased epithelial permeability resulting in increased net fluid movement from interstitial fluid to gut lumen. Diarrhoea is also seen in the functional disorder of IBS. Disorders of motility (e.g. the increased motility that can be associated with diabetic damage to the autonomic nerves supplying the intestine) are uncommon causes of watery diarrhoea. However, any disease that increases the volume of fluid in the intestinal lumen will distend the lumen and stimulate stretch receptors, thereby resulting reflexly in increased smooth-muscle activity. In addition, a specialized motor pattern called power propulsion is triggered as part of an immune response, and results in forceful and rapid propulsion of the luminal contents over long lengths of bowel. Thus watery diarrhoea is often associated with increased frequency of defecation, and cramping abdominal pain.

Whatever the cause, the composition of the diarrhoea fluid is determined by the source of the primary secretion and the time spent in more distal segments of the intestine. For example, the fluid secreted by small intestinal enterocytes in response to cholera toxin is essentially isosmotic NaCl. As this flows through the ileum and colon some Cl^- is exchanged for cell HCO_3^-, and in the colon some Na^+ is exchanged for cell K^+. This results in a faecal fluid that, while still approximately isosmotic, has lower concentrations of Na^+ and Cl^- and higher concentrations of K^+ and HCO_3^- than did the primary secretion. These exchanges mean that a person with chronic watery diarrhoea, as well as being depleted of extracellular fluid volume (with consequent cardiovascular manifestations, if severe), can also develop K^+ depletion, hypokalaemia (p. 581) and a metabolic acidosis (p. 583).

Neoplastic disease

Cancers of the gastrointestinal tract account for at least 25% of all cancer deaths. The incidence of gastrointestinal tumours varies greatly along the length of the gut. Tumours of the colon and rectum (colorectal cancer) are most common, followed by stomach, oesophagus, pancreas, and liver, with very rare occurrence in small intestine. The incidence of **adenocarcinoma** of the oesophagus has risen dramatically in recent years, although the reasons for this are unclear; it is now the most common oesophageal cancer. Risk factors for cancer of the oesophagus include smoking and excessive alcohol consumption, and there is a strong association with GORD and Barrett's oesophagus (p. 534). Incidence of cancer in the most proximal region of the stomach (close to the gastro-oesophageal junction) is also increasing, while more distal gastric cancers are in decline in the developed world. However, gastric cancers, 95% of which are adeno-carcinomas, remain one of the leading causes of cancer mortality worldwide. One of the major risk factors for development of distal gastric cancer is infection of the body (corpus) of the stomach with *H. pylori* (p. 535). The precise mechanisms involved remain to be clarified, but almost certainly include the development of atrophic gastritis, in which the acid producing parietal cells are destroyed. The prevalence of *H. pylori* infection may approach 90% in the developing world, and the organism has been designated a class I carcinogen by the World Health Organization. Other risk factors for gastric cancer include smoking and alcohol consumption, and diets high in salt, nitrates and nitrites or deficient in fresh fruits and vegetables.

The molecular events associated with GI carcinogenesis, i.e. the progression from normal epithel-ium, through adenoma to adenocarcinoma, are perhaps best understood in the case of colorectal cancer. The sequence involves the acquisition of genetic mutations, and one of the earliest events is loss of the *APC* (*Adenomatous polyposis coli*) gene, which encodes a classical tumour suppressor protein. Individuals suffering from familial adenomatous polyposis have germ line mutations in the *APC* gene, develop multiple colorectal polyps (adenomas) and are susceptible to early onset colorectal carcinoma.

Primary cancers of the liver (hepatocellular carcinoma and cholangiocarcinoma) are relatively rare, and most commonly result from cirrhosis or hepatitis, or from environmental toxins or poisons ingested in the diet (e.g. aflatoxin in mouldy nuts and grain). The liver is however a common site for the development of metastatic cancer, secondary to a primary tumour elsewhere. Primary cancers of the GI tract frequently metastasize to the liver, not least because this organ directly receives the entire venous drainage of the gut.

The kidneys are essential for life. Normally more water and ions are ingested than the body requires. This excess intake is excreted in the urine. The kidneys therefore regulate both the volume and the composition of the body fluids. As well as the surplus water and electrolytes, the urine contains metabolic waste products (including inactivated hormones) and foreign substances and their metabolic derivatives.

The kidneys also produce a variety of humoral agents, including erythropoietin, active metabolites of vitamin D, renin and prostaglandins.

Each human kidney has about 1 million functional units—the **nephrons**—arranged in parallel (Fig. 20.1).

The renal regulation of the volume and composition of the body fluids involves each of these nephrons in three processes: (a) **filtration at the glomerulus**; (b) **tubular reabsorption**; and (c) **tubular secretion** (Fig. 20.2).

20.1 Renal blood flow

Organization

Each functional unit of the kidney—the nephron—is supplied with blood by an afferent arteriole that opens into a glomerular capillary bed. This drains into a second, efferent arteriole which supplies the peritubular capillaries and the medullary vasa recta.

Although only a small fraction of the mass of the body (<0.5%), the kidneys receive 20–25% of the cardiac output at rest. The renal arteries arise directly from the abdominal aorta and within the kidney quickly branch into short interlobar, arcuate and then radial arteries, from which arise the **afferent arterioles**. Each nephron is supplied with blood by an afferent arteriole, which opens into a **glomerular capillary bed**. In turn this drains into an **efferent arteriole**, which then breaks up into a second capillary bed that supplies blood to the rest of the nephron—the **peritubular capillaries**. In the juxtamedullary nephrons (p. 541) the efferent arterioles also supply the long capillary loops—the **vasa recta**—that pass deep into the medulla. Blood then drains into veins that finally merge to form the renal vein that enters the inferior vena cava.

Glomerular capillaries are thus unlike others in that they form a capillary bed in the course of an arteriole. This means that the hydrostatic pressure in these capillaries is determined by both afferent and efferent arteriolar resistances. This allows very precise regulation of capillary pressure and therefore of the driving force for glomerular filtration. The pressure profile of the renal vessels is illustrated in Fig. 20.3. Note that there is little pressure drop along the glomerular capillaries.

Regional variations in renal blood flow

Total renal plasma flow (RPF) and renal blood flow

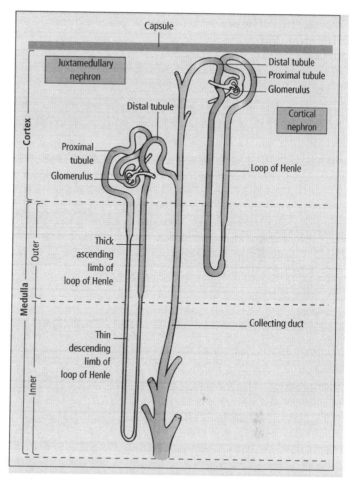

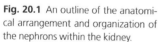

Fig. 20.1 An outline of the anatomical arrangement and organization of the nephrons within the kidney.

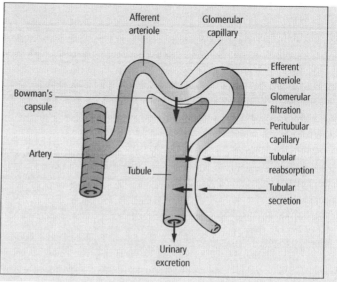

Fig. 20.2 A summary of the three basic functions of the nephron.

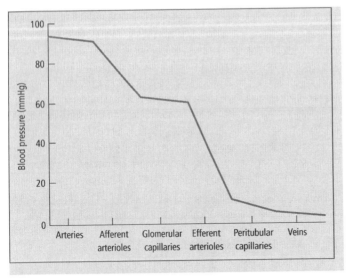

Fig. 20.3 The pressure profile of the renal vessels.

Table 20.1 Distribution of blood flow within the kidney.

	Weight (% total)	Vascular volume (mL per 100 g kidney)	Blood flow (% total)	Transit time (min)	P_aO_2 (mmHg)
Cortex	70	13.5	92.5	0.021	50–70
Outer medulla	20	03.8	06.5	0.086	20–30
Inner medulla	10	02.2	01.0	0.37	05–15

1 Although small in comparison with the flow in the cortex, outer medullary flow in absolute terms, approximately 30 mL per 100 g min^{-1}, is 10 times or more greater than the flow in resting muscle and about half that in brain.
2 The relatively low rate of flow in the inner medulla is important to the role of medullary circulation in preserving the osmotic gradient in the medulla and therefore in H_2O conservation by the kidneys.
3 Reflecting the low P_aO_2, some 70% of the inner medullary metabolism may be anaerobic.

(RBF) can be estimated in humans by measuring the clearance of para-aminohippurate (PAH) (p. 552). The kidney is not all perfused equally; experiments measuring transit times of dyes, wash-out of gases like ^{85}Kr, and the lodgement of microspheres in the renal vessels in experimental animals, suggest that, of the total RBF, the cortex receives 90%, the outer medulla 7% and the inner medulla 1% (Table 20.1).

Control of renal blood flow

Intrinsic control—autoregulation—holds the glomerular filtration pressure relatively constant despite variations in mean arterial blood pressure

over the range 80–180 mm Hg. Superimposed on this is extrinsic control through the sympathetic nervous system, noradrenaline and angiotensin II. When recumbent at rest, extrinsic control is minimal.

Intrinsic control

Mean arterial blood pressures between about 80 and 180 mm Hg have little effect on RBF, which remains relatively constant over this range (Fig. 20.4).

This control of RBF, termed **autoregulation**, is independent of extrinsic nerve supply or extrinsic hormones. It is largely a consequence of afferent

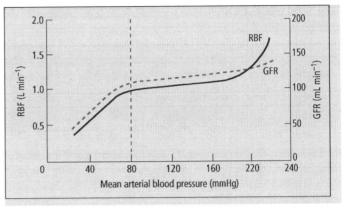

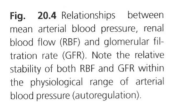

Fig. 20.4 Relationships between mean arterial blood pressure, renal blood flow (RBF) and glomerular filtration rate (GFR). Note the relative stability of both RBF and GFR within the physiological range of arterial blood pressure (autoregulation).

glomerular arteriolar resistance increasing as blood pressure increases. Autoregulation may be **myogenic**, the arterioles contracting when transmural pressure increases, as occurs in arterioles in other organs. However, **tubuloglomerular feedback** through the juxtaglomerular apparatus (p. 544) may play the more important role in this. For example, any tendency for increased delivery of NaCl to the distal tubule will be sensed by the macula densa cells and will result in increased afferent arteriolar resistance. Thus, glomerular hydrostatic pressure will fall, glomerular filtration rate (GFR) will decrease, and the load delivered to the distal nephron will return towards normal. The precise nature of the link between the macula densa and the alterations in arteriolar resistance is unclear. Possible mediators include the renin–angiotensin system acting locally, adenosine, cyclic adenosine monophosphate (cAMP) and prostaglandins.

Extrinsic control

Sympathetic vasoconstrictor activity is minimal at rest (i.e. when warm, recumbent, relaxed), but increases with changes of posture, cold, pain, emotion and exercise and so reduces RBF. The reductions associated with the erect posture and exercise are often exaggerated in patients with cardiac failure. Severe reductions of arterial blood pressure, as in shock, will depress RBF and may precipitate acute renal failure. Chronic pathological processes that destroy nephrons reduce RBF.

20.2 Structure and organization of the nephron

Nephrons are tubes lined with epithelial cells supported on a basement membrane. In the renal cortex, the glomerular capillary bed is invaginated into the start of the nephron. In this region, specialized epithelial cells—the podocytes—form **Bowman's capsule** lining Bowman's space (Fig. 20.5). Together with the glomerulus these form the **renal corpuscle**.

Bowman's space drains into the **proximal convoluted tubule** within the renal cortex, then to the proximal straight tubule that runs from the cortex to the outer medulla. This leads within the medulla to the **thin descending** and **thin ascending limbs**, then the **thick ascending limb** of the **loop of Henle**. The thick ascending limb returns to the cortex as the **distal straight tubule** and makes contact with the afferent arteriole of its glomerulus, forming the **juxtaglomerular apparatus** (Fig. 20.5). The distal tubule has several cell types and is heterogeneous in both structure and function. The distal straight tubule is followed by the **distal convoluted tubule** and then the **connecting segment** that joins with six to eight connecting segments from other nephrons to form a **cortical collecting duct**. This runs into the medulla and becomes the **medullary collecting duct**. In the inner medulla these ducts merge, become progressively larger and finally terminate in the **ducts of Bellini** which drain into the ureter.

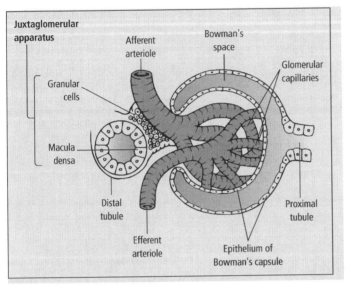

Fig. 20.5 The organization of the glomerulus. The juxtaglomerular apparatus includes modified smooth muscle cells (granular cells) in the wall of the afferent arteriole and specialized epithelial cells (the macula densa) in the distal straight tubule.

Nephrons are similar but not identical; the chief variants (Fig. 20.1) are:

1 superficial, **cortical nephrons**. These have short loops of Henle reaching only into the outer medullary zone and their efferent glomerular arterioles supply their peritubular capillaries. About 80% of the nephrons in the human kidney belong to this group;

2 deeper, **juxtamedullary nephrons**. These have long loops of Henle, which plunge deep into the inner medulla. Their efferent glomerular arterioles supply peritubular capillaries and also capillary loops (vasa recta) which course among the long loops of Henle and the collecting tubules deep in the medulla.

Note that all renal tubules receive only postglomerular blood, and that the vasa recta carry the sole blood supply to the inner medulla.

20.3 Glomerular structure and function

Structure

The glomerulus consists of a fenestrated capillary endothelium supported by a basement membrane which sits on the foot processes of the podocytes lining Bowman's space. The major barrier to convective flow is the basement membrane; solutes of M_r below 10 000 are freely filtered. With larger molecules movement is increasingly restricted and ceases at around 70 000 for negatively-charged albumin to 100 000 for neutral solutes. For the same head of hydrostatic pressure, an ultrafiltrate passes through this barrier about 100 times faster than through capillaries elsewhere.

The energy required for filtration is supplied by the heart, not by the kidney. In the glomerular capillary tufts, blood, at a pressure of about 60% of mean aortic pressure, is exposed to a filtering membrane of over $1\,m^2$ (more than half the external surface area of the body) that separates the plasma from Bowman's space (Fig. 20.5). The capillary endothelium is **fenestrated**; it lies on a basement membrane (0.2–0.3 µm thick) composed of loose fibrillar glycoproteins with fixed negative charges. The foot processes (**pedicels**) of the specialized epithelial cells (**podocytes**) contact the other surface of this basement membrane, which is synthesized by both the capillary endothelial cells and the podocytes. Interstitial contractile **mesangial cells** and the extracellular **mesangial matrix** support the glomerular capillaries and basement membrane. The mesangial cells may have a role in adjusting capillary blood flow and thereby affect glomerular filtration. Slit pores between the foot processes of investing podocytes provide a pathway for convective flow from plasma to Bowman's space that passes between cells. Thus the major barrier to this flow is the basement membrane. Substances up to 10000 M_r pass through the filter freely. For these solutes, which include the ions and metabolites of the extracellular fluid, the concentrations in the filtrate in Bowman's space equal those in the plasma. With larger molecules, diffusion is increasingly restricted and ceases around 70000 M_r (for albumin—an elongated molecule with negative charge) to 100000 M_r (for uncharged molecules).

For the same hydrostatic pressure difference across the same filtration area, an ultrafiltrate passes through this barrier about 100 times faster than through capillaries elsewhere.

The **GFR** is equivalent to the net flow of water across a membrane per unit time (J_v), given on p. 16 as

$$J_v = AL_p(\Delta P - \Delta \pi)$$

where A is the area of the membrane available for flow, L_p is the hydraulic conductivity which is a measure of the ease with which water flows through the membrane, and ($\Delta P - \Delta \pi$) is the driving force which is dependent on the differences in hydrostatic pressure (ΔP) and effective osmotic pressure ($\Delta \pi$) across the membrane.

When applied to GFR, ΔP is the difference between the hydrostatic pressures in glomerular capillaries (P_{gc}) and in Bowman's space (P_t). Since normally only negligible amounts of protein are filtered, $\Delta \pi$ is the colloid osmotic pressure in glomerular capillaries (π_{gc}). Thus

$$GFR = AL_p[(P_{gc} - P_t) - \pi_{gc}]$$

Because it is difficult to estimate the area of the glomerular capillary bed with sufficient accuracy, AL_p is usually represented as K_f, the ultrafiltration coefficient and

$$GFR = K_f[(P_{gc} - P_t) - \pi_{gc}]$$

Representative values for the human are P_{gc} 60 mmHg (with little drop from the afferent to the efferent end), P_t 20 mmHg, and, at the afferent end of the capillary, π_{gc} 25 mmHg. However, as fluid is

filtered the concentration of plasma proteins rises and π_{gc} approximates 35 mmHg by the end of the capillary. The average for π_{gc} is therefore ~30 mmHg. Substituting these values in the equation, the average driving force for fluid movement from capillary to Bowman's space is 9 mmHg.

Measurement of GFR

GFR can be measured using the relationship GFR = UV/P for any substance that is freely filtered and not reabsorbed or secreted. Inulin fulfils these criteria. Clinically the GFR is estimated using creatinine.

Assume that a solute is freely filtered at the glomerulus but is subsequently neither reabsorbed nor secreted. Let P and U be the concentrations of the solute in plasma and urine in the same units, and V be the volume of urine produced per minute.

Then, amount excreted per minute in urine (UV) = amount entering Bowman's space per minute from plasma (i.e. the amount filtered per minute across the glomerulus). Since, for a freely filtered solute, concentration in Bowman's space = concentration in plasma (P), amount filtered per minute at the glomerulus = GFR × P. Therefore, GFR × P = UV, or

$$GFR = \frac{UV}{P}$$

What properties are required in a substance to be used for measurement of GFR? The substances must be:

1 freely filtered at the glomerulus (therefore M_r << 50000–60000);

2 not reabsorbed or secreted (i.e. not able to permeate the tubules in any part of the tubular nephron);

3 not metabolized by the kidney;

4 not toxic; and

5 easily measured in blood and urine.

Classically, inulin (polyfructosan, M_r 5000) is used to measure GFR. But accurate measurement needs continuous infusion to establish a steady state with constant plasma concentration and rate of excretion. Since the amount of inulin excreted is directly proportional to the plasma concentration

(Fig. 20.6a), the plot of UV/P against plasma concentration gives a line parallel to the x axis (Fig. 20.6b). That is, UV/P for a substance which is filtered and neither reabsorbed nor secreted is independent of its concentration in the plasma.

Clinically, creatinine, which is produced by metabolism from creatine, is often used to measure GFR. In the human there is a little proximal tubular secretion of creatinine, but the usual method for measuring plasma concentration overestimates creatinine because plasma contains a non-filtered chromogen which reacts as creatinine, and these errors tend to cancel. The best results are obtained by measuring the amount of creatinine excreted over 24 h. Since plasma creatinine concentration stays relatively constant throughout the day, one plasma sample is usually all that is taken.

A representative value for GFR in adults is about $125 \, \text{mL} \, \text{min}^{-1}$ or $180 \, \text{L} \, \text{day}^{-1}$, of the order of 50 times the volume of plasma in the body. This value represents the sum of the contributions of the individual nephrons from both kidneys. GFR is better related to body surface area than to weight. Even so, it is quite variable from person to person. From about two years of age until after middle-age, when the GFR declines slowly, the average value is $120 \, \text{mL} \, \text{min}^{-1}$ for each $1.73 \, \text{m}^2$ (average body surface area). With 1 million nephrons in each kidney, the average filtration rate per nephron (**single nephron GFR**) comes to $60 \, \text{nL} \, \text{min}^{-1}$ or $90 \, \mu\text{L} \, \text{day}^{-1}$.

Filtered load

If the GFR is known, it is a simple matter to calculate the amount of any solute filtered per minute — the **filtered load**.

Filtered load = GFR × plasma concentration

e.g. filtered load of glucose = $0.125 \, \text{L} \, \text{min}^{-1} \times 5 \, \text{mmol} \, \text{L}^{-1} = 0.625 \, \text{mmol} \, \text{min}^{-1}$.

Filtration fraction

About 650 mL of plasma flows through the kidneys each minute (RPF, p. 552). Of this, about one-fifth is filtered; the remaining four-fifths pass into the peritubular capillaries. That is, the ratio GFR/RPF, called the **filtration fraction**, is about 0.20. Contrast this with the ratio of ultrafiltration to flow through typical systemic capillaries, which is about 0.005.

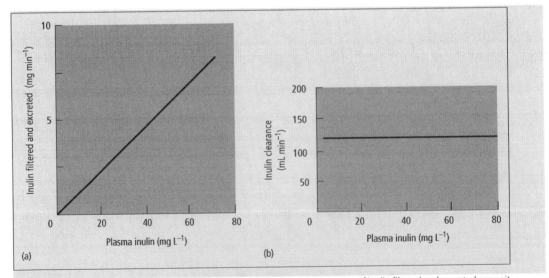

Fig. 20.6 (a) The relationship between plasma inulin concentration and the amounts of inulin filtered and excreted per unit of time. (b) The relationship between plasma inulin concentration and the clearance (UV/P) of inulin.

Variations in GFR

Results from early measurements with inulin probably overemphasized the constancy of GFR. Nevertheless, autoregulation of RBF (p. 542) results in a relatively stable glomerular hydrostatic pressure and therefore GFR. However, if arterial blood pressure falls below about 60 mmHg, as in shock, GFR ceases, leading to anuria. The erect posture, emotion, pain, cold, exercise, and loss of blood are all associated with reductions in GFR, especially the erect posture and exercise in some patients with cardiac failure. Pathological processes which destroy nephrons reduce GFR, and GFR may increase when blood and extracellular fluid volumes are expanded, especially with saline, which dilutes plasma protein and lowers colloid osmotic pressure.

20.4 Clearance

The relationship UV/P can be estimated for any substance. It is referred to as the renal plasma clearance, or clearance for short. With inulin or creatinine, this relationship provides a good estimate of GFR. Any substance that is freely filtered and has a clearance value less than that of inulin must have been reabsorbed. Any substance with a clearance greater than that of inulin must have been secreted.

The expression UV/P can be calculated for any substance and is called **renal plasma clearance** or **clearance** for short. This has the dimensions of volume per unit of time. In general, clearance allows comparison of the renal handling of different substances. However, in two situations where the clearance of substances with special properties is determined, it allows the calculation of a real rate of volume flow—GFR as discussed above, and RPF (p. 552).

The clearance of inulin, as we have seen, estimates GFR. If a substance that is filtered has a clearance less than that of inulin, then there must be a net reabsorption of that substance in the renal tubules. For example, a substance such as glucose that is freely filtered at the glomerulus but is normally completely reabsorbed from the tubules, will have a clearance of 0. If the clearance of a substance is greater than that of inulin, then there must be a net secretion by the tubular cells into the tubular fluid.

This comparison can be made formally by calculating the **clearance ratio**, i.e. clearance of $X(C_X)$/clearance of inulin (C_{In}), which compares the amounts of a substance in the urine and in the glomerular filtrate from which that urine was formed.

$$\frac{C_X}{C_{In}} = \frac{U \times V}{P \times GFR} = \frac{\text{amount of } X \text{ excreted}}{\text{amount of } X \text{ filtered}}$$

If $(C_X)/(C_{In})$ is less than 1.0, there is less X in the urine than was filtered, i.e. X is reabsorbed; while if $(C_X)/(C_{In})$ is greater than 1.0, there is more X in the urine than was filtered, i.e. X is secreted by the tubules as well as being filtered.

20.5 Tubular function

Reabsorption and secretion occur in the tubules. Both processes may be either active or passive. The rate of epithelial transport is determined by surface area multiplied by flux. In the kidney, the available surface area is enormous and there is a very favourable ratio of surface area to volume. Normally, GFR is adjusted to allow adequate contact time with the epithelial cells in the different parts of the nephron. The flux of solutes depends upon the properties of the membranes of the epithelial cells and of the tight junctions between them. The proximal tubule is lined by a typical 'leaky' epithelium and is specialized for the bulk reabsorption of filtered solutes and water. The epithelia lining more distal portions of the nephron show various degrees of 'tightness'.

The whole volume of plasma is filtered many times daily. This effectively removes waste products from the blood, but in so doing removes water and all solutes of low M_r at the same time. Hence a major task of the tubules must be recovery of water and solutes needed by the body.

Reabsorption and secretion occur in the tubules. Both processes may be either active or passive. Before discussing some examples of each, the main factors affecting tubular function need to be summarized.

As discussed in Chapter 1, the rate of epithelial transport is determined by surface area × flux, where flux is defined as amount moved per unit of time per unit area. In the kidney, the available surface area is enormous and offers a very favourable ratio of surface area to volume (each tubule handles only about $1/(2 \times 10^6)$ of the total volume filtered per minute—about 60 nL). In addition, especially in the proximal tubules, there is a very extensive brush border on the luminal surface. In contrast to the situation in the gut, there is no motility to control contact time. Instead, the rate of filtration is such that normally the load presented to the tubules does not exceed their capacity to deal with it. This may be accomplished, in part, through the juxtaglomerular apparatus (p. 544), which senses the load delivered to the distal tubule and alters afferent arteriolar resistance appropriately. However, if more solute than normal is filtered, or if tubular reabsorption is depressed, the increased flow rate downstream may overload the reabsorptive mechanisms for Na^+ in the distal nephron and result in an increased excretion of sodium chloride and water (an example of **osmotic diuresis**).

The flux of solutes depends upon the properties of the membranes of the epithelial cells and of the tight junctions. The proximal tubule is lined by a typical 'leaky' epithelium (p. 20). Glucose, amino acids, organic acids, phosphate, sulphate and some other solutes are co-transported across the luminal membrane coupled to Na^+ transport and driven by the energy inherent in the electrochemical gradient for Na^+ (Fig. 20.7). They pass across the basolateral membrane by either simple or facilitated diffusion. Isosmotic absorption occurs in this segment, as expected for 'leaky' epithelia. The epithelia lining more distal portions of the nephron show various degrees of 'tightness' as will be discussed later. It is important to realize that because of the very leaky junctions between the proximal tubular cells, it is impossible for the proximal tubule to generate major transepithelial ionic gradients. This is crucially important for understanding osmotic diuresis (see next section).

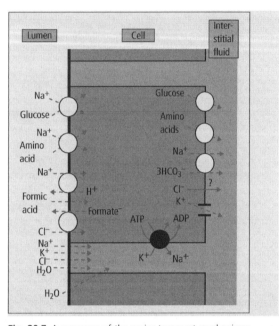

Fig. 20.7 A summary of the major transport mechanisms of solute movements across renal proximal tubules. The cell formate exchanged for luminal Cl^- reacts with H^+ in the lumen to form the weak, lipid-soluble formic acid which then diffuses back into the cell. Although Cl^- entering the cells from the lumen must be lost across the basolateral membrane, the pathways for this loss are ill-defined. Hence the question mark in the figure. Note that there are significant movements of ions and water through the paracellular pathway. ADP, adenosine diphosphate; ATP, adenosine triphosphate.

The gradient for reabsorption reflects, in part, the rate of removal of reabsorbed solutes by the peritubular capillaries. This is rapid and effective in the cortex but the arrangement of the vasa recta in long loops results in accumulation of reabsorbed solutes within the medulla (p. 563).

The same general principles apply to tubular secretion. Secreted solutes may be removed from the peritubular plasma or be synthesized within the tubular epithelial cells and transferred to the luminal fluid.

Some solutes are only reabsorbed, some are only secreted, some undergo both processes.

Organic solutes that are reabsorbed

Glucose, amino acids, organic acids, phosphate,

sulphate and some other solutes are co-transported across the luminal membrane coupled to Na^+ transport and driven by the energy inherent in the electrochemical gradient for Na^+. They pass across the basolateral membrane by either simple or facilitated diffusion. A variety of smaller molecular weight proteins and peptides cross the glomerular filter. Most enter the proximal tubular cells by endocytosis and are then degraded to amino acids which are returned to the plasma. Urea is absorbed passively. Antidiuretic hormone (ADH) increases the permeability of the medullary collecting ducts to urea; hence less urea is excreted at low urinary flow rates.

Glucose

Normally, all of the filtered glucose is reabsorbed and there is no glucose in the urine. Reabsorption involves co-transport with Na^+ at the luminal membrane (Fig. 20.7). The characteristics of glucose handling are illustrated in Fig. 20.8.

If the filtered load is increased by raising the plasma glucose concentration, the transport mechanism in some tubules becomes saturated and glucose begins to appear in the urine. The plasma glucose concentration at which glucose first appears is called the **plasma threshold**, and in the human is some $10–12\,mmol\,L^{-1}$ when GFR is normal at about $125\,mL\,min^{-1}$. Hence the trans-

port mechanism begins to be saturated in some tubules when the filtered load reaches $10 \times 0.125 = 1.25\,mmol\,min^{-1}$. At plasma glucose concentrations of about $15\,mmol\,L^{-1}$, the transport mechanism in all the tubules is saturated, and the maximal reabsorptive capacity of the tubules (**tubular maximum**, T_m) has been reached. This is thus about $1.9\,mmol\,min^{-1}$ ($15\,mmol\,L^{-1} \times 0.125\,L\,min^{-1}$). Note that the plasma threshold reflects the limit of the rate of tubular reabsorption, it is not a fixed plasma concentration. Because filtered load equals $P_{glucose} \times GFR$, threshold concentration is inversely proportional to GFR. With GFR reduced from 125 to $60\,mL\,min^{-1}$ it would take 20 not $10\,mmol\,L^{-1}$ of plasma glucose to reach the threshold load of $1.25\,mmol\,min^{-1}$.

The commonest cause of glycosuria is **diabetes mellitus**, in which the plasma glucose concentration is abnormally high. This will give rise to osmotic diuresis, which is an important symptom often leading to diagnosis of this common disease (**diabetes**—increased flow of urine, **mellitus**—sweet; i.e. an important symptom of diabetes mellitus is excess flow of sweet (glucose-containing) urine). The osmotic diuresis arises because of the inability of the proximal tubule to support a transtubular Na^+ gradient, which is due to the very leaky junctions in this part of the nephron. When more glucose is filtered than can be reabsorbed in the proximal tubule, the excess glucose will

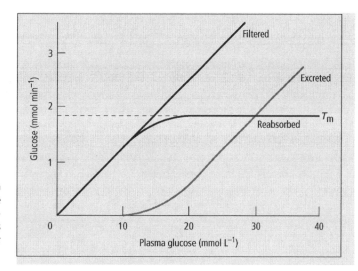

Fig. 20.8 Relationships between plasma glucose concentration and the amount of glucose filtered, reabsorbed and excreted by the kidneys per unit of time. T_m, tubular maximum.

osmotically hold on to water. This is because glucose can only permeate the tubular membrane via its specific transporter. When the Na^+–glucose cotransporter is saturated, the excess glucose cannot permeate the tubular wall and will inevitably exert an osmotic effect. Even though glucose-independent Na^+ transport mechanisms continue to operate in this condition, their ability to cause net Na^+ reabsorption will be severely diminished due to back diffusion across the leaky junctions. Thus excess glucose by osmotically holding on to water will also hold on to Na^+ and decrease both salt and fluid absorption. This increases the delivery of salt and fluid to the distal tubules, which may not cope with this extra load and therefore we observe increased urine flow.

Renal glycosuria occurs as an uncommon anomaly when tubular reabsorptive capacity is subnormal. Here plasma threshold will be low so that glucose appears in the urine though its concentration in the blood is not abnormally high.

Note that the co-transporter is highly selective. It accepts D-glucose but not the L-isomer. It will also accept D-galactose.

Amino acids

About 98% of the filtered load of amino acids is reabsorbed from the proximal convoluted tubules (Fig. 20.7). At least five transport systems—(a) neutral amino acids; (b) imino acids; (c) basic amino acids and cystine; (d) glutamic and aspartic acids; and (e) glycine—exist. Neutral and acidic, but possibly not basic, amino acids are co-transported with Na^+ across the luminal membrane.

Normally about 0.5–2% of the filtered load is lost in the urine but **aminoacidurias**, in which large amounts of particular amino acids are excreted, result from deficiencies in specific enzymes or transport processes, often genetically determined and frequently associated with abnormal metabolism of the amino acids that are being excreted.

Organic acids

Metabolic substrates such as acetate, lactate, citrate, oxalate and keto acids (β hydroxybutyrate and acetoacetate) are normally filtered in small quantities and reabsorbed in the proximal tubule. Again, they enter the cells from the lumen co-transported with Na^+.

In ketoacidosis and lactic acidosis, when plasma concentrations of the relevant organic acids are high, the T_m can be exceeded and these solutes are then lost in the urine. Under such conditions, they provide additional urinary buffer.

Peptides and proteins

Although little plasma protein is filtered, there are a variety of smaller molecular weight proteins and peptides that do cross the glomerular filter. Most (including the very small quantity of albumin that leaks across) are recaptured by endocytosis by the proximal tubular cells and then degraded; only their constituent amino acids are restored to the plasma. Hence the kidney effectively eliminates these substances without excreting them in the urine. The continuous removal of freely filtered peptide hormones (e.g. insulin, glucagon, ADH, parathyroid hormone and gut hormones) at rates proportional to their concentrations in the plasma ensures that their concentrations are largely determined by the rates at which they are released into the circulation.

In some situations plasma concentrations of specific low molecular weight proteins are elevated (e.g. release of myoglobin from damaged muscles or haemoglobin during excessive breakdown of red blood cells). The filtered load then exceeds reabsorptive capacity and, as fluid is removed, tubular concentration rises and protein precipitates causing blockage of the lumen. If extensive this can result in acute renal failure.

Urea

Normally about $0.6\,mmol\,min^{-1}$ ($5\,mmol\,L^{-1} \times 0.125\,L\,min^{-1}$) or $900\,mmol\,day^{-1}$ of urea is filtered at the glomerulus. By the end of the proximal tubule, some two-thirds of the filtered water has been reabsorbed. This raises the urea concentration in the tubular fluid and, since the proximal tubule is permeable to urea, about 50% of the filtered urea diffuses passively from the higher concentration in the tubular fluid to the lower concentration in the plasma.

In the absence of ADH, the urea permeability of the remainder of the nephron is low (although some urea enters the thin ascending limb of the loop of Henle driven by the high medullary interstitial fluid concentration, p. 563). Thus at high urine flow rates (low levels of circulating ADH) up to 60–70% of the urea that enters the tubular fluid may be excreted in the urine. ADH increases the permeability of the medullary collecting ducts to urea, so at low urine flow rates (high levels of circu-lating ADH) net reabsorption of urea in this nephron segment can result in excretion of only about 30% of the filtered load of urea. (Recycling of urea in the medulla is discussed on p. 563.)

At urine flow rates greater than about $2\,\mathrm{mL}$ min^{-1}, the clearance of urea is relatively independent of flow rate and is about two-thirds of the inulin clearance (Fig. 20.9).

Plasma urea concentration does not necessarily provide a good indication of renal function as it depends upon the rate of production of urea (reflecting protein intake and catabolism) as well as its renal excretion (Fig. 20.10).

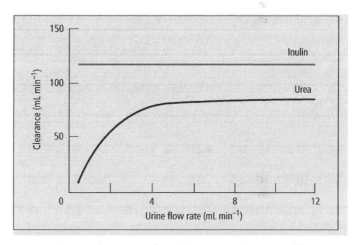

Fig. 20.9 Relationship between urine flow rate and clearance of inulin and urea.

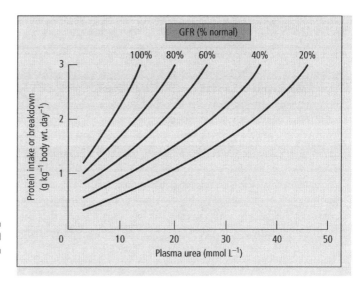

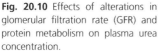

Fig. 20.10 Effects of alterations in glomerular filtration rate (GFR) and protein metabolism on plasma urea concentration.

Organic solutes that are secreted

The kidney excretes a variety of metabolic end-products and potential toxins. Two distinct pathways have been identified—one for organic anions (acids), the other for organic cations (bases). Up to 90% of some such solutes (e.g. PAH) can be removed in one passage through the kidneys. The clearance of PAH can therefore be used to estimate RPF. As well as secreting organic solutes removed from the blood, renal proximal tubular cells secrete ammonium ions—an essential process in the maintenance of acid–base balance.

The kidney, together with the liver, plays an essential role in removing from the circulation a variety of metabolic end-products as well as chemicals that would be toxic if allowed to accumulate in the body. In the kidney, these are taken up from the peritubular blood by the proximal tubular cells and then secreted into the tubular fluid. One system handles the organic anions (acids), the other organic cations (bases). These systems can be extraordinarily effective in removing organic solutes from the plasma, with up to 90% of some solutes being removed in one passage through the kidneys.

Organic acids

A variety of chemicals (e.g. **para-aminohippuric acid (PAH)**) and drugs, including diuretics (e.g. frusemide and ethacrynic acid), penicillin, sulphonamides and salicylates, are secreted by the proximal tubule almost as rapidly as the plasma presents them to the epithelial cells. Secretion is active, steeply 'uphill', and shows saturation, competition between substrates, and inhibition, all typical of carrier-mediated transport (p. 8). A model of the pathways involved in organic anion secretion is illustrated in Fig. 20.11. The very rapid excretion of penicillin is a potential problem for the practical use of this antibiotic; this can be overcome by giving together with penicillin a substance that competes for transport by the same carrier (probenicid).

Use is made of this secretory pathway in estimat-

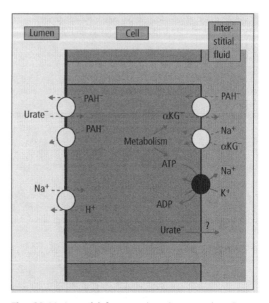

Fig. 20.11 A model for organic anion secretion. Para-aminohippurate (PAH⁻) is shown as a representative compound. In this model, α ketoglutarate (αKG⁻) produced by metabolism exchanges for PAH⁻ across the basolateral membrane and is recycled via a Na⁺-coupled basolateral co-transporter. Other metabolic intermediates may substitute for αKG⁻. At the luminal membrane PAH⁻ leaves the cell either by facilitated diffusion or in exchange for urate or other anions. Probenecid, which inhibits organic anion secretion, and also urate reabsorption, blocks this exchanger. (Adapted from Pritchard, J.B. & Miller, D.S. (1992) Proximal tubular transport of organic anions and cations. In: Seldin, D.W. & Giebisch, G. (eds) *The Kidney: Physiology and Pathophysiology*, 2nd edn, pp. 2921–45. Raven Press, New York.) ADP, adenosine diphosphate; ATP, adenosine triphosphate.

ing RPF with the organic anion **PAH**, which is removed avidly from the plasma.

Use of PAH to measure RPF

For any substance that is transferred from plasma to urine but is not produced, destroyed or stored within the kidney, the amount entering the kidney in the renal artery each minute must equal the amounts leaving the kidney each minute in the renal vein and in the urine. (This ignores the small amount that may leave through the lymphatic system.) These amounts are $P_a \times V_a$ for the renal artery,

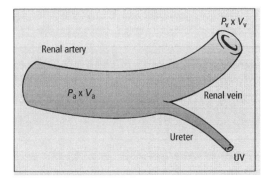

Fig. 20.12 Amount of a substance entering and leaving the kidney each minute. See text for symbols.

$P_v \times V_v$ for the renal vein and UV for the urine (Fig. 20.12), where P_a is the plasma concentration of such a substance entering the kidneys in the renal arteries, P_v is the concentration of the same substance leaving the kidneys in the renal vein, U is the concentration in the urine, V_a is the volume of plasma entering the kidneys in the renal arteries per minute (the **RPF**), V_v is the volume of plasma leaving the kidneys in the renal vein per minute and V is the volume of urine leaving the kidneys per minute.

Thus

$$(P_a \times V_a) = (P_v \times V_v) + UV$$

or

$$(P_a \times V_a) - (P_v \times V_v) = UV$$

The volume of the urine per minute (about 0.5–$1\,mL\,min^{-1}$) is so much smaller than that of the plasma entering the kidneys each minute (about $650\,mL\,min^{-1}$), that V_v can be taken as equal V_a. Therefore

$$V_a(P_a - P_v) = UV$$

and

$$V_a \text{ or RPF} = \frac{UV}{(P_a - P_v)}$$

This is an example of the use of the Fick principle (p. 460) to measure plasma flow rate in an organ. However, it has limited practical application, for although the amount of substance excreted in the urine is readily determined and plasma for measurement of arterial concentration can be obtained from any systemic artery (or vein), a sample of renal venous plasma is not easily obtained. However, if the kidneys could completely remove all of a substance entering each minute, then P_v would be zero and the equation would reduce to the familiar clearance equation,

$$\text{RPF} = \frac{UV}{P_a}$$

Proximal tubular secretion of PAH is so efficient that at low plasma concentrations (that do not saturate the transport system) it is nearly completely removed from the plasma passing through the kidneys. Therefore P_v for PAH approximates to zero, and the clearance of PAH approximates to the RPF.

The renal handling of PAH is summarized in Figs 20.13 and 20.14; note that PAH is filtered at the glomerulus as well as being secreted. Thus, with a filtration fraction of 0.2, 20% of the PAH that enters the kidney each minute in the plasma is removed by filtration and much of the remaining 80% that flows into the peritubular capillaries is then removed by secretion. In reality, the removal of PAH is never complete and values for RPF and RBF obtained from PAH clearance in a person with normal renal function are approximately 90% of the true value. If renal tubular function is impaired, less PAH may be secreted and an erroneous estimate of RPF will be obtained. In practice, PAH clearances are rarely measured clinically. An estimate of RPF can be obtained by following the time course of the removal of an injected bolus of Diodrast, which is also secreted by the organic anion system and (because of its high content of iodine) is opaque to X-rays.

RBF is readily estimated from the RPF if the haematocrit (haem) is known.

$$\text{RBF} - (\text{haem} \times \text{RBF}) = \text{RPF}$$

Therefore, RBF $(1 - \text{haem}) = \text{RPF}$, or

$$\text{RBF} = \frac{\text{RPF}}{(1 - \text{haem})}$$

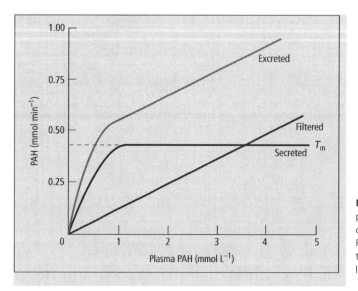

Fig. 20.13 Relationship between plasma para-aminohippurate (PAH) concentration and the amounts of PAH filtered, secreted and excreted by the kidneys per unit of time. T_m, tubular maximum.

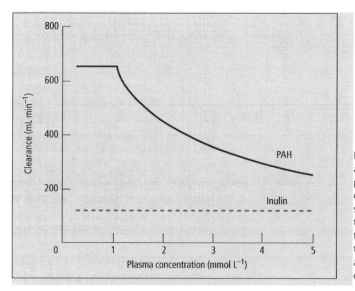

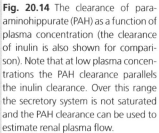

Fig. 20.14 The clearance of para-aminohippurate (PAH) as a function of plasma concentration (the clearance of inulin is also shown for comparison). Note that at low plasma concentrations the PAH clearance parallels the inulin clearance. Over this range the secretory system is not saturated and the PAH clearance can be used to estimate renal plasma flow.

Values obtained in normal people are RPF, 650 mL min⁻¹; RBF, 1200 mL min⁻¹. Thus, the kidneys, which constitute 0.5% body weight but account for nearly 10% of the total oxygen consumption of the body, receive about 20% of the resting cardiac output. Renal arteriovenous difference for oxygen is low. The high rate of flow is required not to supply O_2 for renal metabolism but to provide the volume to be filtered.

Organic bases

A model of the pathways involved in organic cation secretion is illustrated in Fig. 20.15 using

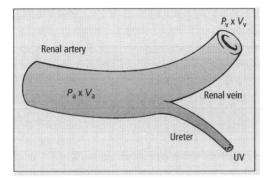

Fig. 20.12 Amount of a substance entering and leaving the kidney each minute. See text for symbols.

$P_v \times V_v$ for the renal vein and UV for the urine (Fig. 20.12), where P_a is the plasma concentration of such a substance entering the kidneys in the renal arteries, P_v is the concentration of the same substance leaving the kidneys in the renal vein, U is the concentration in the urine, V_a is the volume of plasma entering the kidneys in the renal arteries per minute (the **RPF**), V_v is the volume of plasma leaving the kidneys in the renal vein per minute and V is the volume of urine leaving the kidneys per minute.

Thus

$$(P_a \times V_a) = (P_v \times V_v) + UV$$

or

$$(P_a \times V_a) - (P_v \times V_v) = UV$$

The volume of the urine per minute (about $0.5–1\,\mathrm{mL\,min^{-1}}$) is so much smaller than that of the plasma entering the kidneys each minute (about $650\,\mathrm{mL\,min^{-1}}$), that V_v can be taken as equal V_a. Therefore

$$V_a(P_a - P_v) = UV$$

and

$$V_a \text{ or } RPF = \frac{UV}{(P_a - P_v)}$$

This is an example of the use of the Fick principle (p. 460) to measure plasma flow rate in an organ. However, it has limited practical application, for although the amount of substance excreted in the urine is readily determined and plasma for measurement of arterial concentration can be obtained from any systemic artery (or vein), a sample of renal venous plasma is not easily obtained. However, if the kidneys could completely remove all of a substance entering each minute, then P_v would be zero and the equation would reduce to the familiar clearance equation,

$$RPF = \frac{UV}{P_a}$$

Proximal tubular secretion of PAH is so efficient that at low plasma concentrations (that do not saturate the transport system) it is nearly completely removed from the plasma passing through the kidneys. Therefore P_v for PAH approximates to zero, and the clearance of PAH approximates to the RPF.

The renal handling of PAH is summarized in Figs 20.13 and 20.14; note that PAH is filtered at the glomerulus as well as being secreted. Thus, with a filtration fraction of 0.2, 20% of the PAH that enters the kidney each minute in the plasma is removed by filtration and much of the remaining 80% that flows into the peritubular capillaries is then removed by secretion. In reality, the removal of PAH is never complete and values for RPF and RBF obtained from PAH clearance in a person with normal renal function are approximately 90% of the true value. If renal tubular function is impaired, less PAH may be secreted and an erroneous estimate of RPF will be obtained. In practice, PAH clearances are rarely measured clinically. An estimate of RPF can be obtained by following the time course of the removal of an injected bolus of Diodrast, which is also secreted by the organic anion system and (because of its high content of iodine) is opaque to X-rays.

RBF is readily estimated from the RPF if the haematocrit (haem) is known.

$$RBF - (haem \times RBF) = RPF$$

Therefore, RBF $(1 - haem) = RPF$, or

$$RBF = \frac{RPF}{(1 - haem)}$$

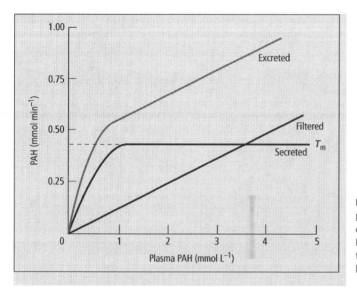

Fig. 20.13 Relationship between plasma para-aminohippurate (PAH) concentration and the amounts of PAH filtered, secreted and excreted by the kidneys per unit of time. T_m, tubular maximum.

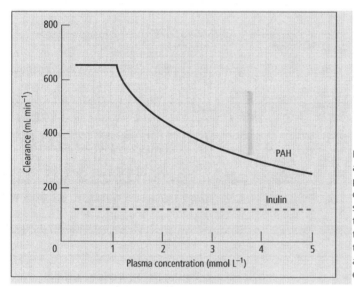

Fig. 20.14 The clearance of para-aminohippurate (PAH) as a function of plasma concentration (the clearance of inulin is also shown for comparison). Note that at low plasma concentrations the PAH clearance parallels the inulin clearance. Over this range the secretory system is not saturated and the PAH clearance can be used to estimate renal plasma flow.

Values obtained in normal people are RPF, 650 mL min^{-1}; RBF, 1200 mL min^{-1}. Thus, the kidneys, which constitute 0.5% body weight but account for nearly 10% of the total oxygen consumption of the body, receive about 20% of the resting cardiac output. Renal arteriovenous difference for oxygen is low. The high rate of flow is required not to supply O_2 for renal metabolism but to provide the volume to be filtered.

Organic bases

A model of the pathways involved in organic cation secretion is illustrated in Fig. 20.15 using

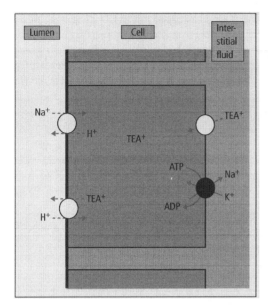

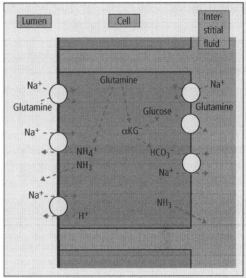

Fig. 20.15 A model for organic cation secretion. Tetraethyl-ammonium ion (TEA$^+$) is shown as a representative compound. In this model, TEA$^+$ enters the cells from the plasma across the basolateral membrane by facilitated diffusion and leaves the cell across the luminal membrane in exchange for H$^+$. The H$^+$ is then recycled through the Na$^+$–H$^+$ exchanger. (Adapted from Pritchard, J.B. & Miller, D.S. (1992) Proximal tubular transport of organic anions and cations. In: Seldin, D.W. & Giebisch, G. (eds) *The Kidney: Physiology and Pathophysiology*, 2nd edn, pp. 2921–45. Raven Press, New York.) ADP, adenosine diphosphate; ATP, adenosine triphosphate.

Fig. 20.16 The production and secretion of NH$_4^+$ by proximal tubular cells. αKG$^-$, α ketoglutarate.

tetraethylammonium ion as an example. For the most part these are amines, and both endogenous substances (e.g. acetylcholine, adrenaline, histamine and some vitamins—riboflavin, thiamin) and a variety of drugs (e.g. amiloride, morphine, quinine) are secreted by this mechanism.

Ammonium ions

As well as secreting organic solutes removed from the blood, renal proximal tubular cells secrete ammonium ions (Fig. 20.16). This is an integral part of the role of the kidney in maintaining extracellular pH, discussed in Chapter 21. Ammonium is generated in the proximal tubular cells largely from glutamine, which enters the cells by Na$^+$-dependent

co-transport across both luminal and basolateral membranes. Glutamine is supplied to the kidneys by the liver. Breakdown of amino acids yields NH$_4^+$ and HCO$_3^-$. In the liver urea synthesis consumes almost all of these ions.

$$\text{Amino acid} + O_2 \rightarrow NH_4^+ + HCO_3^-$$

then

$$NH_4^+ + HCO_3^- \rightarrow \text{urea} + CO_2 + H_2O$$

However, a small fraction of the NH$_4^+$ reacts with glutamate to yield glutamine. The relative amount of glutamine formed by the liver is influenced by liver pH. Acidosis favours production of glutamine rather than urea synthesis and thus under this condition more glutamine is available to the kidneys for NH$_4^+$ production. In the kidneys, metabolism of glutamine produces α ketoglutarate and NH$_4^+$. In turn, metabolism of α ketoglutarate consumes H$^+$ ions, leaving HCO$_3^-$. Effectively, 2 NH$_4^+$ and 2 HCO$_3^-$ are produced for each glutamine metabolized. Since the pK of the reaction NH$_3$ + H$^+$ ⇌ NH$_4^+$ is 9.3, at pH 7.4, most of the ammonium is in the form NH$_4^+$. However, NH$_3$ is much more lipid soluble than NH$_4^+$ and therefore, although the concentration of NH_3 is much lower, non-ionic diffusion of NH_3 also contributes to renal ammonium secretion.

Ammonium leaves the proximal tubular cell across the luminal membrane, either as NH_4^+ substituting for H^+ on the Na^+-H^+ exchanger or by non-ionic diffusion of NH_3, with the associated H^+ leaving on the Na^+-H^+ exchanger. Some NH_3 diffuses from the cell across the basolateral membrane and is removed in the peritubular blood. The HCO_3^- passes across the basolateral membrane. Several pathways may be involved, including a $Na^+-HCO_3^-$ co-transporter (Fig. 20.16). Under normal conditions, most of the NH_4^+ synthesized by the proximal tubular cells passes into the luminal fluid. In the ascending thick limb of the loop of Henle, NH_4^+ is reabsorbed, probably by substituting for K^+ on the luminal $Na^+-K^+-2Cl^-$ co-transporter (see Fig. 20.21). As a consequence of the renal counter-current system, this reabsorbed NH_4^+ is accumulated in the medulla and concentrated towards the papilla. As fluid flows through the collecting ducts, the epithelial cells secrete H^+ into the lumen (p. 558). This lowers luminal pH so that NH_3 diffusing from the medullary interstitium is converted to NH_4^+ and trapped in the lumen.

Organic solutes that are reabsorbed and secreted

Urate

Urate, the final product of purine degradation, is filtered at the glomerulus and both reabsorbed and secreted by proximal tubular cells. In the human, the balance between these processes is such that there is normally net reabsorption. A possible mechanism for reabsorption is illustrated in Fig. 20.11. In some species, urate is secreted by the same mechanisms as PAH (Fig. 20.11) but there may be a separate secretory pathway in the human.

Failure to excrete sufficient urate to balance production can result in precipitation of uric acid crystals in joints—gout. Among agents used to treat this disease is probenecid, which blocks urate reabsorption.

Inorganic ions that are reabsorbed

In addition to sodium and chloride, the reabsorption by the kidneys of magnesium, calcium, phosphate, sulphate and bicarbonate is of physiological importance. Magnesium, calcium and phosphate handling are all affected by parathyroid hormone. For phosphate and sulphate, the renal threshold is a little below the normal plasma concentration. Thus any increased production will result in increased excretion. The actual HCO_3^- ions that are filtered are not reabsorbed. Instead HCO_3^- reacts with secreted H^+ in the tubular lumen to form H_2O and CO_2. However, for every H^+ secreted a HCO_3^- is formed in the cells and returned to the plasma, so the effect is to return to the plasma the same amount of HCO_3^- as was filtered.

Sodium and chloride represent the bulk of the filtered inorganic ions. Their renal handling is discussed in section 20.6.

Magnesium

About one-third (or $0.3\,mmol\,L^{-1}$) of plasma Mg^{2+} is bound to proteins and cannot be filtered. The remainder, mostly ionized, is filtered. Of this, 25% is reabsorbed in the proximal tubule and 65% in the thick ascending limb. A further 5% is reabsorbed more distally. Mg^{2+} reabsorption is thought to occur through both cellular and paracellular pathways. In the thick ascending limb, Mg^{2+} reabsorption (and also Ca^{2+} reabsorption) is stimulated by **parathyroid hormone, glucagon, calcitonin** and **ADH**.

Calcium

About 50% (or $1.25\,mmol\,L^{-1}$) of Ca^{2+} is bound to plasma proteins and cannot be filtered. The remainder, mostly ionized, is filtered. Of the filtered load of about $200\,mmol\,day^{-1}$, less than $5\,mmol$ is usually excreted. Some 60% is reabsorbed proximally, most of the remainder in the ascending limbs of the loop of Henle, distal tubules and collecting duct. Both cellular and paracellular routes are involved. In the proximal tubule and loops of Henle, alterations in Na^+ transport result in parallel changes in Ca^{2+} reabsorption. **Parathyroid hormone** stimulates reabsorption in the distal tubule although it inhibits reabsorption proximally; but, since it raises plasma ionized Ca^{2+}, its net effect is often to promote urinary Ca^{2+} excretion.

Phosphate

Some 95% of the filtered inorganic phosphate is reabsorbed, predominantly in the proximal convoluted tubule, with the threshold a little below the normal plasma concentration. Thus there is normally some phosphate, which is an important buffer, in the urine. Reabsorption involves luminal co-transport with Na^+; the mechanisms of basolateral exit are ill-defined. Reabsorption is inhibited by **parathyroid hormone**.

Sulphate

As with phosphate, most of the filtered sulphate is reabsorbed predominantly in the proximal convoluted tubule by a mechanism that includes luminal co-transport with Na^+. Again, the threshold is a little below the normal plasma concentration. Thus there is normally some sulphate in the urine and changes in plasma sulphate concentration will result in appropriate alterations in renal excretion. There is no known hormonal control over sulphate reabsorption.

Bicarbonate

Normally, about 4500 mmol of HCO_3^- are filtered each day ($24\,mmol\,L^{-1} \times 180\,L\,day^{-1}$). Throughout the nephron, secretion of H^+ from the tubular cells into the lumen results in the conversion of filtered HCO_3^- to H_2O and CO_2 (Fig. 20.17). However, for every H^+ secreted into the lumen, a HCO_3^- is returned to the plasma across the basolateral membrane. Several transporters, including a Na^+—HCO_3^- co-transporter (which may shift three HCO_3^- for each Na^+) appear to be involved in this basolateral movement.

Although the HCO_3^- filtered from the plasma is actually destroyed in the tubular lumen, the effect is to replace it with an equivalent amount of

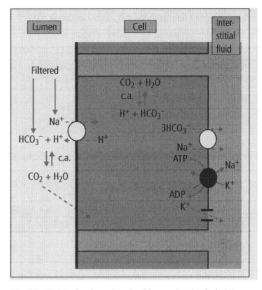

Fig. 20.17 Mechanisms involved in proximal tubule H^+ secretion and HCO_3^- reabsorption. Note the presence of carbonic anhydrase (c.a.) on the luminal membrane as well as intracellularly. ADP, adenosine diphosphate; ATP, adenosine triphosphate.

HCO_3^- synthesized by the renal tubular cells, and the overall process therefore represents net reabsorption of HCO_3^-. Of this reabsorption, 70–85% takes place in the proximal tubule (where the presence of carbonic anhydrase in the luminal membrane catalyses the conversion of H^+ and HCO_3^- to H_2O and CO_2 in the lumen and the production of H^+ and HCO_3^- from CO_2 and H_2O inside the cell), 10–20% in the loop of Henle (mostly in the thick ascending segment), 3–5% in the distal tubule and 1–2% in the collecting ducts. Under alkalotic conditions, when plasma HCO_3^- concentration is elevated, the reabsorptive capacity of the nephrons is exceeded and HCO_3^- appears in the urine.

In the distal part of the nephron (late distal tubule and collecting duct) specialized type B intercalated cells may contribute to this HCO_3^- excretion by secreting HCO_3^- into the lumen via a coupled Cl^-—HCO_3^- exchanger. The regulation of HCO_3^- reabsorption is discussed as part of acid–base balance in Chapter 21.

Inorganic ions that are secreted

Hydrogen ions

Renal epithelial cells secrete H^+ as an integral part of their role in maintaining extracellular pH, discussed in Chapter 21.

In the proximal tubule, luminal Na^+-H^+ exchange mainly contributes to this secretion (Fig. 20.17), which results in HCO_3^- reabsorption, as discussed above. Although the capacity for H^+ secretion is relatively large, the leaky nature of the epithelium limits the H^+ gradient that can be established in this nephron segment.

The thick ascending limb cells appear to secrete some H^+ by the same mechanisms as above. In the relatively tight distal part of the nephron (late distal tubule and collecting ducts), there is primary active transport of H^+ across the luminal membrane of specialized type A intercalated cells (Fig. 20.18). This combination of a tight epithelium and

primary active H^+ transport enables the urine to be acidified to as low as pH 4.4, which, when the plasma remains at pH 7.4, is a ratio $[H^+]_{urine}/[H^+]_{plasma}$ of $1000:1$.

Inorganic ions that are reabsorbed and secreted

Potassium

About 800 mmol of K^+ are filtered at the glomerulus each day. In the proximal convoluted tubule much of this filtered K^+ is reabsorbed. Some of this reabsorption may be a passive consequence of the absorption of NaCl and other solutes together with water, which concentrates luminal K^+ and creates a favourable gradient for diffusion through the paracellular pathway.

In the medullary part of the proximal straight tubule and in the thin descending limb, there is K^+ secretion. This, combined with reabsorption of K^+ by the thick ascending limb (which involves co-transport across the luminal membrane with Na^+ and Cl^-), results in recycling of K^+ within the medulla.

The most distal parts of the nephron (late distal tubule and collecting duct) contain the **principal cells** that secrete K^+ (Fig. 20.19). In addition, K^+ reabsorption occurs in the medullary collecting duct, possibly via an H^+,K^+–ATPase in type A intercalated cells (Fig. 20.18). Thus it is possible to remove much of the filtered K^+ from the urine when body K^+ content needs to be conserved, or to secrete K^+ into the urine when K^+ intake exceeds K^+ losses through other routes—the normal situation.

Figure 20.19 illustrates a model for K^+ secretion by the principal cells. Activity of the basolateral Na^+, K^+–ATPase keeps cell K^+ concentration high. Na^+ entry to the cells through luminal Na^+ channels depolarizes the luminal membrane and thereby increases the electrical potential driving force for diffusion of K^+ from cell to lumen through luminal K^+ channels. Thus, if the luminal Na^+ concentration is increased, there is increased K^+ secretion. There is also a neutral K^+–Cl^- co-transporter in the luminal membrane. Thus reduction in luminal Cl^- concentration will result in

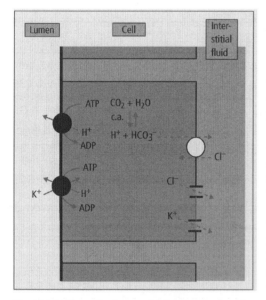

Fig. 20.18 H^+ secretion by type A intercalated cells in the distal nephron. As well as an H^+–ATPase, an H^+,K^+–ATPase, similar to that found in the gastric mucosa, is also shown and would contribute to K^+ reabsorption in this portion of the nephron. (For clarity, the basolateral membrane Na^+,K^+–ATPase is not shown.) ADP, adenosine diphosphate; ATP, adenosine triphosphate; c.a., carbonic anhydrase.

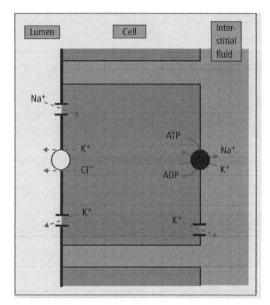

Fig. 20.19 Membrane pathways involved in K+ secretion by principal cells in the distal nephron. ADP, adenosine diphosphate; ATP, adenosine triphosphate.

increased K+ (and Cl−) secretion. Note that the luminal Na+ channels are blocked by the diuretic amiloride. This, therefore, also inhibits K+ secretion in this segment.

20.6 Renal handling of sodium and water

The human kidney can produce a urine ranging in volume from 0.5 to 20 L or more per day, and containing from 5–10 to 600 mmol or more of Na+ per day, with an osmolarity of from 1200 mosmol L−1 (at the lowest volumes) to 50 mosmol L−1 with large volumes. This unique ability requires that about a quarter of the filtered NaCl is reabsorbed in the medulla while the water associated with it returns to the cortex and is reabsorbed there. Urea is also accumulated within the medulla. The combination of medullary NaCl reabsorption and the arrangement of the vasa recta in loops results in the creation and maintenance of an osmotic gradient in the medullary interstitium. The collecting ducts are relatively impermeable to water in the absence of ADH. Under these conditions, a large vol-

ume of a dilute urine is produced (water diuresis). With ADH, water is free to move from lumen to interstitial fluid driven by the osmotic gradient and a small volume of concentrated urine is produced (antidiuresis). Under these conditions, urea recycles between medullary interstitium and tubular fluid and this helps to preserve medullary hyperosmolarity.

Filtration

With a GFR of 125 mL min−1, a plasma Na+ concentration of 150 mmol L−1 and a plasma Cl− of 110 mmol L−1, 180 L of H_2O are filtered by the kidneys each 24 h and the filtered load of Na+ is some 19 mmol min−1 (27 000 mmol per 24 h) and of Cl− some 14 mmol min−1 (19 800 mmol per 24 h). Clearly, changes in either GFR or plasma concentration will change the load presented to the tubules. Figure 20.20 provides a summary of the handling of water and Na+ in the different nephron segments.

Proximal tubules

About two-thirds of the filtered H_2O, Na+ and Cl− (i.e. 120 L H_2O, 18 000 mmol Na+ and 13 200 mmol Cl−) are reabsorbed from the proximal tubules per 24 h. The Na+ enters the cells across the luminal membrane down its electrochemical potential gradient in association with either co-transported solutes or counter-transported H+ or NH_4^+ ions, and is extruded across the basolateral membrane against its electrochemical gradient by the Na+,K+−ATPase (Fig. 20.7). Some Cl− is reabsorbed through the cells, luminal entry being effected by a Cl−−formate exchanger (Fig. 20.7). In addition, the reabsorption of solutes (glucose, amino acids, HCO_3^-) with water early in the proximal tubule increases tubular Cl− concentration. This favours paracellular passive diffusion of Cl− and contributes to salt absorption in this segment.

The Na+ accumulated locally in the lateral intercellular spaces (with Cl− to maintain electroneutrality) assists isosmotic water reabsorption. The hydraulic conductivity of this segment of the nephron is so large that an osmotic imbalance as

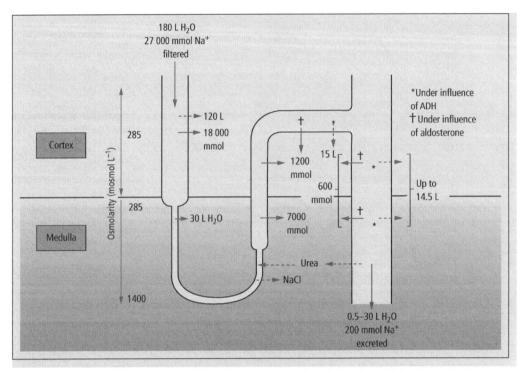

Fig. 20.20 A summary of the contribution of the various segments to the daily handling of Na$^+$ and water by the human kidney. Note that antidiuretic hormone (ADH) promotes water reabsorption in the last part of the distal tubule as well as in the collecting ducts. It therefore affects the reabsorption of up to about 30 L.

little as 1–10 mosmol L^{-1} can account for the observed rate of reabsorption. H$_2$O follows both cellular and paracellular routes in moving from lumen to interstitium.

The amounts of salt and H$_2$O reabsorbed from the proximal tubule are also influenced by the balance of hydrostatic and osmotic forces in the peritubular capillaries. An increased colloid osmotic pressure or a decreased hydrostatic pressure in peritubular capillaries favours uptake of interstitial fluid into capillaries and assists reabsorption. Conversely, decreased colloid osmotic pressure or increased hydrostatic pressure hinders reabsorption. For example, if GFR increases with constant RPF, the filtration fraction will increase and the increased colloid osmotic pressure in the peritubular capillaries will assist in reabsorbing the increased volume of filtrate. Proximal tubular fluid reabsorption matches GFR closely over a wide range of GFR

and such adjustments of capillary forces help to account for this '**glomerulotubular balance**'.

Loops of Henle

A volume of about 60 L containing 9000 mmol Na$^+$ leaves the proximal tubules and enters the **descending limbs** of the loops of Henle each day as an isosmotic solution. Those loops from the juxtamedullary nephrons which run deep into the medulla (some 20% in the human kidney) pass through a region in which the interstitial fluid osmolarity increases progressively from isosmotic (285 mosmol L^{-1}) at the corticomedullary junction to some 1200–1400 mosmol L^{-1} at the tip of the renal papilla in the human. NaCl and urea contribute in similar proportions to this gradient. The mechanism by which it is generated and sustained is discussed later. The epithelium lining

this segment is quite permeable to water, but much less so to Na$^+$, Cl$^-$ and urea. Therefore, H$_2$O moves passively and progressively from the descending limb to the interstitium as fluid flows along the tubules. It is also possible that a little Na$^+$ and Cl$^-$ enter the tubule. Each day there is a net removal of about 30 L of H$_2$O from this tubular segment, much of it from the short descending limbs of cortical nephrons, which penetrate only into the outer medulla. There is probably no active transepithelial transport of solutes in the descending limbs.

In the medullary descending limbs, fluid has equilibrated with the adjacent interstitial fluid and at the tips of the loops now has an osmolarity of some 1200 mosmol L^{-1}. But, whereas NaCl and urea contribute equally (600 mosmol L^{-1} each) to the interstitial osmolarity, in the tubular fluid about 1150 mosmol L^{-1} is contributed by NaCl and only about 50 mosmol L^{-1} by urea.

The **thin ascending limb** of the loop differs significantly from the thin descending limb in its permeabilities, being impermeable to H$_2$O, highly permeable to Na$^+$ and Cl$^-$ and somewhat permeable to urea. Consequently, Na$^+$ and Cl$^-$, which are at much higher concentrations in the tubular fluid, diffuse from the tubules to the interstitium as the fluid flows back towards the cortex, and some urea enters the tubules down its concentration gradient. The loss of NaCl greatly exceeds the gain in urea so that, by the time that the thick ascending segment is reached, the tubular fluid has become hypo-osmotic compared with the adjacent interstitial fluid.

Unlike the thin ascending limb, the **thick ascending limb**, and its continuation in the cortex as the first part of the distal tubule, avidly reabsorb NaCl from the tubular fluid by the process illustrated in Fig. 20.21. This involves co-transport of Cl$^-$ with Na$^+$ and K$^+$ (Na$^+$, K$^+$, 2Cl$^-$ co-transport) at the luminal membrane and passive diffusion at the basolateral membrane. K$^+$ recirculates via K$^+$ channels in the luminal membrane (Fig. 20.21), so that the net process is NaCl absorption. The impermeability to H$_2$O means that the removal of NaCl dilutes the luminal fluid. By the time this fluid enters the distal tubule in the cortex, it has lost about

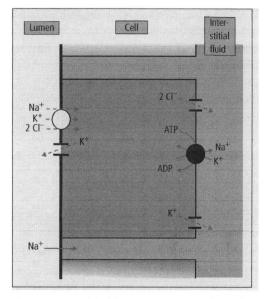

Fig. 20.21 A model of the major transport pathways for ions across the cells in the thick ascending limb of the loop of Henle. Note that the Na$^+$–K$^+$–2Cl$^-$ co-transporter is specifically inhibited by the 'loop diuretics' such as bumetanide and frusemide. ADP, adenosine diphosphate; ATP, adenosine triphosphate.

7000 mmol day^{-1} of Na$^+$, much of this from the ascending thick limb, and has become hypo-osmotic to cortical plasma. In 24 h, 60 L of fluid with 9000 mmol of Na$^+$ entered all of the loops of Henle and 30 L with 2000 mmol returned to the distal tubules. The Na$^+$ concentration is now about 60 mmol L^{-1}, urea concentration is 25 mmol L^{-1} and osmolarity about 150 mosmol L^{-1}. The important diuretic frusemide acts by inhibiting the Na$^+$, K$^+$, 2Cl$^-$ co-transporter. It thereby markedly increases salt delivery to the distal tubules causing excess urinary salt excretion.

Distal tubules

It is now appreciated that the distal tubule is not a homogeneous segment. The first part is lined by an epithelium of the same type as the adjacent ascending limb of the loop of Henle, and the two together comprise the **diluting segment** of the nephron. The last part, the connecting segment, is analogous in its properties to the collecting tubule

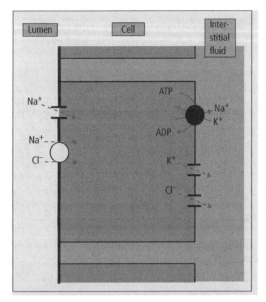

| Lumen | Cell | Interstitial fluid |

Fig. 20.22 A model for Na$^+$ reabsorption by the distal convoluted and connecting tubules. Note that the Na$^+$–Cl$^-$ cotransporter is specifically inhibited by thiazide diuretics whereas the luminal membrane Na$^+$ channels are blocked by the diuretic amiloride. ADP, adenosine diphosphate; ATP, adenosine triphosphate.

which it joins. NaCl is reabsorbed throughout the length of the distal tubule, some 1200 mmol of Na$^+$ (5% of the filtered load) being removed from the tubular fluid each day. Figure 20.22 illustrates one possible model for Na$^+$ reabsorption in the distal convoluted and connecting tubules.

The permeability of the distal tubule to H$_2$O reflects its heterogeneity. While the early part is impermeable to H$_2$O, the permeability of the last part is determined by the level of circulating **ADH**. With normal hydration, of the 30 L of water entering the distal tubule some 10–20 L is absorbed, leaving 10–20 L containing some 800 mmol of Na$^+$ to pass through the collecting ducts. The distal tubule is impermeable to urea. Therefore urea entering the thin ascending limb of the loop of Henle is retained within the tubule in this portion of the nephron.

Collecting system

Though only about 20% of the loops of Henle run deep into the medulla, all of the fluid remaining at the end of the distal tubule enters the collecting duct system which runs through the hyperosmotic medulla to drain into the renal pelvis and ureters. The cells lining the collecting ducts form a 'tight' epithelium. Active Na$^+$ reabsorption continues here and the Na$^+$ concentration in the urine may fall to as low as 10 mmol L^{-1}. On a normal diet, about 600 mmol are reabsorbed each day and this reabsorption is largely independent of water handling in this segment.

Water diuresis (the production of a large volume of a dilute urine) is associated with low circulating levels of ADH. In the absence of this hormone (as in the rare disease **diabetes insipidus**), the water permeability of the collecting duct epithelial cells is very low, little water absorption will occur and some patients have been known to excrete as much as 30 L of urine per day (a flow rate of ~20 mL min^{-1}) with a urine osmolarity lower than 50 mosmol L^{-1}.

ADH increases water permeability of both the cortical and medullary portions of the collecting ducts, as well as of the most distal portion of the distal tubules (the **collecting tubule**). ADH acts via adenylate cyclase, cAMP and protein kinase A and causes cytoplasmic vesicles that contain water channels (aquaporins) to fuse with the luminal membrane, thus increasing its water permeability. Water is then free to move through the cell down the osmotic gradient from tubular lumen to interstitial fluid.

Under these conditions much of the water is reabsorbed from the cortical collecting ducts. With maximal plasma concentrations of ADH (**maximal antidiuresis**), as little as 0.5 L of urine is excreted per day (about 0.3 mL min^{-1}) with a urine osmolarity up to 1200 mosmol L^{-1}. In addition, ADH increases the permeability of the **inner medullary collecting ducts** to urea and promotes its reabsorption in this segment only. Therefore, in antidiuresis, any urea that passes from the medulla into the thin ascending limb of the loop of Henle then diffuses back into the inner medullary interstitium. Its recycling between medullary interstitium and tubular fluid helps to preserve medullary hyperosmolality. During water diuresis, the loss in the urine of much of the urea passing into the ascending limb contributes substantially to the reduction in the medullary osmotic gradient under these conditions.

Generation and maintenance of the medullary hyperosmotic gradient

Generation of the gradient of medullary hyperosmolality requires that about one-quarter of the filtered NaCl is reabsorbed in the medulla while the water associated with it returns to the cortex and is reabsorbed there. Urea is also accumulated within the medulla. The combination of medullary NaCl reabsorption, recycling of urea between medullary interstitium and tubular fluid, and the arrangement of the vasa recta in loops results in the creation and maintenance of an osmotic gradient in the medullary interstitium.

The generation of the gradient of medullary hyperosmolality depends primarily upon the energy-dependent reabsorption of 25% of the filtered load of NaCl in a water-impermeable region of the tubule—the thick ascending limb of the loop of Henle, which is mediated by the Na^+, K^+, $2Cl^-$ cotransporter and the Na^+, K^+ pump.

The solute so reabsorbed would be washed away from the medulla were it not for the fact that the capillaries within the medulla are arranged in loops—the vasa recta—the descending and ascending limbs of which are close to each other and to the adjacent loops of Henle. Reabsorbed solute diffusing into an ascending capillary loop will tend to increase the concentration of NaCl in the capillary at that point. As it is carried towards the cortex, it flows past plasma in the adjacent descending capillary loop in which the NaCl concentration is lower. At every level there will be a tendency therefore for NaCl to diffuse from the ascending to the descending capillary loop and thus to be retained within the renal medulla rather than be lost to the cortex (Fig. 20.23).

Similarly, at every level, plasma in the descending limb coming from a more dilute region of the medulla will be slightly less hyperosmotic than plasma in the ascending limb which is emerging from the deeper, more hyperosmotic medulla.

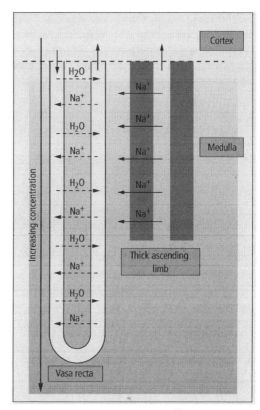

Fig. 20.23 The role of the vasa recta and thick ascending limb of Henle in generating and maintaining the medullary interstitial concentration gradient. For convenience the only solute shown is Na^+.

Thus, in contrast to solute, H_2O will tend at every level to pass from the descending to the ascending limb driven by the osmotic gradient and, thereby, be shunted away from the deeper medulla. Urea, passing from the medullary collecting ducts into the interstitium during antidiuresis, will also be trapped within the medulla by diffusion from ascending to descending vasa recta. These diffusional movements between the two limbs of the vasa recta are often described as **counter-current exchange**.

The arrangement of the vasa recta allows the medullary gradient to be maintained but, were it not for the sources of water-free solute (from energy-dependent NaCl reabsorption in the thick ascending limb and from urea diffusion from the collecting ducts into the medulla during antidiuresis), the large osmotic gradient could not be created. This process is often referred to as **counter-current multiplication**. In effect, what happens is that some of the solute filtered at the glomerulus as an isosmotic solution with H_2O has been trapped in the medulla while its associated H_2O is either lost from the distal tubule in the cortex or excreted in the urine.

Diuresis

There are two types of diuresis: water and osmotic. Water diuresis occurs whenever water intake exceeds body needs; it results from suppression of ADH secretion. Osmotic diuresis results when more solute is presented to the tubules than can be reabsorbed.

An increased rate of production of urine (diuresis) can be of two types: water diuresis and solute or osmotic diuresis. **Water diuresis** results when water is ingested or administered in excess of the body's requirements. ADH secretion is suppressed (p. 572), the collecting ducts become relatively impermeable to water and the excess water is lost without solute. A typical water diuresis is illustrated in Fig. 20.24. There is an inverse relationship between urine osmolarity and urine flow rate; flow rate × osmolarity (the amount of solute excreted per minute) is relatively constant and independent of flow rate. Thus the kidney can adjust its excretion of water without markedly affecting its handling of solutes.

Osmotic diuresis results when more solute is presented to the tubules than they can reabsorb.

For example, an osmotic diuresis occurs if: (a) a non-reabsorbable solute, e.g. mannitol, is filtered; (b) the concentration of glucose in the plasma in diabetes mellitus rises so that the filtered load exceeds the tubular maximum (see p. 549); or (c) tubular function is inhibited (e.g. by drugs which block reabsorption of NaCl in one or more nephron segments). A typical osmotic diuresis is illustrated in Fig. 20.25. In contrast to water diuresis, urinary flow rate depends upon urinary solute content. Moreover, the greater the rate of solute excretion, the lower is the maximal attainable urinary concentration even with maximal concentrations of ADH (Fig. 20.26), for the larger volume of water reabsorbed from the collecting ducts dilutes the medullary interstitial fluid. Faster flow through the ascending limbs of loops of Henle, especially combined with a decreased concentration of Na^+ when glucose or mannitol is present, may also decrease reabsorption so that less Na^+ is deposited to maintain the medullary osmotic gradient. This gradient cannot be demonstrated in kidneys removed during osmotic diuresis.

The roles of the different segments of the nephron are summarized in Table 20.2. If the body needs to retain water, ADH secreted from the neurohypophysis into the blood increases the permeability of the collecting duct luminal membrane to water, and more water is retained. Urinary volume may be only about $0.5\,mL\,min^{-1}$. Therefore, more than 99.5% filtered water has been reabsorbed. Conversely, in the absence of ADH, urinary volume can be as much as $20\,mL\,min^{-1}$ or about 17% of GFR.

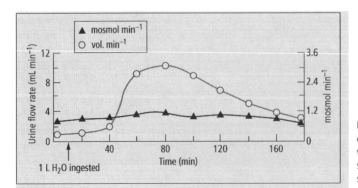

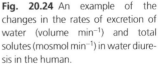

Fig. 20.24 An example of the changes in the rates of excretion of water (volume min^{-1}) and total solutes (mosmol min^{-1}) in water diuresis in the human.

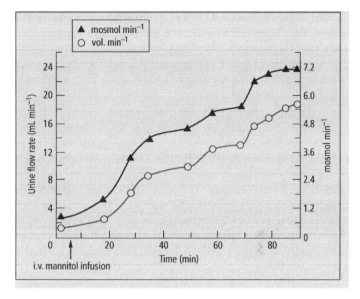

Fig. 20.25 An example of the dependence of the rate of water excretion on solute excretion in osmotic diuresis by the intravenous (i.v.) infusion of mannitol.

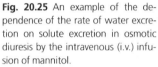

i.v. mannitol infusion

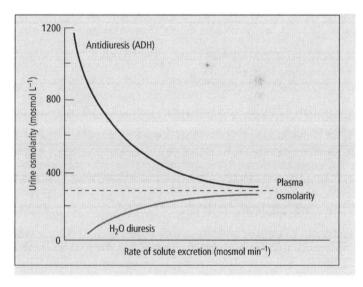

Fig. 20.26 The relationship between the rate of solute excretion and urine osmolarity. As solute load increases, urine osmolarity approaches that of plasma. See text for further explanation. ADH, antidiuretic hormone.

20.7 Function in diseased kidneys

Damaged kidneys may fail to maintain the normal composition and volume of the body fluids because they lose or excessively retain natural constituents of the body or else because they fail to remove waste products.

Disturbances of glomerular function

In the nephrotic syndrome there is damage to the glomerular basement membrane with consequent leakage of protein into the tubular fluid. In chronic renal failure, glomeruli are progressively destroyed. Decreased GFR results in retention of

Table 20.2 Summary of the functions of the different segments of mammalian nephrons (parentheses indicate very small effect under normal conditions).

Segment of nephron	Functions
Renal corpuscle	Ultrafiltration: 125 mL min^{-1}, approx. 20% RPF
Proximal tubule	
reabsorbs	Two-thirds filtered Na$^+$, Cl$^-$ and H$_2$O; most of the HCO$_3^-$, glucose, K$^+$, HPO$_4^{2-}$, amino acids, uric acid; 50% urea
secretes	Organic acids and bases, H$^+$ and some NH$_4^+$
Loop of Henle	
reabsorbs	H$_2$O (descending limb); Na$^+$ and Cl$^-$ (ascending limb); (also, some K$^+$, Ca^{2+} and Mg^{2+})
Distal tubule	
reabsorbs	Na$^+$, Cl$^-$, (HCO$_3^-$), (K$^+$), H$_2$O
secretes	H$^+$, NH$_4^+$, K$^+$
Collecting duct	
reabsorbs	Na$^+$, Cl$^-$, H$_2$O, (K$^+$), urea
secretes	H$^+$, NH$_4^+$, (K$^+$)

urea and creatinine in the body with increased plasma concentrations of these solutes.

The glomeruli may leak protein or may fail to produce their normal daily quota of 180 L of protein-free filtrate for the following reasons.

Protein loss from the kidney

In the nephrotic syndrome, an abnormal glomerular basement membrane allows plasma proteins, especially albumin, to escape; the urine may contain from 5 to as much as 30 g of protein per day. When synthesis in the liver fails to keep up with renal loss, there is less circulating albumin and its concentration in the plasma falls, so that the volume and the colloid osmotic pressure of the plasma tend to be reduced. There is a body-wide disturbance of the Starling equilibrium (p. 394), with gross generalized oedema, caused and sustained by excessive retention of Na$^+$ by the kidneys.

Failure to produce enough glomerular filtrate

In chronic renal failure, destruction of nephrons gradually reduces GFR (Fig. 20.27).

About three-quarters of a person's nephrons can be destroyed before renal function is obviously impaired. The remaining nephrons hypertrophy and adapt so that total function is surprisingly well maintained. For substances excreted primarily by the glomeruli, excretion depends upon filtered load, not upon GFR as such. Consequently, for creatine or urea, the rate of excretion will be maintained if plasma concentration increases in proportion to dwindling GFR (Fig. 20.27). The normal amount of creatinine can be eliminated in one-quarter as much glomerular filtrate if each volume of filtrate contains four times as much creatinine, i.e. if plasma creatinine concentration is four times normal. Similarly, the rising plasma urea concentration with advancing renal failure is not merely a sign of falling GFR; it is an effective compensating mechanism that allows the excretion of urea to be maintained.

In a steady state, the rate of excretion of urea must equal the rate of production. If GFR suddenly falls to half, excretion will at first lag behind production and plasma urea concentration will increase until it reaches twice normal, when excretion will catch up with production. The body's urea pool will then have doubled, but retention of urea will no longer be increasing. If GFR

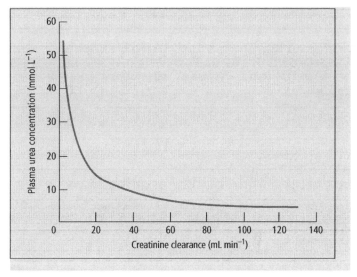

Fig. 20.27 The relationship between plasma urea concentration and the clearance of creatinine, which estimates GFR. In renal failure GFR is reduced and this is reflected in an increased plasma urea concentration.

falls to $12\,mL\,min^{-1}$ (10% of normal), plasma urea will have to rise to 40 mmol instead of 4 mmol and the body will contain 1700 mmol instead of a normal 170 mmol of urea, but the rates of production and of excretion will again be equal and normal at about 500 mmol or $30\,g\,day^{-1}$.

Disturbances of tubular function

Because glomerular capillaries are damaged in chronic glomerular disease, peritubular capillaries are deprived of blood, and the associated tubules are therefore also destroyed. Each functional nephron that remains handles a greater load than normal and operates in a state of osmotic diuresis. The ability to concentrate or dilute the urine is lost progressively. Na^+ balance is often maintained until late in the disease process partly at least because, although less Na^+ can be filtered, the osmotic diuresis means that less can be reabsorbed distally. This means that a greater fraction of the filtered load is excreted. Loss of functional renal mass results eventually in too little K^+ secretion so that the body retains K^+. It will also result in a metabolic (renal) acidosis when HCO_3^- synthesis becomes insufficient to replace HCO_3^- consumed in buffering the H^+ ions produced by metabolism.

In chronic destructive diseases, renal tissue gradually disappears, but the amount of solute to be excreted is not diminished. The hypertrophied and adapted nephrons that are left have to do all the work that was formerly done by a full complement of normal nephrons. If 10% of the nephrons remain, each one of these must on average handle 10 times as much solute as a nephron in a normal kidney. Under such conditions of permanent osmotic diuresis, the urine cannot be concentrated to any extent. During water deprivation, normal kidneys can make urine concentrated to four times the osmolarity of the plasma, but only at rates less than $\sim0.6\,mL\,min^{-1}$ (Fig. 20.26). The attainable concentration falls as flow rate increases during osmotic diuresis, and at $15\,mL\,min^{-1}$ urine can be little more than isosmolar. With only 10% of the nephrons remaining, the urine cannot be more concentrated than the plasma if the rate of production exceeds $1.5\,mL\,min^{-1}$. This is about 2000 mL day^{-1}, the volume of isosmolar urine required to contain the daily output of urinary solutes, which explains the fixed osmolarity and specific gravity of 1010 (isosthenuria) characteristic of renal failure.

Inability to concentrate and to reduce the volume of the urine also accounts for the **nocturia** with may be an early sign of renal damage. Note that a simple test of the power of the kidneys to concentrate the urine (such as the urinary osmolarity or specific gravity after 12 h overnight without fluid) is both the simplest and the most sensitive test for detecting early impairment of renal function, especially in diseases like pyelonephritis, which attack the medulla. Note too that the increased urinary volume that results from the kidneys' loss of concentrating power promotes the excretion of urea; for the clearance of urea increases with rising flow rate and becomes maximal above about $2\,mL\,min^{-1}$ (Fig. 20.9).

Handling of sodium

In contrast to urea, retention of Na^+ with increasing concentration in the plasma would disturb the balance between cells and extracellular fluid. Retention is avoided by reabsorbing a smaller fraction of filtered Na^+ and since normally more than 99% of filtered Na^+ is reabsorbed, there is a large margin of safety. If GFR fell to $12\,mL\,min^{-1}$ (one-tenth of normal), Na^+ balance could still be maintained by reabsorbing 97.5% of the filtered load of $2500\,mmol\,day^{-1}$. Even with GFR reduced to $3\,mL\,min^{-1}$ (one-fortieth of normal), the filtered load would be $600\,mmol\,day^{-1}$ and balance could be maintained by reabsorption of five-sixths of the filtered Na^+. Possible causes of reduced fractional reabsorption include:

1 osmotic diuresis, which decreases contact time for distal reabsorption;

2 reduced availability of NH_4^+, which means that Na^+ must accompany conjugate bases of urinary acids; and

3 the action of natriuretic substances.

Sometimes, and especially when tubular functions have been damaged more than glomerular, too much Na^+ may be lost, with depletion of the volume of extracellular fluid which further depresses GFR and aggravates retention of nitrogenous substances.

Handling of potassium

As nephrons are lost, there are fewer cells in total capable of secreting K^+. This, together with increased catabolism of tissues in uraemia which releases K^+ from broken-down cells, may lead to a dangerous elevation of plasma K^+ concentration requiring treatment by dialysis.

Handling of hydrogen ions

Renal acidosis is a metabolic acidosis arising from impaired capacity of the renal tubular cells to secrete H^+ ions and add HCO_3^- to the plasma, and is accordingly often characterized as **renal tubular acidosis**. Possible causes include:

1 failure to secrete H^+ into the urine and add HCO_3^- to the plasma at a sufficient rate;

2 failure to bring urine to a sufficiently low pH, so that less H^+ can be excreted as titratable acid and ammonium;

3 failure to supply sufficient NH_4^+ to carry H^+ ions into the urine; and

4 shortage of filtered buffer to make into titratable acid.

Only the last of these depends primarily upon GFR. The rest depend upon metabolic failure to transport H^+ ions against gradients or to provide NH_4^+. The biggest single factor is usually the inadequate supply of NH_4^+ from the dwindling of the mass of metabolizing tubular tissue as nephrons are destroyed.

In summary, patients with failing kidneys have an undiminished need for the services of their kidneys, and so must overload a dwindling population of functioning nephrons. Nitrogenous end-products accumulate in the blood (**azotaemia**) because there are too few glomeruli, and GFR falls. Lack of tubular tissue leads to failure to secrete sufficient K^+, H^+ and NH_4^+, and sometimes to retention of Na^+. The overloaded remaining nephrons, possibly with a disorganized medulla with its counter-current arrangements wrecked, cannot concentrate the urine; and so the patient must live with an increased turnover of water or risk dehydration.

20.8 Micturition

The bladder can accommodate up to about $300–400\,mL$ of urine with little increase in tension. As volume increases further and wall tension rises, this is appreciated as a sensation of fullness. If appropriate, an autonomic spinal cord reflex—the micturition reflex—is triggered and urination occurs. This involves a coordinated relaxation of internal and external sphincters, contraction of the bladder muscle and of the abdominal wall and pelvic floor musculature.

Autonomic reflexes, under the control of higher centres, bring about the emptying of the bladder. This hollow organ has stretch receptors in its wall which signal the wall tension and thus the organ volume. The signals are appreciated consciously as a sensation of fullness and they also activate reflex connections in the spinal cord.

The smooth muscle of the bladder wall (the **detrusor muscle**) and neck (the **internal sphincter**) is innervated by sympathetic fibres (inhibitory) from the lumbar segments of the spinal cord and by parasympathetic fibres (excitatory) from sacral segments two to four. The **external sphincter** is a striated muscle with a somatic innervation. When bladder-wall tension reaches a certain level, the detrusor contracts reflexly and the internal sphincter relaxes. It should be noted, however, that the bladder wall can accommodate increasing volumes of urine with very little alteration in tension. Only when the volume reaches 300–400 mL is there

normally an appreciable degree of discomfort associated with a steeper rise in tension and triggering of the **micturition reflex**. That this emptying reflex can be facilitated from the brain is shown by the fact that the bladder can be emptied at any volume. More often, however, these spinal reflexes are inhibited by cerebral activity, until either it is appropriate to urinate or the sensations become insistent. The reflex activity is then augmented and the external sphincter relaxed. The flow of urine then begins. This is facilitated by ancillary reflexes from the urethra that are stimulated by flow of urine and whose efferent activity reinforces bladder muscle contraction and sphincter relaxation. Contraction of the abdominal wall and the pelvic floor also aid the complete emptying of the bladder.

Following transection of the spinal cord and the onset of spinal shock, the bladder wall is inert and the sphincter closed, resulting in urinary retention with overflow. As the shock wears off and detrusor muscle tone returns, reflex emptying can be brought about by, for example, cutaneous stimulation, which may at the same time cause defecation and other evidence of widespread autonomic activity ('**mass' reflex**).

Chapter 21

Fluid and Electrolyte Balance

21.1 Body water

Total body water

Water is the must abundant substance in the body. In young healthy adult men, about 60% of the body mass is water. A normal 70-kg man, therefore, contains about 42 L of water. The percentage of water in the body depends on age and sex. In infants and adult females, body water contents typically are 75% and 50% of body mass, respectively; the relative low value for women is related to body composition. Only approximately 20% of adipose tissue is water. Generally, the fat content of the body is relatively larger in women than in men; therefore, fractional water contents are also different.

Distribution of body water

Approximately two-thirds of the total body water (40% of body mass) is intracellular (Table 21.1). The extracellular water (20% of body mass) is located in different compartments: three-quarters resides in the extravascular, extracellular space as interstitial water, while some 3 L (4.5–5% of body mass) circulates as plasma and lymph water. Small amounts of water are found in other cavities as cerebrospinal, ocular, pleural, peritoneal and synovial fluid; these so-called transcellular fluid volumes are small, relatively stable, and usually

ignored in quantitative considerations of the body fluids.

The distribution of water between the fluid compartments is a dynamic process determined exclusively by prevailing physical forces. With regard to distribution between intra- and extracellular compartments, only osmotic forces are involved (see Chapter 1). The total number of solutes (osmolytes) in the compartments determines the distribution of water, because any difference in compartment osmolalities is equalized quickly by movement of water, cf. 'the water follows the solutes'; however, the regulation of the amount of intracellular solutes is poorly understood. The distribution between intra- and extravascular volumes is determined by the balance between colloid osmotic and hydrostatic pressures (Starling forces, Fig. 16.15).

Water turnover

Despite highly variable intake of fluids, total body water remains remarkably constant. Representative figures of water turnover under sedate conditions in a temperate climate are given in Fig. 21.1. Loss of water through perspiration, sensible or insensible, is highly dependent on environmental conditions and on body temperature regulation. Loss of water via faeces is normally small, but is dependent on the efficiency of intestinal water absorption. Faecal water losses may rise dramatically

Table 21.1 Body water compartments in infants and young adults (percentage of body mass).

Compartment of body water	Infants	Adult women	Adult men
Total body	75	50	60
Intracellular	40	30	40
Extracellular	35	20	20
Interstitial	30	15	15
Intravascular	5	5	5

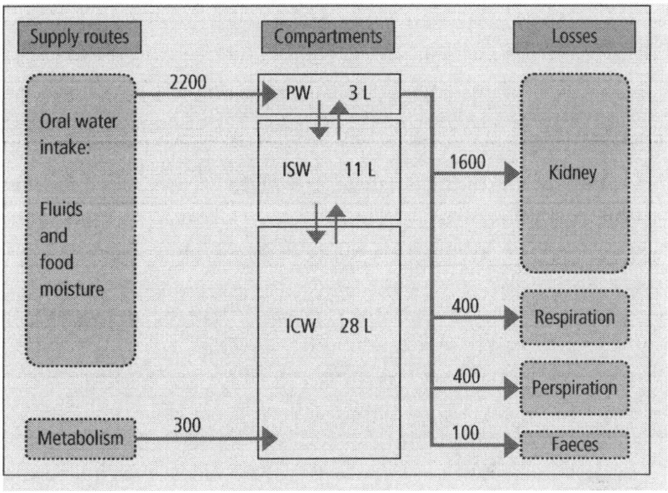

Fig. 21.1 Representative data for water intake and water loss during minimal physical activity, under thermoneutral environmental conditions. Compartment volumes in litres (L). Other figures indicate water transfers in mL day^{-1}. PW, plasma water; ISW, interstitial water; ICW, intracellular water.

in association with diarrhoea. Intake of electrolytes and metabolic end-products constitute an osmotic input of about 600 mOsm day^{-1}. Maximal urinary concentration is about 1200 mOsm kg^{-1}. Therefore, a diuresis of 0.5 L is required to maintain osmotic balance. Normally, urinary output is 1–3 L day^{-1}. After total cessation of vasopressin secretion (p. 562), urine flow may increase to more than 30 L day^{-1}.

Regulation of body water

Water balance is a situation where, over a given time period, the sum of water losses is identical to the amount of water gained by ingestion and metabolic processes. Intake and excretion of water are regulated by thirst and renal water excretion, respectively. Similar to other homeostatic processes, each control system consists of a controlled variable, a specific sensing organ, and an effector

mechanism correcting primary deviations in the controlled variable.

Thirst is a complex sensation leading to the search for, and intake of water. In man, the thirst sensation is generated almost exclusively by an increase in effective plasma osmolality, i.e. an increase leading to a reduction in cell volume. The controlled variable is therefore plasma osmolality. The specific sensory mechanism is located to circumscript areas of the hypothalamus; without proper function of these areas, thirst is absent. The effector system is a characteristic behaviour leading to intake of water, which is absorbed by the gut. In other species, thirst may be generated or modulated by other events such as decreases in blood volume and increases in plasma angiotensin II concentrations. In humans, the importance of such mechanisms is unclear.

Water is lost by several routes (Fig. 21.1), but only renal water excretion is part of the regulation of body water. Respiratory, transcutaneous, and faecal losses vary according to ventilation, temperature control, and intestinal absorption, respectively, without direct feedback links to body water. Effective plasma osmolality is the **controlled variable**; normally, plasma osmolality is 290 mOsm kg⁻¹ water, and is regulated very efficiently—deviations of more than a few mOsm kg⁻¹ are rare. The **sensors** (osmoreceptors) are located in the hypothalamus, in the vicinity of the anterior part of the third ventricle. The osmoreceptors control the activity of the neurones of the neurohypophysis, and thereby the rate of secretion of vasopressin (Fig. 21.2a) which, together with the renal concentrating mechanism (Chapter 20), constitutes the **effector mechanism** (Fig. 21.2). Excretion of concentrated urine will decrease plasma osmolality, while passing of dilute urine elevates plasma osmolality. The osmoregulatory system is precise, mainly because of the high sensitivity of the osmoreceptors, which respond to increases in osmolality of a few per cent by causing a several-fold increase in plasma vasopressin (Fig. 21.2a). In addition, the normal kidney is sensitive to small increases in plasma vasopressin (Fig. 21.2b). Osmoregulatory changes in water excretion are rapid;

a sudden surplus of body water is excreted quantitatively within a couple of hours.

The receptors for thirst and vasopressin secretion are separate entities although both are located in the hypothalamus. Both types of receptors are sensitive to changes in the concentrations of solutes that do not easily permeate cell membranes, i.e. changes in 'effective' osmolality. Urea and glucose are not able to activate thirst or osmoreceptors. Appropriately, the receptor systems have different thresholds so that thirst is elicited at a plasma osmolality about 10 mOsm kg⁻¹ higher than the level that triggers the secretion of vasopressin. Therefore, thirst appears only under conditions where vasopressin has already activated the renal concentrating mechanism.

Osmolality-driven vasopressin secretion is the main determinant of renal water excretion. However, the secretion of vasopressin is modulated by other factors, notably central venous pressure signalled via stretch receptors in the atria and the great veins (Fig. 21.2a), arterial pressure signals mediated via aortic and carotid baroreceptors, and circulating plasma angiotensin II concentrations. In this way, stretch receptors activated by increases in blood volume can influence the excretion of

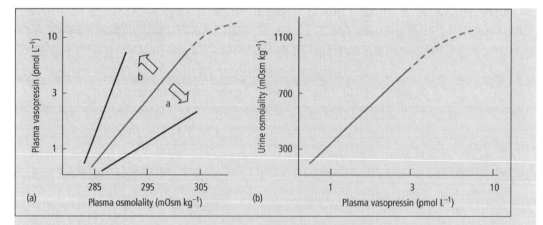

Fig. 21.2 Functional relations of osmoregulation. (a) Plasma vasopressin concentration as a function of plasma osmolality. The slope represents the sensitivity of the osmoreceptor mechanism. Normal values are 290 mOsm kg⁻¹ and 1.3 pmol L⁻¹. Arrows indicate modulation by **a** increased blood volume and **b** decreased blood volume. (b) Urine osmolality as a function of plasma vasopressin. The slope depicts renal sensitivity to vasopressin, which is subject to modulation by other factors.

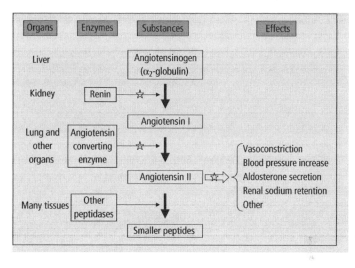

Fig. 21.3 Components of the renin system. The star indicates the location of possible pharmacological inhibition. The smaller peptides may possess some bioactivity, but the significance of this is not evident. Some organs, notably the kidney, have been shown to contain angiotensinogen and the enzymes required to synthesize angiotensin II, but the functional implications of this are unclear. ACE, angiotensin converting enzyme.

volume through the kidneys (Fig. 21.3, left hand side). The influence of the arterial baroreceptors is evident only at substantial decreases in arterial pressure. However, once activated by hypotension, the increase in vasopressin secretion is dramatic and may override any signal from the osmoreceptors; i.e. during hypotension water is retained by the kidney, irrespective of body fluid osmolality (osmocontrol is sacrificed in favour of volume control).

21.2 Body sodium

Distribution of sodium ions

The total body content of Na^+ is approximately 4000 mmol for a 70-kg man. Isotope studies have shown that the majority—some 3000 mmol—mixes readily with injected isotope, thus forming a pool of 'exchangeable Na^+'. This includes Na^+ of the extracellular compartment (2000 mmol), bone (700 mmol) and the intracellular volume (300 mmol). The remaining 1000 mmol is bound mainly in the crystal structures of bone and is therefore non-diffusible and non-exchangeable, and hence not part of the free solutes of the body fluids. Sodium ions are by far the most abundant cations of the extracellular fluid. Sodium salts, mainly Cl^- and HCO_3^-, account for some 92% of the total extracellular osmolality.

Sodium balance

In industrialized societies, daily Na^+ intake is 100–300 mmol (2.3–7 g of Na^+, equivalent to 6–18 g of NaCl), mostly from the salt in processed food. Practically all ingested Na^+ is absorbed, together with the much larger amounts of Na^+ secreted to the gut; 90–95% is excreted in the urine, the rest is lost via faeces. Sodium intake varies with food habits, and large differences occur between individuals, and within individuals on a day-to-day basis.

Sodium is lost in the urine and through sweating. As a result of a primary isoosmolar secretion and subsequent reabsorption of salt, the concentration of Na^+ in sweat (10–50 mmol L^{-1}) is proportional to the rate of sweating. However, the sweat is always hypo-osmolar to plasma, therefore sweating tends to increase body fluid osmolality. The rate of Na^+ loss via sweating is highly variable, as it depends on physical activity and environmental conditions.

The mechanisms of renal and intestinal Na^+ conservation are very efficient. Practically any combination of energy-sufficient food items contains adequate amounts of NaCl; i.e. intakes are easily matched by adjustment of renal function. During a low-Na^+ diet, the urine may become virtually Na^+-free, while Na^+-loading may increase Na^+ excretion to rates well above 500 mmol day^{-1}.

Regulation of sodium balance

The regulation of Na+ excretion is based on the extracellular fluid volume (in contrast to the excretion of water, which is determined by the body fluid solute concentration). Changes in Na+ intake tend to change plasma Na+ concentration and osmolality. However, osmotic regulation via vasopressin is rapid; therefore, changes in Na+ intake are associated with parallel changes in extracellular fluid volume and body mass. Volume is a suitable indication of total body Na+ if the concentration of Na+ does not change, and if the distribution between the different compartments of distribution for Na+ remains constant. Normally, the former assumption is valid, and the latter a good approximation. Relative to the regulation of body water, the regulation of total body Na+ is slow. A sudden step-up in Na+ intake, e.g. from 50 to 200 mmol day^{-1}, will increase fluid volume and body mass over 3–4 days until Na+ balance is again achieved. Usually, this occurs without measurable changes in plasma osmolality or arterial blood pressure. The **regulated variable** is therefore volume. The **receptors** include stretch receptors in the walls of the central veins and the atria, providing cardiovascular centres in the brain stem with necessary information. The role of other putative sensors, such as cardiac ventricular receptors, is unclear. Large deviations in total body Na+ may change blood volume to the extent that arterial blood pressure is affected. In this situation, arterial baroreceptors may contribute to the regulation of Na+ excretion (see Fig. 21.4).

The **effector system** is multifactorial and not fully elucidated. The regulation of Na+ excretion is mainly a renal process. The overall regulation of renal Na+ excretion is complex, being dependent on a number of mediators and modulators. In this context, a mediator is able to cause graded changes in Na+ excretion, while itself being a function of total body Na+—i.e. a mediator is part of a feedback mechanism. A modulator may affect Na+ excretion similarly, but its level of activity, and thus its influence, is apparently unrelated to total body Na+—i.e. a modulator is not part of a feedback system.

The most important mediators are the hormones angiotensin II and aldosterone, which are elements of the renin system (Fig. 21.3). Renin is an enzyme secreted from the granular cells of the juxtaglomerular apparatus. The rate of secretion is regulated via the sympathetic tone of the renal nerves (Fig. 21.4), the level of renal arterial pressure (Fig. 21.4), atrial natriuretic peptide concentration (Fig. 21.4), and through the electrolyte concentration at the macula densa. In addition, the concentration of circulating angiotensin II has a pronounced, direct, negative effect on the secretion of the granular cells, forming a so-called short-loop feedback. Renal sympathetic nerve activity and renal arterial pressure are most directly coupled to total body Na+. A primary increase in Na+ intake will increase extracellular volume, activate low-pressure volume receptors, and—to the extent that the increased preload augments cardiac output—activate arterial pressure receptors. Even large increases in Na+ intake do not elevate arterial pressure measurably; therefore renal arterial pressure remains essentially unchanged. Stretch receptor activation reduces renal sympathetic nerve activity and increases Na+ excretion. In addition, several humoral mechanisms are involved.

The concentration of NaCl in the tubular fluid passing the macula densa, normally approximately 30–40 mmol L^{-1}, is a co-determinant of renin secretion; a decrease in NaCl concentration increases renin secretion. The concentration of NaCl at the macula densa is determined by the end-proximal tubular fluid flow, which is isotonic, and by the rate of NaCl reabsorption occurring without water reabsorption in the ascending loop of Henle. The end-proximal flow is a result of glomerular filtration and proximal reabsorption. In addition to controlling renin secretion, the concentration signal at the macula densa is a critical component of the tubulo-glomerular feedback mechanism (see below). Therefore, the concentration signal at the macula densa is a complex function of multiple haemodynamic events and tubular reabsorption processes. Some of the reabsorption processes, notably proximal reabsorption, may themselves be modulated by intrarenal messengers. The regulatory importance of the macula densa-driven

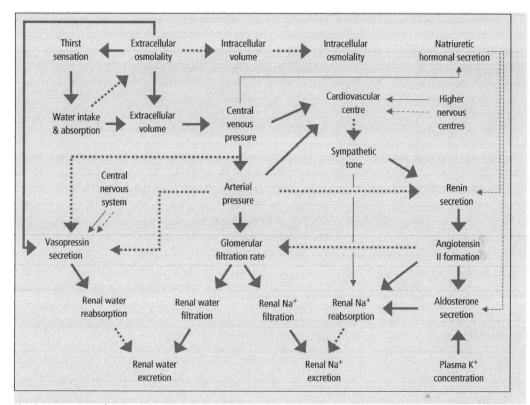

Fig. 21.4 Overview of the main mechanisms regulating renal water and Na$^+$ excretion. Full lines indicate direct (positive) relationship, i.e. stimulation/augmentation. Dashed lines indicate inverse relationship, i.e. inhibition/reduction. Thin lines represent interactions that at present seem less important. For reasons of simplicity, the feedback loops have not been completed. To complete the feedback loops, excretion of water decreases (dashed line to) extracellular volume and increases (full line to) extracellular osmolality. Excretion of Na$^+$ decreases (dashed line to) extracellular osmolality. Large doses of atrial natriuretic peptide decrease tubular reabsorption of Na$^+$, but the regulatory importance of this effect is less clear.

control of renin secretion, relative to renal sympathetic tone and renal arterial pressure, is not clear.

The atrial natriuretic peptide system seems to play only a minor role in the regulation of Na$^+$ excretion. However, the natriuretic peptides may be important for the long-term regulation of body fluids and blood pressure.

Homeostatic renal sodium reabsorption

The rate of excretion of Na$^+$ in the kidney is very small compared to the rate of filtration. Changes within the range of 0.2–0.8% of filtered load are needed to balance Na$^+$ intakes of 50–200 mmol day^{-1}. Reabsorption of Na$^+$ takes place in most segments of the renal tubule. The majority of the filtered load is absorbed in the proximal tubules (65–70%) and the thick ascending limb of the loop of Henle (25%), leaving 5–10% to be reabsorbed in the distal tubular system. Normally, the renal blood flow and the glomerular filtration rate (GFR) are autoregulated; i.e. within a wide range of blood pressures around normal resting pressure, deviations in pressure are not followed by changes in perfusion or filtration flows. Tubulo-glomerular feedback is a mechanism by which the degree of afferent arteriolar contraction is coupled to the ion concentration (particularly Cl$^-$ of the tubular fluid passing the macula densa (see also Chapter 20). An increase in ion concentration causes arteriolar contraction, and thereby increases afferent vascular resistance and decreases GFR. The action of tubuloglomerular feedback stabilizes the delivery of fluid to the distal tubular segments. Functional changes in GFR and proximal, as well as loop of Henle reabsorption rates, do occur and may be important to Na^+ excretion under certain conditions. In addition, resetting of the feedback system occurs, permitting slow changes in the distal inflow of electrolytes. However, normally most of the adjustment of Na^+ reabsorption needed to maintain Na^+ balance occurs in the distal tubular segments, i.e. segments beyond the macula densa. Only 5–10% of filtered Na^+ load enters these segments, but the degree to which this amount is reabsorbed determines the excretion rate.

Transcellular reabsorption in the principal cells of the cortical collecting ducts is most important. The ubiquitous, basolateral Na^+,K^+–ATPase actively transfers Na^+ out of the cell and, together with luminal ion permeabilities, sets up the electrochemical gradient, including a –40 mV lumen negative potential. This drives luminal Na^+ ions into the cell through an epithelial Na^+ channel (ENaC). The ENaC is inhibited by the diuretic amiloride. Aldosterone stimulates principal cell Na^+ reabsorption and K^+ excretion by increasing Na^+,K^+–ATPase pump activity and ENaC efficiency. In addition, luminal K^+ conductance is increased (see below). Aldosterone acts by binding to the mineralocorticoid receptor within the cell. Remarkably, cortisol, which is present in concentrations much greater than those of aldosterone, binds to the mineralocorticoid receptor with similar affinity. However, aldosterone is the principal ligand as cortisol is enzymatically converted to inactive cortisone before it can reach the receptor. The enzyme responsible for this is isoform two of 11β-hydroxy steroid dehydrogenase (11β-HSD-2), which is expressed mainly in aldosterone target tissues (epithelia of kidney, colon, sweat and salivary glands). Glycyrrhetinic acid, found in liquorice, is an inhibitor of 11β-HSD-2; excessive intake of liquorice may reduce renal 11β-HSD-2 activity to the extent that cortisol escapes conversion, activates the miner-

alocorticoid receptor, and causes Na^+ retention and hypertension (so-called apparent mineralocorticoid excess).

A major fraction of the distal load of Na^+ is reabsorbed by the distal convoluted tubule. In the cells of this segment, luminal influx of Na^+ occurs together with Cl^- through an electroneutral Na^+–Cl^- co-transporter (NCC). The basolateral transfer and the necessary gradients are provided by basolateral Na^+,K^+–ATPase in combination with a basolateral Cl^- channel. The NCC may be inhibited specifically by diuretics of the thiazide family.

The medullary collecting duct cells reabsorb only a few per cent of the filtered load of Na^+. However, with regard to Na^+ homeostasis, they are placed in a strategic position; the final excretion rate of Na^+ being a tiny fraction of filtered load, small increases in the rate of inner-medullary reabsorption of Na^+ may result in large decreases in Na^+ excretion. A number of ion pumps and transporters are present in the cell membranes of inner-medullar collecting ducts: Na^+,K^+–ATPase is located basolaterally, together with several ion exchangers (Na^+–H^+ and Cl^-–HCO_3^-); in the luminal membrane, a non-selective (Na^+–K^+) cation channel and K^+,H^+–ATPase are present. Normally, the electrolyte transport is primarily that of Na^+ reabsorption and K^+ secretion, but their participation in the regulation of Na^+ balance is not well-described.

The amount of intrarenal modulators of Na^+ excretion is large. A number of potent signal molecules, such as nitric oxide, endothelins, kallikreins, kinins, dopamine, prostaglandins and other eicosanoids, may influence the rate of Na^+ excretion. Feedback mechanisms have not been identified; however, abnormal levels of one or more modulators may be important in the analysis of patho-physiological conditions. The circulating hormones vasopressin and noradrenaline do not seem to play important roles in Na^+ homeostasis.

21.3 Body potassium

The high intracellular concentration of K^+ contributes to the optimal environment for cell

functions, including enzyme activities and cell growth. The ubiquitous Na^+,K^+–ATPase maintains the intracellular K^+-to-Na^+ concentration ratio at approximately 15, and intracellular K^+ is quantitatively the most important in the regulation of cell volume. In excitable tissues, the resting membrane potential is close to the diffusion potential for K^+; therefore, maintenance of the gradient across the cell membrane is important for the resting potential and for tissue excitability.

Distribution of potassium ions

The total body content of K^+ is approximately 3600 mmol for a 70-kg man. The vast majority of total body K^+ mixes readily with injected K^+ tracer; therefore, almost all K^+ is 'exchangeable'. Potassium is the primary cation of the intracellular fluid; a proximately 98% of total body K^+ is located intracellularly and, together with phosphates, accounts for most of the total intracellular osmolality. Some 80 mmol (~2%) resides in the extracellular fluid. Of the K^+ in the intracellular fluid, 300 mmol is in the skeleton while most (approximately 2700 mmol) is in skeletal muscle. Exchangeable K^+ is about 50 mmol kg^{-1} in men and 40 mmol kg^{-1} in women, the difference mainly being due to the relatively large muscle mass in men.

The concentration of K^+ in the extracellular fluid is 4–5 mmol L^{-1}, and changes of a few mmol L^{-1} have important implications for the function of excitable tissues, notably the heart. Plasma K^+ concentrations outside the range of 2–7 mmol L^{-1} are life-threatening (see below).

Potassium balance

The normal intake of K^+ is in the order of 100 mmol day^{-1}, i.e. more than the amount present in the extracellular fluid. Some 10% is lost via faeces and the remainder is excreted in the urine. Because the extracellular amount of K^+ constitutes a very small fraction of total body K^+, the distribution of body K^+ between the intra- and extracellular volumes is important. This distribution is modulated by hormones, notably insulin, adrenaline, and aldosterone, all of which promote translocation into the cells. Intracellular acidosis leads to loss of cell K^+ and hyperkalaemia, probably because of an inhibitory effect on the Na^+,K^+–ATPase and, when present, on the Na^+–K^+–$2Cl^-$ co-transporter (NKCC2). Loss of a few per cent of the intracellular K^+ to the extracellular space changes plasma K^+ dramatically. Therefore, the concentration of K^+ in plasma reflects the distribution within the body and does not constitute an indicator of total body K^+.

Regulation of potassium balance

The kidney adjusts K^+ excretion to match K^+ intake, less the amount excreted via faeces. In the kidney, K^+ undergoes filtration, reabsorption and secretion. The rate of excretion of K^+ is usually 10–20% of filtered load, but may vary from 1% to 160% under conditions of K^+ depletion and loading, respectively. Some 90% of the filtered K^+ is always reabsorbed before the tubular fluid reaches the distal tubules, illustrating the important position of these in the control of K^+ excretion. During K^+ depletion, the distal nephron segments may reabsorb almost all of the K^+ presented to them; conversely, in the case of K^+ excess, they mediate secretion of K^+ in large quantities.

In the nephron segments proximal to the macula densa, K^+ reabsorption is obligatory and occurs mainly in the proximal tubule and in the thick ascending loop of Henle (Chapter 20). In the former, reabsorption is achieved primarily by solvent drag and by diffusion down the favourable electrochemical gradient, through the low-resistance paracellular pathway. In the thick ascending loop, K^+ reabsorption is driven paracellularly by the lumen-positive potential, and transcellularly by secondary-active luminal NKCC2 transporter, dependent on the concentration gradients created by the basolateral Na^+,K^+–ATPase. Most of the K^+ entering the cell via NKCC2 is reabsorbed to the interstitium via the basolateral K^+ channel. The remainder is returned to the lumen by the ROMK channel of the luminal membrane, thus maintaining the luminal K^+ concentration at levels that allow the continued function of the NKCC2 channel. In the descending and thin ascending segments of the loop of Henle K^+ is secreted and reabsorbed, respectively, by passive mechanisms.

So-called loop-diuretics block the NKCC2 channel (i.e. the transcellular pathway) directly, and eliminate the paracellular pathway indirectly by abolishing the lumen positive potential. The resulting blockade of thick ascending limb electrolyte transport generates: a dramatic increase in Na^+ excretion, as more distal segments are now presented with much more Na^+ than they can handle; a secondary increase in K^+ excretion, as distal Na^+–K^+ exchange is augmented by the massive supply of Na^+; and an impressive diuresis, due to the augmented distal tubular solute load and the breakdown of the renal concentrating mechanism.

The regulatory K^+ transport mechanisms (reabsorption or secretion) of the distal tubular segments occur predominantly in the intercalated cells of the collecting tubules, in the medullary collecting ducts (reabsorption), and in the principal cells of the collecting duct (secretion).

The K^+ **reabsorption by the intercalated cells** (α-intercalated cells) is a result of the action of a luminal adenosine triphosphate (ATP)-driven K^+–H^+ exchange pump (acting similarly to that of the gastric mucosa), and a basolateral K^+ channel allowing intracellular K^+ to drain into the interstitium. During K^+ depletion this process is up-regulated, which explains the concomitant augmentation in the rate of H^+ secretion and the development of the hypokalemic alkalosis associated with this condition.

K^+ **secretion by the principal cells** consists of passive transport across the luminal membrane through two pathways: a K^+ channel, and a K^+–Cl^- co-transporter, through which K^+ transfer is driven by a favourable electrochemical gradient (a lumen negative potential and an outward concentration gradient). Intracellular K^+ is provided by the basolateral Na^+,K^+–ATPase. Aldosterone stimulates principal cell Na^+ reabsorption and K^+ excretion by increasing basolateral Na^+,K^+–ATPase activity and thus uptake of K^+, which in turn is mediated by: increasing luminal Na^+ channel (ENaC) density and activity so that the basolateral Na^+,K^+–ATPase is

able to provide K^+ at an elevated rate continuously; and by increasing luminal K^+ conductance, therefore allowing an augmented rate of passive cell-to-lumen transport of K^+. This means that the coupling between Na^+ reabsorption and K^+ secretion is indirect and subject to the action of a number of modulators affecting K^+ secretion. The activity of the basolateral Na^+,K^+–ATPase is influenced by changes in extracellular K^+ concentrations; a physiological elevation in the extracellular K^+ concentration increases the supply of intracellular K^+ to the principal cells, and consequently augments K^+ secretion. An increase in **tubular flow rate** accelerates K^+ secretion because the passive cell-to-lumen transport of K^+ is normally diffusion-limited; an increased flow of tubular fluid with low concentrations of K^+ removes the self-limiting effect of passive K^+ secretion and elevates the rate of secretion. Other factors that increase K^+ secretion include any **decrease in the lumen negative potential**, as a more negative potential increases the rate of transfer through both luminal transporters, and a reduction in luminal Cl^- concentration, which increases the driving force through the K^+–Cl^- co-transporter. In addition, deviations from normal **acid–base status** influences K^+ transfer by principal cells; acidosis diminishes and alkalosis elevates K^+ secretion.

The renal excretion of the dietary K^+ input is adaptive; i.e. during sustained exposure to either high or low intake of K^+, functional and even morphological changes occur over a period of days as the kidney develops the mechanisms suitable to handle the new dietary situation. Potassium loading increases the activity of the basolateral Na^+,K^+–ATPase and leads to an expansion of the basolateral membrane area of the principal cells in the cortical collecting duct segments. Potassium loading also stimulates aldosterone secretion and thereby accelerates basolateral Na^+,K^+–ATPase, as well as luminal ENaC and K^+ channel conductances. During K^+ depletion, these processes are reversed—basolateral K^+ uptake and aldosterone secretion are both reduced—thus inhibiting the tubular Na^+-for-K^+ exchange normally carried out by the principal cells. In addition, K^+ reabsorption by the intercalated cells is stimulated by activation of the K^+–H^+ pump following the decrease in extracellular K^+ concentration. Potassium depletion leads to changes in the apical membrane structure of the intercalated cells; the membrane area is increased and the number of active pumps in the membrane is probably also increased.

It is difficult to envisage the control system for total body K^+ in terms of controlled variables, sensors, and effectors. Rather, the extracellular K^+ concentration seems to represent a point of balance between first, the mechanisms of distribution between the extra- and intracellular compartments, mainly by modulation of Na$^+$,K$^+$–ATPase activity by hormones and electrolyte concentrations, and second, by the mechanisms of renal excretion controlled by the above-mentioned mediators and modulators. The lack of knowledge regarding the regulation of the mass of intracellular K^+, and the significant interaction between K^+ turnover and acid–base metabolism, make a quantitative approach difficult. Clinical guidelines for handling of K^+ disturbances are most often empiric.

21.4 Magnesium

Magnesium is an important enzyme cofactor and, as such, an important intracellular ion. A number of enzymes using ATP require that it is present in the form of a Mg^{2+} complex; in addition, adequate intracellular levels of ionized Mg^{2+} are important for neuromuscular function. In body fluid compartments divalent cations are present as ions (ionized concentration), in complexes with other small solutes (and thus ultrafiltrable), and bound to proteins.

Distribution of magnesium ions

The total body Mg^{2+} is in the order of 800 mmol. Over 60% (approximately 500 mmol) is found in the skeleton and most of the reminder is within the cells, where 90–95% of the total amount is bound to proteins. The intracellular concentration of ionized Mg^{2+} is in the order of 1 mmol L^{-1}. The total concentration in plasma is around 0.9 mmol L^{-1}, and about one-third of this is protein-bound, so

that the concentration of ultrafiltrable Mg^{2+} is around 0.6 mmol L^{-1}.

Magnesium balance

Ordinary diets supply about 20 mmol day^{-1}, of which about 40% (8 mmol) is absorbed from the gut; the rest is excreted in the faeces. The mechanisms of absorption are largely unknown, but appear to be distinct from those controlling the absorption of Ca^{2+} ions. Absorbed Mg^{2+} is excreted in the urine.

Regulation of magnesium balance

The renal excretion of Mg^{2+} is important for the maintenance of normal physiological levels in plasma. Of the amount of Mg^{2+} filtered into the proximal tubules, 5–10% is excreted. Reabsorption occurs in most segments of the tubules, but mainly in the ascending loop of Henle, where the process is under the influence of parathyroid hormone and other hormones, and is indirectly coupled to salt and water transport. Magnesium reabsorption is inhibited by loop diuretics, volume expansion, and metabolic acidosis.

21.5 Disturbances in fluid and electrolyte metabolism

Abnormalities in Na$^+$ and water turnover are often composite and affect the distribution of total body water between the major fluid compartments. It is useful to describe such abnormalities together, and to identify a number of simple disturbances to provide the basis for the evaluation of clinical situations, which are usually more complex.

Abnormal water and sodium contents

The concepts of body fluid disturbances includes several approximations: first, osmotic equilibrium is assumed to exist throughout the body; i.e. all compartments of body water posses the same osmolality (approximation i); second, deviations of total body Na$^+$ are taken as deviations in extracellular exchangeable Na$^+$; that is, acute changes in intracellular Na^+ and non-exchangeable Na^+ are considered to be negligible (approximation ii).

Losses and gains in total body water and Na^+ occur to and from the extracellular space. Deviations in total body contents of either water or Na^+, change extracellular osmolality and lead to rapid and complete secondary alterations in the intracellular volume-restoring osmotic equilibrium. The osmotic gradients are transient and quantitatively very small (approximation i). It is only the losses and gains of isotonic solutions that are not associated with secondary changes in intracellular volume; it is important to distinguish between fluid disturbances with and without changes in intracellular volume.

Simple dehydration (hypertonic dehydration) is the condition arising from inadequate availability of fresh water, inadequate administration of electrolyte-free water or inappropriate excretion of dilute urine (e.g. diabetes insipidus). The normal, obligatory losses of dilute solutions or water through sweating and breathing, respectively, increase the solute concentration in all body fluids (approximation i). Thirst is an early symptom and a very powerful sensation. If for any reason water ingestion does not occur, the osmolality of all body fluid compartments continues to increase. The central nervous system is most sensitive to hyperosmolality, and confusion and coma develop. Death from simple dehydration is due to intracellular dehydration leading to respiratory paralysis.

Simple overhydration (hypotonic overhydration) due to ingestion of excessive amounts of water is very rare. The renal capacity for excretion of solute-free water is large. However, inappropriate secretion of vasopressin occurs in a number of clinical settings, is difficult to detect, and may inadvertently be combined with administration of isosmolar (5%) dextrose solution, leading to a surplus of water. In the context of fluid balance, dextrose solution is equivalent to pure water as long as the fuel metabolism is normal. Administered dextrose is either metabolized to water and CO_2, or stored as elements of glycogen. In both cases, the dextrose disappears from the body fluids and the water remains. Symptoms are predominantly neurological, reflecting brain oedema, which is the result of osmotic shifts of water into the brain, and range from dizziness, headache, and confusion, to coma, seizures, and death.

Sodium deficiency may occur because of specific disease (hypoaldosteronism) or in situations where losses of Na^+-containing fluids (profuse sweating, intestinal drains, and use of diuretics) have been replaced by electrolyte-free solutions or water. A decrease in the amount of extracellular solute reduces extracellular osmolality (approximation ii), and redistribution of water to the intracellular takes place (approximation i), so the intracellular volume increases at the expense of the extracellular volume. Notably, this redistribution may occur at normal levels of total body water, i.e. without any change in body mass. The principal finding is hyponatraemia. Symptoms are primarily orthostatic hypotension due to the hypovolaemia. Generally, orthostatic hypotension in the absence of specific diseases (neurological disease, deconditioning or sepsis) is indicative of Na^+ depletion. Activation of vasopressin by the hypovolaemia may accelerate water reabsorption, resulting in overhydration.

Sodium excess with hypernatraemia due to acute ingestion of Na^+ is rare; salt is aversive and thirst is a powerful regulator. Sodium retention is commonly associated with renal insufficiency and with inappropriately increased aldosterone activity, either with or without activation of other elements of the renin system. Such slowly-developing retention of Na^+ is followed by water retention, leading to extracellular volume expansion with little increase in plasma Na^+ concentration. Therefore, a slowly developing excess of Na^+ will, when vasopressin-mediated water retention is intact, resemble **isotonic overhydration (extracellular overhydration)**. The latter is also known as 'Na$^+$ retention', a feature of several common diseases (e.g. heart failure). Symptoms include increased vascular filling, possibly developing into peripheral and pulmonary oedema.

Isotonic dehydration (extracellular dehydration) is characterized by loss of fluid containing considerable concentrations of Na^+. Water and Na^+ are rarely lost in proportions identical to that of

plasma, but profuse watery diarrhoea (often of infectious aetiology) approximates this situation. When water and Na^+ salts are excreted in concentrations similar to those of plasma, the loss is predominantly from the extracellular fluid, and therefore each litre of deficit represents a decrease of one-fourteenth (7%) in this compartment. Extracellular dehydration may develop into circulatory insufficiency and shock.

The assessment of fluid disturbances is difficult, partly because the magnitude of the actual body fluid volumes must be estimated by clinical examination, which is not a reliable method. Hyponatraemia may be caused by simple overhydration, but can also result form Na^+ depletion; the former situation is associated with overhydration, including extracellular overhydration, the latter with extracellular dehydration. In addition, several tissues, particularly the central nervous system, are able to counteract primary changes in effective osmolality by adjusting the intracellular amount of osmolytes; if extracellular hypertonicity develops over time, the brain adapts by raising the intracellular levels of substances like amino acids, myoinositol and methylamines (previously called idiogenic osmols). Symptoms may therefore be mild, and correction of the disturbance must allow for reversal of the adaptation.

Disturbances in potassium content

Severe alterations in plasma K^+ are dangerous. Generally, the conditions are considered severe when plasma K^+ is less than half, or more than double, the normal value of approximately $4\,mmol\,L^{-1}$.

Excessive loss of cellular K^+ in connection with cell damage, such as extensive crush damage, may result in hyperkalaemia, particularly in combination with reduced renal function (e.g. as result of shock). If severe and protracted, the condition of shock itself may induce hyperkalaemia due to tissue hypoperfusion, liberation of K^+ from hypoxic cells, and decreased renal function. In these conditions, hyperkalaemia is generated because cellular K^+ is lost faster than the (failing) kidney is able to excrete it; thus total body K^+ may actually be de-

creasing. In addition, chronic K^+ depletion may be associated with hyperkalaemia if present together with metabolic acidosis. In this situation, cell K^+ is exchanged for extracellular H^+. Conversely, metabolic alkalosis may give rise to a condition in which hypokalaemia occurs concomitant with body K^+ levels greater than normal. Chronic K^+ excess and hyperkalaemia are rarely caused by high intake of K^+, but are the result of impaired renal excretion, due sometimes to hypoaldosteronism, but most frequently because of chronic renal failure. Hyperkalaemia affects the electrocardiogram (ECG): the P wave is reduced and the T wave tall and tent-shaped, while widening of the QRS complex may become remarkable (Fig. 21.5). Changes in ECG caused by hyperkalaemia may progress into arrhythmias and ventricular fibrillation and may, therefore, require immediate attention. Temporary measures include intravenous administration of Ca^{2+} salts to reduce muscle cell excitability, and administration of glucose and insulin simultaneously to move K^+ from the extracellular to the intracellular compartment. Permanent reduction of plasma K^+ may require dialysis.

Chronic K^+ losses (through hyperaldosteronism or use of loop diuretics) can be associated with hypokalaemia. If so, ECG changes also occur (Fig. 21.5), including increased QT interval and flattening of the T wave. In addition, muscular weakness increasing to paralysis and impaired urinary concentrating ability, with vasopressin-insensitive polyuria, are characteristics of hypokalaemia.

The relationship between K^+ and acid–base metabolism is described on p. 577.

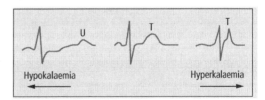

Fig. 21.5 Characteristic changes in an electrocardiogram (ECG) produced by alterations in plasma K^+ concentration. Hypokalaemia results in a reduction in amplitude or reversal in amplitude or reversal of the T wave and the appearance of a U wave; hyperkalaemia results in a reduced P wave, a bizarre QRS complex and a tall, narrow T wave.

Disturbances in magnesium content

The vast majority of body Mg^{2+} is bound to intracellular proteins, and Mg^{2+} deficiency may occur in the presence of normal plasma concentrations. Symptoms may include anorexia, vomiting, and muscular weakness, developing into a syndrome resembling tetany with mental rather than physical irritability. Hypocalcaemia contributes to the hyperirritability, as severe hypomagnesaemia inhibits both the release of parathyroid hormone and the effect of this hormone on the release of Ca^{2+} in skeletal muscle. The major risks in Mg^{2+} depletion are cardiac arrhythmias and cardiac arrest.

Magnesium depletion has been described in chronic diarrhoea, steatorrhoea, and severe chronic alcoholism. It may also be due to sustained renal loss (e.g. due to chronic administration of diuretics). When present, Mg^{2+} deficiency is most often associated with deficiencies in K^+ and phosphorus.

The opposite condition—hypermagnesaemia— is rare, but may occur in relation to end-stage renal disease. Muscle paralysis and coma can result if plasma concentrations exceed $5–7\, mmol\, L^{-1}$.

21.6 Acid–base metabolism and regulation of pH

Biological buffers and the Henderson–Hasselbalch equation

A great number of cell functions, including enzymes, receptors, ion channels and transporters, are pH sensitive, so that small changes in pH are associated with large changes in activity. Therefore, maintenance of pH within a narrow range is important. The pH of arterial blood averages 7.40 ($[H^+] = 39.8\, nmol\, L^{-1}$), and is usually maintained within 7.36–7.44. Values outside the range of 7.0–7.8 are usually lethal. This means that the $[H^+]$ in arterial blood is normally kept within the narrow range of $36–44\, nmol\, L^{-1}$, and that values outside the range $16–100\, nmol\, L^{-1}$ are incompatible with life. In comparison, the pH of gastric juice may fall below 1.0 ($[H^+] = 0.1$ molar $= 100\,000\,000$ $nmol\, L^{-1}$, more than 10^6 times that of blood). Basic

concepts of acid–base reactions are described in Appendix 2.

The pH values of the body fluid compartments (except gastric juice) correspond to H^+ concentrations in the **nanomolar** range. The intracellular fluid is slightly more acidic than blood; normally the pH of the intracellular fluid is about 7.10, corresponding to a $[H^+]$ of approximately $80\, nmol\, L^{-1}$. In very acidic urine (pH = 4.5), the concentration of H^+ may fall to **micromolar** levels. However, metabolism of food constituents from usual diets leaves many **millimoles** of H^+ to be excreted in 1–2 L of urine every day (in addition to other waste products). This excretion of acid takes place concomitant with the excretion of many **moles** of CO_2 per day. CO_2 is the equivalent of acid, because in the body the equilibrium between CO_2 and H_2CO_3 is catalysed by the enzyme carbonic anhydrase. Therefore, the most important equilibrium of acid–base metabolism is that between H^+/HCO_3^- and H_2CO_3/CO_2:

$$H^+ + HCO_3^- \rightleftharpoons H_2CO_3 \rightleftharpoons CO_2 + H_2O \qquad (i)$$

The handling of the large quantities of acid and CO_2 at very low H^+ concentrations would be prone to cause substantial deviations in pH were it not for the additional buffering effects of proteins and phosphates. Proteins, including haemoglobin, are multivalent anions at physiological pH and possess buffer capacity:

$$H^+ + Prot^{n-} \rightleftharpoons HProt^{(n-1)-} \qquad (ii)$$

Such buffers are important due to the large amounts of protein present. In blood, haemoglobin plays a major role in the transport of H^+ (see below). The important phosphate buffer system is:

$$H^+ + HPO_4^{2-} \rightleftharpoons H_2PO_4^{2-} \qquad (iii)$$

as buffer reactions involving phosphoric acid (H_3PO_4) and tertiary phosphate (PO_4^{3-}) are quantitatively negligible.

The buffer systems codetermine a common pH:

$$pH = pK_1 + \log\frac{[HCO_3^-]}{[H_2CO_3]} = pK_2 + \log\frac{[HPO_4^{2-}]}{[H_2PO_4^-]}$$
$$= pK_X + \log\frac{[Prot^{n-}]}{[HProt^{(n-1)-}]}$$

where pK_1 relates to carbonic acid (H_2CO_3), pK_2 to phosphoric acid, and pK_X to proteins. When analysing a mixture, the pH value is determined, and the ratio of base to acid of the individual buffer system is then calculated. The term pK_X is used here only to symbolize the pK values for the individual acid groups of the proteins; it is not feasible to calculate the acid–base behaviour of multiple proteins this way. The titration curve is linear as the pK values of the individual acid groups are rather evenly distributed over the pH scale. The pK_2 for phosphoric acid is about 6.8. At a pH value identical to the pK, the buffer capacity of the system is maximal. Body fluid pH values are relatively close to this pK_2: blood pH falls within 0.6 units, and the pH of urine is frequently between 6.0 and 7.0. Therefore, this buffer system is functionally important. As indicated by reaction (i), the H_2CO_3 system is special to body fluid regulation because H^+ excretion is controlled by the kidneys, at the same time as CO_2 excretion is regulated by the lungs in equilibrium with H_2CO_3, due to the action of the enzyme carbonic anhydrase. In the organism, the [H_2CO_3] is very small, but dissolved CO_2 represents 'functional' H_2CO_3 due to action of the enzyme. Therefore, functionally the correct denominator is the sum of CO_2 and H_2CO_3 which, due to [H_2CO_3] being extremely low, is virtually identical to [CO_2]. The latter is calculated in mmol L^{-1} from P_{CO_2} by means of:

$$[CO_2] = 0.030\, P_{CO_2}$$

where 0.030 is the absorption coefficient for CO_2 in plasma at 38°C (mmol L^{-1} (760 mmHg)$^{-1}$) and P_{CO_2} is in mmHg. The value of pK_1 for H_2CO_3 (6.36) must also be adjusted, partly because the value is relevant only for molar quantities of HCO_3^- and CO_2, and partly because of technical considerations with regard to the measurement of HCO_3^-, including the ionic strength of plasma. The pK value appropriate for plasma concentrations at 38°C is $pK_1' = 6.10$. Often the correction of pK_1 is implicit so that the equation describing the relations between H^+ concentration, HCO_3^- concentration and CO_2 tension most often takes the form of:

$$pH = pK_1 + \log\frac{\left[HCO_3^-\right]}{0.03 \times P_{CO_2}}$$

This equation is called the Henderson–Hasselbalch equation. It is crucially important because kidney function determines the numerator, while alveolar ventilation controls the denominator, and because the balance between the two is constantly challenged by the metabolism, via net production, of H^+ (most often) or OH^- (occasionally).

In the following, the usual situation of net excretion of H^+ will be described first as **metabolic impact, buffering, transport and excretion**. Figure 21.6 gives a simple overview of the essential components of acid–base metabolism. Ingestion and metabolism are summarized in the lower right section. The centre part represents the reactions and transfers of the extracellular compartment, including blood. The process of respiratory excretion of CO_2 is indicated in the top part, while the most important processes of renal excretion of H^+ are summarized to the left. The measures used in the characterization of acid–base metabolism will now be applied to the **acid–base status of the blood**. The four stereotypic anomalies of acid–base metabolism are considered in the following section.

Normal metabolic impact on acid–base balance

The products of cellular metabolism are constantly affecting the acid–base balance. Except for rare occasions, the sum of the metabolic processes is not pH neutral. On a usual mixed diet, including dairy products and meat, metabolic energy is provided concomitant with production of CO_2, H^+, and other waste products, i.e. there is a net gain in H^+. Other diets may result in a net loss of H^+, i.e. a net gain in OH^- (see below). The net gain of H^+ under normal conditions is the result of breakdown of amino acids providing strong acid at a rate 50–80 mmol day^{-1} above the rate by which H^+ is consumed by the metabolic processes, mainly the metabolism of ingested organic anions. This 50–80 mmol of H^+ must be eliminated by the kidneys. In metabolic steady-state, the rate of catabolism of

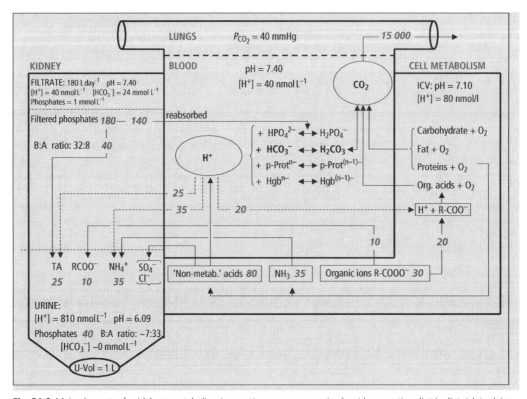

Fig. 21.6 Main elements of acid–base metabolism in a resting person on a mixed, acid-generating diet (a diet rich in dairy products and meat). Ingested carbohydrate, fat, protein, and organic acids are oxidized to yield energy, CO_2, H^+, other waste products, and metabolic water. Blue digits indicate representative steady-state rates of turnover in mmol day^{-1}. The amount of acid ('metabolic H^+') is 80 mmol day^{-1}. CO_2 is produced and excreted via the lungs at a rate of 15 000 mmol day^{-1}. Here, respiration is a mechanism by which arterial P_{CO_2} is maintained at 40 mmHg at all CO_2 production rates. Non-metabolizable acid provides an input of 80 mmol day^{-1} to the extracellular pool of H^+. This H^+ gain is buffered, so that pH deviations remain small at all times, but in terms of input/output the gain is balanced mainly by three processes reducing the extracellular pool of H^+. **(1)** Metabolism of organic acids (OA) ingested and absorbed as anions (OA$^-$ = 20 mmol day^{-1}), but eliminated by oxidation of acid (OA$^-$H$^+$) to CO_2 and water. **(2)** Urinary excretion as titratable acid (TA = 25 mmol day^{-1}) in the form of filtered phosphates. Most of the filtered phosphates (140 of 180 mmol day^{-1}), and notably all of the filtered HCO_3^-, are reabsorbed and returned to the extracellular compartment. Urinary excretion of TA is mainly due to phosphates, which are filtered at base:acid ratio of 4 : 1, but excreted at a ratio of approximately 1 : 5. That is, 80% (4/5) of the filtered, but only 17% (1/6) of the excreted phosphates are present as primary phosphate ($H_2PO_4^{2-}$). This means that the increase in intratubular $[H^+]$ from 40 to 810 nmol L^{-1} has changed the phosphate base:acid ratio, so that 63% of the excreted phosphate ions has accepted a H^+ ion on its way from filtration to final urine. The increase in $[H^+]$ accounts for excretion of 810 − 40 = 770 nmol or 0.77 μmol $[H^+]$ per day; the buffering of filtered phosphate accounts for 25 mmol (25 000 μmol $[H^+]$ per day), or some 32 500 times the amount excreted as H^+. **(3)** Urinary excretion as part of ammonium ion (NH_4^+ = 35 mmol day^{-1}) after binding of H^+ to ammonia (NH_3), which is secreted into the tubular fluid as such. The pK value for NH_4^+/NH_3 is so high (pK$_A$ = 9.2) that the concentration of NH_3 is small at all urine pH values. Practically all the NH_3 secreted into the tubular fluid is excreted as NH_4^+, and is, therefore, accounting for excretion of H^+ in amounts (35 mmol day^{-1}) some 45 000 times that of excretion of free H^+ (0.77 μmol day^{-1}).

To maintain perspicuity, a number of elements have been excluded. These include: (i) the ingestion and metabolic production of phosphoric acid and phosphates contributing to the phosphate buffering; (ii) renal reabsorption of HCO_3^-, which usually is almost complete on an acid-generating diet, and consuming most of the secreted H^+ secreted by the tubules; (iii) the role of urate, oxalate and creatinine in the renal acid excretion; (iv) the intracellular and bone buffers; and (v) the loss of HCO_3^- in faeces (10–20 mmol day^{-1}) equivalent to an input of H^+ ions of similar magnitude. Common to all these mechanisms is that they normally provide minor contributions to the overall acid–base regulation; in special situations, such as very acidic urine (pH < 5.0), base-generating diets, and pathological disturbances, they may be more important. B:A, ratio of concentrations of base and acid form of buffer system; ICV, intracellular volume; non-metab. acids, non-metabolizable acids, including strong inorganic acids from intake and from metabolism of phospholipids and sulphur-containing proteins, and non-metabolizable organic acids (urate, oxalate, creatinine, etc.); TA, titratable acid.

amino acids is identical to the input of amino acids from intestinal absorption. It can be seen from Fig. 21.6, that under conditions of constant protein turnover, the only way to reduce the H^+ load to the kidney is to increase the rate of intake of HCO_3^- (which is normally negligible) or organic acid anions; the latter varies considerably.

Immediate buffering occurs intracellularly, mainly by the actions of proteinate and phosphate. In general terms, the transfer of H^+ across cell membranes is rather slow; however, over time exchange of substantial amounts of H^+ may take place with the cations of bone, such as Na^+, K^+, Ca^{2+} and Mg^{2+}. This is particularly important in situations where there is a chronic disturbance in acid–base balance.

Buffering and transport in the extracellular space

Arterial pH and arterial blood CO_2 tension are normally kept close to 7.40 and 40 mmHg, respectively, and the buffering capacity of blood is considerable. The addition of 28 mmol H^+ to one litre of water lowers the pH from 7.0 to 1.6. However, when added to one litre of blood the same amount of H^+ would lower pH from 7.4 to 7.0 (provided that the P_{CO_2} is maintained at 40 mmHg). In this situation the H^+ concentration increases by only 60 nmol L^{-1}. Almost all of the H^+ ions (27 940 out of the 28 000 nmol) are removed from solution by the four major buffers of the blood—HCO_3^-, haemoglobin, plasma protein, and phosphate. In this example, these buffers neutralize 18, 8, 1.7 and 0.3 mmol of H^+, respectively. However, the concentration of HCO_3^- would be reduced from the normal 24 to 6 mmol L^{-1}. In the interstitial fluid, the buffer capacity is smaller because haemoglobin is absent and plasma proteins are present in much smaller concentrations. Therefore, buffering of this compartment is mainly achieved by HCO_3^-. It is estimated that the capacity of both intracellular and bone buffers is similar to the combined capacity of the extracellular buffer systems.

In peripheral capillaries, O_2 level falls and CO_2 content increases. Carbonic anhydrase is present in erythrocytes. Therefore, reaction (i):

$$H^+ + HCO_3^- \rightleftharpoons H_2CO_3 \rightleftharpoons CO_2 + H_2O$$

proceeds to the left. Buffering, partly by haemoglobin (see Fig. 21.6), maintains the concentration of H^+ at an almost constant level. The arterio–venous increase is about 3 nmol L^{-1} (pH falls from 7.40 to 7.37). In addition, reduced haemoglobin is a stronger base than oxyhemoglobin. Therefore, deoxygenation of haemoglobin increases its efficacy as a physiological buffer. Some two-thirds of the CO_2 in blood is transported as HCO_3^-, the rest as carbamino compounds with haemoglobin (20%) and as dissolved CO_2 (10%). Chloride–bicarbonate exchangers are abundant in the erythrocyte membrane. Intracellular HCO_3^- formed because of CO_2 uptake, therefore exchanges with Cl^- (the Cl^- or Hamburger shift). The increase in intracellular solute content (HCO_3^- or Cl^-) causes redistribution of water by osmosis; thus the haematocrit increases slightly as the blood passes into the capillaries.

Excretion of carbon dioxide (acid equivalents, 'volatile acid') by the lungs

Peripheral arterio–venous differences are reversed in the pulmonary capillaries. Equilibration of O_2 and CO_2 tensions between blood and alveolar compartments is complete, and the gas tensions of arterial blood are very similar to those of alveolar gas. Alveolar gas tensions are regulated via chemoreceptors sensitive (mainly) to arterial P_{CO_2}, which therefore controls alveolar ventilation. This regulation is so efficient that the arterial P_{CO_2} is normally very close to 40 mmHg, irrespective of moderate activity or everyday changes in metabolism (see Chapter 18). Primary changes in alveolar ventilation and inadequate regulation lead to so-called respiratory changes in acid–base balance driven by changes in P_{CO_2} (see below). Alveolar ventilation eliminates CO_2 which, although not an acid, is an acid equivalent because of reaction (i) — if not appropriately excreted, the increase in P_{CO_2} would augment H_2CO_3 levels, increase H^+ concentration and decrease pH.

Excretion of H⁺ by the kidney

Urinary pH may vary between 4.5 and 7.8; however, renal excretion is normally acidic (Fig. 21.6). Net acid excretion is a result of the tubular modification of the glomerular ultrafiltrate, which is similar to plasma water. The essential process is tubular secretion of H^+ and there is considerable interaction between the factors influencing the rate of excretion of K^+ and those affecting H^+ excretion.

Bicarbonate

With regard to HCO_3^-, the reabsorption resulting from tubular luminal secretion of H^+ ions is virtually complete. The reabsorption of HCO_3^- can occur following:

1 H^+ secretion from cells into the lumen by either the Na^+–H^+ exchanger (proximal tubule), the H^+–ATPase (α-intercalated cells), or by the K^+–H^+ exchange pump (cortical and outer medullar collecting duct);

2 combination with filtered HCO_3^- to form H_2CO_3 and CO_2 (with or without the action in the lumen of carbonic anhydrase);

3 diffusion of CO_2 across the luminal membrane, which is highly permeable to CO_2;

4 regeneration of HCO_3^- inside the cell, catalysed by carbonic anhydrase; and

5 basolateral transfer of HCO_3^- (electrogenic Na^+–HCO_3^- co-transporter or anion exchanger) into the interstitial fluid and plasma.

The molecular details vary between tubular segments, but the overall result is that on a normal diet filtration of HCO_3^- does not contribute to the acid–base balance because it is (almost) totally reabsorbed. The situation is quite different where the net result of cellular metabolism is OH^- instead of H^+ (see below).

Phosphate

The tubular luminal secretion of H^+ lowers intratubular pH and changes the ratio of secondary to primary phosphate (base:acid ratio); i.e. reaction (iii, see p. 582) proceeds to the right, and H^+ is removed from solution by the phosphate buffer system. Phosphate ions are filtered at a base:acid ratio of 4:1 because the pK_2 of phosphoric acid is about

6.8 and the pH is 7.4. Most of the filtered phosphate is reabsorbed and returned to the extracellular fluid; this amount does not participate in the regulation of the acid–base balance. The excreted amount (a total of 40 mmol day⁻¹; Fig. 21.6) is excreted at a different base:acid ratio (approximately 1:5; Fig. 21.6). The amount of phosphate ions filtered as secondary phosphate (HPO_4^{2-}) and excreted as primary phosphate ($H_2PO_4^-$), is the buffer effect of phosphate systems at the actual pH change (~25 mmol day⁻¹; Fig. 21.6). Titratable acid (TA) is the amount of strong base that must be added to a sample of urine to bring the pH back to 7.40. Phosphate is by far the most important contributor to TA; minor contributors are creatinine, uric acid and organic acids.

Ammonium ion

Ammonia/ammonium ion is a buffer system that is an important contributor to the renal excretion of H^+. Ammonia (NH_3) is secreted into the renal tubular lumen as such, but is excreted in the urine predominantly as ammonium ion (NH_4^+). Urinary pH may vary between 4.5 and 7.8. The pK_A of NH_3/NH_4^+ is 9.2 and is thus considerably greater than the highest possible urinary pH. From the buffer equation (pH = pK_A + log NH_3/NH_4^+), it is evident that at a representative urinary pH of 6.1 (see Fig. 21.6), log NH_3/NH_4^+ is < –3.0, meaning that more than 99.9% of the secreted NH_3 is present as NH_4^+. Therefore, NH_3 secreted by the tubules is excreted almost quantitatively as NH_4^+, constituting a major pathway for excretion of H^+.

Renal tubular synthesis of NH_3 is based on amino acid metabolism—mainly on conversion of glutamine to glutamate, which may be further deaminated to form α-keto-glutaric acid. The latter reaction may be reverted in the liver, which also synthesizes glutamine, and the glutamate/α-keto-glutaric acid system can be considered as a hepato–renal transfer system for NH_3. Both the hepatic and renal enzyme activities responsible for these reactions adapt markedly to chronic changes in acid–base status. In the case of chronic acidosis, the rate of excretion of NH_4^+ may increase to more than 10-fold that of the normal rate of 30–50 mmol day⁻¹.

Organic anions

Organic acids (R-COOH) are generally relatively weak acids. They may be ingested *per se* or as acid salts (R-COO-), or may arise from the breakdown of larger organic molecules, notably carbohydrates. The latter contribution consists of dissociable acid (R-COOH). Ultimately, the acid form is metabolized to CO_2 and water; therefore there is no overall effect on acid–base balance, apart from the need of buffering in case the intake and/or synthesis of H^+ differs transiently from its breakdown. A minor quantity of organic anions filtered in the kidney is excreted in the urine as such, thereby accounting for a loss that may be considered as a strong base (Fig. 21.6, at the level of 10 mmol day^{-1}); had all organic anions been metabolized, this would have consumed H^+ at a rate of 10 mmol day^{-1}. However, the net effect on acid–base metabolism depends on the form in which these substances were introduced into the body fluids, i.e. anionic or acid form. Organic acids constitute part of the TA of the urine. Conventionally 'net acid excretion' (NEA) is determined by TA, NH_4^+ and HCO_3^- excretion rates (NAE = TA + NH_4^+ – HCO_3^-)—in Fig. 21.6 this amounts to 60 mmol day^{-1} (i.e. 25 + 35 – 0 mmol day^{-1}).

Acid–base status of the blood

The acid–base status of the blood and the extracellular fluid is described in terms of the arterial pH, the arterial CO_2 content (P_{CO_2}), and the base excess (mmol L^{-1}). The base excess is defined as the amount of titratable base on titration to normal pH (7.40) under standard conditions (P_{CO_2} = 40 mmHg, temperature 38°C), but at actual O_2 concentration and saturation. If actual pH values are below 7.40, acid must be titrated to increase the pH to 7.40, and base excess is negative. Base excess in arterial blood is normally zero. However, reduced haemoglobin is a stronger base than oxyhemoglobin, i.e. dexoygenation increases the binding of H^+. In a venous blood sample, base excess is slightly positive (approximately 2 mmol L^{-1}) even though the actual pH is marginally reduced (0.03 units). The reason is the 'standard conditions' under which base excess is determined—the equilibration of venous blood at P_{CO_2} = 40 mmHg (i.e. a reduction of P_{CO_2} by some 6–7 mmHg) elevates pH to values slightly above 7.40, because some 30% of the haemoglobin is present in a reduced, more basic form.

As the H^+ excretion rate by the kidneys and the CO_2 excretion by the lungs are regulated independently, pH and P_{CO_2} are truly independent variables. Both are subject to patho-physiological changes. Base excess provides an estimate of the metabolic (non-respiratory) component of an acid–base disturbance, but a change in base excess may represent either a primary metabolic change or the result of a compensatory reaction to a primary respiratory change (see below). In a clinical situation, the latter is addressed by additional analyses of blood, notably of electrolytes (Na^+, K^+, Cl^- and HCO_3^-), and of O_2 transport parameters including haemoglobin concentration, O_2 saturation, and total O_2 content.

Other concepts of acid–base balance include the so-called 'strong ion difference' defined as the difference between selected cation and anion concentrations ($Na^+ + K^+ + Ca^{2+} + Mg^{2+} – Cl^- – lactate$), and the sum of weak acids. When used, the strong ion difference and total weak acid concentration are considered independent variables. As neither of the variables is independently regulated, this approach may seem less rational physiologically.

Adjustments to changes in dietary load

From day-to-day, regulation of the acid–base balance takes place because dietary and metabolic inputs of H^+ and metabolizable base (organic anions) vary, while lung function (in terms of mean arterial P_{CO_2}) remains approximately constant. That is, physiological adjustments are triggered by changes in 'metabolic' input, rather than by respiratory changes.

Ingestion of acid, or acid-generating compounds such as ammonium chloride, are models of increased non-respiratory acid loads. Such procedures elicit an acceleration in the normal pattern of net acid excretion (Fig. 21.6). The rate of input of strong acid is increased in contrast to the rate of removal of H^+, through the metabolism of organic anions. The excess H$^+$ is buffered almost quantitatively by the extracellular buffer systems, including HCO$_3^-$, thereby elevating Pco$_2$ and increasing alveolar ventilation. The cost of this buffering includes a small decrease in pH and abnormal base:acid ratios of the buffer systems. Both are returned to normal by increased renal excretion of H$^+$. The respiratory excretion is part of the buffering process only; all excess intake of H$^+$ must eventually be excreted by the kidney. Excretion of H$^+$ in the form of ammonium ion is controlled by inducible enzymatic machinery capable of raising the excretion rate of NH$_4^+$ many fold (see above).

The intake of base may increase with certain diets that also tend to be relatively low in meat and milk, while rich in fruit and vegetables. The input of base is mainly as organic anions capable of neutralizing H$^+$ upon conversion to CO$_2$ and water. If protein intake, amino acid turnover, and thus acid production is low, and the intake of organic anions high, the net result may be a negative H$^+$ balance; i.e. cell metabolism eliminates more acid than it produces (see Fig. 21.6). Reaction (i) proceeds to the left because H$^+$ is lost through cell metabolism. Maintenance of pH by buffering is associated with an increase in the HCO$_3^-$ concentration. This leaves the kidney with the task of excreting base instead of acid. Tubular H$^+$ secretion is diminished, and urinary pH increases, so that the rates of excretion of TA (mainly phosphates) and NH$_4^+$ drop sharply. A continuing tendency towards alkalinization (increase in HCO$_3^-$ concentration and pH) leads to excretion of HCO$_3^-$ ions. The renal tubular mechanisms consist mainly of a decrease in renal proximal tubular H$^+$ secretion and a conversion of α-intercalated cells of the cortical collecting duct cells to β-intercalated cells; the latter results in the opposite luminal-to-basolateral distribution of HCO$_3^-$ and H$^+$ transporters and, therefore, secretion of HCO$_3^-$ into the lumen. Quantitatively, extreme alkalinization of the urine (to pH 8.2) decreases urinary H$^+$ concentration by less than one order of magnitude compared to plasma; extreme acidification represents an increase in H$^+$ concentration by a factor of almost 1000 (pH from 7.4 to 4.5).

21.7 Acid–base disturbances

Acidosis and alkalosis are conditions defined by the presence of excess acid and excess base, respectively. By definition (see above), base excess provides a measure of the non-respiratory component of an acid–base disturbance. The deviation in Pco$_2$ reflects the respiratory component of the disease. The 'H$_2$CO$_3$ system' (reaction (i)) plays a key role in controlling the acid–base balance. The reason for this is that the main components of the system, [H$^+$] and Pco$_2$, are regulated independently by different organs, although with highly different rates of change. Disturbances may therefore also arise independently.

An acute decrease in arterial pH may arise for two very different reasons. First, ingestion and/or cell metabolism (non-respiratory pathways) provides additional input into the H$^+$ pool with inverse changes in [HCO$_3^-$] and an altered base:acid ratio for the other buffers; active compensation includes an increase in the alveolar ventilation-normalizing Pco$_2$. Second, a primary increase in Pco$_2$ causes a parallel increase in H$^+$ and HCO$_3^-$; active compensation involves upregulation of a number of enzymes and transporters, thus increasing renal H$^+$ excretion. Analogous considerations apply for increases in arterial pH. Therefore, an abnormal blood pH value indicates the presence of an acid–base disturbance, but is not specific. Furthermore, an acid–base imbalance may also be present at arterial pH values within the normal range when the primary deviation has been (almost) fully compensated for.

The two basic acid–base disorders, acidosis and alkalosis, may both be of respiratory or non-respiratory origin. The term 'metabolic' is often used synonymously with non-respiratory, although only the latter term is technically correct. An overview of simple disturbances is given in Table 21.2. If present for hours and days, compensatory mechanisms will correct the primary deviation, albeit to a variable extent. It may take several weeks for these mechanisms to be fully activated. Therefore, the degree of compensation depends not only on the duration of disease, but also on the primary insult. For example, respiratory

Table 21.2 Simple acid–base disturbances. BE, base excess.

Acid–base disturbance		Primary change	Prototype situation	Acute changes	Chronic compensation	Compensated acid–base disturbance
Acidosis	metabolic	Surplus of H^+	Increased H^+ production (diabetic ketoacidosis)	pH ↓ [HCO_3^-] ↓ P_{CO_2} normal, BE ↓ plasma K^+ ↑	Ventilation ↑, P_{CO_2} ↓ Renal upregulation of enzymes and transporters, H^+ secretion ↑, NH_4^+ excretion ↑	pH partially compensated P_{CO_2} ↓ plasma HCO_3^- ↓ hyperkalaemia
	respiratory (hypercapnia)	Increase in P_{CO_2}	Inadequate alveolar ventilation (poisoning, drugs)	pH ↓ [HCO_3^-] ↑ P_{CO_2} ↑ BE normal plasma K^+ ↑	Renal upregulation of enzymes and transporters, H^+ secretion ↑, NH_4^+ excretion ↑	pH almost normal, plasma HCO_3^- ↑ hyperkalaemia
Alkalosis	metabolic	Loss of H^+	Loss of H^+ (severe vomiting)	pH ↑ [HCO_3^-] ↑ P_{CO_2} normal BE ↑ plasma K^+ ↓	Renal: H^+ secretion ↓, α to β conversion of intercalated cells → HCO_3^- secretion ↑	Often incomplete: pH increased but compensated hypokalaemia
	respiratory (hypocapnia)	Decrease in P_{CO_2}	Hyperventilation (acclimatization, artificial ventilation)	pH ↑ [HCO_3^-] ↓ P_{CO_2} ↓ BE normal plasma K^+ ↓	Renal: H^+ secretion ↓, α to β conversion of intercalated cells → HCO_3^- secretion ↑	pH almost normal, plasma HCO_3^- ↓ hypokalaemia

compensation of metabolic alkalosis is less efficient than respiratory compensation of metabolic acidosis. Simultaneous determinations of pH, P_{CO_2}, and base excess are used to characterize acid–base disturbances. In a specific clinical situation, the acid–base disorder may be uncompensated, partially compensated, or fully compensated. In addition, the underlying disease may influence the relationship between the primary insult and the results of physicochemical analyses. As mentioned above, haemoglobin concentration and saturation determines its acid–base behaviour, as deoxygenated haemoglobin is a stronger base than oxyhaemoglobin. The complexity of a given clinical situation is often considerable.

Chapter 22

Energy Metabolism

22.1 Energy, thermodynamics and animals

The term 'energy' comes from the Greek words en (meaning in, within) and ergon (meaning work) and is thus an apt description of the effort required to stay alive and to grow. The word 'metabolism' is also derived from Greek (metabole, meaning change) and describes the chemical reactions (i.e. changes) that take place within a living organism to maintain life. Energy metabolism is a property of every living cell and to say an organism is 'alive' is to say it has an energy metabolism. To measure the rate of this energy metabolism (metabolic rate) is to measure the 'cost of living'.

Animals are descended from bacteria that obtained their energy and carbon skeletons by feeding on other organisms. Humans are classified as obligate aerobic heterotrophs, which means that during metabolism, the carbon and hydrogen atoms in food molecules are combined with oxygen atoms to produce CO_2 and H_2O. The chemical energy contained in the food molecules is released during metabolism and used to do work, with most of it eventually being converted to heat.

Early investigations into energy metabolism showed that animals obey the laws of thermodynamics and the amount of energy released during metabolism is the same as that released by the combustion or 'burning' of the same foodstuffs. Although food is a complex mixture of molecules, for the purposes of this chapter, the most important components of food are **carbohydrates**, **fats** (or **lipids**) and **proteins**. Digestion is covered in Chapter 19. Energy metabolism has been called the 'fire of life' and can be described by the following equation:

$$\text{nutrients (carbohydrate, fat, protein)} + O_2$$
$$\rightarrow CO_2 + H_2O + \text{nitrogenous waste} + \text{energy}$$

Metabolism is divided into **catabolism** and **anabolism** (Table 22.1 and Fig. 22.1) Catabolism comprises the pathways where complex nutrient macromolecules are broken down to simple, smaller molecules with the release of chemical free energy. Anabolism comprises the metabolic pathways involved in the synthesis of complex molecules from simpler ones and requires the input of energy. Catabolic pathways deliver chemical energy in the form of adenosine triphosphate (ATP), nicotinamide adenine dinucleotide (reduced) (NADH), nicotinamide adenine dinucleotide phosphate (reduced) (NADPH), and flavin adenine dinucleotide (reduced) ($FADH_2$), and these energy carriers are used to run anabolic pathways. In the process of releasing their energy during anabolism, these carriers are converted to adenosine diphosphate (ADP), NAD^+, $NADP^+$ and FAD, respectively, and are then regenerated following catabolism.

Table 22.1 Definition of some key metabolic processes. ATP, adenosine triphosphate; NADH, nicotinamide adenine dinucleotide (reduced).

CATABOLIC	
Glycogenolysis:	breakdown of glycogen to produce glucose-1-phosphate (which can then enter glycolysis).
Glycolysis:	conversion of glucose to pyruvate in living cells, with the accompanying synthesis of ATP and NADH. It does not require the presence of oxygen.
Lipolysis:	breakdown of triglycerides to glycerol and fatty acids. It occurs primarily in adipose cells during the mobilization of energy reserves.
ANABOLIC	
Gluconeogenesis:	metabolic pathway by which glucose is synthesized from non-carbohydrates such as lactate, some amino acids, and glycerol. It occurs primarily in liver and kidney.
Glycogenesis:	synthesis of glycogen from glucose.
Lipogenesis:	synthesis of fatty acids and other lipids from acetyl-CoA.
Ketogenesis:	synthesis of ketone bodies (e.g. acetoacetate, acetone and other) formed in the liver from excess acetyl-CoA, which occurs especially during fasting and starvation. They can be used as a fuel by other cells.

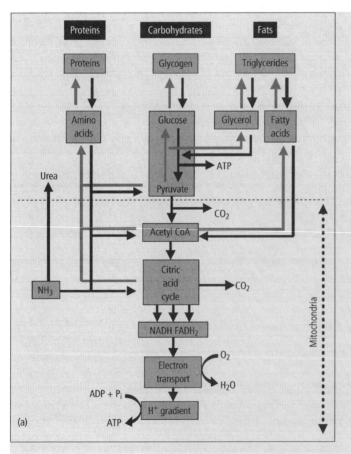

Fig. 22.1 (a) An outline of the main metabolic pathways and key intermediates involved in the metabolism of proteins, carbohydrates and fats in cells. The black lines and arrows represent catabolic (energy-producing) pathways, while the blue lines and arrows represent anabolic (energy-consuming) pathways. All the processes below the dashed line take place in the mitochondria of cells. (b) (*facing*) The relationship of the high-energy intermediates to the link between anabolism and catabolism. ADP, adenosine diphosphate; ATP, adenosine triphosphate; FAD(H$_2$), flavin adenine dinucleotide (reduced); NAD(H), nicotinamide adenine dinucleotide (reduced); NADP(H$_2$), nicotinamide adenine dinucleotide phosphate (reduced); P$_i$, inorganic phosphate.

The concentration of high-energy intermediates in cells is not great, but metabolism is organized to rapidly regenerate them once used. Resting cells, such as liver and nerve cells, contain ~3 mmol ATP and ~1 mmol ADP, while a muscle cell might have ~8 mmol ATP and ~1 mmol ADP. The basic structure of cellular energy metabolism is illustrated in Fig. 22.1. As can be seen, the pathways responsible for metabolizing carbohydrates, fats and proteins are all linked, and thus all three types of nutrients can be used to produce ATP. Although energy can be obtained from the catabolism of proteins and fats, some cell types (notably nerve cells and red blood cells) primarily use glucose as their source of energy, and for this reason the blood glucose concentration is maintained at a relatively constant level.

During catabolism, electrons and hydrogen atoms are removed and CO_2 is released from these molecules before the consumption of O_2, with the last part of aerobic catabolism essentially being when electrons and H^+ ions are combined with O_2 to form H_2O molecules. An important aspect of metabolism is that electron transport in the mitochondria is organized such that H^+ ions (protons) are pumped out of the mitochondrial matrix and a large H^+ ion gradient is created across the mitochondrial inner membrane. The return of these protons to the mitochondrial matrix (down the proton gradient) via ATP synthase (a protein embedded in the mitochondrial inner membrane) results in ATP synthesis from ADP and inorganic phosphate (P_i). The chemical energy in the initial metabolic fuel is thus temporarily stored as energy in an electrochemical gradient (the H^+ gradient) before being converted back to usable chemical energy in the form of ATP.

The production of ATP is not very energy efficient. For example, the complete metabolism of glucose to CO_2 and H_2O releases ~2850 kJ mol^{-1} of free energy and only about 40% is converted to chemical energy in the form of ATP; the remaining 60% is released as heat and is thus not 'usable' energy. The catabolism of fats produces ATP with similar energy efficiency, while ATP production from protein is less efficient (25–35%, depending on the protein).

The 'usable' energy conserved in ATP can be used in cellular work of three types:

1 **transport work**, to move molecules across membranes;

2 **mechanical work**, to create movement by causing intracellular fibres and filaments to move in relation to one another; and

3 **chemical work**, for the synthesis of other molecules (i.e. anabolism).

At the level of the whole organism, if this cellular work is not converted to work on the external environment, or into growth of the organism, the energy consumed from the ATP will eventually be released as 'heat'.

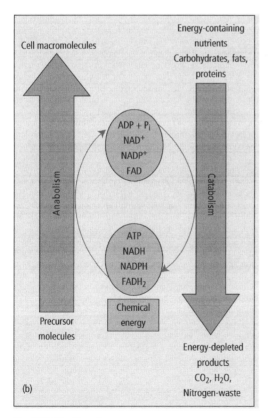

Fig. 22.1 *Continued*

22.2 Metabolic rate: the measurement of energy metabolism

The rate of energy metabolism is called the metabolic rate and can be determined by measuring the rate of change in any of the individual components of the equation describing energy metabolism (see above). Metabolic rate can be measured as the rate of any of the following:

1 food energy consumption (less energy excreted in the faeces);
2 oxygen consumption;
3 carbon dioxide production;
4 metabolic water production; and
5 heat production.

Each technique for measuring metabolic rate has both advantages and disadvantages. Measurement of **heat production** requires a calorimeter (named after the calorie, an early unit of energy; 1 calorie = 4.2 J). This is a sophisticated and expensive piece of equipment in which the organism must be completely enclosed. Measurement of the amount of new **water production** from metabolism is difficult because it is not possible to separate it from the preformed water molecules taken in. For this reason it is never used to measure the metabolic rate of humans. However, it has been used to measure the metabolic rate of animals (such as desert rodents) that do not have access to free water and consume dry food. Measurement of **carbon dioxide production** is technically possible but has two disadvantages. The first is that the amount of CO_2 produced varies significantly depending on which fuel is being metabolized (see Table 22.2). The second disadvantage is that body fluids contain large amounts of HCO_3^- ions and in some situations

(such as changes in the acid–base balance of the body) CO_2 excretion rates are not related to metabolic rate. Measurement of **oxygen consumption** is technically easy, although it normally has to be done in a laboratory setting. Determining metabolic rate by the measurement of **food energy consumption** has a number of disadvantages: it is only a measure of metabolic rate if there are no changes in energy storage (i.e. no change in body mass); and it is necessary to know both the amount and composition of the food consumed (and thus its energy content) as well as the amount (and energy content) of the faeces excreted. These can be difficult to determine. However, it does have the advantage that it can be used to approximate metabolic rate over extended periods outside of a laboratory setting.

In recent years, the **doubly-labelled water** technique has been used to assess the metabolic rate of free-ranging individuals over extended periods. The individual is injected with water molecules made from the non-radioactive isotopes ^{18}O and ^2H and, after allowing a few hours for equilibration with body fluids, a sample of body water is taken (blood, urine, saliva, or even tears) and the concentration of ^{18}O and ^2H measured. The individual is allowed to go about their normal activities and another sample of body water is taken several days later and the concentrations of ^{18}O and ^2H measured again. During this period ^2H leaves the body as ^2H_2O; however the ^{18}O atoms in H_2O molecules exchange with the oxygen atoms in CO_2 and leave the body as both $H_2^{18}O$ and $C^{18}O_2$. The difference in the loss of ^{18}O and ^2H can be used to calculate CO_2 excretion, and thus metabolic rate during the period between the two body water samples. This technique has been used to measure the metabolic

Table 22.2 Energy content, oxygen consumed, and carbon dioxide produced when either carbohydrate, protein or fat are the sole nutrients being metabolized.

	$kJ g^{-1}$	$L O_2 g^{-1}$	$L CO_2 g^{-1}$	RQ[#]	$kJ L^{-1} O_2$	$kJ L^{-1} CO_2$
Carbohydrate	17.5	0.83	0.83	1.00	21.1	21.1
Protein*	18.6	0.97	0.78	0.81	19.3	23.6
Fat	39.6	2.02	1.43	0.71	19.6	27.7

[#] Respiratory quotient (RQ) = CO_2 produced/O_2 consumed.

* The nitrogenous excretory product is urea.

rate of individual humans undergoing their normal daily activities.

Carbohydrates, fats and proteins release different amounts of energy per gram when metabolized, and also result in different amounts of O_2 consumed and CO_2 produced (Table 22.2). As metabolic fuels, carbohydrate and fat have different properties, with protein being intermediate. There is much less variation in the $kJ L^{-1} O_2$ consumed ($\pm 4\%$) with the different metabolic fuels compared to the $kJ L^{-1} CO_2$ produced ($\pm 13\%$) (see Table 22.2). Thus if the fuel being metabolized is unknown then less error results if the measure is oxygen consumption. This is one reason why oxygen consumption is generally the preferred measure of metabolic rate. The respiratory quotient (RQ) is the ratio of CO_2 produced:O_2 consumed, and this equals 1.0 if carbohydrate is the metabolic fuel, and 0.7 if fat is being metabolized for energy. Measuring both O_2 consumed and CO_2 produced is the most accurate method for assessing energy metabolism and can normally indicate the fuel an individual is metabolizing.

Metabolic rate varies according to the work being done. **Basal metabolic rate (BMR)** is the minimal rate of energy metabolism. The **maximal metabolic rate** that can be sustained is called the maximal aerobic capacity and is also known as VO_2max. Although individuals can work at rates greater that this maximum for short periods using

anaerobic metabolism, such work rates cannot be sustained (see Chapter 24). **Daily metabolic rate** falls somewhere between these two extremes, depending on the activity of the individual.

Basal metabolic rate (BMR)

The BMR is the rate of energy metabolism of a post-absorptive, resting adult in a thermoneutral environment. As these conditions indicate, the main factors resulting in an elevated metabolic rate are processing a meal, muscular activity, growth, and maintaining a constant body temperature in a cold environment. We will deal with each of these influences later but will first examine the cellular activities responsible for the BMR. For a 65-kg human, BMR is about $14 L O_2 h^{-1}$ or $\sim 290 kJ h^{-1}$ (i.e. $6900 kJ day^{-1}$). Since $1 W = 1 J s^{-1}$, this is about the same energy consumption as an 80 W light bulb!

During the resting state associated with BMR, most of the energy metabolism and thus heat production occurs in the internal organs (Table 22.3). These internal organs (liver, heart, lungs, kidneys, brain, etc.) make up about 8% of total body mass but are responsible for more than 70% of the heat produced and O_2 consumed during rest.

The cellular processes that use this energy include ion transport, mechanical work, and the biosynthesis of molecules. The relative importance of these processes however varies between tissues.

Table 22.3 The relative size of the major organs of a 65-kg human and their energy metabolism (heat production) at rest.

Organ	Mass (kg)	% total mass	Heat production (kJ h⁻¹)	% total
Brain	1.35	2.1	52.3	16.0
Heart	0.29	0.45	35.1	10.7
Lungs	0.60	0.9	14.2	4.4
Kidneys	0.29	0.45	25.1	7.7
Splanchnic organs*	2.50	3.8	110.0	33.6
Summed organs		**7.7**		**72.4**
Skin	5.00	7.8	6.3	1.9
Muscle	27.00	41.5	51.0	15.7
Other	27.97	43.0	32.6	10.0
Total	65.00	100.0	326.6	100.0

* Abdominal organs not including kidneys (i.e. includes liver).

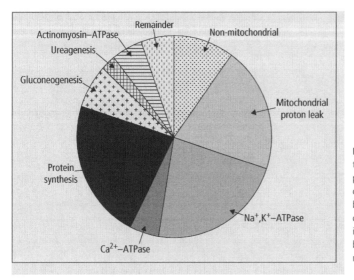

Fig. 22.2 An estimation of the relative contribution of various cellular processes to basal metabolic rate. The contribution of these processes varies between tissues, and the relative size of tissues has been taken into account in these estimations. The blue contributions are those associated with membranes.

For example, the membrane pump responsible for maintaining a low intracellular Na^+ concentration (the Na^+,K^+–ATPase; see Chapter 1) is responsible for ~60% of energy consumption of neurones and kidney cells but only ~10% in liver cells. This is because the Na^+ gradient across the plasma membrane of cells is the immediate source of energy for action potentials, as well as being intimately involved in ion transport across cells, and both cellular ion homeostasis and volume control. Thus the activity of the Na^+ pump is a major activity in neurones and kidney cells but not as important in liver cells.

Similarly, even when they are not making ATP, mitochondria maintain a proton gradient across the mitochondrial inner membrane, which is continually being dissipated by a leak of protons back into the mitochondrial matrix. The activity of the mitochondrial respiratory chain to counteract this proton leak is also a significant part of the energy turnover of resting cells.

Ion gradients can be expressed as electrical potentials across membranes. For example, the ion gradients across the plasma membrane represent a membrane potential of ~90 mV in neurones and muscle cells and ~40 mV in liver cells. The potential across the mitochondrial inner membrane is approximately 160–200 mV.

When the contributions from various tissues are summed, it is estimated that ~10% of mammalian BMR is non-mitochondrial O_2 consumption. Approximately 20% constitutes O_2 consumed by mitochondria to maintain the proton gradient against mitochondrial proton leak, and the remaining 70% is consumed by mitochondria to manufacture ATP. This provides energy for protein synthesis (~20–25%), maintenance of the trans-plasma membrane Na^+ gradient by the Na^+ pump (~20–25%), maintenance of trans-membrane Ca^{2+} gradients (~5%), gluconeogenesis (~7%), ureagenesis (~2.5%) and actinomyosin–ATPase activity (~5%), with activities such as nucleic acid synthesis and substrate-cycling accounting for the remainder of ATP turnover (Fig. 22.2).

Body size and BMR

Small mammals have a much higher BMR per kg of body mass than larger mammals. The BMR of a 3800-kg elephant is 0.4 W kg^{-1}, while the BMR of a 5-g shrew is 40 W kg^{-1}. This represents a 100-fold difference in metabolic intensity! The reason why we don't find mammals smaller than shrews, is that in order to service such high rates of energy metabolism, mammals of this size have heart rates and respiratory rates of ~1000 min^{-1}. This is a cycle time of ~60 ms, which is similar to the duration of an action potential and thus represent the highest possible respiratory and heart rates.

Mammals, irrespective of size, have essentially the same body temperature, but larger species have a much smaller surface area per kg of body mass. For this reason it is essential that metabolic rate per kg must decrease with increasing body size. It has been calculated that if a mouse-sized mammal was scaled up to a horse-sized mammal without a change in its BMR per kg body mass, then this horse-sized mouse would need a surface temperature of > 100°C just to rid itself of the heat produced by its BMR. A self-cooking mammal!

Although this mouse-to-elephant BMR relationship has been known for a long time, the cellular basis for this variation in BMR has been described only recently. As noted above, membrane-associated processes constitute a large component of BMR. In small mammals such as mice, cellular membranes are highly polyunsaturated (especially with the omega-3 polyunsaturates) and with increases in body size, the degree of polyunsaturation of membrane lipids decreases in a systematic way. It seems that polyunsaturated membrane lipids can increase the activity of enzyme proteins in membranes and in this way increase BMR. When the membrane lipids surrounding Na^+ pumps from one species are replaced with more polyunsaturated membrane lipids from a species with a high BMR, the pumps increase their activity. If the membrane pumps are surrounded by less polyunsaturated lipids from a species with a lower BMR, pump activity decreases.

This association of polyunsaturated membranes with high BMR has also been observed in bird species, ranging from finches to emus, and in comparison of cold-blooded (ectothermic) species with warm-blooded (endothermic) species. Whether such membrane differences can explain some of the variation in BMR of humans is currently being investigated.

Specific dynamic action: effect of a meal on energy metabolism

Metabolic rate is increased for several hours follow-ing a meal. This effect is called **specific dynamic action** (**SDA**). The period following a meal, when the products of digestion are being absorbed, used and stored is called the **fed** or **absorptive state**. The period after this is called the **fasting** or **post-absorptive state**. SDA was initially thought to be the 'work of digestion', representing the costs associated with mastication, muscle movements to transport food through the gut, secretion of digestive fluids and enzymes, as well as the cost of nutrient absorption. However, these processes represent only a small part of SDA, as most SDA occurs even when the digestive system is by-passed and nutrients are provided intravenously. SDA is largely due to the metabolic processing of food, especially protein, after it has been absorbed.

The intensity of SDA varies according to both the size and type of a meal. The larger the meal the larger the SDA and the longer it lasts after the meal. A meal high in protein can result in SDA of ~30% BMR, while a meal with the same total energy content, but as fat, will result in a SDA of ~13% BMR, and a carbohydrate meal will have an SDA of ~6% BMR. The time-course for the heat produced from SDA following a meal coincides with the time-course of increased urinary nitrogen excretion. This observation, together with the large influence of protein content on the magnitude of the SDA, and the fact that mammals do not have a system for storing excess protein, suggests that the predominant part of SDA is the metabolic processing of protein. This includes the deamination of individual amino acids, the consequent synthesis of urea molecules for nitrogen excretion and the synthesis of carbohydrate and fat energy stores from the carbon skeletons of the amino acids.

Activity and energy metabolism

When BMR is being measured, the only significant muscle actions are those of the heart and respiratory muscles. The use of skeletal muscles to do work has the greatest effect on metabolic rate. The more intense the activity, the greater the metabolic rate. A range of human activities and their associated metabolic rates are listed in Table 22.4. This demonstrates that during intense activity or heavy

Table 22.4 Metabolic rate (kJ h^{-1}) of humans during various activities. BMR, basal metabolic rate.

Activity	kJ h^{-1}
BMR	290
Standing at ease	425
Walking at 1 km h^{-1}	500
Driving a car	700
Walking at 4 km h^{-1}	850
Cricket batting	1500
Playing tennis	1780
Rapid marching	2400
Playing squash	2560
Axe work (51 blows min^{-1})	6000
Carrying 60 kg upstairs	7700

work metabolic rate can be up to 27-times the BMR. Daily activity and work vary dramatically among humans, depending on their occupation. On average, up to 70% of a person's daily energy requirements is determined by their BMR. Exercise is covered in more detail in Chapter 24.

Growth and energy metabolism

Growth is a form of work. In humans it is the biosynthesis of new body constituents. In agricultural animals growth includes the production of meat, eggs, milk, fat, wool, etc.

At birth, a human baby's metabolic rate is lower than expected for its body mass, but within 18–30 h, it increases dramatically to be more than twice the metabolic rate of an adult human per kg of body mass. During the first year of human life, the metabolic rate in relation to body mass increases more rapidly than predicted from the increase in mass. After the first year the rate of increase slows. During this first year the metabolic demands of the brain accounts for more than 50% of the total metabolic rate of the baby. This is because the brain is a metabolically expensive tissue and makes up a much larger percentage of the body mass (~14%) than in an adult human (~2%).

During growth, metabolic rate is high for two reasons: first, because of the cost of synthesizing new tissue; and second, because the metabolically-expensive tissues (e.g. brain, liver) make up a greater percentage of the body.

Thermoregulation and energy metabolism

The final product of energy metabolism is heat. In cold environments (i.e. at temperatures below thermoneutrality) mammals, including humans, use involuntary micro-contractions of antagonistic muscles, not to do work, but to create heat (**thermogenesis**). This is called shivering and is covered in more detail in Chapter 23. Since all metabolic activity produces heat, even the heat produced processing a meal (SDA) can be used for thermoregulation, and this substitutes for the heat produced by shivering in cold environments. After a meal, shivering thermogenesis will be activated at a lower ambient temperature than is the case in the fasting state. Similarly the heat produced by activity can be used for thermoregulation but activity has the disadvantage of often increasing the loss of body heat.

22.3 Energy balance and the storage of metabolic energy

Energy balance is the difference between energy intake and energy output (metabolic rate). If the rate of metabolism exceeds the food energy intake, the subject is in a state of **negative energy balance** and the energy deficit is provided by the body's energy stores. If food energy intake exceeds the metabolic rate, a state of **positive energy balance** ensues and the excess energy taken in is stored. Energy storage differs from growth in that excess energy is stored as either carbohydrate or fat molecules, but not protein molecules; whereas growth involves the synthesis of all the molecules that make up body tissues, and thus includes the synthesis of proteins and nucleic acids.

The storage form of carbohydrates in animals is the polymer **glycogen**, which consists of long branched chains of glucose molecules. In plants, the storage carbohydrate is **starch**, which also consists of chains of glucose, but these are less branched than in glycogen. Glycogen is especially abundant in the liver where it is used to maintain blood glucose levels relatively constant. It is also present in muscle.

In animals fat is stored in the form of **triglycerides** (also called **triacylglycerols**), which consist of three fatty acid chains (normally containing 16–20 carbon atoms), each linked to the three-carbon backbone of a glycerol molecule. Triglycerides are stored in adipose tissue, which consists of **adipocytes** (fat cells) and is amorphous and widely distributed throughout the body.

Fat contains more than twice the energy per gram than carbohydrate. Fat has another advantage over carbohydrate as an energy store; carbohydrates are hydrophilic molecules and are therefore stored hydrated, while fat molecules being hydrophobic are stored without additional water molecules. When these differences are combined, the storage of metabolic energy as fat is almost 10-times more efficient than the storage of carbohydrate, in terms of the additional body tissue that must be carried. In most animals, metabolic energy is almost always stored as fat.

Storage of energy as carbohydrate, however, does have two advantages. The energy stored in carbohydrates can be accessed more quickly than from fat. In addition, it is available anaerobically, whereas energy stored as fat is only available via aerobic metabolism. It is thus advantageous to make sure muscles have a source of intracellular glycogen for rapid bursts of activity.

Hormonal control of food intake and energy metabolism

The maintenance of energy balance is normally achieved by the regulation of food energy intake. The brain integrates long-term energy balance in response to both hormonal and neural input. The status of long-term energy stores is signalled by the hormones **leptin** (produced from adipose tissue) and **insulin** (from the endocrine pancreas). Recent nutrisional state is signalled both hormonally, by various gut peptides, and neurally via the vagus nerve, which relates information about stomach distension as well as the chemical and hormonal status of the upper small intestine. These act as

satiety signals (i.e. the feeling of having enough) by inhibiting appetite-stimulating neurones in the hypothalamus that contain **neuropeptide Y (NPY)**. The NPY neurones in turn act on second-order neurones in the brain to stimulate eating, and regulate both the timing and the size of meals.

Ghrelin is a hormone released by the stomach that stimulates appetite by activating the NPY-expressing neurones in the hypothalamus. The control of food intake is currently an area of intense research activity in an attempt to develop anti-obesity drugs that act as satiety signals and thus control excessive eating. These pathways are illustrated in Fig. 22.3.

Several hormones influence metabolism and are described in more detail in Chapter 11. Most affect the availability of various fuels; some stimulate anabolism (e.g. insulin), others stimulate catabolism (e.g. glucagon, noradrenaline, glucocorticoids), while some have both anabolic and catabolic effects (e.g. thyroxine, growth hormone). The thyroid hormones (thyroxine, triiodothyronine) increase BMR, and prior to the availability of hormone assays, measurement of BMR was the method used clinically to determine thyroid status. A high BMR indicated hyperthyroidism and a low BMR indicated a hypothyroid state. Some hormonal influences on metabolism are listed in Table 22.5.

Starvation

Total starvation results in eventual death. Without food the chemical energy required to run the body comes from the metabolism of body substance (Fig. 22.4). Carbohydrate stores (liver and muscle glycogen) are the first energy stores to be metabolized. Because they are stored with water, the loss of body mass following the metabolism of these glycogen stores is many times the loss if the same amount of energy had been provided by fat metabolism. The human body has less than one day's energy requirements stored as carbohydrate. Individuals that either fast or commence an energy-restriction diet lose a large amount of body weight in the first days (which is mainly water loss), but then often become disheartened when

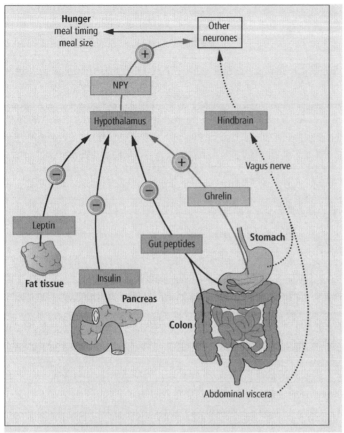

Fig. 22.3 Summary of the inputs controlling food intake. The hormonal inputs include adiposity signals (leptin and insulin) and satiety signals (various gut peptides) that inhibit neuropeptide Y (NPY)-containing neurones in the hypothalamus, as well as the hunger signal (ghrelin) from the stomach that stimulates these neurones. The NPY-containing hypothalamic neurones together with neural inputs from the vagus nerve act on second order neurones in the brain, which then controls the timing and size of meals via the 'hunger' drive.

Table 22.5 Hormones and their effects on metabolism.

Hormone	Blood glucose	Carbohydrate metabolism	Protein metabolism	Lipid metabolism
Insulin	decreased	↑ glycogen formation ↓ glycogenolysis ↓ gluconeogenesis	↑ amino acid transport	↑ lipogenesis ↓ lipolysis ↓ ketogenesis
Glucagon	increased	↓ glycogen formation ↑ glycogenolysis ↑ gluconeogenesis	no direct effect	↑ lipolysis ↑ ketogenesis
Growth hormone	increased	↑ glycogenolysis ↑ gluconeogenesis ↑ glucose utilization	↑ protein synthesis	↓ lipogenesis ↑ lipolysis ↑ ketogenesis
Glucocorticoids	increased	↓ glycogen formation ↑ gluconeogenesis	↓ protein synthesis	↓ lipogenesis ↑ lipolysis ↑ ketogenesis
Noradrenaline	increased	↓ glycogen formation ↑ glycogenolysis ↑ gluconeogenesis	no direct effect	↑ lipolysis ↑ ketogenesis
Thyroxine	no effect	↑ glucose utilization	↑ protein synthesis	no direct effect

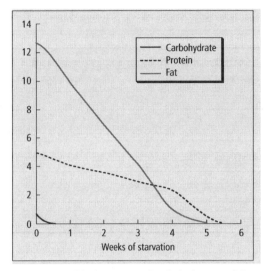

Fig. 22.4 Initial body reserves of carbohydrates, mobilizable proteins, and fats of a typical human, and their changes during total starvation.

the rate of weight loss rapidly diminishes as they move into the fat metabolism stage that follows.

Following the initial stage, body fat is metabolized as the primary source of energy. The length of this second stage of starvation depends largely on the initial level of body fat stores. Body triglyceride stores in a typical human would be ~12.5 kg and this is enough to fuel BMR for more than a month. A moderately obese individual may have 15–20 kg of fat which is enough energy to fuel the BMR for approximately 3 months. However, a disadvantage of fat metabolism is that gluconeogenesis is not adequately supported by fat catabolism (see Fig. 22.1) and thus blood glucose cannot be maintained solely by fat catabolism. Body protein is also catabolized during this second stage of starvation as gluconeogenesis is possible from some amino acids.

Loss of body mass during starvation is not shared equally among the tissues. Adipose tissue can lose ~97% of its initial mass, whereas the brain and heart lose only negligible mass. Liver can lose 50–70% of its original mass, while skin and hair, intestinal tract, and skeletal muscle can lose 20–30% of their initial weight. The loss of proteins from the digestive tract means that recovery from severe starvation requires provision of food that requires little digestion.

Obesity and the metabolic syndrome

When energy intake exceeds energy output for an extended period, then the quantity of body adipose tissue increases. Lack of exercise coupled with excessive intake of high-energy food is an obvious cause of obesity. Body mass index (BMI) has been used to quantify this:

$$BMI = mass\ (kg)/height\ (m)^2$$

Obesity is increasing in incidence in the developed world, and although the above scenario can result in excessive obesity, it appears that the problem may have other possible causes.

In the 1980s, it was realized that obesity, hypertension, type II (or mature onset) diabetes, and blood dyslipidaemias, as well as some other conditions, often occurred together. The primary cause was unknown and their co-occurrence was initially described as 'syndrome X'. More recently it has been renamed the 'metabolic syndrome' and it has become apparent that **insulin-resistance** is basic to this condition. Animal studies have shown that the syndrome can be induced by dietary change and that the insulin-resistance appears very early after implementing this change, preceding obesity and the development of hypertension. It has been documented that ~25% of the US population currently suffers from metabolic syndrome. The reason for the recent increase in incidence is the subject of intense research.

One possible, intriguing explanation is the suggestion that the balance between omega-6 and omega-3 polyunsaturates in the modern human food chain has changed. Both types of fatty acids cannot be synthesized by animals and are essential dietary components, as well as being important constituents of cell membranes. Human diets have generally had approximately equal amounts of both types of fat; however, recently the human food chain in the developed world has increased in omega-6 fats, at the expense of omega-3. Plants make omega-3 fats in the chloroplasts in their leaves (the site of photosynthesis), yet they store fats in their seeds as omega-6. Fish are an excellent source of omega-3 fats but do not synthesize them—they obtain them from the algae at the base of the marine food chain. Changing the balance of these fats to favour omega-6 in the diet of animals can both decrease metabolic rate and result in insulin-resistance. If this hypothesis turns out to be correct, it will justify the parental advice most of us received as children: "eat your greens!"

Chapter 23

Temperature Regulation

23.1 Temperature and life

Life exists in a universe with temperatures ranging from near absolute zero (–273°C) to greater than 1 000 000°C. However, temperatures inside most living organisms fall into a much narrower range— from 0 to 45°C. At the lower end of this range, water freezes; at the higher end, enzymes that catalyse living reactions start denaturing. Because 'lower' animals have a body temperature at the lower end or in the middle of this range they are **cold-blooded**. They are also **poikilothermic**, i.e. their body temperature changes with a change in ambient temperature, **bradymetabolic**, (their metabolic rate is low and does not increase in response to cold), and **ectothermic**, (their major source of heat is their external environment). In contrast, 'higher' animals (mammals and birds) have a body temperature close to denaturing temperatures and are therefore **warm-blooded**. These animals are classed as being **homeothermic**, as their body temperature is maintained at a relatively constant level and is largely independent of ambient temperature. They achieve warm-bloodedness and homeothermy because they can readily generate heat. They have a high metabolic rate and can further increase it in response to cold, i.e. they are **tachymetabolic**, and they are **endothermic** because their major source of heat is inside their body. Based on the above, man can be looked upon as a warm-blooded, homeothermic,

tachymetabolic, and endothermic animal. By using powerful autonomic and even more powerful behavioural means, man can survive at ambient temperatures ranging from –110°C (the surface of the Moon) to 2000°C (the air around a space shuttle as it re-enters the atmosphere), while maintaining deep body temperature within a few tenths of a degree Celsius. This chapter analyses how man exchanges heat with the environment. It then discusses what the temperature of the human body is, how it is regulated, and how its regulation changes in disease.

23.2 Heat exchange between the body and the environment

The body exchanges heat with the environment through **conduction**, **convection**, **radiation** and **evaporation**. Heat loss from the body that occurs via the first three mechanisms is called **sensible** (or Newtonian). A thermal environment in which body temperature regulation is achieved only by control of sensible heat loss (without regulatory changes in metabolic heat production or evaporative heat loss) is **neutral**.

Conduction

Heat transfer between objects in direct contact is conduction. The heat flow between such objects is proportional to the difference in their surface temperatures (temperature gradient) and is directed from the higher to the lower temperature. Materials differ in their thermal conductivity, or capacity to conduct heat. For example, water is a relatively good heat conductor (bad heat insulator): its conductivity is 25-times greater than that of dry air. Materials also differ in the quantity of heat needed to increase the temperature of 1 kg of the material by 1°C—the specific heat. The higher the specific heat of the material surrounding the body, the more heat this material can withdraw from (give to) the body before the temperature gradient between the body and the material is reduced to zero. The specific heat of water is 1000-times greater than that of air. Together with the fact that water has a higher thermal conductivity, this explains why hypothermia is a major problem for people submerged in water (e.g. victims of sea catastrophes). The same characteristics of water explain why both heat and cold are felt more severely when air humidity (water content of the air) is high. Not only can the conductivity of the environment change, but the conductivity of bodily tissues can also change with changes in blood perfusion. In a cool environment, blood perfusion of subcutaneous fatty tissue is low, and this tissue has a rather low thermal conductivity (three-times lower than that of muscle). However, subcutaneous blood flow can increase ten-fold at elevated body or ambient temperatures, thus increasing heat conductivity substantially and accelerating heat exchange with the environment. The total amount of heat exchanged between the body and the environment also depends on their area of contact. The surface of the human body (even naked) is not entirely in contact with the environment: the effective surface area depends on body posture. A person feeling cold tends to curl up, because the sphere is the geometric shape with smallest surface area for a given volume. A person feeling hot often presents postural extension.

Convection

Because the body is always submerged in fluid (gas or liquid), heat exchange between the body and the environment is affected by convection. Con-

vection is the motion of a thermally heterogeneous fluid. It can be driven by a temperature gradient or by temperature-independent factors. The former type occurs when the fluid (e.g. air) surrounding the body warms up, expands, and ascends. The latter type occurs due to movement of the body or wind. In either case, layers of fluid that are adjacent to the body and have their temperature close to that of the body surface get replaced with new, remote layers that have the temperature of the environment at large. Hence, heat exchange between the body and the environment via conduction intensifies in the presence of convection: if the body is exposed to cold, it cools down faster; if the body is exposed to heat, it heats up faster too. Convection, therefore, is often referred to as facilitated conduction. The effectiveness of convection is well-known to people living in hot climates: depending on how warm it is inside their house, they may or may not turn on the air conditioner, but they will always turn on the more economical fan, either as a sole or an additional 'cooling' device. Convection is also the basis for the popular term, 'wind-chill factor'. Heat exchange occurs constantly, not only between the body and the environment, but also between different organs and tissues within the body. As body tissues have relatively low thermal conductivity, the core would easily overheat if the heat were not redistributed by blood flow. Haemodynamic changes have a drastic effect on the distribution of bodily heat. For example, the initial, rapid cooling of the body core in surgical patients is due to a sudden increase in blood flow in peripheral tissues caused by the removal of vasoconstrictor tone by general anaesthesia. Heat transfer within the body also occurs via conduction, and the counter-current heat exchange between the many adjacent arteries and veins throughout the body provides an example of effective synergy between conduction and convection.

Radiation

The role of radiation in heat exchange between the body and the environment is often underestimated. All objects continuously emit and absorb energy in the form of electromagnetic waves. The quantity of the radiated energy is proportional to the fourth power of the absolute temperature (measured in degrees Kelvin), and also to the emissivity (ability to emit or absorb radiation) of the object surface. An object that absorbs and emits heat perfectly (a black body, or full radiator) has an emissivity of one; a perfect mirror has an emissivity of zero. Having an emissivity of 0.95 in the infrared range, human skin behaves like a black body. As any other object, the human body both emits radiant energy into the environment and absorbs it from external objects. The net energy exchange by radiation is thus related to the temperature difference between the emitting and receiving surfaces. Radiation from the Sun explains why a person feels warmer in an open area than in the shade, even though both areas may have the same air temperature. Naked human skin emits and absorbs infrared radiation regardless of skin colour. A clothed body also emits and absorbs radiant heat, but it is the surface temperature of the clothing, not the skin temperature, that determines the direction and intensity of the exchange between the clothed body and the environment.

Evaporation

Heat loss from the body via 'dry' mechanisms (conduction, convection, and radiation) is called sensible (or Newtonian). Heat can also be lost via a 'wet' (or insensible), evaporative mechanism. Because the amount of energy it takes to vaporize water is so high ($0.58\,\text{kcal}\,\text{g}^{-1}$), evaporation of water from skin or lungs is the most efficient way to lose bodily heat and cool the surface at which evaporation occurs. To put it into perspective, it takes nearly six-times more energy to evaporate water at 100°C than to heat the same amount of water from 0 to 100°C. Importantly, evaporation is not only the most efficient mechanism to lose heat, but also the only mechanism that can work even when ambient temperature is higher than skin temperature. Not surprisingly, evaporative cooling is widely spread in nature, as different animals use sweating (horses), panting (dogs), thermoregulatory saliva-

tion and spreading saliva over the bodily surface (rats), or even defecation on their feet (some African birds) to cool themselves. In a cool environment, humans do not sweat, and evaporation accounts for ~15% of the total heat loss from the body. Approximately one-third to one-half of this fraction is due to evaporation from the respiratory tract, while the rest comes from water that passively diffuses through the skin and evaporates from its surface. In a warm environment and during exercise, a substantially larger fraction of heat loss (30–70% and higher) occurs via evaporation, and 80–90% of this fraction is due to sweating. It should be noted, however, that sweating becomes less efficient at high air humidity, because water evaporation slows down. If the air is saturated with water (has a relative humidity corresponding to 100% at skin temperature), sweating becomes completely inefficient as an evaporative mechanism (but it will still increase the thermal conductivity of the skin). Another notion of practical concern is that heat exposure results in loss of water from the skin and lungs, and compensating for this loss by drinking enough water is probably the most important measure in preventing overheating.

Thermoneutrality

All animals search for a thermally non-stressful environment, one in which thermal balance can be maintained without expending too much energy (i.e. without activation of metabolism) or losing too much water (i.e. without activation of evaporative heat-loss mechanisms). Such an environment is called thermoneutral. It is often described as a range of ambient temperatures—the **thermoneutral zone** (TNZ). However, ambient temperature is only one of several physical factors determining heat exchange with the environment. Other factors include air humidity, air velocity, barometric pressure, contact area with materials in the environment, thermal conductivity of these materials, and radiant field. Depending on these factors, the same ambient temperature (e.g. 18°C) can be sub-neutral (a naked man standing on a windy beach after swimming), neutral (the same man lying in bed under a down quilt), or supraneutral (the same man walking indoors while dressed in heavy winter clothes). Whether the environment is neutral can be determined by measuring metabolic rate (which is minimal within the TNZ), by assessing skin vasomotor tone (which continuously switches between mild constriction and mild dilation inside the TNZ, but shows marked, steady vasoconstriction or vasodilation outside), or by using other, indirect methods. For example, paradoxical (rapid-eye-movement, REM) sleep occurs only when internal and external conditions, including thermal, are favourable. Accordingly, REM sleep is maximally expressed inside the TNZ. People try to avoid shivering or sweating and, in modern society, they spend most of their lives under thermally neutral conditions.

23.3 Body temperature

Body core temperature is one of the clinical vital signs. It is monitored in all hospitalized patients and is included in every medical history. There are only small (a few tenths of a degree Celsius) temperature differences between the main internal organs (thoracic and abdominal viscera and the brain), and it is their temperature that is referred to as body core (or deep) temperature. Traditionally, body core temperature was measured by a mercury thermometer (and later by an electronic thermometer) in the mouth (e.g. in North America), axilla (e.g. in Eastern Europe), or rectum (in young children all over the world). Nowadays, infrared tympanic thermometry is becoming common, especially in outpatients and paediatric patients. For rough comparison, body temperatures obtained from the ear are up to 1°C lower than axillary or oral temperatures, and 0.5–1.5°C lower than rectal temperatures. In patients with appropriate catheters, core temperature can be reliably determined at the pulmonary artery or distal oesophagus; it can also be estimated from nasopharyngeal or bladder measurements. There is a diurnal variation in core temperature with a zenith (37.2°C, rectal) in the early evening and a nadir (35.7°C, rectal) in the early morning. The amplitude of diurnal changes in deep body temperature is between 0.5°C (oral) and 1.5°C (rectal). In women, core temperature varies throughout the menstrual cycle, being about 0.5°C higher in the luteal phase. Because the main purpose of clinical thermometry is not to miss fever (an early symptom of infection), it is important to define the upper limit of normal core temperature. As a rule of thumb, this limit is somewhere between 37.2 and 37.7°C, regardless of which site and at what time of day the temperature is obtained. Deep body temperatures above 41°C are rare (especially in adults) and often indicative of a serious condition. Deep temperatures of 42°C are considered lethal, although there are recorded cases of people surviving short-lasting elevations of body temperature to even higher values. Because normal body temperature is much closer to the deadly temperature of enzyme denaturation than to that of water crystallization, low body temperatures are less dangerous than high ones. Although core temperatures below 34°C give rise to amnesia, and temperatures below 30°C can cause arrhythmia and cardiac arrest, the whole body can be cooled to 10°C or even lower (if the circulation is externally supported) with a very high probability of surviving the rewarming without suffering any damage.

Whereas the body core is thermally homogeneous and its temperature is maintained within a couple of degrees Celsius throughout a person's life, temperatures of the shell (peripheral tissues) vary widely, by a few-tens of degrees Celsius. **Body shell temperatures** can be anywhere between core temperature and skin temperature. Skin temperature depends on the skin blood flow: if blood flow is low (cutaneous vasoconstriction), skin temperature is close to ambient; if blood flow is high (cutaneous vasodilation), skin temperature is close to core temperature. The latter situation is often referred to as an extension of the core, because the homogenous area of high temperature inside the body increases.

23.4 Regulation of body temperature

The body actively modifies its heat exchange with the environment in order to maintain constant

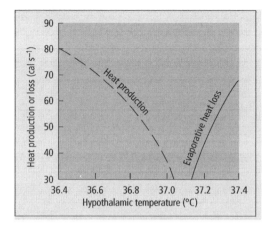

Fig. 23.1 Dependence of heat production and evaporative heat loss on hypothalamic temperature in man. (Adapted from Benzinger, T.H. (1969) *Physiol Rev*, **49**, 671–759.)

core temperature (Fig. 23.1). When, due to any reason, core body temperature (hypothalamic temperature in Fig. 23.1) increases above its basal level (~37°C in Fig. 23.1), evaporative heat loss is activated to bring the temperature back to normal. Importantly, the greater the increase in body temperature, the greater is the increase in heat loss. When core body temperature decreases, heat production is activated, and the greater the decrease in body temperature, the greater is the increase in heat production. To regulate deep body temperature, the body uses **temperature sensors** and heat-loss and heat-production mechanisms (**thermoeffectors**). The sensors and thermoeffectors are connected by **neural pathways**. Circuitries of different effectors form independent **thermoeffector loops**. While affecting each other's activity (by changing body temperature on which activity of the effectors depends), thermoeffector loops are recruited in various **thermoregulatory responses** in what looks like a coordinated fashion.

Thermosensors

Brain (core) temperature is detected by **central thermosensory neurones** (central thermoreceptors). Most of them are **warm-sensitive**, i.e. they increase their activity with an increase in brain temperature. The abundance of warm-sensitive

central sensors can be explained by two facts. First, core overheating is very dangerous (p. 606). Second, humans are endothermic animals, and their principal source of heat is located inside their body. Although much less common, **cold-sensitive** neurones (i.e. those that increase their activity with a decrease in brain temperature) also exist. However, the cold sensitivity of most of them seems to be due to inhibitory synaptic input from nearby warm-sensitive neurones. Furthermore, cold-sensitive neurones have little role in triggering thermoeffector responses. It appears that heat-loss responses are triggered primarily by activation of warm-sensitive neurones, whereas heat-production responses are triggered primarily by inhibition of warm-sensitive neurones. Thermoregulatory responses in a variety of animal species can be elicited by local thermal stimulation of various areas in the central nervous system, including the medulla oblongata and midbrain reticular formations and the spinal cord, but warm-sensitive neurones of the preoptic anterior hypothalamus (POA) are the most important for triggering autonomic thermoeffectors. The location of thermosensitive neurones triggering behavioural responses is largely unknown. Warm-sensitive POA neurones are characterized by the horizontal orientation of their dendrites: towards the third ventricle medially and the medial forebrain bundle laterally. Such an orientation seems ideal for receiving input from neurones bringing information on shell temperatures (p. 610). Because warm-sensitive POA neurones display spontaneous membrane depolarization, they are pacemakers. Their thermosensitivity is due to currents that determine the rate of spontaneous depolarization between successive action potentials.

Most **peripheral thermosensory neurones** (peripheral thermoreceptors) are **superficial sensors**: they detect shell temperatures in the skin and in the oral and urogenital mucosa. Most superficial sensors are cold-sensitive. Because central thermosensors are concerned mainly with warmth, specialization of peripheral sensors in cold sensitivity is expected. Skin cold sensors are located immediately beneath the epidermis. Their signals are conveyed by thin myelinated Aδ fibres. The less common warm sensors are located slightly deeper in the dermis; their signals travel via unmyelinated C fibres. Mechanisms of peripheral thermosensitivity are thought to involve changes in the resting membrane potential. Importantly, the response of most peripheral thermosensors shows a powerful dynamic (phasic) component: these cells are very active when the temperature is changing, but quickly adapt to a stable temperature. Such a response enables the organism to rapidly react to environmental changes. In addition to superficial cold- and warm-sensitive neurones, there are peripheral **deep-body sensors**, which respond to the core body temperature. They are located in the oesophagus, stomach, large intra-abdominal veins, and other organs. Although these deep-body sensors are different from superficial sensors, they also mainly detect cold rather than warmth.

A recent advance in the understanding of temperature sensation has come from the cloning and characterization of a subclass of transient receptor potential (TRP) ion channels known as **thermoTRP channels**. Although each of these channels is specific for a distinct temperature range, all of them convert thermal information into electrical signals by increasing the inward non-selective cationic current and, consequently, the resting membrane potential. This mechanism of action agrees more readily with the mechanism of peripheral thermosensitivity rather than with that of hypothalamic thermosensitivity. For some of these channels (such as TRP vanilloid 4), a physiological role has been established; other thermoTRP channels are currently under investigation.

Thermoeffectors

Behavioural strategies ranging from primitive responses (e.g. postural changes) to complex programs (e.g. maintaining temperature inside a space shuttle) are the most powerful means to defend body temperature, and it is primarily behavioural defences that allow humans to live and work in extreme environments. Selection of clothing and bedding is almost automatic, and artificial control of the environment, e.g. by opening and shutting windows, is accurate even in the absence of appropriate gauges.

The principal **autonomic** (or physiological) heat defences are sweating and skin vasodilation. The principal autonomic cold defences are skin vasoconstriction, shivering, and non-shivering thermogenesis. Other thermoeffector mechanisms (e.g. piloerection) also exist, but their significance in humans is limited. **Sweating** (sudation) is the excretion of sweat, a hypo-osmotic ultrafiltrate of plasma, produced by exocrine glands that are widely, but unevenly, distributed over the skin. Because sweat glands are controlled by cholinergic sympathetic nerves, their activity can be blocked by atropine. The maximum sweating rate in most adults is ~0.5 L h^{-1}, and it is several-fold greater in trained athletes and people acclimatized to a hot environment. Hence, sweating can rapidly diminish not only body water but also electrolyte content. If these are severely depleted, the rate of sweating decreases, and body temperature can rise to fatal levels. As discussed on p. 605, sweating is most efficient in a dry environment.

The efficacy of sweating is augmented by precapillary thermoregulatory **vasodilation**, as a brisk blood flow is needed to deliver the heat (to be dissipated) and water (to be vaporized) to the skin. Cutaneous vasodilation in palms and feet is especially important. These hairless body parts serve as heat exchangers with the environment and are characterized by a high surface:volume ratio, high density of blood vessels, and the presence of arterio–venous shunts. When dilated, the shunts have a diameter of ~100 μm; consequently, a shunt carries 100 times as much blood as a common 10-μm capillary of the same length. The magnitude of skin vasodilation is striking: during hyperthermia, the skin can receive blood at a rate as high as 8 L min^{-1}. Cutaneous vasodilation initially occurs as **passive** vasodilation; it results from the withdrawal of the noradrenergic sympathetic vasoconstrictor activity. The sympathetic **active** vasodilator system is activated later, when core temperature increases further. This active vasodilation involves cholinergic sympathetic nerves, but it is disputed whether these nerves are vasomotor (and cause vasodilation directly) or sudomotor (and cause vasodilation via release of bradykinin from sweat glands). Local temperature is also important: local warming can induce maximal skin vasodilation in humans.

When active vasodilation ceases, the diameter of arterio–venous shunts decreases, and such a decrease can be viewed as passive vasoconstriction. Active thermoregulatory **vasoconstriction** occurs via activation of the adrenergic sympathetic control. Skin vasoconstriction is triggered by local α_2-adrenoreceptors, central α_1-adrenoreceptors, and local hypothermia.

Shivering is an increased contractile activity of skeletal muscles not involving voluntary movements or external work. In humans, shivering can raise the metabolic rate about three-fold. Initially, the tone of skeletal muscles throughout the body increases without causing actual shaking. As shivering progresses, thermoregulatory muscle tone changes to microvibrations and then to clonic contractions of both flexors and extensors. Shivering involves activation of anterior motor neurones (γ-neurones are thought to be affected first) and oscillation of the spindle stretch reflex mechanism. All shivering thermogenesis is blocked by curare.

Non-shivering thermogenesis is a cold-defence mechanism associated primarily with brown adipose tissue (BAT), a highly vascularized fatty tissue located between the scapulas and around large intra-abdominal blood vessels. BAT owes its brown colour to its enormous mitochondrial density. The mitochondria are equipped with unique proteins, uncoupling proteins (UCP), primarily UCP1. By collapsing the electrochemical proton gradient generated by oxidation, UCP prevent adenosine triphosphate (ATP) synthesis, thus effectively dissociating mitochondrial respiration and oxidative phosphorylation and transforming substrate energy into heat. BAT thermogenesis is activated by sympathetic nerves via the β_3 adrenoreceptor. BAT is well developed in many animal species, including small rodents, throughout their lifespan. In humans, however, BAT plays a significant role only during the neonatal period; thereafter, it undergoes involution (replacement with white fat) and contributes little to thermoregulation. Other tissues, especially those having high metabolism (brain, liver, skeletal muscles, heart) also generate heat and, hence, possess non-shivering thermogenesis—if the term is taken literally. However, if the body of an adult human is cooled, its core temperature continues dropping until the shivering response is activated. This suggests that the thermogenic properties of tissues other than BAT are not used for active thermoregulation in man.

Thermoregulatory pathways

Afferent pathways start with primary thermosensory neurones located in the dorsal root ganglia. These bipolar cells project to the dorsal horn of the spinal cord (mostly lamina I), where they synapse with secondary monopolar neurones. Axons of these secondary neurones cross the midline and ascend in the lateral funiculus of the spinal cord. This crossover explains why unilateral lesions of the spinal cord in man may cause contralateral thermosensory deficiencies. It was believed for a long time that the secondary neurones project directly to the ipsilateral ventrobasal complex of the thalamus, from where their signals are conveyed to the ipsilateral somatosensory cortex (postcentral gyrus) by tertiary neurones. However, this pathway, which is involved in tactile sensation, seems uninvolved in temperature sensation. Instead, the lamina-I neurones carry temperature signals to the insular cortex via either a monosynaptic (relay in the posterolateral thalamus) or bisynaptic (relays in the parabrachial nucleus and ventrobasal thalamus) pathway. These two spino–thalamo–cortical pathways are involved in **discriminative** temperature sensation. Temperature information is transmitted by these pathways at a high spatial resolution (e.g. temperature of the surface under the tip of an individual finger can be assessed). This information is important for making decisions about a wide range of issues related to interactions with the environment, but it has little to do with body temperature regulation. Temperature information that is important for thermoregulatory purposes is **integrated**, so that it represents areas large enough to affect heat exchange between the body and the environment. This information is generated in the spino–reticulo–hypothalamic pathway, in which the secondary lamina-I neurones project to the reticular formation of the medulla and pons in such a way that a single tertiary neurone receives convergent inputs from multiple lamina-I cells. The tertiary neurones then project to hypothalamic structures (including the POA) either via the periventricular stratum, passing along the wall of the third ventricle, or via the more laterally-passing medial forebrain bundle. As described on p. 607, warm-sensitive POA have a dendrite orientation ideal for collecting integrated information from both the periventricular stratum and the medial forebrain bundle.

Surprisingly, **efferent pathways** from the brain to thermoeffectors have not been well-characterized in humans. The overall organization of the thermoeffector pathways in the rat is shown

in Fig. 23.2. Both skin vasculature and BAT are controlled by sympathetic ganglia, with the bodies of preganglionic neurones located in the intermediolateral column of the spinal cord. These spinal neurones receive direct input from cells located primarily in the raphé/peripyramidal area of the medulla. These medullary cells are under the control of hypothalamic (dorsomedial and paraventricular nuclei) and midbrain (periaqueductal grey matter, retrorubral field, and ventral tegmental area) neurones that receive input from warm-sensitive POA cells. Although the efferent pathways for skin vasomotor tone and non-shivering thermogenesis have some similarities, they are not identical, and both differ substantially from the pathway controlling shivering. Within the shivering pathway, anterior motor neurones (γ and α) of the ventral horn receive direct and indirect inputs from the midbrain and brainstem. Axons of the midbrain neurones descend the ventrolateral column with the reticulospinal and rubrospinal tracts. These midbrain neurones are under control

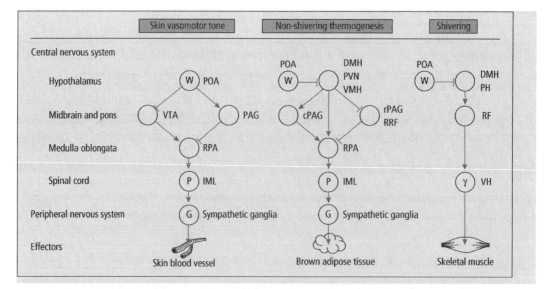

Fig. 23.2 Efferent pathways for control of skin vasomotor tone, non-shivering thermogenesis in brown adipose tissue, and shivering in the rat. (Adapted from Nagashima, K., *et al.* (2000) *Auton Neurosci*, **85**, 18–25. ◯ neuronal body; ⓦ warm-sensitive neurone; ⓟ preganglionic neurone; ⓖ postganglionic neurone; ⓨ γ-motorneurone; ⟶ excitatory projection; ⊣ inhibitory projection; DMH, dorsomedial hypothalamus; IML, intermediolateral column; PAG, periaqueductal grey matter; cPAG, caudal PAG; rPAG, rostral PAG; PH, posterior hypothalamus; POA, preoptic anterior hypothalamus; PVN, paraventricular nucleus; RF, reticular formation; RPA, raphé/peripyramidal area; RRF, retrorubral field; VH, ventral horn; VMH, ventromedial hypothalamus; VTA, ventral tegmental area.)

of posterior hypothalamic neurones, which in turn receive inhibitory input from warm-sensitive POA cells. The efferent pathways described are to a large extent inhibitory. Consequently, thermoeffector activation involves disinhibition of tonically-inhibited neurones.

Thermoeffector loops and coordination

Thermoregulatory pathways form distinct **thermoeffector loops**. The efferent parts of the loops clearly differ, because each effector has its own efferent pathway. The afferent parts are also not identical, as each effector receives a unique combination of signals from peripheral and central thermosensors. In general, behavioural responses of man depend more on signals from peripheral thermosensors (shell temperatures) than central thermosensors (core temperature), whereas core temperature is approximately five-times more important than shell temperatures for triggering autonomic responses. Such an organization reflects the fact that behaviour often acts as the first echelon of defence against cold or heat: behavioural responses are often aimed at escaping the forthcoming thermal insult. In contrast, autonomic cold-defence responses (energetically expensive) and heat-defence responses (water-consuming) are often recruited only when deep body temperature starts changing because behavioural mechanisms were ineffective or could not be used (e.g. due to competing behavioural demands). All autonomic responses involve warm-sensitive POA neurones and do not occur in experimental animals with POA lesions. This is not the case with thermoregulatory behaviours, many of which are unaffected by POA lesions. Even within the autonomic responses, different effectors receive different signals. Because peripheral thermosensors are mostly cold sensors, information from peripheral sensors is relatively more important for triggering cold-defence effectors than heat-defence ones. Because central thermosensors are mostly warm sensors, information from central sensors is relatively more important for triggering heat-defence responses.

Being anatomically distinct, thermoeffector loops function largely independently, and **effector coordination** is achieved mainly through their dependence on a common variable: body temperature. Because autonomic responses depend mostly on body core temperature, the analysis below ignores their dependence on shell temperatures. Such simplification approximates a situation when the body is exposed to constant ambient temperature. Under such conditions, each effector mechanism is activated when core temperature reaches a certain value, **threshold**. For example, heat production in Fig. 23.1 increases (due to triggering of shivering) when core temperature decreases below the threshold temperature of 37.0°C. Although thresholds for activation of different thermoeffectors are normally close (tenths of a degree Celsius) to each other, they are not identical. Those thermoeffectors that do not consume a lot of energy or water are usually recruited in the response first; their thresholds are the closest to the normal value of deep body temperature. More 'expensive' effectors have their thresholds further from the normal value of body temperature; they are activated only if the first line of effectors fails, and body temperature continues decreasing or increasing. As a rule, the order of recruitment of autonomic thermoeffectors in response to cold is: skin vasoconstriction (passive then active), non-shivering thermogenesis (if available), and shivering (from thermoregulatory muscle tone to active contractions). In response to heat, skin vasodilation (passive then active) is recruited followed by sweating. For a long time, such coordination was explained with the help of a single command centre. This centre was thought to collect information about all temperatures in the body, compare it with the desired value (reference signal, or set point), and then send individually tailored commands to thermoeffectors. However, the single command centre model of temperature regulation has not been confirmed experimentally. Figure 23.3 shows how four independent thermoeffectors, each having a distinct threshold, function in a highly coordinated way without having a single controller. When body temperature decreases, effectors 1 (Fig. 23.3a) and 2 (Fig. 23.3b) are subsequently recruited

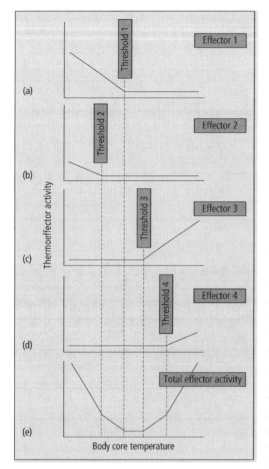

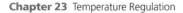

Fig. 23.3 Coordinated recruitment of independent thermoeffectors to control body temperature.

in cold defence; when body temperature increases, effectors 3 (Fig. 23.3c) and 4 (Fig. 23.3d) are subsequently recruited in heat defence.

Thermoregulatory states

Figure 23.3e shows the total activity of all cold-defence effectors (left branch of the graph) and heat-defence effectors (right branch). The threshold of cold defence is the threshold of effector 1; the threshold of heat defence is the threshold of effector 3. In the normal state (Fig. 23.4a), body temperature balances in a narrow zone between these two thresholds, the **interthreshold zone**. The **balance point** (or equilibrium point) is the value at

which body temperature would stabilize if the activity of thermoeffectors and other factors affecting heat exchange between the body and the environment would remain the same. In many situations, body temperature is either increased or decreased compared to its normal level. Regardless of the causes or underlying mechanisms, any increase in body temperature is **hyperthermia**, and any decrease is **hypothermia**. Some cases of hyperthermia or hypothermia involve no changes in thermoeffector thresholds and no primary changes in the balance point. In these cases, body temperature is temporarily brought above or below its balance point as a result of an internal (e.g. extensive muscle activity) or external (e.g. immersion in cold water) heat disturbance uncorrected by thermoeffector activity. When the disturbance is removed or when the effectors 'catch up' with the task, body temperature returns to normal. In other cases, thresholds of thermoeffectors change, which then changes either the level at which body temperature is regulated (balance point), or the precision of its regulation (interthreshold zone), or both. Hence, all thermoregulatory states are classified based on whether the interthreshold zone remains narrow or becomes wide, and whether the balance point is increased or decreased. States with a narrow (a few tenths of a degree Celsius) interthreshold zone are **homeothermic**; states with a wide (a few degrees Celsius) interthreshold zone are **poikilothermic**. (Compare these terms with the ones highlighted on p. 603.) States with an increased balance point are called **fever**; states with a decreased balance point are called **anapyrexia**.

The large variety of thermoregulatory states can be explained by only two **thermoeffector threshold mechanisms**, which can act either separately or jointly. The **first type** occurs when the threshold body core temperatures for activation of cold and heat defences are shifted upwards by the same extent (Fig. 23.4b). These shifts result in fever (increased balance point) associated with homeothermy (narrow interthreshold zone), and are characterized by precise regulation of body temperature and its relative independence of ambient temperature. The **second type** occurs when the threshold for cold defence is drastically de-

Fig. 23.4 Changes in thermoeffector thresholds and the balance point of body temperature in different thermoregulatory states (responses). (Adapted from Romanovsky, A.A. (2004) *Am J Physiol Regul Integr Comp Physiol*, **287**, R992–5. ◇ Threshold body temperature for activation of cold-defense effectors; ◆ Threshold body temperature for activation of heat-defense effectors; ↔ Wide interthreshold zone; | Balance point; ↞ Environmental cooling 'pressure'; ↠ Environmental warming 'pressure'.)

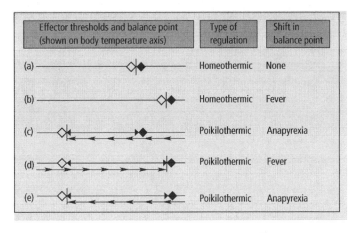

Effector thresholds and balance point (shown on body temperature axis)	Type of regulation	Shift in balance point
(a)	Homeothermic	None
(b)	Homeothermic	Fever
(c)	Poikilothermic	Anapyrexia
(d)	Poikilothermic	Fever
(e)	Poikilothermic	Anapyrexia

creased, while the threshold for heat defence remains more or less the same (Fig. 23.4c). Such threshold dissociation creates a poikilothermic state, in which body temperature is regulated with greatly reduced precision and strongly depends on ambient temperature. In fact, within the new, wide interthreshold zone, body temperature is the result of passive heat exchange between the body and the environment. In a subneutral environment, or when associated with cold-seeking behaviour (which is often the case), such a response results in a decreased balance point, i.e. anapyrexia. This mechanism (decrease in the threshold body temperature for activation of cold defence) is exactly opposite to what occurred during the transition from poikilothermy to homeothermy in the course of evolution. In evolution, homeothermy appeared when tachymetabolism replaced bradymetabolism, thus effectively increasing the threshold body temperature for activation of cold defence. High heat production explains the high energetic demand of mammals and birds. It is no surprise, therefore, that anapyrexia occurs in homeothermic animals when they either need to save energy in the normal course of life (REM sleep, hibernation), or when they face a threat of energy deficit due to severe disease, intoxication, shock of any etiology, or exposure to extreme environmental conditions. Because autonomic thermoregulation is to a certain extent turned off in poikilothermic states, behavioural thermoregula-

tion becomes predominant in these states. **The first and second types** of threshold changes described above (Figs 23.4b and 23.4c) can overlap; i.e. a decrease in the threshold body temperature for cold defence can occur after both thresholds are already increased. Such effector shifts result in poikilothermy and either fever (in a supraneutral environment or when accompanied by warmth-seeking behaviour; Fig. 23.4d), or anapyrexia (in a subneutral environment; Fig. 23.4e). The potential adaptive value of such overlapping shifts is discussed on p. 615.

23.5 Pathophysiology of thermoregulation

In many clinical situations, regulation of body temperature is affected by both thermal and non-thermal factors. While analysing these situations from the thermoregulatory point of view, the following questions should be answered. Does hyperthermia or hypothermia occur? How is heat balance changed, and what thermoeffectors are involved? Is the type of body temperature regulation homeothermic or poikilothermic? Is this fever? Is this anapyrexia? Below, the results of such analyses are presented for one situation (heat stroke) in which thermoregulation is affected primarily by a thermal factor, and for another situation (systemic inflammation) in which thermoregulation is affected primarily by non-thermal factors.

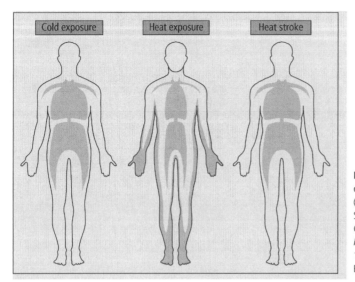

Fig. 23.5 Blood distribution under different thermal conditions. (Adapted from Rowell, L.B. (1983) In: Shepherd, J.T., Abboud, F.M. and Geiger, S.R. (eds) *Handbook of Physiology*, sect. 2, vol. 3, pp. 967–1023. American Physiological Society, Bethesda, USA.)

Heat stroke

Heat stroke is circulatory collapse (shock) due to excessive heat accumulation in the body. **Exertional heat stroke** occurs after strenuous physical activity and results from increased heat production overwhelming the body's ability to dissipate heat; it rarely occurs in its pure form. **Classical heat stroke** occurs as the result of exposure to a hot environment and reflects a failure of heat-loss mechanisms to dissipate heat at a sufficient rate; it occurs more often. As heat is lost from the body due to sweating and cutaneous vasodilation, heat exposure causes dehydration and redistribution of blood flow from the abdominal viscera to the skin (Fig. 23.5). Cardiovascular adjustments to thermal stress are discussed in Chapter 15. The high cutaneous blood flow results in an extension of the core (p. 606). If heat exposure continues, and the water loss due to sweating is not compensated by increased water intake, then hypovolemia, dehydration, and eventually cardiovascular collapse occur. Hypovolemia and decreased central venous pressure increase threshold body temperatures for skin vasodilation and sweating. Vasodilation of skin changes to vasoconstriction (Fig. 23.5) and sweating ceases, thus decreasing the already insufficient heat loss and resulting in a further increase in body temperature. Typically, deep-body temperature in heat-stroke victims exceeds 41°C. Cardiovascular collapse may also cause a decrease in the threshold for heat production, thus resulting in the poikilothermic type of body temperature regulation. Therefore, if a heat-stroke patient was exposed to a cool environment shortly after heat exposure, the patient's body temperature may not be high (and may be even lower than normal) upon admittance to a medical facility. Nevertheless, in a typical case of heat stroke (i.e. with a very high body temperature), caution should be exercised not to trigger heat production while attempting to cool the patient. It was found empirically that spraying the skin of a patient with warm water often provides efficient cooling without causing shivering.

Systemic inflammation

Systemic inflammation and related syndromes (including sepsis and septic shock) are leading causes of hospital mortality. Whenever inflammatory agents (mostly of bacterial origin) enter the bloodstream, they cause production of cytokines, prostanoids (including prostaglandin E_2, PGE_2), nitric oxide, and other inflammatory mediators. These mediators cause body temperature to either increase or decrease, and all clinically used definitions of the systemic inflammation-associated syndromes include both hyperthermia and hypothermia as symptoms. Hyperthermia in systemic inflammation is fever. The principal distal extracellular mediator of this response is PGE_2. This agrees with the fact that the principal mechanism of action of common antipyretics is inhibition of cyclooxygenase-2, a PGE_2-synthesizing enzyme. Febrigenic PGE_2 is produced both in the brain (mostly by endothelial and perivascular cells) and in the periphery (liver and lungs). Whether of central or peripheral origin, PGE_2 gains access to warm-sensitive POA neurones and increases threshold body temperatures of all autonomic effectors by about the same degree. Such changes result in an increased balance point, while the type of body temperature regulation remains homeothermic. Increased body temperature aids many immune functions, including neutrophil migration, phagocytosis, interferon production, and T-cell proliferation. These benefits, however, come at substantial metabolic costs and cannot be afforded if the energy supply is compromised. In more severe cases, a decrease in the threshold temperature for heat production (shivering) occurs, while the threshold for heat loss stays increased (Figs 23.4d and 23.4e). These changes lead to poikilothermy. In poikilothermy, a high body temperature (and its immuno-stimulating effects) can be achieved via energetically inexpensive mechanisms—by using warmth-seeking behaviour and utilizing environmental heat (Fig. 23.4d). On the other hand, if the environment is subthermoneutral, body temperature decreases in a poikilothermic state (Fig. 23.4e). Low body temperature also has an adaptive value—it decreases tissue metabolic demands and possibly possesses an anti-inflammatory action. Finally, in most severe cases of systemic inflammation, the threshold body temperature for heat production decreases drastically; the threshold body temperature for heat loss shows little change, and strong cold-seeking behaviour occurs (Fig. 23.4c). The balance point shifts downwards (anapyrexia) and body temperature decreases (hypothermia). Because hypothermia is associated with the most severe cases of systemic inflammation, it is a sign of poor prognosis. However, it is probably still an adaptive response, because animal experiments suggest that the deleterious effects of systemic inflammation would likely be even more severe if body temperature were higher. What causes the threshold body temperature for cold defence to decrease in inflammation is unknown, but prostanoids other than PGE_2 are likely to be involved. There is no consensus among clinicians as to whether and how to treat hypothermia in systemic inflammation.

Chapter 24

Exercise

Exercise consists of voluntary activation of skeletal muscle. This chapter deals first with the accompanying increased metabolic activity in the muscle, then the changes that occur in the circulatory and respiratory systems to meet the needs for supply of more O_2 and for removal of CO_2, heat and metabolites. Finally, some aspects of performance and training are dealt with in a section on applied aspects of exercise physiology.

24.1 Energetics

Muscles convert about 20% of the energy of adenosine triphosphate (ATP) to external work, the remaining energy appearing as heat. The demand for ATP is met by anaerobic and aerobic metabolism. Consumption of oxygen by the aerobic system takes time to develop and continues for some time after exercise stops.

The energy for muscular work is derived from the breakdown of ATP and creatine phosphate (p. 105). As stores of ATP are limited, exercise lasting for more than a few seconds demands an increased supply from **aerobic** and **anaerobic metabolism**. In mild exercise ATP is produced by the aerobic pathway by oxidation of fatty acids and ketones, while in more vigorous exercise glycogen is utilized. At higher levels of exercise the additional demand for ATP is met by the anaerobic pathway, which produces ATP more rapidly by converting glycogen to lactic acid. The relative contributions

from the aerobic and anaerobic pathway depend on the duration of the exercise. Aerobic metabolism contributes very little of the total energy utilized during brief explosive exercise. The contribution increases to about 50% for events such as a 400-m race lasting under 1 min, and exceeds 90% in events lasting 10 min or more.

Fatigue in a muscle is the failure to maintain the required force or power output. In comparison with rested muscle, fatigued muscle fibres develop a lower peak tetanic tension, contract at a lower velocity, have a reduced maximal velocity of contraction, and have a prolonged relaxation time. Fatigue is a complex phenomenon with many contributing factors. The relative importance of each factor may depend on the fibre-type composition of the muscle, the intensity, type and duration of activity, and the individual's degree of physical fitness. Current evidence suggests that the mechanism of fatigue lies within the muscle itself and that any one or more of the following factors could contribute: (a) altered sarcolemma excitability; (b) altered T-tubule excitability; (c) uncoupling of the T-tubule charge sensor and the Ca^{2+}-release channel (ryanodine receptor) in the sarcoplasmic reticulum; (d) inhibition of the Ca^{2+}-release channel in the sarcoplasmic reticulum; (e) impaired Ca^{2+} reuptake by the Ca^{2+}-activated ATPase in the sarcoplasmic reticulum; (f) impaired Ca^{2+} binding to troponin; and (g) changes to actin–myosin binding, ATP hydrolysis and the cross-bridge cycle.

Fatigue develops more rapidly as the intensity of exercise increases, apparently because of the increased contribution of anaerobic pathways to the production of ATP. The concomitant production of lactic acid lowers the intracellular pH, which changes the kinetics of many cellular processes, including those responsible for fatigue.

The **efficiency** of exercise is a measure of the conversion of chemical energy into external work. In estimating efficiency, the exercise physiologist is usually content to measure the steady-state O_2 consumption ($\dot{V}o_2$) of a subject in conditions where the rate of external work can be estimated with reasonable accuracy. It is assumed either that aerobic metabolism is the sole source of power, or that any products of anaerobic metabolism are oxidized. (The latter usually does not occur within the time frame of a bout of exercise and may lead to an overestimation of efficiency during anaerobic metabolism.) The efficiency can then be calculated after converting the O_2 cost of exercise ($\dot{V}o_2$ in exercise–$\dot{V}o_2$ at rest) measured, for example, in millilitres per second, into units of power. On a mixed diet, $1\,mL\,s^{-1}$ of oxygen (standard temperature and pressure, dry; STPD) yields $20\,W$ of total power (determined using whole-body calorimetry), and therefore:

$$\% \text{ efficiency} = \frac{\text{rate of external work}}{\left(\dot{V}o_2 \text{ in exercise} - \dot{V}o_2 \text{ at rest}\right) \times 20} \times 100$$

The external work of exercise may be very difficult to estimate, as for example where work is done to accelerate and decelerate the limbs and to raise and lower the centre of gravity with each step. On the other hand, the external work of cycling is easily determined with a cycle ergometer, and the efficiency of cycling is found to be 20–25%. This means that someone doing $200\,W$ of external work on a cycle ergometer is also generating about $800\,W$ of heat, which must be transferred to the skin from where it can be dissipated (p. 608).

If exercise is started abruptly and a constant moderate work output is maintained, the O_2 uptake takes several minutes to reach a steady state (Fig. 24.1). The missing O_2 that would have been consumed, if the body's response to the O_2 demand of exercise was immediate, is known as the **oxygen deficit**. For mild to moderate exercise the oxygen deficit is accounted for by:

1 the lower content of ATP and creatine phosphate in the active muscles;

2 the reduction in O_2 content of myoglobin in the active muscles; and

3 the reduction in O_2 content of the venous blood leaving the muscles.

The **oxygen debt** or **excess post-exercise oxygen consumption** represents repayment of the O_2 deficit (Fig. 24.1). When the exercise is vigorous or prolonged the debt is considerably greater than the deficit. Following such exercise the ATP and creatine phosphate stores and the O_2 content of myoglobin and venous blood return to normal within a minute or two, but there is a residual elevated O_2 consumption that can last for minutes to hours depending on the intensity and duration of the exercise. This extra O_2 consumption is attributed to the energy needed to dissipate heat and

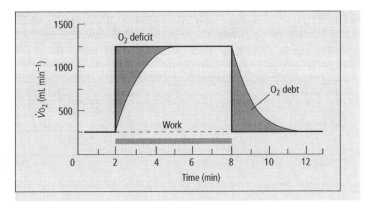

Fig. 24.1 Time course of O_2 consumption ($\dot{V}o_2$) during moderate exercise, illustrating the O_2 deficit and debt.

restore intracellular electrolytes to normal concentrations, and to the higher metabolic rate caused by the increase in body temperature and in circulating levels of catecholamines and thyroxine. Regeneration of intramuscular glycogen stores also produces a very small increase in O_2 consumption over a period of a day or two following the exercise. Lactate produced by the anaerobic pathway is metabolized within 30 min after exercise.

24.2 Circulatory responses in exercise

Blood flow to muscles increases during exercise as a result of vasodilation caused primarily by local metabolic factors. Activity in the sympathetic nervous system also increases cardiac output and reduces flow to other tissues to meet the demand for increased muscle blood flow.

Rhythmic exercise produces an increase in blood flow in the active muscles, which at maximum can reach 20 times the resting blood flow. The initial increase in blood flow is probably a consequence of the muscle pump increasing pressure gradients for flow and producing passive dilation within the muscle vasculature; some of it may also be due to increased activity of the cholinergic sympathetic nerves. The sustained increase in blood flow, however, is caused by local metabolic factors, such as the decrease in Po_2 and pH, the increase in Pco_2, extracellular $[K^+]$ and temperature, and release of other metabolites such as adenosine (p. 388). The

exercise-induced vasodilation results in a large increase in the number of capillaries carrying blood through the muscle; this shortens the mean path length between capillaries and mitochondria in the muscle fibres, allowing a greater extraction of O_2 from the haemoglobin. Off-loading of O_2 from haemoglobin is also assisted by the increased Pco_2, temperature and acidity in the working muscles (p. 473), resulting in the extraction of about 90% of the O_2 from blood perfusing muscles at maximum exercise.

Changes in blood flow to the rest of the body during exercise are shown in Table 24.1. Blood flow to heart muscle increases, meeting the extra O_2 demand of the increased cardiac work; as in skeletal muscle this flow is under local control, although circulating adrenaline may also contribute to the dilation of the coronary vessels via activation of β_2 receptors. Blood flow to the gut and kidney is reduced by sympathetic activity, making more blood available for the exercising muscles. Blood flow to the skin increases as the need to dissipate heat increases, but at maximum exercise skin flow decreases, giving the subject a pale or ashen pallor just before exhaustion; this indicates that heat dissipation is compromised when cardiac output cannot be increased further to meet the demands of exercise. The constancy of blood flow to the brain reflects the unchanged metabolic rate of the brain whatever the level of exercise, and there appears to be no reserve here that can be drawn upon for the exercising muscles.

Table 24.1 Changes in blood flow distribution during exercise.

| | Rest | | Exercise | | | |
| | | | Light | Medium | Heavy | |
	(mL min^{-1})	(%)	(mL min^{-1})	(mL min^{-1})	(mL min^{-1})	(%)
Cerebral	750	13.0	750	750	750	3.0
Coronary	250	4.5	350	650	1000	4.0
Renal	1100	19.0	900	600	250	1.0
Splanchnic	1400	24.0	1100	600	300	1.2
Skin	500	8.5	1500	1800	600	2.4
Others	600	10.5	400	300	100	0.4
Skeletal muscle	1200	20.5	4500	10800	22000	88.0
Cardiac output	5800	100.0	9500	15500	25000	100.0

Table 24.2 Changes in blood flow distribution during exercise.

	Rest	Exercise		
		Light	Medium	Heavy
Oxygen consumption (mL min^{-1})	250	1500	2800	3500
Oxygen consumption of muscles (mL min^{-1})	50	1250	2200	3150
Cardiac output (L min^{-1})	5	13	16	21
Arteriovenous oxygen difference (mL L^{-1})	50	100	127	130
$P_{v}O_2$ (mmHg)	40	26	23	20
Heart rate (beats min^{-1})	72	144	160	190
Diastolic filling time (ms)	500	200	170	150
Stroke volume (mL)	70	90	100	110
Mean blood pressure (mmHg)	85	90	95	100
Pulse pressure (mmHg)	40	60	90	120
Systolic/diastolic pressure (mmHg)	110/70	130/70	155/65	180/60

The effects of exercise on circulatory and respiratory variables are summarized in Table 24.2 and Fig. 24.2. The increase in O_2 consumption (about 15-fold at maximum in a young adult) is accommodated by an increase in the arteriovenous O_2 concentration difference (up to threefold) and an increase in cardiac output (up to fivefold). The increase in cardiac output results from venoconstriction, vasodilation and increased myocardial contractility and heart rate, as well as from the maintenance of right atrial pressure (pp. 400–401) by an increase in venous return due to the repeated squeezing of the veins by the active muscles (the muscle pump). The increase in heart rate limits the increase in stroke volume to a factor of 1.5. Most of this increase in stroke volume occurs at light to moderate levels of exercise and results from an increase in end-diastolic volume (increased filling due to higher central venous pressure) and from a decrease in end-systolic volume (increased emptying due to sympathetically increased contractility). At high levels of exercise the end-diastolic volume is no greater than at rest, and all the increase in stroke volume is due to a greater emptying (p. 367). Systolic pressure increases and diastolic pressure decreases during exercise, resulting in a pronounced increase in pulse pressure; however, in healthy young people mean blood pressure increases only slightly during moderate dynamic exercise. The crucial point is that over a wide range of exercise intensities the mean pressures in the various vascular compartments and the arterial partial pressures of O_2 and CO_2 as well as pH are kept relatively constant.

The nature of the primary signal activating the sympathetic nervous system during exercise is still not entirely clear, but it is probably due to commands from the motor cortex and activity in sensory nerves that detect movement and those metabolic factors inducing vasodilation in the active muscles (p. 388). The baroreceptor reflex (p. 403) helps to buffer changes in mean arterial blood pressure resulting from mismatch of cardiac output and peripheral resistance in dynamic exercise. The set-point at which arterial pressure is regulated is reset to higher levels in severe exercise. Note, however, that in exercise where perfusion of muscles is absent or limited (e.g. sustained static contractions, or arm work with arms raised above the head), vasodilator factors accumulate in the muscles, stimulate sensory nerves and produce dramatic increases in blood pressure.

The time course of the changes in cardiac output during a bout of moderate exercise is shown in Fig. 24.3. There is a sudden increase in cardiac output at the start of exercise, followed by a gradual exponential rise to the steady state; when exercise is stopped, there is a sudden decrease in cardiac output, then an exponential fall. The increase in heart rate at the onset of exercise is due to the rapid withdrawal of vagal tone rather than to the increase in sympathetic nerve activity to the sinoatrial node,

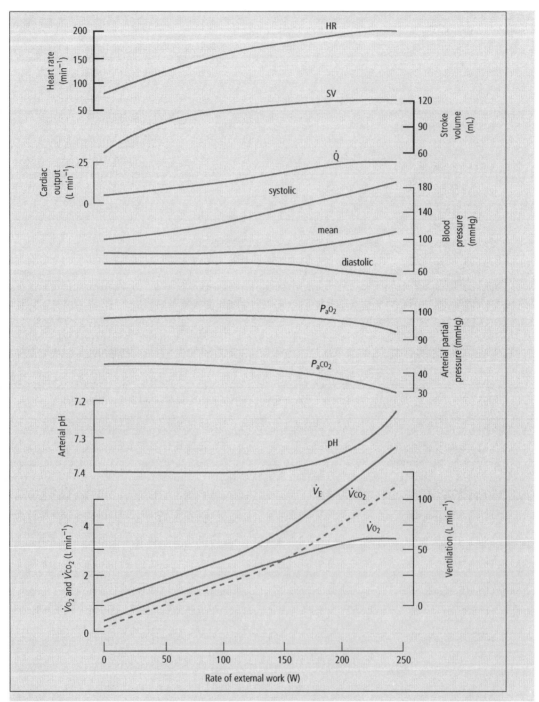

Fig. 24.2 Changes in metabolism, ventilation, arterial pH, arterial gases and cardiovascular variables of a healthy male subject as a function of steady-state work on a cycle ergometer. HR, heart rate; $\dot{Q}$, cardiac output; SV, stroke volume (see also Glossary of symbols, p. 427).

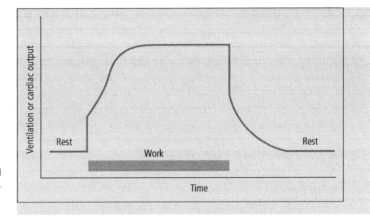

Fig. 24.3 Time course of abrupt and slow changes in ventilation and cardiac output during exercise.

which takes 10–20 s to occur. The sudden changes at the onset and cessation of exercise are also attributed to the effect of the muscle pump on venous return and its effect on stroke volume, as well as to sensory nerve activity associated with movement and to commands from the motor cortex. The slower changes in cardiac output reflect the time course of vasodilation in active muscles and the stimulation of the cardiovascular system in response to activation of the sensory nerves that detect vasodilator factors in the muscles.

24.3 Respiratory responses in exercise

The increase in pulmonary ventilation that occurs during exercise clears CO_2 from the venous blood and maintains arterial Po_2 and Pco_2 at the normal level.

Pulmonary ventilation ($\dot{V}_E$) increases with light to moderate exercise in proportion to the increased demand for the supply of O_2 and the excretion of CO_2 (Fig. 24.2). This involves increases in both the frequency of breathing and tidal volume. The transient response of $\dot{V}_E$ during a bout of exercise (Fig. 24.3) shows rapid and gradual changes similar to those for cardiac output.

The nature of the stimuli that produce the increase in ventilation with exercise is still uncertain. The sudden changes in $\dot{V}_E$ at the beginning and end of exercise appear to result from neuronal input to the respiratory centre from neural activity

in the motor cortex and possibly also from movement receptors in the exercising limbs (p. 482). However, this neural drive appears to play only a minor role in the steady-state response, which has been shown to be coupled very closely to the delivery of CO_2 to the lungs. Detection of CO_2 by a chemoreceptor is therefore implicated, but a venous or pulmonary CO_2 receptor driving ventilation has not been clearly demonstrated. Arterial chemoreception also seems to be ruled out, because an increase in mean arterial Pco_2 or a decrease in Po_2 would be necessary to provide the stimulus for the increased $\dot{V}_E$, and these are not observed (Fig. 24.2). The sensitivity of chemoreception by the carotid bodies may be altered during exercise, and/or the increase in venous CO_2 load increases the rate of change of arterial pH associated with the breath-to-breath oscillations in arterial Pco_2. This could be sensed by the carotid bodies and provide the primary stimulus to ventilation.

At higher levels of exercise there are disproportionate increases in $\dot{V}_E$ and $\dot{V}co_2$ compared with increases in $\dot{V}o_2$ (Fig. 24.2). This hyperventilation appears to arise from additional stimulation of the carotid bodies, because it is virtually absent when the carotid bodies are denervated. The stimulus is usually taken to be the fall in arterial pH that occurs when lactic acid is released by the muscles and starts to accumulate in the blood; the hyperventilation is viewed as an additional buffering mechanism that lowers arterial Pco_2 and thereby prevents arterial blood from becoming too acidic. However, other substances released by active muscles, for example K^+ may also stimulate the carotid chemoreceptors and contribute to the hyperventilation response.

At the most intense levels of exercise, O_2 consumption begins to reach a plateau that defines its maximum value, the $\dot{V}_{O_{2max}}$ (Fig. 24.2). Utilization of O_2 by muscles (oxidative capacity) is not considered to be a limiting factor for $\dot{V}_{O_{2max}}$, and in most people the limitation appears to be the supply of O_2 to muscles by cardiac output. However, in some highly trained athletes, significant arterial hypoxaemia (P_{O_2} <70 mmHg) develops as $\dot{V}_{O_{2max}}$ is approached, indicating that for these individuals the limitation may be in the lungs. The hypoxaemia results from a combination of a reduced hyperventilation response and a reduced transit time for blood in the pulmonary capillaries (p. 460).

24.4 Physiological indices of performance

The only useful physiological indices of physical performance are maximum oxygen consumption and the anaerobic threshold.

Some measurements made by the physiologist in the laboratory under defined conditions can be useful indices of the current performing ability of athletes. However, in sprint or power events the relationship between physiological measures and physical performance is not good. For example, oxygen deficit, oxygen debt and blood lactate concentration in short-term maximal exercise tests might be expected to be related to performance in sprint or power events, but the correlation turns out to be poor. On the other hand, the performance of endurance athletes correlates well with several physiological measures. One of these is $\dot{V}_{O_{2max}}$, which is usually determined by exercising the subject gradually to maximum on a treadmill or cycle ergometer over a 5–15-min period. An even better measure is the so-called **anaerobic threshold**. This is the workload above which the concentration of

lactic acid in the blood builds up rapidly. The high correlation between the anaerobic threshold and endurance performance arises most probably because the anaerobic threshold represents the highest level of exercise that can be performed without fatigue occurring from the accumulation of acid in the muscles. Muscle cells can produce ATP and lactic acid via anaerobic metabolism, even when aerobic metabolism is not limited by the supply of O_2, so the anaerobic threshold is not necessarily a threshold for the onset of hypoxia.

Training can be for strength or short-term power (anaerobic training) or for endurance (aerobic training). The various changes that occur can be regarded as adaptations to the stress of exercise, but the mechanisms that bring about the changes are poorly understood. Anaerobic training, which consists of many repetitions of brief, intense exercise, results in increases in muscle-fibre diameter and activities of enzymes of anaerobic metabolism. Increases in blood pressure during anaerobic training may also produce thickening of the left ventricular wall of the heart. Aerobic training is achieved by exercising at moderate to high intensity for at least 20 min several times per week. The most well-known adaptation to such training is an increase in the maximum $\dot{V}_{O_2}$, which is attributed to an increase in maximum cardiac output and maximum blood flow to the muscles. The increase in cardiac output is itself a consequence of an increased stroke volume with no change in maximum heart rate. The stroke volume is increased at all workloads, including rest, as a result of an increase in circulating blood volume and in the volume of the ventricles. Cardiac output at rest does not change, so the increased stroke volume entails a reduced resting heart rate. Endurance-trained muscles have significant increases in the concentration of oxidative enzymes and myoglobin, and in the density of mitochondria and of capillaries (p. 111); these changes probably contribute to the increase in the maximum $\dot{V}_{O_2}$ and anaerobic threshold.

Appendix 1

Units of Measurement

Throughout this text the units are those commonly used by physiologists. Unfortunately, physiologists and their clinical colleagues have been slow to adopt the now accepted SI units familiar to chemists and physicists. To assist readers trained in this system (and those who believe that physiology should use a logical and consistent system), a summary of SI units and conversion for common units used by physiologists follows.

Basic SI units.

	Unit
Length	metre (m)
Mass	kilogram (kg)
Time	second (s)
Electric current	ampere (A)
Thermodynamic temperature	kelvin (K)
Amount of substance	mole (mol)
Luminous intensity	candela (cd)

Derived SI units and relationships to other units in common use.

	Unit	Definition	Other units
Area		m^2	
Volume		m^3	1 litre (L) = 1 dm^3
Velocity		$m\,s^{-1}$	
Concentration		$mol\,dm^{-3}\,(mol\,L^{-1})$	
Density		$kg\,m^{-3}$	
Force	newton (N)	$m\,kg\,s^{-2}$	1 dyne (dyn) = 10^{-5} N
Pressure	pascal (Pa)	$N\,m^{-2}\,(m^{-1}\,kg\,s^{-2})$	1 atmosphere (atm) = 101.3 kPa
			= 760 mmHg
			1 mmHg = 1 torr = 133.3 Pa
			1 cmH$_2$O = 98.07 Pa
Energy	joule (J)	$N\,m\,(m^2\,kg\,s^{-2})$	1 calorie (cal) = 4.19 J
Power	watt (W)	$J\,s^{-1}\,(m^2\,kg\,s^{-3})$	
Dynamic viscosity		$Pa\,s\,(m^{-1}\,kg\,s^{-1})$	1 poise (P) = 10^{-1} Pa s
Surface tension		$N\,m^{-1}\,(kg\,s^{-2})$	1 dyne cm^{-1} = 10^{-5} N cm^{-1}
Electric charge	coulomb (C)	$A\,s$	
Electric potential difference	volt (V)	$J\,C^{-1}\,(m^2\,kg\,A^{-1}\,s^{-3})$	
Electric resistance	ohm (Ω)	$V\,A^{-1}\,(m^2\,kg\,A^{-2}\,s^{-3})$	
Electric conductance	siemens (S)	$\Omega^{-1}\,(A^2\,s^3\,m^{-2}\,kg^{-1})$	
Electric capacitance	farad (F)	$C\,V^{-1}\,(m^{-2}\,kg^{-1}\,A^2\,s^4)$	
Frequency	hertz (Hz)	s^{-1}	

Appendix 1 Units of Measurement

Physical constants.

Name	Symbol	Numerical value
Gravitational constant	G	$6.67 \times 10^{-11} \, N \, m^2 \, kg^{-2}$
Universal gas constant	R	$8.314 \, J \, K^{-1} \, mol^{-1}$ (at atmos press and 0°C, i.e. $P_o = 101.3 \, kPa$, $T_o = 273.15 \, K$)
Molar volume of ideal gas	V_O	$2.24 \times 10^{-2} \, m^3$ (22.4 L) (at $P_o = 101.3 \, kPa$, $T_o = 273.15 \, K$)
Avogadro constant	N_A	$6.02 \times 10^{23} \, mol^{-1}$
Faraday constant	F	$9.65 \times 10^4 \, C \, mol^{-1}$

Note: R is also sometimes expressed as $8.206 \times 10^{-2} \, L \, atm \, K^{-1} \, mol^{-1}$

Decimal multiples and submultiples of units.

kilo	(k)	for 10^3
hecto	(h)	for 10^2
deca	(da)	for 10^1
deci	(d)	for 10^{-1}
centi	(c)	for 10^{-2}
milli	(m)	for 10^{-3}
micro	(μ)	for 10^{-6}
nano	(n)	for 10^{-9}
pico	(p)	for 10^{-12}
femto	(f)	for 10^{-15}
atto	(a)	for 10^{-18}

Note: 1 angstrom (Å) = 10^{-10} metre

Appendix 2

Basic Concepts of Acid–Base Chemistry

Electrolytes

Electrolytes are atoms or small molecules that exist in solution as electrically charged particles, anions carrying one or more negative charges, and cations carrying positive charge(s), e.g. amino acids, various metabolites, Na^+, K^+, Ca^{2+}, Cl^-, HCO_3^-, NH_4^+.

Acids and bases

An acid is a potential proton donor, and a base is a potential proton acceptor. Ampholytes are components, which—depending on actual conditions—may behave as either acids or bases (water, amino acids, proteins, etc.). Aprotes are substances that are neither acids nor bases. Under physiological conditions, several important organic and inorganic substances, such as glucose, urea, Na^+ and Cl^- are essentially aprotes.

In principle, acid–base reactions are reversible and the protolytic reaction between an acid, HB, and its corresponding base, B^- (a conjugated acid–base pair), is given by:

$$HB \rightleftharpoons H^+ + B^- \qquad (i)$$

Protolytic reactions imply exchange of H^+ between two corresponding acid–base pairs. When the acid HB is dissolved in water, the following reaction will proceed until chemical equilibrium is attained:

$$HB + H_2O \rightleftharpoons H_3O^+ + B^- \qquad (ii)$$

In aqueous solutions, 'free' H^+ exist only in hydrated forms, mainly as 'hydroxonium ions' (H_3O^+), but in the following text, like most other texts, these ions will be described only by the symbol H^+.

In dilute solutions, strong acids are fully dissociated, i.e. the concentration of B^- is very much larger than the concentration of HB ($[B^-] \gg [HB]$), and eqn. (ii) is shifted to the right. The strength of an acid is defined by its ability to give off H^+ and hence by the concentration of H^+ ($[H^+]$). By applying the law of mass action to the concentrations of eqn. (ii) we get:

$$K = \frac{[H^+] \times [B^-]}{[H_2O] \times [HB]} \qquad (iii)$$

The equilibrium constant, K and the water concentration ($[H_2O] \sim 55\,mol\,L^{-1}$) is often combined into a new dissociation constant, K_A which represents a (relative) measure of the strength of the acid (HB) in water:

$$K_A = \frac{[H^+] \times [B^-]}{[HB]} \qquad (iv)$$

In the case of a weak acid, the K_A is low. The weak acid will remain almost undissociated in the form HB, whereas a strong acid, being completely dissociated in dilute solutions, has a high K_A.

Buffers

A buffer reduces the deviations in pH generated by addition of strong acid or strong base. In solution, a buffer consists of a buffer pair: a weak acid and its conjugate base. When the buffer acid, HBuf, is mixed ('titrated') with a strong base (OH⁻ together with an aprote, e.g. Na⁺), or the corresponding buffer base, Buf⁻ (together with an aprote, such as Na⁺), is titrated with strong acid (H⁺ together with an aprote, e.g. Cl⁻) the following reactions take place:

$$HBuf + NaOH \rightarrow H_2O + Buf^- + Na^+ \qquad (v)$$

$$NaBuf + HCl \rightarrow HBuf + Na^+ + Cl^- \qquad (vi)$$

The HBuf/Buf⁻ system is a closed buffer system, in which the total amount of buffer is constant ([HBuf] + [Buf⁻] = k). When a strong base (NaOH) or a strong acid (HCl) is added, the chemical reactions proceed until HBuf is converted to Buf⁻ or vice versa. However, the physiological buffer reactions taking place in the body fluids include open systems as well as closed buffer systems.

In an open buffer system (such as the H_2CO_3/HCO_3^- system), the amounts of buffer acid (CO_2/H_2CO_3) and buffer base (HCO_3^-) can be exchanged independently with the surroundings in a regulated manner; this will further reduce the changes in pH induced by addition of strong acid and strong base (see below).

The titration curve

In Fig. A2.1, the titration curve of a closed buffer system (HBuf/Buf⁻) is outlined showing that the change in pH is minimized (but not prevented) as the amounts of added H⁺ or OH⁻ are 'tied up' by the buffer system.

The buffer equation

Defining pH as the negative logarithm to [H⁺] (i.e. $pH = -\log_{10}[H^+]$), and pK_A as the negative logarithm to K_A, and substituting and rearranging eqn. (iv), we get the buffer equation:

$$pH = pK_A + \log \frac{[B^-]}{[HB]} \qquad (vii)$$

In a homogenous solution containing two or more buffer pairs, these are exposed to the same pH (the isohydric principle) with buffer ratios depending on the individual pK values:

$$pH = pK_1 + \log \frac{[B_1^-]}{[HB_1]} = pK_2 + \log \frac{[B_2^-]}{[HB_2]}$$
$$= pK_3 + \log \frac{[B_3^-]}{[HB_3]} \qquad (viii)$$

In the body, buffer systems may be separated by membranes creating pH gradients due to the differences in ionic composition of the various body fluid compartments.

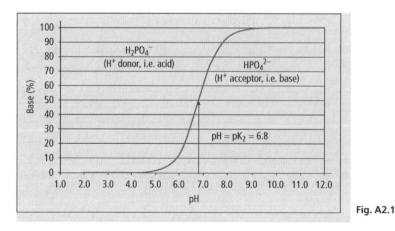

Fig. A2.1

Carbonic acid

The equilibrium between H_2CO_3 and HCO_3^- is peculiar because the pK value is influenced by the presence of CO_2. The pK_1 of H_2CO_3 in the complete absence of CO_2 is 3.60. However, CO_2 is always present in biological systems, and the levels of H_2CO_3 are always very low. In the presence of CO_2, the equilibrium is rather that of:

$$CO_2 + H_2O \rightleftharpoons HCO_3^- + H^+$$

and this has a pK value of 6.36 ('the acidity constant of CO_2'). In biological systems other — mostly technical — considerations warrant minor adjustments of this value, and the pK value usually applied in the analysis of blood gases is 6.10.

Buffer capacity

The buffer capacity of the weak acid–base system is defined as: $\beta = \dfrac{dOH^-}{dpH} \, mmol \, L^{-1} \, pH^{-1}$, which is identical to the slope of the titration curve shown in Fig. A2.1. In the case of $[B^-] = [HB]$, $\log [B^-]/[HB]$ is zero and therefore, pH = pK and the slope of the titration curve attains its maximum value.

Index

Printed and bound by CPI Group (UK) Ltd, Croydon, CR0 4YY